Oxford Textbook of

Nature and
Public Health

Oxford Textbooks in Public Health

Oxford Textbook of
Nature and Public Health

The role of nature in improving the health of a population

Edited by

Matilda van den Bosch
Assistant Professor
The University of British Columbia, Vancouver
Canada

William Bird
Honorary Senior Lecturer,
European Centre for Environment and Human Health Truro, UK
Family Doctor and CEO Intelligent Health, Reading, UK

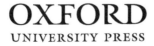

OXFORD
UNIVERSITY PRESS

OXFORD
UNIVERSITY PRESS

Great Clarendon Street, Oxford, OX2 6DP,
United Kingdom

Oxford University Press is a department of the University of Oxford.
It furthers the University's objective of excellence in research, scholarship,
and education by publishing worldwide. Oxford is a registered trade mark of
Oxford University Press in the UK and in certain other countries

Published in the United States of America by Oxford University Press
198 Madison Avenue, New York, NY 10016, United States of America

British Library Cataloguing in Publication Data
Data available

Library of Congress Control Number: 2017948318

ISBN 978–0–19–872591–6

Printed in Great Britain by
Ashford Colour Press Ltd.

Dedication

Anthony J. McMichael: a champion for environmental health

Tony McMichael died soon after writing Chapter 7.5 in this book. Born 1942, he was inspired by microbiologist turned planetary health ecologist René Dubos to 'think global act local'. Best known for his leadership in global ecology, climate change, and health, McMichael also pioneered the harm done by lead. He was prolific: 300+ papers, 160+ chapters, 3 sole-authored books, and 9 that were co-edited.

After graduating in medicine, McMichael was elected president of the Australian National Union of Students in 1968. By 1994, he was Epidemiology Professor at the London School of Hygiene and Tropical Medicine. He instigated and led the health chapter in the second report of the Intergovernmental Panel on Climate Change.

If we are to survive as an advanced and compassionate species, the work of people like McMichael will be recognized as fundamental to the shift that we must accelerate.

Dr Colin Butler
Visiting Fellow NCEPH
Australian National University, Australia

Dedication

Stephen R. Kellert

Nature lost an important friend and advocate with the passing of Stephen R. Kellert on 27 November 2016. Kellert was a pioneering scholar in exploring the biological origins of our environmental values, and the many important ways children and adults interact with, and benefit from, contact with the natural world. He is probably best known for his work in support of the concept of biophilia: the belief that humans have an innate connection and need to affiliate with nature.

Kellert was not simply an academic, but one who cared deeply about seeing these biophilic principles put into practice and utilizing them to improve design of the built environment.

Kellert leaves behind both a biophilic design movement, and a cadre of friends and colleagues who he helped to infect with his enthusiasm for biophilia. Kellert organized the first major national meeting on biophilic design, later leading to the important book, *Biophilic Design: Theory, Science, and Practice of Bringing Buildings to Life* (2008). Many of us who attended that meeting began to see our own work through a biophilic lens, and we became Kellert disciples on a mission to foster a renewed sense of the wonder and beauty of nature, and its special power to heal and to bring meaning and rootedness in a turbulent world. His passion, intellect, and vision for what might be, will be missed by us all.

Tim Beatley
Teresa Heinz Professor of Sustainable Communities
Department of Urban and Environmental Planning
School of Architecture
University of Virginia, USA

Foreword

We live in epochal times.

The origins lie far back in time. Our genus, *Homo*, dates back more than two million years, our species roughly 200,000. Through evolutionary time, we have outlasted many of our Homo cousins—neanderthalensis, heidelbergensis, floresiensis, and more (Harari, 2014). That long process shaped us in complex ways, including endowing us with a deep connection to nature (Wilson, 1984). But we may not fully understand and appreciate that connection; we are arguably wired more for fight or flight than for foresight and wisdom (Buss, 2015; Kahneman, 2011).

Cultural history provides further context. Our civilization arose roughly 13,000 years ago, when the Younger Dryas cooling at the end of the Pleistocene gave way to post-glacial warming, marking the beginning of the Holocene. Our ancestors shifted from hunting and gathering to what we recognize as modern life—agriculture and manufacturing, art and culture, towns and cities. Human well-being improved in many ways, although there were also costs, such as less diverse diets and less contact with nature (McMichael *et al.*, 2017).

Recent industrial history provides still further context. The current human predicament dates from just a few hundred years ago, when we learned how to unleash vast amounts of energy that had been locked in fossil fuels over geologic time. This ushered in the Great Acceleration (Steffen *et al.*, 2015)—a time of unprecedented growth in population, urbanization, manufacturing, and of ecological degradation. So great was the impact that we have destabilized the very systems that maintain our planet. Rising atmospheric concentrations of greenhouse gases, especially carbon dioxide, are altering the climate. Biodiversity is diminishing as species go extinct at alarming rates. The pH of the ocean is falling. In many parts of the world, nitrogen and phosphorus cycles have been profoundly altered, soil degraded, forests extirpated, river flows interrupted, fresh water supplies depleted. Human impacts on earth systems define the epoch in which we live: the Anthropocene (Steffen *et al.*, 2007).

In many ways, the Anthropocene has been good to us. Our numbers have grown, as has our life expectancy. We have conquered ancient health problems such as polio, and we have limited the damage done by many diseases, from leprosy to tuberculosis to syphilis. But the story is not all rosy. Deep disparities persist; the wealthy enjoy far better health than the poor. And the Great Acceleration brought with it an epidemiologic transition, in which chronic and degenerative diseases supplanted infectious diseases around the world (Barrett *et al.*, 2015; Omran, 1971; Zuckerman *et al.*, 2014). Cardiovascular diseases, chronic respiratory diseases, and cancers—the so-called 'non-communicable diseases'—became the predominant killers. The factors that contribute to these conditions—obesity, high blood pressure, unhealthy diets, sedentary lifestyles, stress—became routine realities for far too many people.

Other conditions have also become common, causing suffering if not death, and the explanation is not always clear. Allergies, asthma, and autoimmune diseases such as lupus are on the rise, and may reflect, at least in part, an alteration of the human relationship with the microbial world (Versini *et al.*, 2015; Velasquez-Manoff, 2012). Back pain, neck pain, and headaches are disturbingly common (Vos *et al.*, 2016). So are autism, attention deficit-hyperactivity disorder (Vos *et al.*, 2016), anxiety, depression, and substance abuse (Whiteford *et al.*, 2015). In a world of increasing plenty, even in the wealthiest and most peaceful countries, large proportions of people report being unhappy and unsatisfied with their lives (Helliwell *et al.*, 2016).

Part of the solution can be found in this book.

We humans have a longstanding affiliation with the natural world, one embedded in evolutionary time (Wilson, 1984). Like all deep, authentic relationships, it is not always happy: sabre-toothed tigers chased us, snakes bit us, bees stung us, storms lashed us. But the natural world has also been a source of sustenance, succour, and inspiration. And now, it is increasingly clear that a feature of modern life—indeed, a corollary of our frenzied charge into the Anthropocene—is the breaching of this relationship.

The litany of problems is familiar. Urbanization has reduced opportunities for nature contact—not urbanization per se, but bad urbanization, featuring sterile, lifeless settings, and vast distances between where people live and where they can access greenspace. People in 'developed' nations spend the vast majority of their time indoors—in the United States, more than 90% (Klepeis *et al.*, 2001). Technology has taken centre stage in many people's lives, supplanting nature contact; children younger than age eight have an average of almost two hours of screen time each day (Rideout, 2013), a figure that nearly quadruples, to more than 7.5 hours, during their teenage years (Rideout *et al.*, 2010). Adults go even further, averaging a stunning 10 hours and 39 minutes of 'total media consumption' each day (Nielsen, 2016). Park visitation, hunting, fishing, camping, and children's outdoor play have all declined substantially over recent decades (Pergams and Zaradic, 2008; Clements, 2004;

Frost, 2010). 'Nature deficit disorder', while not a formal diagnostic term, denotes a widespread ailment (Louv, 2005).

Nature contact offers an astonishingly wide range of benefits for human health and well-being, from improving birth outcomes and reducing obesity, relieving depression to prolonging life. The relevant body of science is growing rapidly, and many published reviews have summarized it (Bowler *et al.*, 2010; Lee and Maheswaran, 2011; Russell *et al.*, 2013; Martens and Bauer, 2013; Hartig *et al.*, 2014; James *et al.*, 2015; Seymour, 2016). It is essential to document these benefits, and there is no more comprehensive collection of that documentation than in this book.

It is also essential to understand how nature benefits health and well-being—through what biomedical, social, and cultural pathways it operates. As with pharmaceuticals, this biomedical understanding will enable us to provide the most effective 'doses' of nature, in the most effective ways, to those who will benefit the most. Innovative science, from brain imaging to immune function tests, is propelling the needed research. This book admirably summarizes what we now know about the mechanisms that underlie nature benefits.

But scientific understanding is not enough. We need to implement what we know. We need to apply evidence to designing, creating, and maintaining opportunities for nature contact in ways that demonstrably make people healthier, happier, and more self-actualized. This is a task for the design professions—architects, urban planners, and landscape architects. It is a task for educators, school board members, and child care professionals. It is a task for parks and recreation professionals. It is a task for health professionals. It is a task for parents, and for elected officials. This book offers a rich selection of strategies and tactics for translating research into action.

We need a moral dimension to this work. In far too many ways, modern societies are stratified and unequal. Small minorities in most societies control vastly disproportionate shares of resources, and large numbers of people live in deprivation. Nature contact is not just an amenity; it is a birthright. Moreover, given evidence that nature contact disproportionately benefits those who are less well-off (Mitchell and Popham, 2008; Mitchell *et al.*, 2015), it may be an effective way to help rectify health disparities.

And cradling all of this—the science, the implementation, the social justice—we need culture change. A deeply felt appreciation of the natural world and of the human place in it, a sense of reverence and humility, an openness to awe and wonder, the ability to think in systems, a commitment to creating and preserving legacy—these must be promoted as cultural norms. They can be found in the wisdom of indigenous peoples worldwide, in philosophy, art, poetry, and popular culture, from ancient Greece to the New England transcendentalists (McLuhan, 1994). In these troubled times, when planetary health hangs in the balance, when, as Bill McKibben memorably wrote (McKibben, 1989), the 'end of nature' seems possible, may this fine book provide the evidence, the wisdom, and the inspiration to help renew the human relationship with the natural world, enabling health and well-being now and for generations to come.

Howard Frumkin, M.D., Dr. P.H.
Professor of Environmental and Occupational Health Sciences
University of Washington
Seattle, USA

References

Barrett, B., Charles, J. W., & Temte, J. L. (2015). Climate change, human health, and epidemiological transition. *Prev Med*, 70, 69–75.

Bowler, D. E., Buyung-Ali, L. M., Knight, T. M., & Pullin, A. S. (2010). A systematic review of evidence for the added benefits to health of exposure to natural environments. *BMC Public Health*, 10, 456.

Buss, D. M. (2015). *Evolutionary Psychology: The New Science of the Mind*, Boston, MA: Allyn & Bacon.

Clements, R. (2004). An investigation of the status of outdoor play. *Contemporary Issues in Early Childhood*, 5, 68–80.

Frost, J. L. (2010). *A History of Children's Play and Play Environments: Toward a Contemporary Child-Saving Movement*. New York, NY: Routledge.

Harari, Y. N. (2014). *Sapiens: A Brief History of Humankind*. London, UK: Vintage Books.

Hartig, T., Mitchell, R., De Vries, S., & Frumkin, H. (2014). Nature and health. *Annu Rev Public Health*, 35, 207–28.

Helliwell, J., Layard, R., & Sachs, J. (2016). *World Happiness Report 2016, Volume I*. Available at: http://worldhappiness.report/wp-content/uploads/sites/2/2016/03/HR-V1_web.pdf [Online].

James, P., Banay, R. F., Hart, J. E., & Laden, F. (2015). A review of the health benefits of greenness. *Curr Epidemiol Rep*, 2, 131–42.

Kahneman, D. (2011). *Thinking, Fast and Slow*. New York, NY: Farrar, Straus and Giroux.

Klepeis, N. E., Nelson, W. C., Ott, W. R., et al. (2001). The National Human Activity Pattern Survey (NHAPS): a resource for assessing exposure to environmental pollutants. *J Expo Anal Environ Epidemiol*, 11, 231–52.

Lee, A. C. K. & Maheswaran, R. (2011). The health benefits of urban green spaces: a review of the evidence. *J Public Health*, 33, 212–22.

Louv, R. (2005). *Last Child in the Woods: Saving Our Children from Nature-Deficit Disorder*. Chapel Hill, NC: Algonquin Books.

Martens, D. & Bauer, N. (2013). Natural environments: A resource for public health and well-being? A literature review. In: Noehammer, E. (ed.) *Psychology of Well-Being: Theory, Perspectives and Practice*. Hauppauge NY: Nova Science Publishers.

McKibben, B. (1989). *The End of Nature*. New York, NY: Random House.

McLuhan, T. C. (1994). *The Way of the Earth: Encounters with Nature in Ancient and Contemporary Thought*. New York, NY: Simon & Schuster.

McMichael, A. J., Woodward, A., & Muir, C. (2017). *Climate Change and the Health of Nations: Famines, Fevers, and the Fate of Populations*, Oxford and New York, Oxford University Press.

Mitchell, R. & Popham, F. (2008). Effect of exposure to natural environment on health inequalities: an observational population study. *Lancet*, 372, 1655–60.

Mitchell, R. J., Richardson, E. A., Shortt, N. K., & Pearce, J. R. (2015). Neighborhood environments and socioeconomic inequalities in mental well-being. *Am J Prev Med*, 49, 80–4.

Nielsen (2016). *The Nielsen Total Audience Report: Q1, 2016*. Nielsen. Available at: http://www.nielsen.com/us/en/insights/reports/2016/the-total-audience-report-q1-2016.html [Online].

Omran, A. R. (1971). The epidemiologic transition. A theory of the epidemiology of population change. *Milbank Mem Fund Q*, 49, 509–38.

Pergams, O. R. & Zaradic, P. A. (2008). Evidence for a fundamental and pervasive shift away from nature-based recreation. *Proc Natl Acad Sci U S A*, 105, 2295–300.

Rideout, V. J. (2013). *Zero to Eight: Children's Media Use in America 2013*. Common Sense Media. Available at: https://www.commonsensemedia.org/research/zero-to-eight-childrens-media-use-in-america-2013 [Online].

Rideout, V. J., Foehr, U. G., & Roberts, D. F. (2010). *Generation M2: Media in the Lives of 8- to 18-Year-Olds*. Kaiser Family Foundation. Available at: http://www.kff.org/other/poll-finding/report-generation-m2-media-in-the-lives/ [Online].

Russell, R., Guerry, A. D., Balvanera, P., *et al.* (2013). Humans and nature: How knowing and experiencing nature affect well-being. *Annu Rev Environ Resour*, 38, 473–502.

Seymour, V. (2016). The human–nature relationship and its impact on health: a critical review. *Frontiers in Public Health*, 4. Available at: http://journal.frontiersin.org/article/10.3389/fpubh.2016.00260/full [Online].

Steffen, W., Broadgate, W., Deutsch, L., Gaffney, O., & Ludwig, C. (2015). The trajectory of the Anthropocene: The Great Acceleration. *The Anthropocene Review*, 2, 81–98.

Steffen, W., Crutzen, P. J., & McNeill, J. R. (2007). The Anthropocene: Are humans now overwhelming the great forces of nature? *AMBIO: A Journal of the Human Environment*, 36, 614–21.

Velasquez-Manoff, M. (2012). *An Epidemic of Absence: A New Way of Understanding Allergies and Autoimmune Diseases*. New York, NY: Scribner

Versini, M., Jeandel, P. Y., Bashi, T., Bizzaro, G., Blank, M., & Shoenfeld, Y. (2015). Unraveling the Hygiene Hypothesis of helminthes and autoimmunity: origins, pathophysiology, and clinical applications. *BMC Med*, 13, 81.

Vos, T., Allen, C., Arora, M., *et al.* (2016). Global, regional, and national incidence, prevalence, and years lived with disability for 310 diseases and injuries, 1990-2015: A systematic analysis for the Global Burden of Disease Study 2015. *Lancet*, 388, 1545–602.

Whiteford, H. A., Ferrari, A. J., Degenhardt, L., Feigin, V., & Vos, T. (2015). The global burden of mental, neurological and substance use disorders: an analysis from the Global Burden of Disease Study 2010. *PLoS One*, 10, e0116820.

Wilson, E. O. (1984). *Biophilia*. Cambridge, MA: Harvard University Press.

Zuckerman, M. K., Harper, K. N., Barrett, R., & Armelagos, G. J. (2014). The evolution of disease: anthropological perspectives on epidemiologic transitions. *Glob Health Action*, 7, 23303.

Contents

[†] It is with regret we report the death of Anthony J. McMichael during the preparation of this textbook.
[††] It is with regret we report the death of Stephen R. Kellert during the preparation of this textbook.

Abbreviations

AAA	animal-assisted activities	HEAL	Health and Environment Alliance
AAE	animal-assisted education	HEAT	health economic assessment tool
AAI	animal-assisted interventions	HFA	Health For All
AAT	animal-assisted therapy	HGT	horizontal gene transfer
ACT	artemisinin-based combination therapy	HIA	health impact assessment
ADHD	attention deficit and hyperactivity disorder	HL	Hodgkin's lymphoma
AQBAT	Air Quality Benefits Assessment Tool	HRV	heart rate variability
AR	allergic rhinitis	HSE	Health and Safety Executive
ART	Attention Restoration Theory	IAHAIO	International Association of Human–Animal Interaction Organizations
ASD	acute stress disorder		
BDNF	brain-derived neurotrophic factor	IARC	International Agency for Research on Cancer
BFV	Barmah Forest Virus	ICIMOD	International Centre for Integrated Mountain Development
BMI	body mass index		
CBNRM	community-based natural resources management	IPA	International Play Association
CFM	collaborative forest management	ISAAT	International Society for Animal Assisted Therapy
CNS	central nervous system	ITDP	Institute for Transportation and Development Policy
CRED	Center for Research on the Epidemiology of Disasters	LEED	Leadership in Energy and Environmental Design
CRH	corticotropine-releasing hormone	MUS	medically unexplained symptoms
CRP	C-reactive protein	MVPA	moderate-to-vigorous physical activity
DAF	directed attention fatigue	NAI	nature-assisted interventions
DALY	disability-adjusted life year	NBI	nature-based interventions
DHF	dengue haemorrhagic fever	NCD	non-communicable disease
DOHaD	Developmental Origins of Health and Disease	NFC	near field communication
EA	environmental assessment	NGF	nerve growth factor
EE	environmental enrichment	NGO	non-governmental organization
EF	ecological footprinting	NK	natural killer
EIA	environmental impact assessment	NRPA	National Recreation and Park Association
ELC	European Landscape Convention	OFFE	Olfactory Function Field Exam
ELF	early life stress	OPEC	Outdoor Play Environment Categories
EPA	Environmental Protection Agency	PAHO	Pan American Health Organization
ES	ecosystem services	PANIC	Physical Activity and Nutrition in Children
ESS	Emotional State Scale	PAR	predictive adaptive responses
ESSP	Earth Systems Science Partnership	PFA	Perceptual Fluency Account
FAO	Food and Agriculture Organization	PHC	Primary Health Care
FoF	fear of falling	PSR	Physicians for Social Responsibility
FSS	functional somatic syndrome	PTSD	post-traumatic stress disorder
FSSD	Framework for Strategic Sustainable Development	QALY	quality-adjusted life year
GAD	generalized anxiety disorder	QoL	quality of life
GBD	global burden of disease	RMSF	Rocky Mountain spotted fever
GDM	gestational diabetes mellitus	ROS	reactive oxidative species
GI	green infrastructure	RRT	Reward Restoration Theory
HCWH	Health Care Without Harm	RRV	Ross River Virus
HD	Huntington's disease	RSPB	Royal Society for Protection of Birds

SAVE	sociocultural appraisals, values, and emotions	SNS	sympathetic nervous system
SCCYP	Scotland's Commissioner for Children and Young People	SPUGS	small public urban green spaces
		SRT	Stress Reduction Theory
SCI	spinal cord injury	TBE	tick-borne encephalitis
SCL	skin conductance level	TBI	traumatic brain injury
SES	socioeconomic status	TEEB	The Economics of Ecosystems and Biodiversity
SET	Supportive Environment Theory	TWS	tsunami warning system
SETAC	Society of Environmental Toxicology and Chemistry	UHI	urban heat island
SIDS	Small Island Developing States	UNEP	United Nations Environment Programme
SIRCC	Scottish Institute for Residential Child Care	USDA	United States Department of Agriculture
SMR	standardized mortality ratios	WHO	World Health Organization

Contributors

Julia Africa, The Center for Health and the Global Environment, Harvard School of Public Health, Boston, MA, USA

Albert Ahenkan, University of Ghana Business School, Department of Public Administration and Health Services Management, Accra, Ghana

My S. Almqvist, Stockholm Resilience Centre, Stockholm University, Stockholm, Sweden

Silvia Ariccio, Department of Psychology of Development Processes and Socialization, Faculty of Medicine and Psychology, Sapienza University of Rome, Rome, Italy

David J. Ball, Middlesex University, School of Science and Technology Centre for Decision Analysis and Risk Management, London, UK

Laurence N. Ball-King, King's College London, London, UK

Tim Beatley, University of Virginia, Charlottesville, VA, USA

Simon Bell, Department of Landscape Architecture, Estonian University of Life Sciences, Estonia; and OPENspace Research Centre, Edinburgh School of Architecture and Landscape Architecture, University of Edinburgh, Edinburgh, UK

Julie Bernhardt, Florey Institute of Neuroscience and Mental Health, Melbourne, Australia

Jeffrey M. Bielicki, Department of Civil, Environmental, and Geodetic Engineering, The Ohio State University and John Glenn College of Public Affairs, The Ohio State University, Columbus, OH, USA

William Bird, Honorary Senior Lecturer, European Centre for Environment and Human Health, Truro, UK; Family Doctor and CEO Intelligent Health, Reading, UK

Marino Bonaiuto, Department of Psychology of Developmental and Socialization Processes, Faculty of Medicine and Psychology, CIRPA - Interuniversity Research Centre for Environmental Psychology, Sapienza University of Rome, Rome, Italy

Mirilia Bonnes, CIRPA - Interuniversity Research Centre for Environmental Psychology, Sapienza University of Rome, Rome, Italy

Emmanuel Boon, Department of Public Health (BISI), Vrije Universiteit Brussel (VUB), Brussels, Belgium

Fiona Bull, School of Earth and Environment and School of Sport Science, Exercise and Health, Center for Built Environment and Health, The University of Western Australia, Perth, Australia

Cinnamon P. Carlarne, The Ohio State University, Michael E. Moritz College of Law, Columbus, OH, USA

Jack Carman, FASLA, Medford, NJ, USA

Ben Cave, Ben Cave Associates Ltd, Leeds, UK; School of Environmental Sciences, University of Liverpool, Liverpool, UK; and Centre for Primary Health Care and Equity, University of New South Wales, Sydney, Australia

Carolina C. Sgobaro Zanette, Independent Landscape Architect, Curitiba, PR, Brazil

Gunnar Cerwén, Department of Landscape Architecture, Planning and Management, Swedish University of Agricultural Sciences, Uppsala, Sweden

Hayley Christian, School of Population and Global Health, The University of Western Australia, Perth, Australia

George Panagiotis Chrousos, First Department of Pediatrics, National and Kapodistrian University of Athens, Athens, Greece

Germán Tovar Corzo, Secretaría Distrital de Ambiente, Alcaldía Mayor de Bogotá, Bogotá, Colombia

Åslög Dahl, Department of Biological and Environmental Sciences, University of Gothenburg, Gothenburg, Sweden

Michael H. Depledge, European Centre for Environment and Human Health, University of Exeter Medical School, Exeter, Devon, UK

Mark Detweiler, Department of Psychiatry, Edward Via College of Osteopathic Medicine, Blacksburg, VA, USA

Stefano De Dominicis, Department of Psychology of Developmental and Socialization Processes, CIRPA - Interuniversity Research Centre for Environmental Psychology, Sapienza University of Rome; Department of Business and Management, LUISS Guido Carli University, Rome, Italy

Birgit Elands, Forest and Nature Conservation Policy, Wageningen University and Research, Wageningen, the Netherlands

Thomas Elmqvist, Stockholm Resilience Centre, Stockholm University, Stockholm, Sweden

Elissa Epel, University of California, San Francisco, CA, USA

Ana Faggi, Argentine National Council of Research, and School of Ecological Engineering, Flores University, Buenos Aires, Argentina

Cathey E. Falvo, International Public Health, New York Medical College, New York, NY, USA; and North America, International Society of Doctors for the Environment, North America, CA, USA

Aubrey H. Fine, Department of Education, California State Polytechnic University, Pomona, CA, USA

Luke Fortney, Sauk Prairie Healthcare River Valley Clinic, Family Medicine, Spring Green, WI, USA

Billie Giles-Corti, McCaughey VicHealth Community Wellbeing Unit, Centre for Health Equity, Melbourne School of Population and Global Health, The University of Melbourne, Melbourne, Australia

Peter D. Gluckman, Liggins Institute, University of Auckland, Auckland, New Zealand

Patrik Grahn, Swedish University of Agricultural Sciences, Alnarp, Sweden

Leila Haddad, Central Institute of Mental Health, University of Heidelberg, Medical Faculty of Mannheim, Mannheim, Germany

Caroline Hägerhäll, Department of Work Science, Business Economics and Environmental Psychology, Swedish University of Agricultural Sciences SLU, Alnarp, Sweden

Anthony Hannan, Florey Institute of Neuroscience and Mental Health, University of Melbourne, Melbourne, Australia

Mark A. Hanson, Institute of Developmental Sciences, University of Southampton, Southampton, UK

Ben Harris-Roxas, South Eastern Research Collaboration for Health (SEaRCH), Part of the Centre for Primary Health Care and Equity and South Eastern Sydney Local Health District, University of New South Wales, Sydney, Australia

Claire Henderson-Wilson, Faculty of Health, School of Health and Social Development, Deakin University, Melbourne, Australia

Michael T. Hernke, School of Business, University of Wisconsin-Madison, Madison, WI, USA

Paula Hooper, Centre for the Built Environment and Health, School of Earth and Environment and School of Sports Science, Exercise and Health Faculty of Science, The University of Western Australia, Crawley, Australia; and NHMRC Centre for Research Excellence in Healthy Liveable Communities, University of Melbourne, Melbourne, Australia

Eva Bojner Horwitz, Department of Clinical Neuroscience and Center for Social Sustainability CSS, Institution of Neurobiology, Caring Sciences and Society, Karolinska Institutet, Solna, Sweden; and Department of Public Health and Caring Sciences, Uppsala University, Stockholm, Sweden

Jeannette R. Ickovics, Yale University, New Haven, CT, USA

Heidi Janssen, Hunter Medical Research Institute, University of Newcastle, Hunter New England Health Local Health District, Newcastle, Australia

Génon K. Jensen, Health and Environment Alliance, Brussels, Belgium

Francesqca E. Jimenez, HDR, Omaha, NE, USA

Peter H. Kahn, Jr., Department of Psychology, and School of Environmental and Forest Sciences, University of Washington, Seattle, WA, USA

Joshua Karliner, Program and Strategy, Health Care Without Harm, San Francisco, CA, USA

Stephen R. Kellert, Yale University, School of Forestry and Environmental Studies, New Haven, CT, USA

Dacher Keltner, Department of Psychology, University of California, Berkeley, CA, USA

Anas A. Khan, Department of Emergency Medicine, College of Medicine and University Medical City, King Saud University, Riyadh, Saudi Arabia

Cecil Konijnendijk van den Bosch, Department of Forest Resources Management, University of British Columbia, Canada

Mohammad Javad Koohsari, Faculty of Sport Sciences, Waseda University, Tokyo, Japan; and Behavioural Epidemiology Laboratory, Baker Heart and Diabetes Institute, Melbourne, Australia

Raffaele Lafortezza, Dip. Scienze Agro-Ambientali e Territoriali, Università degli Studi di Bari, 'Aldo Moro', Bari, Italy

Florian Lederbogen, Central Institute of Mental Health, University of Heidelberg, Medical Faculty Mannheim, Mannheim, Germany

Evelyne de Leeuw, Centre for Health Equity Training, Research and Evaluation (CPHCE), University of New South Wales, South Western Sydney Local Health District, Ingham Institute for Applied Medical Research, Sydney, Australia

Qing Li, Department of Hygiene and Public Health, Nippon Medical School, Tokyo, Japan

Thomas Linden, Institute of Neuroscience and Physiology, Sahlgrenska Academy, University of Gothenburg, Gothenburg, Sweden; Florey Institute of Neuroscience and Mental Health, and Hunter Medical Research Institute, New South Wales, Melbourne, Australia

Elisabet Lindgren, Stockholm Resilience Centre, Stockholm University, Stockholm, Sweden

Alan Logan, 'In-FLAME' the International Inflammation Network, World Universities Network (WUN), Crawley, Australia

Rebecca Lovell, European Centre for Environment and Human Health, University of Exeter Medical School, Truro, Cornwall, UK

Felicia M. Low, Liggins Institute, University of Auckland, Auckland, New Zealand

Fredrika Mårtensson, Department of Work Science, Business Economics and Environmental Psychology, Swedish University of Agricultural Sciences, Alnarp, Sweden

Erik Martin, School of Medicine, Faculty of Health, Deakin University, Melbourne, Australia

Antony McMichael, Formally of the Research School of Population Health, Australian National University, Acton, Australia

Jonna G. Meinersmann-Detweiler, Geriatric Research Group, Salem VAMC, VA, USA

Andreas Meyer-Lindenberg, Central Institute of Mental Health, University of Heidelberg, Medical Faculty Mannheim, Mannheim, Germany

Steven C. Minta, Consultant, OR, USA

Richard Mitchell, MRC/CSO Social and Public Health Sciences Unit, Institute of Health and Wellbeing, University of Glasgow, Glasgow, Scotland, UK

Sylvie Nail, Faculté des Langues et Cultures Etrangères, Université de Nantes, Nantes, France

Michael Nilsson, University of Newcastle, Hunter Medical Research Institute, Hunter New England Local Health District, New Lambton, New South Wales, Australia

Eric K. Noji, Department of Emergency Medicine, King Saud University Hospitals and College of Medicine, Riyadh, Kingdom of Saudi Arabia

David J. Nowak, Northern Research Station, Syracuse, NY, USA

Thomas Ogren, The Society for Allergy-Friendly Environmental (SAFE) Gardening, North America, CA, USA

Danielle C. Ompad, Department of Epidemiology, College of Global Public Health, New York University, New York, NY, USA

Marla Orenstein, Habitat Health Impact Consulting, Calgary, Canada

Walter Osika, Department of Clinical Neuroscience, Center for Social Sustainability, Karolinska Institute, Stockholm, Sweden

Sabine Pahl, School of Psychology, Faculty of Health and Human Sciences, University of Plymouth, Plymouth, UK

Anna María Pálsdóttir, Swedish University of Agricultural Sciences, Alnarp, Sweden

Panagiota Pervanidou, Unit of Developmental and Behavioral Pediatrics, First Department of Pediatrics, National and Kapodistrian, University of Athens; and Aghia Sophia Children's Hospital, Athens, Greece

Karin Peters, Wageningen University and Research, Cultural Geography Group, Wageningen, the Netherlands

Paul Piff, Department of Psychology and Social Behavior, University of California, Irvine, CA, USA

Rian Podein, Department of Family Medicine and Community Health, University of Wisconsin School of Medicine and Public Health, Madison, WI, USA

Michael Pollack, HNE Health, New Lambton, New South Wales, Australia

Daniel Press, University of California, Santa Cruz, CA, USA

Haywantee Ramkissoon, Department of Marketing and Behaviour Works Australia, Monash University, Victoria, Australia

Karl-Henrik Robèrt, Blekinge Institute of Technology, Karlskrona, Sweden

Graham Rook, Centre for Clinical Microbiology, Department of Infection, UCL (University College London), London, UK

Osama A. Samarkandi, Basic Science Department, College for Emergency Medical Services, King Saud University, Riyadh, Kingdom of Saudi Arabia

Massimiliano Scopelliti, Department of Human Studies, Libera Università Maria Ss. Assunta (LUMSA University), Rome, Italy

Joe Sempik, School of Social Policy, University of Birmingham, Birmingham, UK

Filipe Silva, Public Health by Design, London, UK

Neil J. Spratt, HNE Health, New Lambton, New South Wales, Australia

Henk Staats, Department of Social and Organizational Psychology, Leiden University, Leiden, the Netherlands

Rachel Stancliffe, The Centre for Sustainable Healthcare, Oxford, UK

Linda Steg, Faculty of Behavioural and Social Sciences, University of Groningen, Groningen, the Netherlands

Cecilia Stenfors, Environmental Science Lab, Department of Psychology, University of Chicago, IL, USA; and Department of Neurobiology, Care Sciences and Society, Karolinska Institute, Stockholm, Sweden

Takemi Sugiyama, Faculty of Health Sciences, Australian Catholic University, Institute for Health and Ageing, Melbourne, Australia

Danny Taufik, Wageningen University and Research, Wageningen, the Netherlands

Richard Taylor, Physics Department, University of Oregon, Eugene, OR, USA

Töres Theorell, Department of Neuroscience, Karolinska Institute, Stockholm, Sweden

Mardie Townsend, School of Health and Social Development, Deakin University, Melbourne, Australia

Agnes E. van den Berg, Department of Cultural Geography, Faculty of Spatial Sciences, University of Groningen, Groningen, the Netherlands

Matilda van den Bosch, School of Population and Public Health, Department of Forest and Conservation Sciences, The University of British Columbia, Vancouver, Canada

Leonie Venhoeven, Faculty of Behavioral and Social Sciences, University of Groningen, Groningen, the Netherlands

Francesca Viliani, International SOS, Copenhagen, Denmark

Salim Vohra, Department of Public Health, College of Nursing, Midwifery and Healthcare, University of West London, London, UK

Sebastian Völker, Institute for Hygiene and Public Health, University of Bonn, Germany

Sjerp de Vries, Wageningen Environmental Research (Alterra), Wageningen University and Research, Wageningen, the Netherlands

Peter Währborg, Währborg Research and Consulting AB, Gothenburg, Sweden

Frederick R. Walker, University of Newcastle, School of Biomedical Sciences and Pharmacy, Hunter Medical Research Institute, Newcastle, Australia

Temo Waqanivalu, World Health Organization, Geneva, Switzerland

Catharine Ward Thompson, OPENspace Research Centre, University of Edinburgh, Edinburgh, UK

Greg Watts, Bradford Centre for Sustainable Environments, Faculty of Engineering and Informatics, University of Bradford, Bradford, UK

Shawna J. Weaver, College of St. Scholastica, Duluth, MN, USA

Premila Webster, Nuffield Department of Population Health, University of Oxford, Oxford, UK

Rona Weerasuriya, School of Health and Social Development, Deakin University, Melbourne, Australia

Nancy M. Wells, Design and Environmental Analysis, College of Human Ecology, Cornell University, New York, NY, USA

Benedict W. Wheeler, European Centre for Environment and Human Health, University of Exeter Medical School, Exeter, Cornwall, UK

Mathew P. White, European Centre for Environment and Human Health, University of Exeter Medical School, Knowledge Spa, Exeter, Cornwall, UK

David Wong, U.S. Public Health Service, Epidemiology Branch, Office of Public Health, National Park Service, Albuquerque, NM, USA

Robert Zarr, Park Rx America, Unity Health Care, Inc., US National Park Service, Washington, DC, USA

Jia Wei Zhang, Department of Psychology, University of California, Berkeley, CA, USA

SECTION 1

Why is nature a health factor?

CHAPTER 1.1

Setting the scene and how to read the book

Matilda van den Bosch and William Bird

Healthy nature, healthy people

For virtually all our development humans have been totally dependent on nature. With increasing industrialization and urbanization human beings have become partly disconnected from natural environments, both physically and mentally. The disconnection is now being viewed as a threat to health and this book explains how this disconnection displays through several pathways and eventually defined health outcomes. Equally, contact with natural environments may serve as a remedy for many contemporary health issues.

Public health does not depend only on the health of other human beings, but also on the health of our surrounding natural ecosystems. This notion is, for example, included in the concept of ecological public health (Rayner, 2012). Ecological public health embraces complex and dynamic biological, material, social, and cultural dimensions of the human, living, and physical world. This opens up questions of non-linearity, evolutionary mismatch and biological feedback, and other aspects of nature and human behaviour. To put it simple—it is obvious that we cannot expect to live healthy lives, unless also the ecosystems, on which we depend, are healthy and functional (Lang and Rayner, 2012). To fully acknowledge this, and to create knowledge aimed for action, the various interactions between humans and natural environments must be explored and illuminated. This means all kinds of interactions with all kinds of humans and with all kinds of nature.

This book considers various interactions between humans and nature and the influence on health. This implies all potential health benefits, all trade-offs, all medical and healthcare options, all policies, and all directly and indirectly related topics of the relationship between humans and nature. By presenting the multiple facets of this relationship, a fascinating and challenging complexity will be revealed. This complexity mirrors the kind of health issues we are facing today.

A changing disease scenario

A new disease scenario is challenging global health, due to changes in lifestyles as well as social and environmental conditions. Non-communicable diseases (NCDs) are currently dominating the global disease burden. This means that diabetes, cancer, cardiovascular and chronic obstructive pulmonary diseases, obesity, and mental disorders have surpassed infectious diseases as the main health issues globally (WHO, 2014). However, this obviously varies between populations and regions of the world. In sub-Saharan Africa, infectious diseases, like HIV/AIDS and malaria, are still the major threats to health, though also here the NCDs are rapidly increasing in prevalence (Naghavi and Forouzanfar, 2013). This is, at least partly, a consequence of urbanization, energy consumption, and adoption of Western world lifestyles (Potts, 2012).

Environmental change, sustainability, and public health

Biodiversity loss and climate change have a major impact on human health (Watts et al., 2015) and this demonstrates the complex interdependence between the environment and health and well-being. In order to halt further environmental degradation and climate change we need to change ways of living and find mutual and sustainable solutions for health of people and nature. As part of a new sustainable development agenda from 2015, countries adopted a set of goals to end poverty, protect the planet, and ensure prosperity for all over the coming 15 years. Of the 17 Sustainable Development Goals (SDGs) only one explicitly mentions health (goal no. 3: 'Good health and well-being'), but all goals trespass the traditional disciplinary silos and make it clear that every goal is dependent on the fulfilment of the others (Waage et al., 2015). This means that environmental threats to human health are considered as well as environmental solutions which can reinforce human health and well-being. For example, a subgoal under goal no. 3 declares that by 2030 access to green spaces shall be secured particularly for women, children, and other vulnerable population groups. This is a clear indication that exposure to nature is starting to be recognized as vital for human health.

A guide to the book

Section 1: Why is nature a health factor?

This book seeks to explore how natural environments and ecosystems contribute to human health and well-being. This exploration will start by laying out a foundation of fundamental concepts like system science, the life course approach, the Developmental Origins of Health and Disease (DOHaD), stress, and evolution. While the contents of this first section may at a first glance appear peripheral to the book's topic, outlining these concepts contributes to a more profound understanding of what nature means to human health and how we can approach it in thought and action. It may be possible to exclude this section and go directly to the theories and evidence around nature's impact on health, but for putting theories, evidence, and practice into a conceptual, planetary, philosophical, and outreaching context this foundation will be highly supportive.

In Chapter 1.2, 'A life course approach to public health: why early life matters', Felicia Low and her colleagues describe the full range of early life exposures and the implications for future health. They also explain recent research which expands beyond heritability of disease risk, because genetic variation is a poor explanation for the increasingly common NCDs. In order to promote health we need to understand how and why disease prevalence varies between populations and how the impact of environment contributes to shaping health and disease patterns. As it becomes clear that negative environmental exposures during prenatal and early life determine a person's health development throughout the entire life, it is plausible that early exposure to natural environments, with opportunities for physical activity and recreation, can contribute to healthier and longer lives. Keeping in mind that natural environments may represent ideal settings for healthy behaviours, the DOHaD paradigm is a way to incorporate nature into the life course approach to public health research and actions. It also clarifies the urgent need to consider health and interventions for improving public health from a much wider and more inclusive perspective than what is currently the prevailing situation within many medical curricula.

By introducing systems science in Chapter 1.3, 'Systems thinking for global health and strategic sustainable development', we want to further emphasize how inter- or transdisciplinary thinking is necessary for achieving health for all—both people and planet. By outlining a framework for strategic sustainable development (FSSD), Karl-Henrik Robèrt and his colleagues show how resilient environments and global health are intimately intertwined. In doing so, they provide tools for implementing systems science for efficient solutions in complex systems. As we have already concluded that current health and environmental issues are of increasingly complex characters, such tools are of fundamental value for public health understanding and action, not the least for increasing the understanding of nature's value for health development.

A basic understanding of the stress concept is useful in any work on current diseases and relation to the environment. Particularly when considering how and why nature may have a positive influence on health, stress is a central feature. In Chapter 1.4, 'The physiology of stress and stress recovery' Peter Währborg and colleagues share their experience from lifetime research and work around stress physiology and disease development.

Stress has been defined as a state where our bodily equilibrium is threatened (McEwen, 1998). While this is an evolutionary developed physiological reaction, as we need to respond adequately to acute risks to our survival, the same reactions tend to be harmful if an acute stress reaction is not followed by recovery and return to equilibrium. The further we alienate ourselves from our species' evolutionary origin the risk for such sustained stress states seem to increase.

Many chronic diseases can, at least partly, be attributed to dysfunctional or prolonged stress reactions (McEwen, 2008). While we are developed for a life connected to nature, we are today mostly spending our days in urban indoor settings experiencing stress from factors like economic uncertainties, management of conflicts, or hostile urban realms without opportunities for recovery. None of these situations are likely to be alleviated by physiological stress reactions, such as excretion of stress hormones, increased heart rate

and blood pressure, and redirection of blood flow from brain to muscles. This is one of the basic premises for why nature may play a fundamental role for our health, as it can contribute to recovery and return to a balanced physiological state. While increasing the understanding of this fundament, this text can also work as a reference chapter when the stress concept is mentioned throughout the book.

Building on Chapter 1.4, Chapter 1.5 'Unifying mechanisms: nature deficiency, chronic stress, and inflammation' by William Bird and colleagues develops the theories around the fundamental relevance of chronic stress and chronic inflammation for health and disease. This text brings us further into the role of cell metabolism, mitochondria, and genetic material for understanding linkages between environment, stress, and inflammation. The authors present recent research demonstrating the intricate links between our inner biochemical environments and the outer world and how these links interact to determine various states of health.

Section 2: How nature can affect health—theories and mechanisms

Next section presents the development of the scientific field around nature and health relations; from early theories and hypotheses in, for example, environmental psychology to later research exploring biological mechanisms behind human reactions to nature exposure.

In Chapter 2.1, 'Environmental psychology', Agnes van den Berg and Henk Staats give a broad overview of the topic's rise and progress within the environmental psychology discipline. In this chapter, the historic development of human-nature research is revealed, including theories around aesthetics and preferences. Many of these values tend to be subjectively perceived and are thus important to understand for drawing conclusions on what particular environments may be beneficial across different populations and cultures. While keeping this relative perspective in mind, several of the theories also refer to the concept of biophilia, drawing on human evolution in natural landscapes. Biophilia proposes that there is an inherent human bond to natural environments, recognized for survival, restoration, and protection (Wilson, 1984). The authors describe how the field has developed over time and how empirical findings have spurred new theory advancement, essential for coming research.

Mardie Townsend and her colleagues continue the exploration of psychological concepts of nature and well-being in Chapter 2.2, 'Therapeutic landscapes, restorative environments, place attachment, and well-being'. The historical outlook on these notions dates back to several centuries BC. While therapeutic landscapes and restorative environments may initially appear as abstract models, this chapter defines and explains distinctions between the two and clarifies the relation to theories outlined in the previous chapter. As the authors further illuminate and concretize place attachment, sense of place, and ecopsychology the link to well-being and public health is revealed. Case studies are used to illustrate the concepts. The chapter also describes current challenges to the psychological relation between human and nature, a relation that may be more important to recognize now than ever before.

In Chapter 2.3, 'Microbes, the immune system, and the health benefits of exposure to the natural environment', Graham Rook presents theories on the importance of microbial biodiversity for healthy immune system development. Those theories are supported by findings of differences in immune function depending on childhood exposure to natural and biodiverse environments

(Kondrashova *et al.*, 2013). These ideas thus represent another biological mechanism or pathway between nature and health. It also provides a possible explanation for the rise of autoimmune diseases in later years, correlating in time with increasing urbanization and disconnection from nature.

Following this, Heidi Janssen and her colleagues explain how the expanding research on enriched environments (Chapter 2.4, 'Environmental enrichment: neurophysiological responses and consequences for health') may relate to nature and health mechanisms. While much of the research in this field is based on rat studies and an enriched environment may not fully correspond to a particular natural setting, the intriguing mechanisms occur likely to parallel human reactions to nature. Therefore, it is important to follow this research line and the chapter demonstrates how certain positive clues, providing multisensory stimulation in the environment, affect neuroanatomical and physiological functions, which improve behavioural and health outcomes. For example, neurogenesis and neuronal survival are enhanced by a richness in environmental stimuli (Sale *et al.*, 2009). Certain features of enriched environments, such as complexity and novelty, are abundant in nature and may thus represent an inherently enriched environment.

In Chapter 2.5, 'Biological mechanisms and physiological responses to sensory impact from nature', Caroline Hägerhäll and colleagues take us from psychology to physiology. Drawing on both old and novel theories and hypotheses they describe empirical findings which demonstrate how humans are biologically affected by nature. Adding such findings to epidemiological results on causality provides a firm evidence base for health effects of nature exposure. The authors draw partly on their own research on visual, auditory, and olfactory sensory input from nature, demonstrating specific physiological responses as measured by neuroimaging and other physiological monitoring methods.

Much of our health and well-being is determined by our behaviour. In Chapter 2.6, 'The role of nature and environment in behavioural medicine' Leonie Venhoeven and colleagues describe how input from nature may influence our behaviour and how this affects our health both directly and indirectly. While behavioural medicine has traditionally studied behaviours with direct impact on health, such as physical activity and social interactions, this chapter outlines theories and research around environmentally related behaviour. For example, pro-environmental behaviour is described and how this may be triggered by contact with nature, and the influence this may have on health. This highlights an intriguing chain reaction where pro-environmental behaviour can have an effect on individual well-being, but may also indirectly affect public health through prevention of further environmental degradation and climate change. Once again, the dynamics and interrelatedness in the area of nature and public health are exposed.

Section 3: Public health impact of nature contact—pathways to health promotion and disease prevention

In Section 3, major pathways through which natural environments are in general believed to affect public health, are described. This section provides an abundance of arguments for why investments in green spaces across different populations are necessary for maintaining and improving public health. Such arguments are important in any health policy making and should increase collaboration across environmental and health sectors and disciplines. By providing empirical evidence on the importance of urban greenery for

public health, nature gains a step in the ever increasing competition around urban land.

One mediating factor between nature and health outcomes is physical activity. In Chapter 3.1, 'Promoting physical activity—reducing obesity and non-communicable diseases', Billie Giles-Corti and her colleagues first outline the multiple health risks that are associated with physical inactivity and how this issue has increased over time. By doing so, it becomes obvious that even minor interventions that can promote physical activity are of substantial value in a larger population perspective. It has been recognized that the availability, quality, and design of public green spaces may play an important role for community levels of physical activity (Sallis *et al.*, 2016; Almanza *et al.*, 2012). The chapter presents findings on the value of nature and green spaces for children, adolescents, adults, and elderly in promoting physical activity and thereby preventing obesity and other NCDs. Whether there is a connection between access to green spaces and physical activity or not has recently come to debate. Potential explanations and ideas around some inconsistency in results are presented and discussed by the authors.

Another potential factor contributing to the health and nature relation is stress. This is discussed by Matilda van den Bosch and her colleagues in Chapter 3.2, 'Preventing stress and promoting mental health'. Similar to physical inactivity, stress is a major risk factor in today's disease scenario and often attributed to the increasing prevalence of mental disorders (McEwen, 2012). Early theories from environmental psychology and related disciplines already suggested that restoration and stress recovery may have an important explanatory role to play. The evolutionary fundaments for this are explained in for example Chapter 2.1 and physiological mechanisms are outlined in the chapter on stress (1.4). This chapter explains how nature may affect stress and how this may reduce the prevalence of mental disorders, currently a major public health issue across the world (Vos *et al.*, 2015).

Finally, nature's potential for building social capital is elaborated on in Chapter 3.3, 'Promoting social cohesion and social capital—increasing well-being'. In this chapter Birgit Elands and her colleagues present their own and others' work, demonstrating how green areas seem to facilitate social interactions and thereby creating individual and community well-being. Social isolation is today considered a risk factor of the same magnitude as smoking with similar odds for morbidity and mortality (Holt-Lunstad *et al.*, 2015). Thus, if green spaces encourage social networking there is a vast potential for health gains. Open green spaces are often visited by various population groups, thereby offering opportunities for interactions across cultural and social borders. The authors also discuss how certain types of green spaces, for example community or allotment gardens, are particularly suited for social interactions and how appropriate planning of green spaces is necessary for encouraging social interactions.

Section 4: Public health impact of nature contact—intervention and rehabilitation

The contents of this book are much focused on classical public health approaches, such as health promotion and disease prevention. The following section describes how nature has been incorporated in healthcare for treatment of various conditions. In this context, animal-assisted interventions and other correlating complex interventions are included.

In Chapter 4.1, 'Using nature as a treatment option', Anna María Pálsdóttir and colleagues provide definitions and examples of the broad spanning field of interventions using nature in various forms to treat and cure illnesses. Gardens have traditionally been used in mental healthcare, but many other forms of nature interactions, such as farming and wilderness experiences, exist as therapeutic means. The chapter provides an overview of how nature can be both an arena for interventions and have therapeutic effects in itself. Concepts such as horticultural therapy, green care, and wilderness therapy are described and related to respective diagnoses for which efficiency has been demonstrated.

The human–animal bond is an inherent and profound feature of humankind. Therefore, it is not surprising that interactions with animals may be restorative and help recovering from various diseases. In Chapter 4.2, 'The human–animal bond and animal-assisted intervention', Aubrey H. Fine and Shawna J. Weaver demonstrate how animals and pets can be used in healthcare. They also outline various theories and describe how research has tried to uncover the biological fundaments behind the health effects of, for example, petting an animal. Some of this has been related to release of the hormone oxytocin, which is associated with feelings of happiness and trust (Rodrigues et al., 2009).

Finally, Cecilia Stenfors and her colleagues give an outlook on other non-pharmaceutical or surgical interventions that may be used in healthcare. In the chapter 'Similarities, disparities, and synergies with other complex interventions—stress as a common pathway' (4.3), commonalities between nature therapies and other complex interventions, based on for example meditation or cultural utterances, are revealed. Many parallels, both psychological and physiological, seem to lead back to stress and stress recovery processes. By recognizing both commonalities and distinctions, individually tailored therapies and synergistic effects may be achieved.

Section 5: Public health impact of varied landscapes and environments

In Section 5, various types of nature and respective effects on health and well-being are described. It may appear unnatural to try and divide something as complex and dynamic as nature into separate entities. Obviously, this is a construct far from the real world—urban woodlands dynamically transfer into wilderness, lakes, and seashores are embedded in forests or parks—nature as a whole involves all parts to various extents and in various shapes. The chapters in this section evidently do not ignore this fact, but by a small act of nature dissection some particular features of specific environments can be revealed and our understanding of the whole may thus increase.

First, Simon Bell and Qing Li describe the wonders of 'The great outdoors: Forests, wilderness, and public health' (5.1). Forests may, by some, be considered the ultimate representation of nature—the wild, the untouched, and containing many of the basics for our survival. However, today only very few, if any, forests are untouched by human hand and the health benefits may be of a different, less basic kind, at least in the Western part of the world. In spite of this, forests still seem to be places where people go to search for peace and to find an escape from the hectic daily grind and stress of city living. This chapter draws on theories and research to highlight some particular health benefits that may be achieved by visiting forests; for example, effects on the neuroendocrine immune system and thereby reduced stress by so-called 'forest bathing' (Shinrin-yoku).

Another distinct type of nature is water in its various shapes and forms. Mathew White and his colleagues describe how access to landscapes including water affect health in Chapter 5.2, 'Blue landscapes and public health'. Water continues to have a special value for humankind in terms of survival, culture, and religion. Many symbolic rituals, such as baptism, are centred on elements of water. This may indicate an innate preference for water with an instant well-being effect. Research on blue landscapes has not yet developed as much as for green landscapes (although bearing in mind that green and blue are not always to be considered as separate from each other), but recent studies suggest that health effects of visiting, for example, a seashore, may be even stronger than visiting a merely green landscape. Many effects seem to relate to stress recovery.

In the chapter 'Technological nature and human well-being' (5.3) Peter Kahn shares his view and research on so-called technological nature, to be found in the interface between human dependence on healthy ecosystems and the current exponential growth of technological solutions. Technological nature can take many forms, from nature films on television to geocaching in the woods. Kahn discusses what happens to human beings and our health if we replace real nature with simulated natural settings. It becomes clear that many of the sensory experiences and dynamics gained by interacting with nature in the mountains, the forests, or the water landscapes are falling short in technological nature interactions. And while we may manage to adapt to technological forms of nature, it may not be a beneficial adaptation—neither for us nor the environment.

Section 6: Varied populations and interactions with nature

In the complex landscape of nature and human health associations it is often found that different people react differently to nature. This is fairly evident considering our various backgrounds and various needs across the lifespan. Although individual differences evidently exist, it seems possible to draw some general conclusions on reactions to nature depending on population group. In Section 6, different responses to interactions with nature depending on age, and socioeconomic or cultural belonging are described together with the implications this has for how nature can best be integrated in planning, care, and living environments.

Nancy Wells and her colleagues start this section with Chapter 6.1, 'Children and nature'. Children's relation to nature is of specific value—not only for the developing individual itself, but also for the environment. If no connection to nature is established in early years it will be hard for the growing individual to develop a sense for the environment, which may lead to further environmental destruction and biodiversity loss. For the child itself, outdoor nature exposure contributes to an almost endless line of various benefits—for cognitive, social, and motoric development, for play and physical activity, for concentration capacity and academic performance, and for preventing myopia, vitamin D deficiency, stress, and obesity.

Older people may suffer from anxiety disorders, often aggravated by multimedication. In Chapter 6.2, 'Nature-based treatments as an adjunctive therapy for anxiety among elders', Mark B. Detweiler and his colleagues describe how we can prevent anxiety and reduce pharmaceutical use among older people by increasing access and exposure to nature in daily life. First a general outlook on anxiety among elders and neurobiological mechanisms is provided and this is then linked to how and why nature interactions may be of specific importance for this group.

Difference in health depending on socioeconomic status and general vulnerability is a major public health issue, which requires actions across several disciplines and authorities (Marmot *et al.*, 2012). In Chapter 6.3, 'Vulnerable populations, health inequalities, and nature', Richard Mitchell and his colleagues explain why we need to incorporate measures of particular vulnerability in any public health action and how this may imply an environmental aspect, in particular access to nature. It is generally found that people of less wealth and education respond more positively in terms of improved health outcomes to nature exposure than do already healthy and wealthy populations. This means that nature may counteract some of the health differences determined by socioeconomic group belonging. The chapter presents evidence on the buffering effect of nature on health inequalities and outlines suggestions for environmental justice for public health.

Finally, Caroline Hägerhäll presents a cultural exposé in Chapter 6.4, 'Responses to nature from populations of varied cultural background'. This chapter discusses the topic of whether there is any common preference for nature independent of cultural and ethnical belonging, or whether such preferences are socially determined. The research on this subject is scarce and the chapter is a first scientific attempt to bring together current existing knowledge on definitions and conceptualizations of and preferences for natural environments in a cross-cultural perspective.

Section 7: Threats, environmental change, and unintended consequences of nature—protecting health and reducing environmental hazards

So-called disservices from and harmful effects of nature and ecosystems have recently become a topic in focus. In science it is necessary to be critical and to strive to falsify hypotheses in order to prevent harmful consequences and optimize prioritizations based on research results. From this perspective, it may be possible to understand why a focus on the negative aspects of nature has become relevant. However, nature and healthy ecosystems are the fundaments for our survival and health. Apart from nutrition and other basic provisional needs, this is obvious from the level of microbiota and neurocognitive development to spiritual and emotional well-being (van den Bosch and Nieuwenhuijsen, 2017). Anthropogenic impact on nature, has come to disturb many ecosystem functions, leading to, for example, prolonged seasons of more allergenic pollen grains and harmful effects of various natural disasters, such as hurricanes and vector-borne diseases. Section 7 takes a closer look at these events, showing that while interactions with nature can sometimes be unsafe, the damaging effects are mainly due to human interference with nature in the first place. What we need to do is therefore to prevent further harmful impact on nature by humans and learn to interact with nature in a healthy way. This is different than saying that nature is dangerous and brings disservices to human beings. The section also discusses these issues from the perspective of what we have to lose in terms of health and well-being by further biodiversity loss and climate change, as well as from the perspective of a sometimes unbalanced risk perception.

In Chapter 7.1, 'Allergenic pollen emissions from vegetation—threats and prevention', Åslög Dahl first outlines the biology of pollen and allergenic plant species, pollen counts, and impacts of anthropogenic disturbance by, for example, climate change. Matilda van den Bosch then describes the basics of allergenic diseases and their impact on health. Finally, Thomas Ogren shares insights in how to plan for less allergenic environments by more careful selection of, for example, street trees and by applying more functional botanical sexism.

Another threat that is possible to encounter in nature, and also in urban green and blue spaces, are vector-borne diseases. In Chapter 7.2, 'Vector-borne diseases and poisonous plants', David Wong outlines those threats and includes advice on how we can act sensibly and thereby reduce the risks and prevent harms from such vectors and plants. The chapter's main focus is from an outdoor recreational perspective, as people who engage in such activities are evidently at increased risk. However, by adequate prevention measures and education, the potential risks from these conditions are by far outweighed by the vast amount of health benefits to be achieved from outdoor recreation.

Through unsustainable practices and climate change the incidence of natural disasters has increased globally. In Chapter 7.3, 'The health impact of natural disasters', Eric K. Noji and Anas A. Khan discuss how natural hazards such as earthquakes, hurricanes, floods, droughts, and volcanic eruptions are considered as disasters, while these events are in fact only natural agents that transform a vulnerable human condition into a disaster. Ignorance of, for example, appropriate building codes in combination with poverty and social inequalities, improper land use, rapid population growth in poor regions, and global climate change and biodiversity loss can create a hazardous environment with severe negative impact on health in particularly low- and middle-income countries. This chapter provides the most up-to-date knowledge on natural disasters, evaluation, impacts, risk reduction, and prevention.

David J. Ball and Laurence N. Ball-King provide an overview of how we have, with time, become disconnected from nature and how this has led to a sometimes exaggerated fear of nature in Chapter 7.4, 'Risk and the perception of risk in interactions with nature'. The chapter includes perspectives on risk perception and what may cause unbalance in how we perceive threats versus opportunities. The authors also discuss current impediments for realizing the many benefits of nature and what we can do to act against these streams.

The final chapter of this section is written by the late Anthony McMichael, who completed it in his last days. The devotion of such precious time to authoring the chapter 'Population health deficits due to biodiversity loss, climate change, and other environmental degradation' (7.5) is a symbol of the urgency of the topic. While this book has focused on the many health benefits we can gain from nature, this chapter takes another view by showing all the losses we are indisputably to face by further disconnection from nature and continued destruction of Earth and its ecosystems. By a holistic approach, the text displays how traditional scientific and medical assumptions and methods are no longer appropriate if we aim to avert the multiple catastrophic effects on environment and human health, following climate change and environmental degradation.

Section 8: The nature of the city

We live in a rapidly urbanizing world. This major demographic shift has had and will continue to have wide implications on public health. This perfectly well demonstrates how the environment impacts health in a multitude of ways. Section 8 takes a closer look at the urban environment, how nature is or is not integrated in cities, and the effects on health for various populations.

In Chapter 8.1, 'The shift from natural living environments to urban: population-based and neurobiological implications for public health' Florian Lederbogen and colleagues discuss how the shift from rural to urban environments has equally created a shift in the general disease scenario. This is exemplified by population studies on diabetes prevalence in China and India, and by neuroscientific findings on differences in brain anatomy and function between rural and urban populations.

Timothy Beatley and Cecil Konijnendijk van den Bosch walk us through the city in Chapter 8.2, 'Urban landscapes and public health'. They discuss the challenges and opportunities in creating healthy and resilient urban environments and how various disciplines and sectors must collaborate to reach this goal. This comes together in the socioecological approach, where human behaviour is understood as a factor of interactions with physical and sociocultural surroundings. The authors argue that by strategically implementing a socioecological approach we can come closer to creating urban landscapes that promote public health and well-being. Within this context urban green and blue spaces are considered central, as expressed through concepts like green urbanism and biophilic cities.

This reasoning continues in Chapter 8.3, 'Nature in buildings and health design' by the late Stephen R. Kellert. The chapter draws on the concept of biophilia, the supposed innate connection between humans and nature, based on our evolutionary origin (Wilson, 1984). This means that by incorporating natural features in buildings and design we may foster health and well-being in a largely urbanized world. This may be particularly important in healthcare facilities. Apart from providing an environment which is perceived as pleasant and corresponding to our biological functions, biophilic design may encourage positive interactions with the natural world contributing to the overall coherence of the human ecosystem.

Another concept which is often used in the discussion of creating resilient and healthy cities is green infrastructure (GI). Cecil Konijnendijk van den Bosch and Raffaele Lafortezza go into depth with this topic in Chapter 8.4, 'Green infrastructure—its approach and public health benefits'. GI is commonly understood as an interconnected network of natural areas with various benefits to the society. Although the concept is rooted in planning and environmental sectors, it has a large bearing on public health. The principle of GI is to gain benefits for both people and the environment through pro-active urban planning and management where natural resources are strategically included.

Closely related to the concept of green infrastructure is ecosystem services. Elisabet Lindgren and her colleagues reveal the various benefits and services provided by urban ecosystems in Chapter 8.5, 'Ecosystem services and health benefits—an urban perspective'. Human beings are all part of ecosystems and this fact may be expressed through the terms of ecosystem services, as this clarifies all direct and indirect health benefits we gain from ecosystems. In this chapter the particular challenges of global urbanization to functional ecosystem services are outlined and discussed. This is diversified across different types of urban environments—affluent mature cities, affluent growing cities, and low-income growing cities.

Taking us to the border between environmental health and policy making, Evelyne de Leeuw and Premila Webster give an overview of the WHO Healthy Cities Project in Chapter 8.6, 'The healthy settings approach: Healthy cities and environmental health indicators'. A basic principle of the project is to move health high on social and political agendas in urban policies, sometimes expressed as Health in All Policies. From an urban green planning perspective, this means that environmental workers and policy makers should consider the health aspects of any planning or management strategy around built versus green environments. Equally it would imply that public health workers and decision makers collaborate closely with urban planners and create shared visions and goals for healthy, green, and resilient cities. The Healthy Cities concept draws attention to the close connection between people's health and their surrounding environment and among many other goals, it states that a healthy city should strive to provide ecosystems that are stable and sustainable.

Section 9: Natural public health across the world

Much of the research on associations between public health and nature has been conducted in Western parts of the world with comparatively high resources for both science and development. While low- and middle-income countries are rapidly developing Western-based lifestyles, they are still facing unique issues and challenges in regard to associations between health and nature. It is of particular value to increase the focus on other parts of the world, partly in order to avoid similar mistakes that have been made in the Western world. Such mistakes include, for example, densification of cities at the cost of biodiversity and natural spaces, without considering long-term effects on public health.

In Section 9 we make a first attempt to bring together existing knowledge on nature and public health relations in other parts of the world—Africa, Latin America, and Small Island Developing States.

Emmanuel K. Boon and Albert Ahenkan take us to Africa in Chapter 9.1, 'Africa and environmental health trends'. In Africa, natural resources are central to people's livelihoods and health, especially in the relatively large rural populations. To a higher extent than in, for example, Europe, the provisioning ecosystem services are of strong importance for population health. However, forests and other natural areas also play an important role for cultural services, such as tourism and recreation, spiritual healing, leisure, and religious practices. General natural resource management is becoming an increasing topic of concern in Africa, in the tracks of deforestation, population growth, and urbanization. While threats and opportunities from nature vary across the continent, there are also commonalities, such as increasing beneficiary and community participation, developing and sharing environmental friendly technologies, and formulating appropriate environmental policies for improved public health. Another specific theme of the African region is traditional medicine (also called botanical medicine), which is defined as the use of whole plants or part of plants to prevent or treat illness.

Following this we continue to another continent in Chapter 9.2, 'Latin America and the environmental health movement', authored by Ana Faggi and her colleagues. In Latin America green spaces have by tradition been considered places for everyone to meet and socialize and are associated with healthy environments, as well as culture and multiculturalism. During the influence of French and English models in the late nineteenth century, urban green spaces and large parks were established to prevent health issues associated with city living. Today, Latin America has the most urbanized population in the world—public green spaces are under high pressure and urban development is far from sustainable. The planning of urban green spaces is not coherent and the green infrastructure urgently requires investments for achieving health benefits. Often, deprived neighbourhoods have very poor quality or a complete lack of green spaces. While the health–nature relationship is poorly recognized in policy campaigns and in the grey literature, some recent activities seem to acknowledge the value of green spaces for mental health and other health benefits. This chapter provides a few examples of such activities, including the showcase of Curitiba, Brazil, with 64.5 m^2 of green area per citizen.

Finally, Evelyne de Leeuw and her colleagues take us to Small Island Developing States (SIDS) in Chapter 9.3, 'Healthy islands'. In nation-state islands, nature and ecosystem health meet population health in a particular way. The WHO has initiated a programme which connects SIDS' (in the Pacific Ocean) environmental development with public health, the Healthy Islands programme. The programme has several interconnected priority areas, including ecological sustainability and social and emotional well-being. Apart from NCDs, the most serious threat to health on these islands is climate change.

Section 10: Bringing nature into public health actions

This book seeks to contribute to a paradigm shift in how we look at health in relation to the natural environment. The aim is to provide knowledge in order to create a deeper understanding of what health means, how we can change our approach to current major health issues, and improve public health today and in the future. This knowledge and understanding must be created through a transdisciplinary strategy where scientists from various disciplines collaborate with stakeholders and practitioners, through all phases from the initial research problem identification to the solution. This final section aims to bring us into action by providing a few examples of the roles that various actors can play in distributing and applying the knowledge around nature and public health.

In Chapter 10.1, 'The role of the health professional', the physicians Robert Zarr and William Bird share their experiences from clinical practice where natural spaces have been incorporated in the treatment and care of patients with various chronic conditions. They also provide examples of well-established health promoting programmes, which draw on nature exposure in order to maintain and improve health in a population.

Cinnamon P. Carlarne and Jeffrey M. Bielicki share insights around legal and regulatory strategies related to the environment in Chapter 10.2, 'The role of environmental law'. Many environmental law makers recognize that natural spaces are important for human well-being for several reasons, including recreation and mental health. This is mirrored in for example National Park System and National Forest System in the United States and many other natural resource laws. Similarly, land use laws affect many factors with important ramification for public health, for instance transportation, levels of noise, and ease of access to public green spaces. Environmental lawmakers must continue and increase interactions with other sectors for understanding and improving the interplay between law, nature, and human well-being.

Related to environmental law and policies are impact assessments. In Chapter 10.3, 'Environmental assessment and health impact assessment', Salim Vohra and colleagues provide an overview of how the practice of environmental impact assessments has grown with the recognition of human health impact. While most health impact assessments of planned environmental interferences concern negative health outcomes, recently also health impact assessments of, for example, urban park establishments, have locally been applied while looking at health gains. This can have an important bearing for quantifying the health effects of green spaces and thereby provide a common ground for practical implementation in urban planning.

David Nowak presents a practical ecosystem evaluation tool in Chapter 10.4, 'Quantifying and valuing the role of trees and forests on environmental quality and human health'. While recognizing that not everything can be calculated in money, monetary tools may facilitate practical implementation of environmental strategies for public health. By accounting for the ecosystem services in monetary terms, better planning, design, and economic decisions may be made towards utilizing nature as a means to improve human health.

Finally, Chapter 10.5, 'The role of civil society and organizations', authored by Matilda van den Bosch and colleagues presents a selection of non-governmental and civil society organizations, which through various channels work for improved practice regarding human and nature relationships. The organizations outlined in the chapter are all committed to increasing the awareness of human health and nature relations, from various perspectives. They are non-profit organizations, with independent status, and contribute to engaging civil society and people in putting the important matters of nature and health higher on the political agenda. This may be one tool for indirectly bridging the science–policy gap and to increase the incorporation of positive environmental impact on health in healthcare, and to more strongly prevent the major losses expected by the degradation of natural resources.

Conclusion

The final paragraph of Charles Darwin's *Origin of Species* begins with a beautiful reflection on nature and our dependence of functional interactions between all species: 'It is interesting to contemplate a tangled bank, clothed with many plants of many kinds, with birds singing on the bushes, with various insects flitting about, and with worms crawling through the damp earth, and to reflect that these elaborately constructed forms, so different from each other, and dependent upon each other in so complex a manner, have all been produced by laws acting around us.' (Darwin, 1859)

These laws define numerous rules, including growth and reproduction, and variability. By the latest century's reduced respect for nature and its laws, and by our lost connection to nature, we seem to disrupt or insult those laws. We do so at growing peril to ourselves and to nature itself.

We want this book to challenge the way we view the impact that nature has on human health and why this is so important. Connection, respect, and reverence celebrate the relation between us and nature and represent the interface between science and philosophy. Inherent in the recognition of nature as a public health asset must be a realization of how much we all have to lose by disconnecting from or degrading natural environments. If we realize this, forests, lakes, seashores, urban parks and woodlands may continue to provide settings for recovery and recreation, while simultaneously delivering basic services for our health and survival.

How shall we move forward and who is responsible for increasing the visibility of nature in the public health agenda? We all are. We, the people of the planet Earth, have a responsibility to drive decisions that account for the health of forthcoming generations of human beings and ecosystems. We are the people that must reframe our thinking and our values to change and develop new societies, economies, and policies that embrace an understanding of the inherent beauty of nature and how much we have to lose by destroying her.

References

Almanza, E., Jerrett, M., Dunton, G., Seto, E., & Pentz, M. (2012). A study of community design, greenness, and physical activity in children using satellite, GPS and accelerometer data. *Health Place*, 18, 46–54.

Darwin, C. (1859). *The Origin of Species by Means of Natural Selection or the Preservation of Favoured Races in the Struggle for Life*. London, UK: John Murray.

Holt-Lunstad, J., Smith, T. B., Baker, M., Harris, T., & Stephenson, D. (2015). Loneliness and social isolation as risk factors for mortality: a meta-analytic review. *Perspect Psychol Sci*, 10, 227–37.

Kondrashova, A., Seiskari, T., Ilonen, J., Knip, M., & Hyöty, H. (2013). The 'Hygiene hypothesis' and the sharp gradient in the incidence of autoimmune and allergic diseases between Russian Karelia and Finland. *APMIS*, 121, 478–93.

Lang, T. & Rayner, G. (2012). Ecological public health: The 21st century's big idea? An essay by Tism Lang and Geof Rayner. *BMJ*, 345, e5466.

Marmot, M., Allen, J., Bell, R., Bloomer, E., & Goldblatt, P. (2012). WHO European review of social determinants of health and the health divide. *Lancet*, 380, 1011–29.

McEwen, B. S. (1998). Stress, Adaptation, and Disease: Allostasis and Allostatic Load. *Ann N Y Acad Sci*, 840, 33–44.

McEwen, B. S. (2008). Central effects of stress hormones in health and disease: Understanding the protective and damaging effects of stress and stress mediators. *Eur J Pharmacol*, 583, 174–85.

McEwen, B. S. (2012). Brain on stress: How the social environment gets under the skin. *Proc Natl Acad Sci*, 109, 17180–5.

Naghavi, M. & Forouzanfar, M. H. (2013). Burden of non-communicable diseases in sub-Saharan Africa in 1990 and 2010: Global Burden of Diseases, Injuries, and Risk Factors Study 2010. *Lancet*, 381, S95.

Potts, D. (2012). Viewpoint: What do we know about urbanisation in sub-Saharan Africa and does it matter? *Int Dev Plann Rev*, 34, v-xxii.

Rayner, G. & Langm T. (2012). *Ecological Public Health: Reshaping the Conditions for Good Health*. Oxford UK: Earthscan/Routledge.

Rodrigues, S. M., Saslow, L. R., Garcia, N., John, O. P., & Keltner, D. (2009). Oxytocin receptor genetic variation relates to empathy and stress reactivity in humans. *Proc Natl Acad Sci*, 106, 21437–21441.

Sale, A., Berardi, N., & Maffei, L. (2009). Enrich the environment to empower the brain. *Trends Neurosci*, 32, 233–9.

Sallis, J. F., Cerin, E., Conway, T. L., et al. (2016). Physical activity in relation to urban environments in 14 cities worldwide: a cross-sectional study. *Lancet*, 387, 2207–17.

van den Bosch, M. & Nieuwenhuijsen, M. (2017). No time to lose—Green the cities now. *Environ Int*, 99, 343–50.

Vos, T., Barber, R. M., Bell, B., et al. (2015). Global, regional, and national incidence, prevalence, and years lived with disability for 301 acute and chronic diseases and injuries in 188 countries, 1990-2013: A systematic analysis for the Global Burden of Disease Study 2013. *Lancet*, 386, 743–800.

Waage, J., Yap, C., Bell, S., et al. (2015). Governing the UN Sustainable Development Goals: interactions, infrastructures, and institutions. *Lancet Glob Health*, 3, e251–2.

Watts, N., Adger, W. N., Agnolucci, P., et al. (2015). Health and climate change: policy responses to protect public health. *Lancet*, 386, 1861–914.

Wilson, E. O. (1984). *Biophilia: The Human Bond With Other Species*. Cambridge, MA: Harvard Univ Press.

World Health Organization (WHO) (2014). Global status report on noncommunicable diseases 2014. Geneva, Switzerland: World Health Organization.

CHAPTER 1.2

A life course approach to public health: why early life matters

Felicia M. Low, Peter D. Gluckman, and Mark A. Hanson

Developmental origins of health and disease

Research efforts to illuminate the underlying heritability of disease risk, which had traditionally relied on twin and adoption studies, received a tremendous boost in the early 2000s upon completion of the Human Genome Project. The availability of the full three billion base pair-sequence comprising the human genome was touted as a breakthrough in elucidating the determinants of human disease, and, accordingly, in devising appropriate therapeutic strategies. When applied to common complex non-communicable diseases (NCDs), however, it soon became apparent that such aspirational promises could not be fully met. Genome-wide association studies attempting to identify functional mutations associated with disease found that single nucleotide polymorphisms could be clearly linked to monogenic Mendelian diseases such as cystic fibrosis. However, genetic variation was a poor explanator at the population level for increasingly common disorders involving a non-Mendelian heritable component (Kaiser, 2012; Drong et al., 2012), especially obesity and associated NCDs such as type 2 diabetes (T2D), cardiovascular and chronic lung disease, other components of the metabolic syndrome, and some mental health problems.

With the gradual realization that narratives based solely on a gene-centric viewpoint were no longer viable, greater attention was paid to the mounting interdisciplinary evidence showing that exposures in early life are important influences on an individual's vulnerability to disease risk in later life. Today, a significant corpus of research encompassing epidemiological, clinical, and experimental work, underpinned by a cogent theoretical framework, overwhelmingly supports the integral role of extrinsic factors acting in early life in modulating later life vulnerability to NCDs. This paradigm has been formalized as the Developmental Origins of Health and Disease (DOHaD) concept and is supported by an international learned society and associated scholarly journal (Gluckman and Hanson, 2006b; International Society for Developmental Origins of Health and Disease, n.d.). Cues as varied as maternal and childhood nutrition, stress, and toxins or chemicals have been implicated in an increased risk of a broad range of pathologies, including components of the metabolic syndrome, respiratory disease, atopy, osteoporosis, mood and cognitive disorders, and some types of cancer. While this phenomenon is often referred to as developmental 'programming', we note that such terminology raises connotations of genetic determinism, and that individuals may be more appropriately described as 'primed' or 'conditioned' to respond differently to later environmental exposures (Hanson and Gluckman, 2014).

The modern day epidemics of obesity and other NCDs exert a profound impact on public health in both developed and developing societies, and the magnitude of the problem is only set to grow (Capizzi et al., 2015). In this chapter we provide an overview of DOHaD and discuss the concept of developmental plasticity underpinning it, effected in part by epigenetic processes that serve as a molecular bridge between an inducing cue and later phenotypes. We discuss how a life course approach, which is informed by developmental plasticity and gives particular focus to optimizing early life conditions, presents a fundamentally new and scientifically sound paradigm for reducing both an individual's and a population's risk of obesity and its co-morbidities.

Historical overview

The idea that early life factors could have a delayed, detrimental impact on later life health was mooted as early as the 1930s, when a study reported unusual trends in mortality rates in Great Britain consistent with the hypothesis that poorer conditions during childhood were linked to lower life expectancy (Kermack et al., 1934). However, despite attracting some attention at the time, the clinical significance of the work was underappreciated and this line of enquiry largely languished. Several decades later, in the 1970s–1980s, a number of clinical studies correlating pre and perinatal conditions to risk of obesity, metabolic and cardiovascular disease, were reported (Plagemann, 2005). In rats, experimentally inducing foetal growth restriction or gestational diabetes in the mother induced pancreatic dysfunction and multiple metabolic changes in the pups (Aerts and Van Assche, 1979). Some epidemiological reports in the same period broached the possibility that pregnancy complications such as undernutrition (Ravelli et al., 1976) and pre-eclampsia (Higgins et al., 1980) had effects on offspring adiposity and blood pressure. Then, in the late 1980s–early 1990s, a team led by English epidemiologist David Barker published a series of large-scale analyses showing that low birth weight was associated with increased adult mortality from cardiovascular disease and risk of impaired glucose tolerance or T2D (Barker et al., 1989b; Barker et al., 1989a; Hales et al., 1991; Osmond et al.,

1993). The concerted efforts of Barker and his colleagues to publicize the phenomenon spurred an upsurge of interest in this field of research, his key role being reflected in the eponymous naming of the 'Barker hypothesis' by the *British Medical Journal* in 1995 (Paneth and Susser, 1995).

Further work from epidemiologists, clinicians, and experimental physiologists began to reinforce the validity of the notion that there is indeed an early life component to adult disease risk. Large studies linked lower birth weight with increased risk of hypertension, stroke, and higher body mass index (BMI) (Curhan *et al.*, 1996; Rich-Edwards *et al.*, 2005), while asymptomatic children who had experienced intrauterine growth retardation were shown to be markedly insulin resistant compared to normal birth weight peers (Hofman *et al.*, 1997). Multiple animal models of rats, mice, and sheep provided supportive data by demonstrating that quantitative or qualitative manipulations of maternal diet led to dysregulations in metabolic and cardiovascular physiology (Langley and Jackson, 1994; Vickers *et al.*, 2000; Ozaki *et al.*, 2000; Goyal *et al.*, 2010). However, over time it emerged that the association between low birth weight and disease risk was only part of a broader range of developmental phenomena linking events in early life to later ill health. Birth weight itself was not on the causal pathways involved, except insofar as it was a proxy for conditions that might have affected the developing foetus *in utero*. Indeed, distinct pathways reflecting different mechanisms appeared likely, with the recognition that foetal macrosomia, such as that associated with maternal gestational diabetes, also had long-term consequences for the offspring's later health (van Assche *et al.*, 2001).

Evolution of a conceptual framework

The idea that adverse exposures during development could lead to later disease, without necessarily having immediate manifestations of ill health, was intriguing and well-supported by empirical data. However, it ran counter to prevailing medical belief, which was resistant to making associative connections between prenatal/infant and adult health. Instead, emphasis remained on the combination of genetic risk and unhealthy adult lifestyle as the major contributors to NCDs. It became evident that there was a need to conceptualize the phenomenon of DOHaD within an acceptable framework to engender its greater acceptance. Barker, together with Nicholas Hales, drew an analogy from the 'thrifty genotype' hypothesis that was proposed by James Neel (1962) as one of the first attempts at explaining the growing NCD epidemic in modern environments. Neel had posited that genes promoting metabolic 'thrift' became selected in the course of human evolution as an energy-conserving strategy to cope with famine situations, and that they had repercussions in the modern context of abundant nutrition. In their framework, Hales and Barker hypothesized that poor early life nutrition induces a nutritionally 'thrifty phenotype', resulting in low birth weight and insulin resistance, and placing the individual at greater risk of metabolic disease in an environment of nutritional plenitude (Hales and Barker, 1992, 2001).

Although valuable for bringing evolutionary and adaptive considerations to the fore in the discourse on disease risk, this model had several limitations. It considered birth weight as a causal factor operating on a single 'programming' pathway, and failed to appreciate that the relationship between development and adverse postnatal consequences operated over the full spectrum, rather than operating as a low-versus-normal birth weight dichotomy. However,

available and subsequent datasets documented clear gradation in the relationship, strongly suggesting that foetal insults need not be severe for induction of increased disease risk (Hales *et al.*, 1991; Osmond *et al.*, 1993; Curhan *et al.*, 1996; Rich-Edwards *et al.*, 2005; Harder *et al.*, 2007). Birth weight came to gain undue importance as a proxy for foetal nourishment, leading to scepticism of the validity of DOHaD when data arose of a lack of association between birth weight and some disease markers (Paneth and Susser, 1995). Questions were also raised about its public health importance given the relatively low frequency of low birth weight in Western populations. Yet, importantly, human (Gale *et al.*, 2006; Drake *et al.*, 2012; Heijmans *et al.*, 2008) and animal (Nijland *et al.*, 2010) data have shown that disease susceptibility may be elevated in the absence of birth weight differences or other overt phenotypic outcomes. Furthermore, contrary to the model's assumptions of insulin resistance at birth, clinical data have shown that infants born small are in fact insulin sensitive at birth, and only display insulin resistance at about the age of three years (Mericq *et al.*, 2005). The absence of satisfactory mechanistic and theoretical frameworks by which to interpret the apparently conflicting observations thus remained a major impediment to the widespread acceptance of the DOHaD paradigm and its integration into clinical, medical, and public health domains (Gluckman and Buklijas, 2014).

Peter Gluckman, Mark Hanson, and Patrick Bateson, taking the Hales–Barker model as a starting point, provided further conceptual refinements based on the concept of *predictive adaptive responses* (PARs). PARs refer to a developing organism's capacity to assess the nature of cues to which it is currently exposed in order to predict its later life environment, and tune its phenotype accordingly, for delayed selective advantage (Bateson *et al.*, 2004; Gluckman *et al.*, 2005a, 2005b). Among the key attributes of this model was its differentiation between severe environmental influences that are developmentally disruptive (i.e. teratogenic), and more subtle cues of potentially evolutionarily adaptive value (Gluckman *et al.*, 2005b; Hanson and Gluckman, 2014). The latter invoke an organism's capacity for *developmental plasticity*, which refers to the adaptive responses to environmental cues that enable it to adjust its phenotypic development to match the current external environment. A key underlying principle is that organisms are more plastic in early development. Thus, exposure to exogenous influences in early life affects biological and behavioural development, leading to long-term consequences that become more apparent as the individual ages. The pervasiveness of this capacity throughout the animal kingdom implies that it has been evolutionarily conserved because it may be critical for maximizing survival and reproduction upon exposure to a range of physiologically and ecologically normative cues (Low *et al.*, 2012). As discussed later, there is increasing evidence that the molecular mechanisms underlying developmental plasticity include epigenetic changes that regulate gene expression from development through to maturity (Low *et al.*, 2014).

Another important attribute of the new model was that it further distinguished between responses that were potentially adaptive and induced by ecological cues such as alterations in maternal nutrition and maternal stress, and those associated with evolutionary novelty, which likely involved non-adaptive processes. The latter included cues such as maternal obesity, infant formula feeding, and gestational diabetes mellitus (GDM) (Ma *et al.*, 2013a). The model proposed that among exposures that are not outright teratogens or representative of evolutionary novelty, those that are more severe may induce responses that have immediate phenotypic impact at the expense of longer-term trade-offs. An example is uterine infection-induced premature delivery, which promotes immediate foetal survival at the cost of greater morbidity or mortality in infancy. Cues that are less severe, such as variations in maternal diet and maternal stress, may elicit PARs that confer delayed adaptive advantage by tuning the individual's phenotype to best cope with the forecast postnatal environment (Gluckman et al., 2005a; Bateson et al., 2014). In this way, Darwinian fitness is enhanced even if no phenotypic consequences are outwardly observed. However, the corollary is that inaccurate transduction of cues, arising for example from placental insufficiency, erroneously signalling a low nutrient environment, or exposure to a postnatal environment different from that predicted in utero, then places the individual in a situation of developmental mismatch (Gluckman and Hanson, 2006a), which results in heightened risk of disease later in life. Despite the potentially deleterious effects of PARs, they are thought to have evolved and persisted through our evolutionary history owing to their value in maximizing survival to at least reproductive age. Being a fitness-enhancing strategy, no regard is paid to longer-term impact on health and longevity.

In its initial iteration, the PAR model encountered opposition primarily due to differing interpretations of the available empirical data in relation to maternal–foetal conflict theory; it was argued that protection of maternal fitness was the primary driver of foetal responses (Wells, 2007). This theoretical criticism has been thoroughly addressed (Bateson et al., 2014; Hanson and Gluckman, 2014), and the model now emphasizes that adaptive advantage need only occur in childhood and early adolescence for Darwinian fitness to be promoted. Furthermore, the model explains some of the empirical data that were discrepant with the Hales–Barker model, such as the delayed appearance of insulin resistance until after infancy. An advantage of PARs is that they do not operate in the infant during the postnatal period of high maternal care and lactation, when the infant is somewhat protected from the actual macroenvironment, and when insulin resistance would impede fat deposition needed to buffer the infant brain at the evolved time of weaning (Kuzawa, 2010; Bateson et al., 2014). Rather, insulin resistance only emerges upon cessation of the maternal supply of lipid-enriched milk, which in evolutionary terms signals a less secure nutritional environment. In the predicted nutritionally insecure post-weaning environment, the development of insulin resistance would, as Hales and Barker (2001) had proposed, become advantageous.

The operation of PARs has been experimentally supported by a number of animal studies. For example, rats whose mothers were undernourished during gestation become conditioned to develop obesity, insulin resistance, leptin resistance, hyperphagia (excessive appetite), and sedentary behaviour in adulthood (Vickers et al., 2000). These physiological characteristics represent an integrated manifestation of an energy-conserving phenotype best adapted to a predicted low nutrient postnatal environment. Administering leptin, an anorexigenic hormone, to these offspring within the neonatal period appears to reverse PARs made in utero and abolishes phenotypic priming, restoring physiological settings to resemble those of pups born to adequately nourished mothers (Vickers et al., 2005). PARs have also been reported in the silkworm (Sato et al., 2014) and butterfly (van den Heuvel et al., 2013). The meadow

vole, a small rodent native to North America, provides an excellent ecological example. Maternal melatonin levels, mediated by day length, act as a cue to induce PARs in the foetus such that offspring are born with a thick fur coat in autumn in anticipation of impending cold, or with a thin coat in spring to cope with warmer temperatures (Lee and Zucker, 1988).

While it is more difficult to directly test PARs in humans, it has been shown that being born smaller is associated with less severe morbidity and rates of mortality when exposed to a very low plane of nutrition in childhood (Forrester et al., 2012). This may reflect adoption of an energy-conserving metabolism prompted by in utero predictions of nutritional scarcity, and is the first direct demonstration of the PAR-induced promotion of fitness in humans. As discussed later, there is extensive evidence for developmental mismatch leading to NCDs at the public health level, particularly with respect to migration and socioeconomic advancement.

The role of epigenetics

A major hurdle faced by the DOHaD community was the lack of plausible biochemical explanations to account for the long latency between exposure to a cue which induced a response via developmental plasticity, and onset of adult disease much later in life. Early research, predominantly employing highly artificial models of maternal nutritional or stress manipulation, pointed towards conditioning of physiological systems including the neuro-endocrine-immune system and hypothalamic-pituitary-adrenal (HPA) axis (Plagemann, 2005), and structural alterations such as a reduction in nephron number (Dötsch et al., 2009). Then the advent of the epigenomic era in the 2000s, facilitated by rapid advances in next-generation sequencing technology, began to reveal that epigenetic switches were responsive to external cues and could essentially function as a molecular interface between the genome and the environment. In a molecular context, epigenetic processes refer to the DNA sequence-independent mechanisms that establish and maintain patterns of gene expression that persist through mitosis (Gluckman et al., 2009). These processes, which can sometimes be reversible and may be maintained by stochastic mechanisms, include methylation of specific nucleotides (in mammals, predominantly cytosine that is adjacent to guanine); post-translational modification of the histone proteins around which DNA is packed to form nucleosomes; and transcriptional modulation by noncoding RNAs.

Epigenetic mechanisms had long been known and studied, but mostly in the context of cell differentiation and oncology. It was the recognition that the epigenome is malleable to early environmental influences which persist, that then inspired a raft of studies investigating the epigenetic basis of DOHaD. This has been rigorously demonstrated in animal studies (Seki et al., 2012). For example, in a maternal low-protein diet rat model, in which offspring are conditioned towards hypertension and lipid dysregulation, liver cells of offspring had lower promoter methylation at the gene-encoding PPARα, a transcription factor known to regulate lipid metabolism (Lillycrop et al., 2005). The transcriptional impact of this change was reflected in higher PPARα expression levels. Importantly, maternal folic acid supplementation not only reversed the phenotypic effects of foetal unbalanced nutrition, but also normalized epigenetic regulation to control levels (Lillycrop et al., 2005; Torrens et al., 2006). The maternal hypocaloric diet rat model described earlier has reported greater promoter methylation at offspring hepatic PPARα promoter, an effect ablated by neonatal leptin administration (Gluckman *et al.*, 2007). The bidirectional changes in methylation between the two maternal dietary manipulation models may reflect nuanced responses to different nutritional exposures. Nevertheless, the hormonal or dietary restoration of DNA methylation levels to those of controls, concomitant with phenotypic reversals, strongly supports the epigenetic basis of developmental conditioning. In baboons, mild undernourishment during gestation decreased promoter methylation levels at foetal hepatic *PCK1*, concomitant with elevated mRNA expression, suggesting downstream effects on intermediary metabolism (Nijland *et al.*, 2010).

In humans, initial evidence implicating early life-induced epigenetic dysregulation in disease risk came from studies of populations exposed to extraordinary circumstances. For example, a cohort of Dutch individuals whose mothers were exposed to a short but severe famine during pregnancy in the Second World War has been intensively studied. Comparisons with unexposed siblings revealed that prenatal famine exposure in early gestation is associated with increased risk of coronary heart disease, glucose intolerance, poorer lipid profile and, in female offspring, obesity (Roseboom *et al.*, 2006). These individuals, in about their sixth decade of life, showed differential methylation at multiple candidate genes such as *IGF2*, an imprinted gene involved in foetal growth (Heijmans *et al.*, 2008), and *LEP* and *APOC1*, both involved in lipid metabolism (Tobi *et al.*, 2009). The magnitude of changes was small; they may be real or an artefact of confounding variables that are hard to control in human studies, such as postnatal environmental effects or age-related epigenetic drift. Nevertheless it is interesting that such gene-specific methylation changes were identified against a background of relatively static global DNA methylation levels (Lumey *et al.*, 2012), the latter possibly reflecting a buffering effect within the epigenome. It is also remarkable that a relatively transient exposure may induce epigenetic changes that persist through to late adulthood and which are detectable in peripheral blood. A pilot study examining candidate gene methylation in blood from 40-year-old individuals has uncovered gene-specific correlations of current methylation levels with measures of neonatal anthropometry, current adiposity, and blood pressure, and exposure to a maternal low carbohydrate/high protein diet (Drake *et al.*, 2012). Notably, the effects observed in this and the Dutch famine studies were independent of birth weight.

In the first demonstration that epigenetic status at birth may be associated with later phenotypic variation of clinical relevance, Keith Godfrey and colleagues reported positive correlations between umbilical cord methylation levels in part of the *RXRA* gene and adiposity later in childhood (Godfrey *et al.*, 2011). RXRA is a crucial component of transcriptional regulation of adipogenesis and fat metabolism, underscoring the biological significance of these findings. This association, replicated in a second independent cohort, suggested that at least 25% of the variation had a developmental component, making this the first study to provide a quantitative estimate of early life contribution to a known human disease risk factor. Additionally, a lower proportion of dietary carbohydrate during early pregnancy, previously identified as a risk factor for higher neonatal adiposity (Godfrey *et al.*, 1997), was associated with higher *RXRA* methylation at birth. The detection of these effects in a cohort of uncomplicated pregnancies suggests an exquisite level of epigenetic sensitivity to apparently unremarkable cues operating early in pregnancy.

Other, mostly small sample-size studies, have linked birth weight (Gordon *et al.*, 2012; Zhao *et al.*, 2014) or aspects of maternal nutrition such as intake of the methyl donors folic acid and choline, or micronutrient supplementation, with epigenetic status of candidate genes at birth or in infancy (Hoyo *et al.*, 2011; Jiang *et al.*, 2012; Cooper *et al.*, 2012; Khulan *et al.*, 2012; Dominguez-Salas *et al.*, 2014), although the functional importance of these epigenetic changes for disease risk was not determined. A number of larger, longitudinal cohorts tracking individuals from before conception have recently been established (Soh *et al.*, 2014; Vuillermin *et al.*, 2015), providing a crucial tool for determining directions of causality and giving much needed insights into the effects of exposures within the normal range in normal populations, for greater applicability to the wider population. The fields of developmental epigenetics and epigenetic epidemiology are currently progressing with great vigour.

While much of the DOHaD work has centred on maternal undernutrition, in part as a result of the early focus on low birth weight, there is increasing appreciation that early life overnutrition—experienced via maternal overweight/obesity, excessive gestational weight gain, or GDM—also imposes increased risk of adiposity and metabolic disorders in offspring (Ma *et al.*, 2013b; Gademan *et al.*, 2014; Mitanchez *et al.*, 2014). Unlike maternal undernutrition and stress, which likely operate through adaptive mechanisms, extreme overnutrition—and maternal hyperglycaemia in particular—are proposed to present evolutionarily novel circumstances against which humans have evolved few protective mechanisms, and therefore could be expected to operate through different pathways (Ma *et al.*, 2013a; Hanson and Gluckman, 2014). Thus, in contrast to normative cues and undernutrition, both of which may induce plastic responses for potential adaptive benefit, the adverse consequences of extreme maternal overnutrition represent a pathophysiological (non-adaptive) pathway.

The influence of maternal overnutrition on the epigenome has been studied by analysing DNA methylation levels in placenta, cord blood, or umbilical cord samples. Small studies have detected a link between preconceptional BMI and methylation at the *PPARGC1A* promoter, which encodes a key regulator of gluconeogenesis (Gemma *et al.*, 2009), and a potential effect of maternal obesity, GDM, and pre-eclampsia on global methylation levels in the placenta (Nomura *et al.*, 2014). Genome-wide analyses have uncovered methylation differences in numerous genes in both placenta and cord blood samples from GDM pregnancies, many of which are involved in metabolic disease pathways including disorders of glucose metabolism (Ruchat *et al.*, 2013). GDM has further been associated with *MEST* hypomethylation in placenta and cord blood, an aberration that was similarly found in blood samples from morbidly obese adults (El Hajj *et al.*, 2012). However, of particular concern is that epigenetic changes are apparent even under milder levels of maternal hyperglycaemia (Desgagné *et al.*, 2014). Indeed, the relationship persists in a graded manner from normal through to high blood glucose levels (Bouchard *et al.*, 2010; Bouchard *et al.*, 2012), raising the possibility that even less severe maternal insulin resistance or clinically normal pregnancies may confer some level of risk. This accords with clinical observations that maternal hyperglycaemia and maternal BMI are associated in a continuous manner with risk of certain negative pregnancy outcomes including high birth weight, delivery by caesarean section, and high cord serum C-peptide, a proxy for neonatal hyperinsulinaemia (The

Hyperglycemia and Adverse Pregnancy Outcome (HAPO) Study Cooperative Research Group, 2009; The HAPO Study Cooperative Research Group, 2010).

Some degree of maternal insulin resistance, especially in late gestation (Catalano et al., 1991), is a conserved mechanism to ensure that the foetus receives adequate glucose. Transfer of glucose, unlike that of fatty acids and amino acids, is not saturable and is likely a mechanism to buffer against effects of nutritional scarcity that occurred more frequently in our evolutionary past. Further, moderate foetal hyperinsulinaemia—and hence neonatal adiposity—may have thermogenetic and neuroprotective functions in a harsh postnatal environment (Kuzawa, 2010). However, such a physiology that had initially evolved to be adaptive has become incompatible within the backdrop of the contemporary obesogenic environment, leading to raised GDM risk (Ma et al., 2013a). GDM likely is an evolutionarily new phenomenon in that if untreated it induces foetal macrosomia, putting both mother and infant at risk during delivery.

Other cues representing evolutionary novelty include maternal obesity and formula feeding. Rodent models have shown that a maternal high-fat diet induces an offspring phenotype similar to the metabolic syndrome in humans, including obesity, hyperphagia, hypertension, hepatic steatosis, and insulin resistance (Samuelsson et al., 2008; Bruce et al., 2009). Numerous distinct epigenetic changes have been described, such as hypomethylation at the gene-encoding hepatic Cdkn1a, which modulates liver growth (Dudley et al., 2011), and histone modification at Pck1 which encodes a key enzymatic component of hepatic gluconeogenesis (Strakovsky et al., 2011). In baboons, a maternal high-fat/high-fructose diet induces differential expression of cardiac microRNAs that are also known to be dysregulated in human cardiovascular disease (Maloyan et al., 2013).

Epigenetic basis of other disorders

While most of the studies reviewed here so far have referred to nutritional signals, other environmental cues such as maternal exposure to stress and environmental toxicants have been well studied for their epigenetic and functional impact on offspring. Early life stress is an important determinant of long-term neuropsychiatric outcomes such as mood and anxiety disorders (Gershon et al., 2013), and there is growing evidence for the involvement of epigenetic mechanisms. Several studies have reported associations between maternal depression or anxiety during pregnancy, and differential methylation of the glucocorticoid receptor (GR) gene NR3C1 at birth, with infants displaying altered HPA axis stress responses or other behavioural traits characteristic of impaired neurodevelopment (Oberlander et al., 2008; Conradt et al., 2013). Some work has pointed towards altered neuronal GR methylation in suicide victims who experienced childhood abuse compared to those with no similar history and to non-suicide controls (McGowan et al., 2009; Labonte et al., 2012). A study of adolescents whose mothers were exposed to the physical and emotional effects of a severe ice storm during pregnancy showed distinct methylation differences in genes implicated in immune function (Cao-Lei et al., 2014).

Provocatively, prenatal socioeconomic status has been linked to placental HSD11B2 methylation, which regulates maternal cortisol (Appleton et al., 2013), while other small studies employing a genome-wide approach have detected changes in DNA methylation at adulthood linked to early socioeconomic adversity,

implying persistence of induced changes (Borghol et al., 2012; Lam et al., 2012).

The role of epigenetic mechanisms in early life stress is strongly backed by animal data: in rats, maternal care levels influence methylation and expression levels of the GR, potentially impacting on HPA axis pathway regulation, and drug-induced interference of histone modification restores the epigenetic state and phenotype (Weaver et al., 2004). Mice subjected to early postnatal maternal separation develop depression-like behaviours accompanied by altered candidate gene methylation in sperm (Franklin et al., 2010). In a non-human primate model involving rhesus macaques, being reared by inanimate surrogates, which promotes emotional and social disturbances, was shown to interfere with methylation patterns in the brain and T-cells (Provençal et al., 2012).

Maternal exposure to environmental toxins such as vehicle-emitted polycyclic aromatic hydrocarbons and tobacco smoke increases risk of asthma in offspring. Prenatal exposure to the former perturbs epigenetic regulation at genes encoding the regulatory cytokine IFNγ and the fatty acid metabolism component ACSL3 in cord blood (Perera et al., 2009; Tang et al., 2012). Functional studies on infants prenatally exposed to tobacco smoke revealed blunted stress responses, potentially mediated by epigenetic dysregulation at placental NR3C1 (Stroud et al., 2014). Epigenetic alterations may persist until at least childhood: a study of 5–12-year-old asthmatic children whose mothers smoked during pregnancy showed small but independently replicable changes at two methylation sites in whole blood (Breton et al., 2014). The perturbative effects of environmental pollutants on epigenetic regulation, with potentially adverse impact on disease risk, warrant attention especially as levels of urbanization increase (Klingbeil et al., 2014).

Opportunities arising from DOHaD epigenetic research

Depending on the cue, DOHaD-related pathways may be adaptive or non-adaptive in origin and may invoke differing cellular or physiological mechanisms, even though a common clinical phenotype is induced (Hanson and Gluckman, 2014). While numerous studies are solidifying support for the notion that epigenetic changes can transduce early environmental cues and modulate subsequent disease risk, much of the specific molecular detail on how such variation affects regulation of gene expression and changes developmental trajectory leading to an altered phenotype remains to be explicated. Care also needs to be exercised in interpreting correlation-or-causation effects. Most of the data are correlative, and establishing causality will help to clarify the functional role of disease-associated variations, and inform efforts towards therapeutic purposes (Mill and Heijmans, 2013). Nonetheless, the burgeoning field of developmental epigenomics is starting to highlight the utility of specific epigenetic marks at birth and in childhood as novel prognostic biomarkers of later disease risk. A methodological advantage is that non-invasively sourced tissues, including the umbilical cord, cord blood, and buccal cells, can be used. Advances in imaging techniques have further enabled more accurate assessments of body composition or cardiovascular structure as phenotypic outcomes, even in children. The example of RXRA gene methylation levels linking to unbalanced maternal nutrition and to a prodrome of metabolic disease is an important starting point (Godfrey et al., 2011).

Animal data have provided good evidence that developmentally conditioned phenotypes can be reversed by endocrinological, dietary, or pharmacological means. For example, supplementing a maternal low-protein diet with folic acid prevents cardiovascular dysfunction in offspring (Torrens et al., 2006), and administering leptin (Vickers et al., 2005) or growth hormone (Gray et al., 2013) to offspring of maternally undernourished rats reverts their compromised metabolic and vascular phenotype to that of controls that received adequate nourishment. Reversal of poor metabolic and vascular function has also been achieved through postnatal dietary supplementation of omega-3 fatty acids in offspring born to glucocorticoid-treated mothers, even in those exposed to a high-fat diet (Zulkafli et al., 2013). Of relevance to the modern environment with plentiful food are studies showing that maternal antioxidant or taurine supplementation can ameliorate the effects of maternal diet-induced obesity on offspring phenotype (Sen and Simmons, 2010; Li et al., 2013). While the translational potential of these findings to humans awaits further investigation, they clearly provide strong proof of concept that reversal is possible and can be effected irrespective of whether conditioning has occurred by adaptive or non-adaptive pathways. A key point in common is that treatments were provided sufficiently early in life for plasticity still to operate, and the developmental trajectory is still amenable to change; this point will be revisited in detail later.

Scope of the public health challenge

In recent decades, global rates of overweight, obesity, and related chronic illnesses including T2D and cardiovascular disease have soared (World Health Organization, 2011; Ng et al., 2014; Guariguata et al., 2014b). However, while this epidemic has been observed first in high-income countries, there is particular concern that this is being rapidly mirrored in low- to middle-income countries, on which downstream impact through loss of economic productivity and overburdening of emergent health systems may present an insurmountable problem. The World Health Organization estimates that these and other NCDs account for nearly two-thirds of global mortality, 80% of which occurs in low- and middle-income countries. Secular trends in maternal overweight and obesity, and increased gestational weight gain, are also becoming apparent (Heslehurst et al., 2007; Ferrari et al., 2014). GDM, which occurs in as many as 25% of pregnancies in Southeast Asia (Guariguata et al., 2014a), is a strong risk factor for offspring adiposity and T2D—a disease legacy that may be perpetuated across multiple generations.

Animal evidence is rapidly emerging that early exposures can have transgenerational phenotypic effects on descendants that have been entirely unexposed to the inducing cue (Nilsson and Skinner, 2015). It is also becoming clear that epigenetic marks can pass through meiosis (Borgel et al., 2010; Hackett et al., 2013; Hammoud et al., 2009), with growing evidence suggesting the involvement of noncoding RNAs and other epigenetic changes in the germline (Lane et al., 2014). At present, the evidence base in humans is mostly circumstantial, with the preponderance of data derived from a historical Swedish cohort in which grandparental food supply in childhood associates with a grandchild's mortality in a sex-specific manner (Pembrey et al., 2014).

Globally, the enormity of the challenge of obesity and overweight is well-recognized (Swinburn et al., 2011). Most attention has however focused on adult behaviours, with emphasis on sustained weight loss. The dogmatic view of weight control has focused on the balance of 'energy in' versus 'energy out', whereby greater energy intake results in weight gain while increasing energy expenditure leads to weight loss. However, this perspective is arguably naïve in excluding considerations of other complex biological, psychological, cultural, and socioeconomic determinants that can also make substantial contributions to the development of obesity and related NCDs. The considerable increase in our understanding of, firstly, the importance of developmental influences in setting the stage for later life health; secondly, of the wide range of conditioning factors for obesity risk; and thirdly, of the metabolic and other physiological responses to weight loss which attempt to counteract it; show that a much more nuanced perspective is essential. Yet the DOHaD paradigm has until very recently received little appreciation within the obesity research domain. As a consequence, public health models have mostly been based on the principle of reducing the energy intake:energy expenditure ratio, with appeals to voluntary adult behavioural modification such as dietary change and physical activity (Beaglehole et al., 2011). The sobering statistics on global metabolic health reveal that such approaches are ineffective. Forecasts suggesting that the disproportionate burden on low- and middle-income countries will persist, and that overweight and obesity—including in children—will continue to rise (World Health Organization, 2011; Guariguata et al., 2014b), together present a clear imperative for formulating more effective strategies to address the growing health, economic, and social threat. In 2011, the United Nations General Assembly meeting on the prevention and control of NCDs formally recognized the crucial role of development in NCD risk (see Clause 26 in United Nations General Assembly, 2012), setting the stage for a reassessment of current paradigms for tackling the NCD epidemic.

The public health consequences of the DOHaD concept and of developmental mismatch are manifold. One concerns the increasing rates of obesity and its co-morbidities in low-income countries undergoing intragenerational nutritional transition as a result of rapid economic improvements (Popkin et al., 2012). In this situation, relatively impoverished individuals who may not have been well-nourished in early life find themselves in a nutritionally rich adult environment, and with the economic means to access such nutrition. In a similar vein, rural-to-urban migrants or refugees seeking more prosperous conditions are subjected to a mismatched later life environment to which they are not physiologically well adapted. The adverse health impact of nutritional transition on metabolic health has been well documented in populations from several low-income countries (Jeemon et al., 2009; Ebrahim et al., 2010; He et al., 2014).

A further consequence of developmental mismatch relates to the set of evolved, physiologically normative processes known as maternal constraint that limit foetal growth to match maternal size, thus reducing risk of dystocia (Gluckman and Hanson, 2004). The level of maternal constraint is higher in primiparous mothers, and hence first-born children tend to be born about 0.15 kg lighter than their siblings (Ward, 1993). As predicted by the developmental mismatch model, studies have now shown that first-borns have poorer indices of metabolic health later in life, such as reduced insulin sensitivity and higher blood pressure in childhood (Ayyavoo et al., 2013), and higher adiposity at age 30 (Reynolds et al., 2010). This has great public health importance as progressive decreases in family size in many countries have directly resulted in first-borns comprising a greater proportion of the population. Maternal constraint is also greater in women of short stature, multiple pregnancies, preterm deliveries, and with maternal smoking or drug-taking (Gluckman and Hanson, 2004, 2005). However, more recently it has been shown that perinatal survival is greater in infants with birth weights much higher than the population median, showing that the processes of constraint for maternal advantage operate across the population (Vasak et al., 2014; Francis et al., 2014). It is therefore clear that potential mismatch is not just a feature of the extremes of prenatal development.

Which developmental factors condition later influence NCD risk?

The extensive DOHaD literature has shown that multiple developmental factors operate from early gestation through to infancy to modulate the later risk of obesity and its clinical *sequelae* (Fig. 1.2.1; see World Health Organization, 2014, for comprehensive review). From these factors, three interrelated categories emerge relating to the individual's biology, behaviour, and context. It should be noted that although each is considered separately here next, they are not mutually exclusive.

'Biological' factors

The degree of biological susceptibility towards greater adiposity within an obesogenic environment is fundamentally dependent on an individual's developmental history spanning the preconceptional period to infancy. There are likely also genetic determinants, and indeed there is now growing evidence of powerful genetic-epigenetic interactions (Teh et al., 2014). As previously described, maternal unbalanced nutrition is one major conditioning factor. Offspring relying on such cues to predict a nutritionally scarce postnatal environment are conditioned to develop a metabolic phenotype, appetite, satiety set-point (Ross and Desai, 2014), and possibly food preferences biased towards energy preservation (Bellinger et al., 2004; Bayol et al., 2007). However, developmental mismatch ensues when the predicted *versus* actual postnatal

conditions become discordant (Gluckman and Hanson, 2006a). Maternal overnutrition and hyperglycaemia condition a similar phenotype, likely via pathophysiological, non-adaptive pathways, although the extent of disruption may depend on the degree of the challenge. At a cellular level, experimental studies have suggested multiple effects on neural function and appetite control (Vucetic et al., 2010), mitochondrial function, adipocyte biology (Borengasser et al., 2013; Bruce et al., 2009), as well as increased oxidative stress (Zhang et al., 2011). A recent pilot study of infants prenatally exposed to GDM or growth restraint identified several epigenetic alterations in clinically relevant genes in common, suggesting that different developmental exposures may affect common epigenetic pathways that elevate risk of later disease such as T2D (Quilter et al., 2014). There is now accumulating evidence from animal studies that paternal diet may influence disease risk. Male rats that consume high-fat diets sire daughters that later develop impaired β-cell function (Ng et al., 2010); offspring of male mice receiving a protein-deficient diet develop abnormal cholesterol and lipid metabolism (Carone et al., 2010); and a low-folate paternal diet in mice leads to birth defects in offspring (Lambrot et al., 2013). Multiple studies of paternal dietary manipulation have detected epigenetic dysregulation in sperm of fathers and male offspring, although the specific molecular details of transgenerational transmission remain to be established. In humans, preliminary data suggest the existence of a graded relationship between paternal BMI and methylation at cord blood *IGF2* (Soubry et al., 2013), clearly warranting replication in larger cohorts with follow-up clinical phenotyping.

A further emerging area of research focuses on the role of the gut microbiota—which may be influenced by delivery mode and antibiotic administration in infancy—in mediating risk of obesity and T2D (Ajslev et al., 2011; Karlsson et al., 2013). It seems increasingly likely that metagenomics will form an important component of DOHaD research. Other biological factors operating during infancy include overfeeding through formula use and inappropriate complementary foods, and establishment of inappropriate taste preferences (Beauchamp and Mennella, 2009; Oddy et al., 2014).

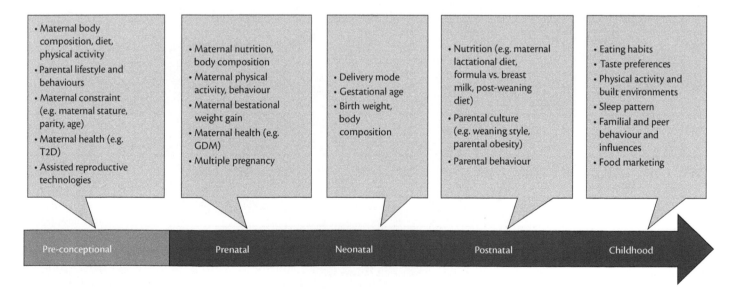

Fig. 1.2.1 Early life influences on obesity and related diseases that encompass biological, behavioural, and contextual domains.

Behavioural factors

Behaviours learnt early in life—moulded and reinforced by family and cultural factors—may become deeply entrenched during the early post-weaning period of continued plasticity. For example, maternal diet during gestation and breastfeeding is an important determinant of food acceptance in infancy, as flavours are transmitted to amniotic fluid and breast milk (Mennella et al., 2001; Forestell and Mennella, 2007). Adopting a baby-led instead of parent-led style of weaning was associated with a preference for carbohydrate over sweet food, and a lower incidence of obesity in early childhood (Townsend and Pitchford, 2012). A small study has suggested that healthful changes in food preference may be encouraged by parental behaviour: repeated exposure of recently weaned infants to an initially disliked vegetable could promote its acceptance to a level equivalent to that of another initially liked vegetable within eight days (Maier et al., 2007).

Other contributing factors include insufficient physical activity, excessive consumption of poor quality food, and even curtailed sleep—a large study has found links between chronic lack of sleep during infancy and early childhood, and levels of central and overall adiposity at age seven (Taveras et al., 2014).

Contextual factors

Every individual lives within the context of his/her culture, community, and wider society. Factors ranging from family and peer behaviour, through to food marketing and food supply, converge to define the overall context in which disease risk is established (World Health Organization, 2014). Thus for example, consistent exposure of a young child to poor familial eating habits, a sedentary lifestyle that is also adopted by other family members and peers, excessive screen time, and an at-home abundance of 'empty' calorie processed snacks high in energy but low in nutritional value, could lead to such an environment becoming erroneously viewed as normative by the impressionable child. Wider issues of socioeconomic status, increased urbanization and digitalization, and aggressive food marketing practices also create

built and social environments that promote obesity (McLaren, 2007; Harris et al., 2009).

A life course approach to reducing disease risk

The DOHaD paradigm forms the conceptual basis of a *life course approach* for addressing obesity and other NCDs. The core principle of this approach is that relatively minor changes in early life become magnified over the life course to have larger effects later in life. Thus, small shifts during the plastic phase of development can have substantial impact on the response of a child, adolescent, or adult to later challenges, such as living in an obesogenic environment (Fig. 1.2.2).

The life course model suggests that at a particular time point, disease risk is determined not only by the level of (say) environmental obesogenicity, but also by the cumulative antecedent life of the individual, their exposure to risks, and the resulting degree to which they are able to cope in adulthood with environmental exposures and challenges to their health. This model relates closely to the economic concept of path dependency, which describes how the range of options available for decision-making for a given circumstance is restricted by previous paths taken and decisions made. Thus from a life course perspective, what happens in early life determines or limits how one can respond to challenges later in the life course. An additional outcome of path dependency and the greater plasticity of early life is that once a situation has become established, costs of switching become greater, leading to a system 'lock in' that takes a major event in order to be shifted. A good example comes from modelling studies of female obesity which show how post-pregnancy weight is dependent on pregravid weight, and that postpartum maintenance of a higher calorie diet (a 'lock in') will result in continued weight gain unless significant changes are made to energy intake and expenditure (Sabounchi et al., 2014).

Developmental plasticity is, unequivocally, an integral element of the life course approach. A core principle of biology is that organisms have high levels of plasticity in early life, when biological and

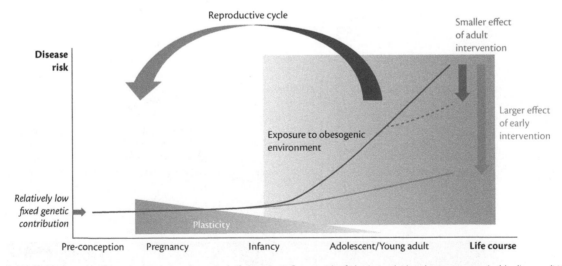

Fig. 1.2.2 An individual's developmental experiences during the period of plasticity influence risk of obesity and related non-communicable diseases (NCDs) on later life exposure to an obesogenic environment. Primary interventions applied early in life have a greater effect on disease risk compared to secondary interventions in adulthood, when levels of plasticity are relatively low. The reproductive cycle highlights important intergenerational considerations, whereby the health status of young adults of reproductive age impacts on the next generation.

behavioural development is affected by exogenous influences with long-term consequences that become more obvious as maturation proceeds. Energetic and other costs of maintaining plasticity, as well as inherent difficulties in reversing developmental pathways, generally limit the phase of plasticity from the preconceptional period until weaning (Fig. 1.2.2), after which an age-related decline occurs (Gluckman *et al.*, 2010). However there may also be certain ontogenic windows of sensitivity during foetal development that give rise to timing-of-exposure-specific differences in risk, depending on the physiological system affected (Roseboom *et al.*, 2006).

Implications for intervention strategies

A life course perspective suggests that any package of measures to address the development of obesity and its attendant health, economic, and social costs will need to take into account the full range of biological, behavioural, environmental, and contextual risk factors. As it is unlikely that a focus on any single component can be efficacious, a holistic approach traversing the whole life course is essential (Fig. 1.2.3).

Reducing risk and enhancing later resilience

The biological plasticity that is inherent in early life affects the sensitivity of the developing individual to the obesogenic environment that will usually be encountered in the current developed and developing world. Within a high nutrition environment, susceptibility towards obesity is underpinned by the individual's developmentally and genetically influenced levels of *risk* and *resilience*. Risk is modulated by physiological changes in the developing foetus/child induced by early life events that make him or her more

or less susceptible to obesity. Resilience—defined in this context as the ability of the phenotype to withstand challenges (Hanson and Gluckman, 2014)—is enhanced when early life events assist the development of behaviours and physiology that reduce the likelihood of obesity in an obesogenic environment. This strategy calls for focus on the conditioning factors operating during the window of developmental plasticity, so as to enhance later resilience and reduce the risk of disease vulnerability later (Hanson and Gluckman, 2015). It directs our attention to the nutritional state, body composition, and behaviours of the future mother and father prior to conception; the nutritional, emotional, and health status, and body composition of the mother during pregnancy and lactation; the development of the foetus; the nature of weaning; and related factors that influence the development of appetite control and food preference (World Health Organization, 2014).

By focusing on the earliest phases of life, this primary prevention strategy entails the reduction of risk factors so as to prevent disease occurrence. It is in contrast to secondary prevention, which aims to control disease progression at the prodromal stage, and to tertiary prevention, which has palliative aims after disease onset. The crux of the life course-based intervention model is that efficacy of efforts later in childhood is contingent on the success of reducing risk and enhancing later resilience during the earlier life phases. The view created by this new knowledge provides a possible explanation of the limited efficacy of adopting a narrower focus on the obesogenic environment alone. Indeed, prevention from the earliest stages of life is crucial, given that an individual may be well on the pathway to obesity and its co-morbidities in the absence of any obvious clinical symptoms. For example, carotid

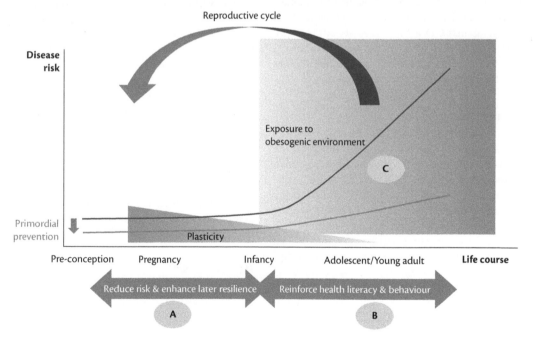

Fig. 1.2.3 A life course-based suite of integrated strategies to reduce risk of obesity and related diseases. The coloured lines represent the potential risk trajectories of individuals who are not (dark blue line) or are (light blue line) subject to appropriate interventions across the life course. (A) The high degree of developmental plasticity in early life can be exploited to achieve a physiology that confers minimum risk of disease vulnerability and maximum later resilience. (B) From the postnatal period, the individual is directly exposed to the obesogenic environment, and thus reinforcement of knowledge and behaviours through to at least the childhood period is crucial for later resilience. Health literacy and other educational measures aid in reinforcement, and additionally can minimize initial risk of the next generation through optimal parental preconceptional health and behaviour to achieve primordial prevention (downward shift from dark blue to light blue line). (C) The severity of the obesogenic environment needs to be addressed to further reduce the divergence between risk trajectories.

intima-media thickening—a prodrome of atherosclerosis—has been observed in otherwise outwardly healthy children independently of birth weight, but is nonetheless related to modifiable risk factors such as maternal nutrition (Gale *et al.*, 2006).

Reinforcement of health literacy and behaviour

Following the establishment of a favourable physiological phenotype, constant *reinforcement* through infancy and childhood may be necessary for later resilience to be maximized. This preschool period is a critical window for consolidation and imprinting of behaviours. This reinforcement phase requires attention to eating and exercise behaviours, and familial health and nutritional literacy in infancy and childhood through to school-age years. Formal school- or hospital-based educational efforts on adolescents have met with success in terms of increased awareness of the impact of personal health on the next generation (Bay *et al.*, 2012; Grace *et al.*, 2012), but these will require integration with other measures to maximize behavioural change.

Targeting young people before they become parents facilitates primordial prevention. This is distinct from primary prevention, as it entails the prevention of risk factors emerging in the first place, rather than their modification once risk factors have been established (Weintraub *et al.*, 2011). For instance, an overweight woman who has successfully reduced her BMI before proceeding with a planned pregnancy has essentially eliminated maternal obesity-associated risk factors for her offspring. A recent British study found low levels of preconception health knowledge among both pregnant women and, of especial concern, their healthcare professionals (Stephenson *et al.*, 2014). Yet many of the women demonstrated motivation to adopt healthier behaviours before pregnancy, especially on the advice of their healthcare professional. Large studies have found that adopting healthy dietary patterns and increasing physical activity prior to pregnancy is substantially protective against GDM (Tobias *et al.*, 2011, 2012). There is clearly ample opportunity to further empower young people and parents-to-be to take greater responsibility and increase self-efficacy for personal health and hence that of their offspring.

Reducing environmental obesogenicity

As a child gains increasing autonomy from its mother, its exposure to the obesogenic environment effectively increases. Reducing the severity of the obesogenic environment, particularly for women and children, will require multilevel behavioural and contextual interventions from the individual and family through to the community and the wider macroenvironment. This will require reassessment of how various stakeholders, including the private sector, are engaged. Regulatory measures such as that undertaken by the New York City government to reduce junk food consumption have met with some success (Farley, 2012). Positive outcomes from constructive engagement with industry are not without precedent—in Denmark, actions of a self-regulatory body comprising food producers, retailers, and media organizations have rapidly led to near negligible levels of advertising of unhealthy foods to children (Peetz-Schou, 2014). There is also growing interest in how the emerging economic concept of social capital, which broadly refers to the resources made available through an individual or group's social networks, may be a useful tool in lowering obesity risk (Holtgrave and Crosby, 2006; Moore, 2010; Yoon and Brown, 2011).

Conclusion

The theoretical basis and mechanistic observations underlying the DOHaD concept suggest that a much broader focus on the life course is needed than has previously been given by the medical and public health communities and policy makers, if the prevalence of conditions such as obesity and NCDs is to be reduced. The DOHaD endeavour has greatly benefited from the rapid progress in developmental epigenetic research, which has helped to illuminate the underlying mechanisms, and this could potentially provide molecular guidance for therapeutic strategies.

A prudent public health approach to the obesity and NCD epidemic will by necessity be context-dependent, taking into account economic, nutrition, environmental, cultural, and policy dimensions. As shown in Figure 1.2.3, a three-pronged, unified approach across the life course is likely to offer optimal efficacy and efficiency. Nevertheless the conditioning phase stands out as a focal point for intervention given that targeting the post-infancy obesogenic environment, while necessary, is plainly insufficient. The evidence further implies that much of the problem extends beyond the control of the individual child or family, which justifies a society-based approach. Counter to the dominant thinking underlying existing methods for tackling obesity, expecting adults to achieve and sustain weight loss, for example, is not feasible as a population-wide measure, especially as there are strong and persistent endocrinological drivers towards increased appetite in response to weight loss (Sumithran *et al.*, 2011). Increasing evidence suggests that the conditioning phase requires a focus on fathers-to-be in addition to mothers, as well as attention to pregnancy care, infant feeding patterns, and weaning. This has important implications for equity and healthcare access.

The indisputable importance of a life course approach for dealing with the contemporary challenge of obesity and other NCDs has been formally endorsed in the 2011 Political Declaration by the United Nations (United Nations General Assembly, 2012). The recently established World Health Organization Commission on Ending Childhood Obesity, which has been tasked with tackling the growing global problems and consequences of child and adolescent obesity, has noted the indispensable contribution of life course concepts towards informing its work (World Health Organization, 2014). Although this chapter has drawn largely on obesity to illustrate the merits of a life course approach, this perspective is generalizable (UK Chief Medical Officer, 2013, New Zealand House of Representatives Health Committee, 2013). The moral, social, and economic arguments for its utility in counteracting other NCDs are compelling, and its greater integration into public health thinking is overdue.

References

Aerts, L. & van Assche, F. A. (1979). Is gestational diabetes an acquired condition?. *J Dev Physiol*, 1, 219–25.

Ajslev, T. A., Andersen, C. S., Gamborg, M., Sorensen, T. I. A., & Jess, T. (2011). Childhood overweight after establishment of the gut microbiota: the role of delivery mode, pre-pregnancy weight and early administration of antibiotics. *Int J Obes*, 35, 522–9.

Appleton, A. A., Armstrong, D. A., Lesseur, C., et al. (2013). Patterning in placental 11-B hydroxysteroid dehydrogenase methylation according to prenatal socioeconomic adversity. *PLoS One*, 8, e74691.

Ayyavoo, A., Savage, T., Derraik, J. G. B., Hofman, P. L., & Cutfield, W. S. (2013). First-born children have reduced insulin sensitivity and higher daytime blood pressure compared to later-born children. *J Clin Endocrinol Metab*, 98, 1248–53.

Barker, D. J. P., Osmond, C., Golding, J., Kuh, D., & Wadsworth, M. E. (1989a). Growth in utero, blood pressure in childhood and adult life, and mortality from cardiovascular disease. *BMJ*, 298, 564–7.

Barker, D. J. P., Winter, P. D., Osmond, C., Margetts, B., & Simmonds, S. J. (1989b). Weight in infancy and death from ischaemic heart disease. *Lancet*, 2, 577–80.

Bateson, P., Barker, D., Clutton-Brock, T., *et al.* (2004). Developmental plasticity and human health. *Nature*, 430, 419–21.

Bateson, P., Gluckman, P., & Hanson, M. (2014). The biology of developmental plasticity and the Predictive Adaptive Response hypothesis. *J Physiol*, 592, 2357–68.

Bay, J. L., Mora, H. A., Sloboda, D. M., Morton, S. M., Vickers, M. H., & Gluckman, P. D. (2012). Adolescent understanding of DOHaD concepts: a school-based intervention to support knowledge translation and behaviour change. *J Dev Orig Health Dis*, 3, 469–82.

Bayol, S. A., Farrington, S. J., & Stickland, N. C. (2007). A maternal 'junk food' diet in pregnancy and lactation promotes an exacerbated taste for 'junk food' and a greater propensity for obesity in rat offspring. *Br J Nutr*, 98, 843–51.

Beaglehole, R., Bonita, R., Horton, R., *et al.* (2011). Priority actions for the non-communicable disease crisis. *Lancet*, 377, 1438–47.

Beauchamp, G. K. & Mennella, J. A. (2009). Early flavor learning and its impact on later feeding behavior. *J Pediatr Gastroenterol Nutr*, 48, S25–S30.

Bellinger, L., Lilley, C., & Langley-Evans, S. C. (2004). Prenatal exposure to a low protein diet programmes a preference for high fat foods in the rat. *Br J Nutr*, 92, 513–20.

Borengasser, S. J., Zhong, Y., Kang, P., *et al.* (2013). Maternal obesity enhances white adipose tissue differentiation and alters genome-scale DNA methylation in male rat offspring. *Endocrinology*, 154, 4113–25.

Borgel, J., Guibert, S., Li, Y., *et al.* (2010). Targets and dynamics of promoter DNA methylation during early mouse development. *Nat Genet*, 42, 1093–100.

Borghol, N., Suderman, M., McArdle, W., *et al.* (2012). Associations with early-life socio-economic position in adult DNA methylation. *Int J Epidemiol*, 41, 62–74.

Bouchard, L., Hivert, M.-F., Guay, S.-P., St-Pierre, J., Perron, P., & Brisson, D. (2012). Placental adiponectin gene DNA methylation levels are associated with mothers' blood glucose concentration. *Diabetes*, 61, 1272–80.

Bouchard, L., Thibault, S., Guay, S.-P., *et al.* (2010). Leptin gene epigenetic adaptation to impaired glucose metabolism during pregnancy. *Diabetes Care*, 33, 2436–41.

Breton, C. V., Siegmund, K. D., Joubert, B. R., *et al.* (2014). Prenatal tobacco smoke exposure is associated with childhood DNA CpG methylation. *PLoS One*, 9, e99716.

Bruce, K. D., Cagampang, F. R., Argenton, M., *et al.* (2009). Maternal high-fat feeding primes steatohepatitis in adult mice offspring, involving mitochondrial dysfunction and altered lipogenesis gene expression. *Hepatology*, 50, 1796–808.

Cao-Lei, L., Massart, R., Suderman, M. J., *et al.* (2014). DNA methylation signatures triggered by prenatal maternal stress exposure to a natural disaster: Project Ice Storm. *PLoS One*, 9, e107653.

Capizzi, S., de Waure, C., & Boccia, S. (2015). Global burden and health trends of non-communicable diseases. In: Boccia, S., Villari, P., & Ricciardi, W. (eds) *A Systematic Review of Key Issues in Public Health*, pp. 19–32. Cham, Switzerland: Springer International Publishing.

Carone, B. R., Fauquier, L., Habib, N., *et al.* (2010). Paternally induced transgenerational environmental reprogramming of metabolic gene expression in mammals. *Cell*, 143, 1084–96.

Catalano, P. M., Tyzbir, E. D., Roman, N. M., Amini, S. B., & Sims, E. A. H. (1991). Longitudinal changes in insulin release and insulin resistance in nonobese pregnant women. *Am J Obstet Gynecol*, 165, 1667–72.

Conradt, E., Lester, B. M., Appleton, A. A., Armstrong, D. A., & Marsit, C. J. (2013). The roles of DNA methylation of *NR3C1* and *11β-HSD2*

and exposure to maternal mood disorder in utero on newborn neurobehavior. *Epigenetics*, 8, 1321–9.

Cooper, W. N., Khulan, B., Owens, S., *et al.* (2012). DNA methylation profiling at imprinted loci after periconceptional micronutrient supplementation in humans: results of a pilot randomized controlled trial. *FASEB J*, 26, 1782–90.

Curhan, G. C., Chertow, G. M., Willett, W. C., *et al.* (1996). Birth weight and adult hypertension and obesity in women. *Circulation*, 94, 1310–5.

Desgagné, V., Hivert, M.-F., St-Pierre, J., *et al.* (2014). Epigenetic dysregulation of the IGF system in placenta of newborns exposed to maternal impaired glucose tolerance. *Epigenomics*, 6, 193–207.

Dominguez-Salas, P., Moore, S. E., Baker, M. S., *et al.* (2014). Maternal nutrition at conception modulates DNA methylation of human metastable epialleles. *Nat Commun*, 5, 3746.

Dötsch, J., Plank, C., Amann, K., & Ingelfinger, J. (2009). The implications of fetal programming of glomerular number and renal function. *J Mol Med*, 87, 841–8.

Drake, A. J., McPherson, R. C., Godfrey, K. M., *et al.* (2012). An unbalanced maternal diet in pregnancy associates with offspring epigenetic changes in genes controlling glucocorticoid action and foetal growth. *Clin Endocrinol*, 77, 808–15.

Drong, A. W., Lindgren, C. M., & McCarthy, M. I. (2012). The genetic and epigenetic basis of type 2 diabetes and obesity. *Clin Pharmacol Ther*, 92, 707–15.

Dudley, K. J., Sloboda, D. M., Connor, K. L., Beltrand, J., & Vickers, M. H. (2011). Offspring of mothers fed a high fat diet display hepatic cell cycle inhibition and associated changes in gene expression and DNA methylation. *PLoS One*, 6, e21662.

Ebrahim, S., Kinra, S., Bowen, L., *et al.* (2010). The effect of rural-to-urban migration on obesity and diabetes in India: a cross-sectional study. *PLoS Med*, 7, 12.

El Hajj, N., Pliushch, G., Schneider, E., *et al.* (2012). Metabolic programming of MEST DNA methylation by intrauterine exposure to gestational diabetes mellitus. *Diabetes*, 62, 1320–8.

Farley, T. A. (2012). The role of government in preventing excess calorie consumption: The example of New York City. *JAMA*, 308, 1093–4.

Ferrari, N., Mallmann, P., Brockmeier, K., Struder, H., & Graf, C. (2014). Secular trends in pregnancy weight gain in German women and their influences on foetal outcome: a hospital-based study. *BMC Pregnancy and Childbirth*, 14, 228.

Forestell, C. A. & Mennella, J. A. (2007). Early determinants of fruit and vegetable acceptance. *Pediatrics*, 120, 1247–54.

Forrester, T. E., Badaloo, A. V., Boyne, M. S., *et al.* (2012). Prenatal factors contribute to emergence of kwashiorkor or marasmus in response to severe undernutrition: evidence for the predictive adaptation model. *PLoS One*, 7, e35907.

Francis, J. H., Permezel, M., & Davey, M. A. (2014). Perinatal mortality by birthweight centile. *Aust N Z J Obstet Gynaecol*, 54, 354–9.

Franklin, T. B., Russig, H., Weiss, I. C., *et al.* (2010). Epigenetic transmission of the impact of early stress across generations. *Biol Psychiatry*, 68, 408–15.

Gademan, M. G. J., Vermeulen, M., Oostvogels, A. J. J. M., *et al.* (2014). Maternal prepregnancy BMI and lipid profile during early pregnancy are independently associated with offspring's body composition at age 5–6 years: the ABCD study. *PLoS One*, 9, e94594.

Gale, C. R., Jiang, B., Robinson, S. M., Godfrey, K. M., Law, C. M., & Martyn, C. N. (2006). Maternal diet during pregnancy and carotid intima-media thickness in children. *Arterioscler Thromb Vasc Biol*, 26, 1877–82.

Gemma, C., Sookoian, S., Alvariñas, J., *et al.* (2009). Maternal pregestational BMI is associated with methylation of the PPARGC1A promoter in newborns. *Obesity*, 17, 1032–9.

Gershon, A., Sudheimer, K., Tirouvanziam, R., Williams, L. & O'Hara, R. (2013). The long-term impact of early adversity on late-life psychiatric disorders. *Curr Psychiatry Rep*, 15, 1–9.

Gluckman, P. & Hanson, M. (2006a). *Mismatch: Why Our World No Longer Fits Our Bodies*. Oxford, UK: Oxford University Press.

Gluckman, P. D. & Buklijas, T. (2014). Developmental Origins of Health and Disease—The Past and the Future. In: Zhang, L. & Longo, L. D. (eds) *Stress and Developmental Programming of Health and Disease: Beyond Phenomenology*, pp. 1–12. Hauppauge, NY: Nova Science.

Gluckman, P. D. & Hanson, M. A. (2004). Maternal constraint of fetal growth and its consequences. *Semin Fetal Neonatal Med*, 9, 419–25.

Gluckman, P. D. & Hanson, M. A. (2005). *The Fetal Matrix: Evolution, Development, and Disease*. Cambridge: Cambridge University Press.

Gluckman, P. D. & Hanson, M. A. (eds) (2006b). *Developmental Origins of Health and Disease*. Cambridge, UK: Cambridge University Press.

Gluckman, P. D., Hanson, M. A., & Buklijas, T. (2010). A conceptual framework for the Developmental Origins of Health and Disease. *J Dev Orig Health Dis*, 1, 6–18.

Gluckman, P. D., Hanson, M. A., Buklijas, T., Low, F. M., & Beedle, A. S. (2009). Epigenetic mechanisms that underpin metabolic and cardiovascular diseases. *Nat Rev Endocrinol*, 5, 401–8.

Gluckman, P. D., Hanson, M. A., & Spencer, H. G. (2005a). Predictive adaptive responses and human evolution. *Trends Ecol Evol*, 20, 527–33.

Gluckman, P. D., Hanson, M. A., Spencer, H. G., & Bateson, P. (2005b). Environmental influences during development and their later consequences for health and disease: implications for the interpretation of empirical studies. *Proc Royal Soc B*, 272, 671–7.

Gluckman, P. D., Lillycrop, K. A., Vickers, M. H., *et al.* (2007). Metabolic plasticity during mammalian development is directionally dependent on early nutritional status. *Proc Natl Acad Sci U S A*, 104, 12796–800.

Godfrey, K. M., Barker, D. J., Robinson, S., & Osmond, C. (1997). Maternal birthweight and diet in pregnancy in relation to the infant's thinness at birth. *Br J Obstet Gynaecol*, 104, 663–7.

Godfrey, K. M., Sheppard, A., Gluckman, P. D., *et al.* (2011). Epigenetic gene promoter methylation at birth is associated with child's later adiposity. *Diabetes*, 60, 1528–34.

Gordon, L., Joo, J. E., Powell, J. E., *et al.* (2012). Neonatal DNA methylation profile in human twins is specified by a complex interplay between intrauterine environmental and genetic factors, subject to tissue-specific influence. *Genome Res*, 22, 1395–406.

Goyal, R., Goyal, D., Leitzke, A., Gheorghe, C. P., & Longo, L. D. (2010). Brain renin-angiotensin system: fetal epigenetic programming by maternal protein restriction during pregnancy. *Reproductive Sciences*, 17, 227–38.

Grace, M., Woods-Townsend, K., Griffiths, J., *et al.* (2012). Developing teenagers' views on their health and the health of their future children. *Health Education*, 112, 543–59.

Gray, C., Li, M., Reynolds, C. M., & Vickers, M. H. (2013). Pre-weaning growth hormone treatment reverses hypertension and endothelial dysfunction in adult male offspring of mothers undernourished during pregnancy. *PLoS One*, 8, e53505.

Guariguata, L., Linnenkamp, U., Beagley, J., Whiting, D. R., & Cho, N. H. (2014a). Global estimates of the prevalence of hyperglycaemia in pregnancy. *Diabetes Res Clin Pract*, 103, 176–85.

Guariguata, L., Whiting, D. R., Hambleton, I., Beagley, J., Linnenkamp, U., & Shaw, J. E. (2014b). Global estimates of diabetes prevalence for 2013 and projections for 2035. *Diabetes Res Clin Pract*, 103, 137–49.

Hackett, J. A., Sengupta, R., Zylicz, J. J., *et al.* (2013). Germline DNA demethylation dynamics and imprint erasure through 5-hydroxymethylcytosine. *Science*, 339, 448–52.

Hales, C. N. & Barker, D. J. (1992). Type 2 (non-insulin-dependent) diabetes mellitus: the thrifty phenotype hypothesis. *Diabetologia*, 35, 595–601.

Hales, C. N. & Barker, D. J. (2001). The thrifty phenotype hypothesis. *Br Med Bull*, 60, 5–20.

Hales, C. N., Barker, D. J. P., Clark, P. M. S., *et al.* (1991). Fetal and infant growth and impaired glucose tolerance at age 64. *BMJ*, 303, 1019–22.

Hammoud, S. S., Nix, D. A., Zhang, H., Purwar, J., Carrell, D. T., & Cairns, B. R. (2009). Distinctive chromatin in human sperm packages genes for embryo development. *Nature*, 460, 473–8.

Hanson, M. A. & Gluckman, P. D. (2014). Early developmental conditioning of later health and disease: physiology or pathophysiology?. *Physiol Rev*, 94, 1027–76.

Hanson, M. A. & Gluckman, P. D. (2015). Developmental origins of health and disease – Global public health implications. *Best Pract Res Clin Obstet Gynaecol*, 29, 24–31.

Harder, T., Rodekamp, E., Schellong, K., Dudenhausen, J. W., & Plagemann, A. (2007). Birth weight and subsequent risk of type 2 diabetes: a meta-analysis. *Am J Epidemiol*, 165, 849–57.

Harris, J. L., Pomeranz, J. L., Lobstein, T., & Brownell, K. D. (2009). A crisis in the marketplace: how food marketing contributes to childhood obesity and what can be done. *Annu Rev Public Health*, 30, 211–25.

He, Y., Lam, T. H., Jiang, B., *et al.* (2014). Changes in BMI before and during economic development and subsequent risk of cardiovascular disease and total mortality: a 35-year follow-up study in China. *Diabetes Care*, 37, 2540–7.

Heijmans, B. T., Tobi, E. W., Stein, A. D., *et al.* (2008). Persistent epigenetic differences associated with prenatal exposure to famine in humans. *Proc Natl Acad Sci U S A*, 105, 17046–9.

Heslehurst, N., Ells, L. J., Simpson, H., Batterham, A., Wilkinson, J., & Summerbell, C. D. (2007). Trends in maternal obesity incidence rates, demographic predictors, and health inequalities in 36 821 women over a 15-year period. *BJOG*, 114, 187–94.

Higgins, M., Keller, J., Moore, F., Ostrander, L., Metzner, H., & Stock, L. (1980). Studies of blood pressure in Tecumseh, Michigan. I. Blood pressure in young people and its relationship to personal and familial characteristics and complications of pregnancy in mothers. *Am J Epidemiol*, 111, 142–55.

Hofman, P. L., W. S. Cutfield, E. M. Robinson, *et al.* (1997). Insulin resistance in short children with intrauterine growth retardation. *J Clin Endocrinol Metab*, 82, 402–6.

Holtgrave, D. R., & Crosby, R. (2006). Is social capital a protective factor against obesity and diabetes? Findings from an exploratory study. *Ann Epidemiol*, 16, 406–8.

Hoyo, C., Murtha, A. P., Schildkraut J. M., *et al.* (2011). Methylation variation at IGF2 differentially methylated regions and maternal folic acid use before and during pregnancy. *Epigenetics*, 6, 928–36.

International Society for Developmental Origins of Health and Disease (n.d.). Available at: https://dohadsoc.org/ (accessed 10 November 2014) [Online].

Jeemon, P., Neogi, S., Bhatnagar, D., Cruickshank, K. J., & Prabhakaran, D. (2009). The impact of migration on cardiovascular disease and its risk factors among people of Indian origin. *Curr Sci*, 97, 378–84.

Jiang, X., Yan, J., West, A. A., *et al.* (2012). Maternal choline intake alters the epigenetic state of fetal cortisol-regulating genes in humans. *FASEB J*, 26, 3563–74.

Kaiser, J. (2012). Genetic influences on disease remain hidden. *Science*, 338, 1016–17.

Karlsson, F., Tremaroli, V., Nielsen, J., & Bäckhed, F. (2013). Assessing the human gut microbiota in metabolic diseases. *Diabetes*, 62, 3341–9.

Kermack, W., McKendrick, A., & McKinlay, P. (1934). Death rates in Great Britain and Sweden: some general regularities and their significance. *Lancet*, 223, 698–703.

Khulan, B., Cooper, W. N., Skinner, B. M., *et al.* (2012). Periconceptional maternal micronutrient supplementation is associated with widespread gender related changes in the epigenome: a study of a unique resource in the Gambia. *Hum Mol Genet*, 21, 2086–101.

Klingbeil, E. C., Hew, K. M., Nygaard, U. C., & Nadeau, K. C. (2014). Polycyclic aromatic hydrocarbons, tobacco smoke, and epigenetic remodeling in asthma. *Immunol Res*, 58, 369–73.

Kuzawa, C. W. (2010). Beyond feast–famine: Brain evolution, human life history, and the metabolic syndrome. In: Muehlenbein, M. P. (ed.) *Human Evolutionary Biology*, pp. 518–27. Cambridge, UK: Cambridge University Press.

Labonte, B., Yerko, V., Gross, J., *et al.* (2012). Differential glucocorticoid receptor exon 1B, 1C, and 1H expression and methylation in suicide completers with a history of childhood abuse. *Biol Psychiatry*, 72, 41–8.

Lam, L. L., Emberly, E., Fraser, H. B., *et al.* (2012). Factors underlying variable DNA methylation in a human community cohort. *Proc Natl Acad Sci*, 109, 17253–60.

Lambrot, R., Xu, C., Saint-Phar, S., *et al.* (2013). Low paternal dietary folate alters the mouse sperm epigenome and is associated with negative pregnancy outcomes. *Nat Commun*, 4, 2889.

Lane, M., Robker, R. L., & Robertson, S. A. (2014). Parenting from before conception. *Science*, 345, 756–60.

Langley, S. C. & Jackson, A. A. (1994). Increased systolic blood pressure in adult rats induced by fetal exposure to maternal low protein diets. *Clin Sci*, 86, 217–22.

Lee, T. M. & Zucker, I. (1988). Vole infant development is influenced perinatally by maternal photoperiodic history. *Am J Physiol*, 255, R831–8.

Li, M., Reynolds, C. M., Sloboda, D. M., Gray, C., & Vickers, M. H. (2013). Effects of taurine supplementation on hepatic markers of inflammation and lipid metabolism in mothers and offspring in the setting of maternal obesity. *PLoS One*, 8, e76961.

Lillycrop, K. A., Phillips, E. S., Jackson, A. A., Hanson, M. A., & Burdge, G. C. (2005). Dietary protein restriction of pregnant rats induces and folic acid supplementation prevents epigenetic modification of hepatic gene expression in the offspring. *J Nutr*, 135, 1382–6.

Low, F. M., Gluckman, P. D. & Hanson, M. A. (2012). Developmental plasticity, epigenetics and human health. *Evol Biol*, 39, 650–5.

Low, F. M., Gluckman, P. D., & Hanson, M. A. (2014). Epigenetic and developmental basis of risk of obesity and metabolic disease. In: Ulloa-Aguirre, A., & Conn, P. M. (eds) *Cellular Endocrinology in Health and Disease*, pp. 111–132. London, UK: Elsevier.

Lumey, L. H., Terry, M. B., Delgado-Cruzata, L., *et al.* (2012). Adult global DNA methylation in relation to pre-natal nutrition. *Int J Epidemiol*, 41, 116–23.

Ma, R. C. W., Chan, J. C. N., Tam, W. H., Hanson, M. A., & Gluckman, P. D. (2013a). Gestational diabetes, maternal obesity and the NCD burden. *Clin Obstet Gynecol*, 56, 633–41.

Ma, R. C. W., Gluckman, P. D., & Hanson, M. A. (2013b). Maternal obesity and developmental priming of risk of later disease. In: Mahmood, T. A. & Arulkumaran, S. (eds) *Obesity—A Ticking Timebomb for Reproductive Health*, pp. 193–212. London, UK: Elsevier.

Maier, A., Chabanet, C., Schaal, B., Issanchou, S., & Leathwood, P. (2007). Effects of repeated exposure on acceptance of initially disliked vegetables in 7-month old infants. *Food Quality and Preference*, 18, 1023–32.

Maloyan, A., Muralimanoharan, S., Huffman, S., *et al.* (2013). Identification and comparative analyses of myocardial miRNAs involved in the fetal response to maternal obesity. *Physiol Genomics*, 45, 889–900.

McGowan, P. O., Sasaki, A., D'Alessio, A. C., *et al.* (2009). Epigenetic regulation of the glucocorticoid receptor in human brain associates with childhood abuse. *Nat Neurosci*, 12, 342–8.

McLaren, L. (2007). Socioeconomic status and obesity. *Epidemiol Rev*, 29, 29–48.

Mennella, J. A., Jagnow, C. P., & Beauchamp, G. K. (2001). Prenatal and postnatal flavor learning by human infants. *Pediatrics*, 107, e88.

Mericq, V., Ong, K. K., Bazaes, R. A., *et al.* (2005). Longitudinal changes in insulin sensitivity and secretion from birth to age three years in small- and appropriate-for-gestational-age children. *Diabetologia*, 48, 2609–14.

Mill, J. & Heijmans, B. T. (2013). From promises to practical strategies in epigenetic epidemiology. *Nat Rev Genet*, 14, 585–94.

Mitanchez, D., Burguet, A., & Simeoni, U. (2014). Infants born to mothers with gestational diabetes mellitus: mild neonatal effects, a long-term threat to global health. *J Pediatr*, 164, 445–50.

Moore, S. (2010). Chapter 54—Social networks, social capital and obesity: A literature review. In: Dubé, L., Bechara, A., Dagher, A., *et al.* (eds) *Obesity Prevention*, pp. 673–85. San Diego, CA: Academic Press.

Neel, J. V. (1962). Diabetes mellitus: a "thrifty" genotype rendered detrimental by "progress"?. *Am J Hum Genet*, 14, 353–62.

New Zealand House of Representatives Health Committee (2013). Inquiry into improving child health outcomes and preventing child abuse, with a focus on preconception until three years of age. Wellington, New Zealand: New Zealand House of Representatives.

Ng, M., Fleming, T., Robinson, M., *et al.* (2014). Global, regional, and national prevalence of overweight and obesity in children and adults during 1980–2013: a systematic analysis for the Global Burden of Disease Study 2013. *Lancet*, 384, 766–81.

Ng, S. F., Lin, R. C., Laybutt, D. R., Barres, R., Owens, J. A., & Morris, M. J. (2010). Chronic high-fat diet in fathers programs β-cell dysfunction in female rat offspring. *Nature*, 467, 963–6.

Nijland, M. J., Mitsuya, K., Li, C., *et al.* (2010). Epigenetic modification of fetal baboon hepatic phosphoenolpyruvate carboxykinase following exposure to moderately reduced nutrient availability. *J Physiol*, 588, 1349–59.

Nilsson, E. E. & Skinner, M. K. (2015). Environmentally induced epigenetic transgenerational inheritance of disease susceptibility. *Transl Res*, 165, 12–17.

Nomura, Y., Lambertini, L., Rialdi, A., *et al.* (2014). Global methylation in the placenta and umbilical cord blood from pregnancies with maternal gestational diabetes, preeclampsia, and obesity. *Reprod Sci*, 21, 131–7.

Oberlander, T. F., Weinberg, J., Papsdorf, M., Grunau, R., Misri, S., & Devlin, A. M. (2008). Prenatal exposure to maternal depression, neonatal methylation of human glucocorticoid receptor gene (NR3C1) and infant cortisol stress responses. *Epigenetics*, 3, 97–106.

Oddy, W. H., Mori, T. A., Huang, R. C., *et al.* (2014). Early infant feeding and adiposity risk: from infancy to adulthood. *Ann Nutr Metab*, 64, 262–70.

Osmond, C., Barker, D. J. P., Winter, P. D., Fall, C. H. D., & Simmonds, S. J. (1993). Early growth and death from cardiovascular disease in women. *BMJ*, 307, 1519–24.

Ozaki, T., Hawkins, P., Nishina, H., Steyn, C., Poston, L., & Hanson, M. A. (2000). Effects of undernutrition in early pregnancy on systemic small artery function in late-gestation fetal sheep. *Am J Obstet & Gynecol*, 183, 1301–7.

Paneth, N. & Susser, M. (1995). Early origin of coronary heart disease (the "Barker hypothesis"). *BMJ*, 310, 411–12.

Peetz-Schou, M. (2014). *Self-regulatory approach for the control of marketing of foods to children. 17th European Health Forum Gastein*. Gastein: International Forum Gastein.

Pembrey, M., Saffery, R., Bygren, L. O., & Network in Epigenetic Epidemiology (2014). Human transgenerational responses to early-life experience: potential impact on development, health and biomedical research. *J Med Genet*, 51, 563–72.

Perera, F., Tang, W.-Y., Herbstman, J., *et al.* (2009). Relation of DNA methylation of 5'-CpG island of ACSL3 to transplacental exposure to airborne polycyclic aromatic hydrocarbons and childhood asthma. *PLoS One*, 4, e4488.

Plagemann, A. (2005). Perinatal programming and functional teratogenesis: Impact on body weight regulation and obesity. *Physiol Behav*, 86, 661–8.

Popkin, B. M., Adair, L. S., & Ng, S. W. (2012). Global nutrition transition and the pandemic of obesity in developing countries. *Nutr Rev*, 70, 3–21.

Provençal, N., Suderman, M. J., Guillemin, C., *et al.* (2012). The signature of maternal rearing in the methylome in rhesus macaque prefrontal cortex and T cells. *J Neurosci*, 32, 15626–42.

Quilter, C. R., Cooper, W. N., Cliffe, K. M., *et al.* (2014). Impact on offspring methylation patterns of maternal gestational diabetes mellitus and intrauterine growth restraint suggest common genes and pathways linked to subsequent type 2 diabetes risk. *FASEB J*, 28, 4868–79.

Ravelli, G. P., Stein, Z. A., & Susser, M. W. (1976). Obesity in young men after famine exposure in utero and early infancy. *N Engl J Med*, 295, 349–53.

Reynolds, R. M., Osmond, C., Phillips, D. I. W., & Godfrey, K. M. (2010). Maternal BMI, parity, and pregnancy weight gain: influences on offspring adiposity in young adulthood. *J Clin Endocrinol Metab*, 95, 5365–9.

Rich-Edwards, J. W., Kleinman, K., Michel, K. B., *et al.* (2005). Longitudinal study of birth weight and adult body mass index in predicting risk of coronary heart disease and stroke in women. *BMJ*, 330, 1115.

Roseboom, T., de Rooij, S. & Painter, R. (2006). The Dutch famine and its long-term consequences for adult health. *Early Human Development*, 82, 485–91.

Ross, M. G. & Desai, M. (2014). Developmental programming of appetite/satiety. *Ann Nutr Metab*, 64 (Suppl 1), 36–44.

Ruchat, S.-M., Houde, A.-A., Voisin, G., *et al.* (2013). Gestational diabetes mellitus epigenetically affects genes predominantly involved in metabolic diseases. *Epigenetics*, 8, 935–43.

Sabounchi, N. S., Hovmand, P. S., Osgood, N. D., Dyck, R. F., & Jungheim, E. S. (2014). A novel system dynamics model of female obesity and fertility. *Am J Public Health*, 104, 1240–6.

Samuelsson, A. J., Matthews, P. A., Argenton, M., *et al.* (2008). Diet-induced obesity in female mice leads to offspring hyperphagia, adiposity, hypertension, and insulin resistance: a novel murine model of developmental programming. *Hypertension*, 51, 383–92.

Sato, A., Sokabe, T., Kashio, M., Yasukochi, Y., Tominaga, M., & Shiomi, K. (2014). Embryonic thermosensitive TRPA1 determines transgenerational diapause phenotype of the silkworm, Bombyx mori. *Proc Natl Acad Sci U S A*, 111, E1249–E55.

Seki, Y., Williams, L., Vuguin, P. M., & Charron, M. J. (2012). Epigenetic programming of diabetes and obesity: animal models. *Endocrinology*, 153, 1031–8.

Sen, S. & Simmons, R. A. (2010). Maternal antioxidant supplementation prevents adiposity in the offspring of Western diet–fed rats. *Diabetes*, 59, 3058–65.

Soh, S.-E., Chong, Y.-S., Kwek, K., *et al.* (2014). Insights from the Growing Up in Singapore Towards Healthy Outcomes (GUSTO) Cohort Study. *Ann Nutr Metab*, 64, 218–25.

Soubry, A., Schildkraut, J., Murtha, A., *et al.* (2013). Paternal obesity is associated with IGF2 hypomethylation in newborns: results from a Newborn Epigenetics Study (NEST) cohort. *BMC Med*, 11, 29.

Stephenson, J., Patel, D., Barrett, G., *et al.* (2014). How do women prepare for pregnancy? Preconception experiences of women attending antenatal services and views of health professionals. *PLoS One*, 9, e103085.

Strakovsky, R. S., Zhang, X., Zhou, D., & Pan, Y.-X. (2011). Gestational high fat diet programs hepatic phosphoenolpyruvate carboxykinase gene expression and histone modification in neonatal offspring rats. *J Physiol*, 589, 2707–17.

Stroud, L. R., Papandonatos, G. D., Rodriguez, D., *et al.* (2014). Maternal smoking during pregnancy and infant stress response: test of a prenatal programming hypothesis. *Psychoneuroendocrinology*, 48, 29–40.

Sumithran, P., Prendergas, L. A., Delbridge, E., *et al.* (2011). Long-term persistence of hormonal adaptations to weight loss. *N Engl J Med*, 365, 1597–604.

Swinburn, B. A., Sacks, G., Hall, K. D., *et al.* (2011). The global obesity pandemic: shaped by global drivers and local environments. *Lancet*, 378, 804–14.

Tang, W. Y., Levin, L., Talaska, G., *et al.* (2012). Maternal exposure to polycyclic aromatic hydrocarbons and 5'-CpG methylation of interferon-γ in cord white blood cells. *Environmental Health Perspectives*, 120, 1195–200.

Taveras, E. M., Gillman, M. W., Peña, M.-M., Redline, S., & Rifas-Shiman, S. L. (2014). Chronic sleep curtailment and adiposity. *Pediatrics*, 133, 1013–22.

Teh, A. L., Pan, H., Chen, L., *et al.* (2014). The effect of genotype and in utero environment on inter-individual variation in neonate DNA methylomes. *Genome Res*, 24, 1064–74.

The HAPO Study Cooperative Research Group (2009). Hyperglycemia and Adverse Pregnancy Outcome (HAPO) study: associations with neonatal anthropometrics. *Diabetes*, 58, 453–9.

The HAPO Study Cooperative Research Group (2010). Hyperglycaemia and Adverse Pregnancy Outcome (HAPO) study: associations with maternal body mass index. *BJOG*, 117, 575–584.

Tobi, E. W., Lume, L. H., Talens, R. P., *et al.* (2009). DNA methylation differences after exposure to prenatal famine are common and timing- and sex-specific. *Hum Mol Genet*, 18, 4046–53.

Tobias, D. K., Zhang, C., Chavarro, J., *et al.* (2012). Prepregnancy adherence to dietary patterns and lower risk of gestational diabetes mellitus. *Am J Clin Nutr*, 96, 89–295.

Tobias, D. K., Zhang, C., van Dam, R. M., Bowers, K., & Hu, F. B. (2011). Physical activity before and during pregnancy and risk of gestational diabetes mellitus: a meta-analysis. *Diabetes Care*, 34, 223–9.

Torrens, C., Brawley, L., Anthony, F. W., *et al.* (2006). Folate supplementation during pregnancy improves offspring cardiovascular dysfunction induced by protein restriction. *Hypertension*, 47, 982–7.

Townsend, E. & Pitchford, N. J. (2012). Baby knows best? The impact of weaning style on food preferences and body mass index in early childhood in a case–controlled sample. *BMJ Open*, 2, e000298.

UK Chief Medical Officer (2013). Annual Report of the Chief Medical Officer 2012, Our Children Deserve Better: Prevention Pays. London, UK: Department of Health.

United Nations General Assembly (2012). Resolution adopted by the General Assembly. 66/2. Political Declaration of the High-level Meeting of the General Assembly on the Prevention and Control of Non-communicable Diseases.

van Assche, F. A., Holemans, K., & Aerts, L. (2001). Long-term consequences for offspring of diabetes during pregnancy. *Br Med Bull*, 60, 173–82.

van den Heuvel, J., Saastamoinen, M., Brakefield, P. M., Kirkwood, T. B. L., Zwaan, B. J., & Shanley, D. P. (2013). The predictive adaptive response: modeling the life-history evolution of the butterfly Bicyclus anynana in seasonal environments. *Am Nat*, 181, E28–E42.

Vasak, B., Koenen, S. V., Koster, M. P. H., *et al.* (2014). Human fetal growth is constrained below optimal for perinatal survival. *Ultrasound in Obstetrics & Gynecology*, doi: 10.1002/uog.14644.

Vickers, M. H., Breie, B. H., Cutfiel, W. S., Hofman, P. L., & Gluckman, P. D. (2000). Fetal origins of hyperphagia, obesity, and hypertension and postnatal amplification by hypercaloric nutrition. *Am J Physiol*, 279, E83–7.

Vickers, M. H., Gluckman, P. D., Coveny, A. H., *et al.* (2005). Neonatal leptin treatment reverses developmental programming. *Endocrinology*, 146, 4211–16.

Vucetic, Z., Kimmel, J., Totoki, K., Hollenbeck, E., & Reyes, T. M. (2010). Maternal high-fat diet alters methylation and gene expression of dopamine and opioid-related genes. *Endocrinology*, 151, 4756–64.

Vuillermin, P., Saffery, R., Allen, R., *et al.* (2015). Cohort profile: the Barwon Infant Study. *Int J Epidemiol*, 44, 1148–60.

Ward, W. P. (1993). *Birth Weight and Economic Growth: Women's Living Standards in the Industrializing West*. Chicago, IL: University of Chicago Press.

Weaver, I. C. G., Cervoni, N., Champagne, F. A., *et al.* (2004). Epigenetic programming by maternal behavior. *Nat Neurosci*, 7, 847–54.

Weintraub, W. S., Daniels, S. R., Burke, L. E., *et al.* (2011). Value of primordial and primary prevention for cardiovascular disease: a policy statement from the American Heart Association. *Circulation*, 124, 967–90.

Wells, J. C. K. (2007). Flaws in the theory of predictive adaptive responses. *Trends Endocrinol Metab*, 18, 331–7.

World Health Organization (WHO) (2011). Global status report on noncommunicable diseases 2010. Geneva, Switzerland: WHO.

World Health Organization (WHO) (2014). Report of the first meeting of the ad hoc working group on science and evidence for ending childhood obesity. Geneva, Switzerland: WHO.

Yoon, J. & Brown, T. T. (2011). Does the promotion of community social capital reduce obesity risk?. *Journal of Socio-Economics*, 40, 296–305.

Zhang, X., Strakovsky, R., Zhou, D., Zhang, Y., & Pan, Y.-X. (2011). A maternal high-fat diet represses the expression of antioxidant defense genes and induces the cellular senescence pathway in the liver of male offspring rats. *J Nutr*, 141, 1254–9.

Zhao, Y., Gong, X., Chen, L., *et al.* (2014). Site-specific methylation of placental HSD11B2 gene promoter is related to intrauterine growth restriction. *Eur J Hum Genet*, 22, 734–40.

Zulkafli, I. S., Waddell, B. J., & Mark, P. J. (2013). Postnatal dietary omega-3 fatty acid supplementation rescues glucocorticoid-programmed adiposity, hypertension, and hyperlipidemia in male rat offspring raised on a high-fat diet. *Endocrinology*, 154, 3110–3117.

CHAPTER 1.3

Systems thinking for global health and strategic sustainable development

Karl-Henrik Robèrt, Michael T. Hernke, Luke Fortney, and Rian J. Podein

Science and decision-making: the tree metaphor

Decision-making for global health builds on information from many specialized fields. All human and natural systems—for example, agriculture, transportation, and energy—influence health.

We can use a tree as a metaphor for the relationship between specialized knowledge, and how it may be structured for decision-making; the foliage and leaves represent details regarding data and information, while the trunk and branches symbolize the overall structure with its principles and relationships. To pay attention only to the former—the detailed information—is reductionism, which is no longer sufficient in a complex world. Only by regarding the whole picture—that is, through systems thinking—do the details begin to make sense, and allow action to be guided by wisdom. The roots, feeding the principles as well as data, would then be *drivers* to create that kind of full comprehension. One branch of the root-system is about humans' desire to survive. This feeds into another branch—the awareness of how our current civilization is threatening the complex web of nature and ecosystems that we are all dependent on. This, in turn, leads to yet another branch of the root-system—that we ask science for help to create the necessary comprehension and structure that is needed for effective cooperation to solve the problems.

To begin, we need basic principles around which data can be structured for comprehension. We need such principles to evaluate what information is needed and not needed for making a decision. And we need such principles to discover when available data is insufficient for making decisions, thus requiring more science. Without an understanding on how to structure data and knowledge, our efforts to acquire wisdom often drown us in information. Integrating scientific details within a broader, coherent framework supports planning, collaboration, and development in complex systems.

Planning in complex systems

It is possible to describe systems on a principle level with relevance to planning. A foundational 'Framework for Strategic Sustainable Development' (FSSD) was created using rigorous peer review to derive scientific consensus around a unifying theory for sustainable development (see Ny et al., 2006; Robèrt, 2000). At the time when this framework began to be explored, a number of frameworks and concepts had already been developed for managing various aspects of sustainable development. Some examples of this are: (i) industrial ecology (Hileman, 1992) and life cycle assessment (Postlethwaite, 1994), which aims to keep track of, and reduce, specific impacts linked to specific material flows; (ii) management systems such as the ISO14001 (Kumar and Kumar, 1997), which represents an administrative vehicle to organize and report challenges, plans, and results around sustainable development; (iii) ecological footprinting (Pandey et al., 2001), a framework to communicate the average impact on nature from any action or organization as expressed in areal units; and (iv) the precautionary principle (Foster et al., 2000; Young, 1995), which is an approach of not taking chances if there are suspected risks of harm to the environment or the public, even if scientific consensus does not yet exist. When in doubt about the link between an action and serious sustainability-related impacts, the action should be phased out or not even started.

How do all those frameworks, concepts, and tools relate to a universal definition of sustainability, and to each other? The FSSD is the only framework *designed* to be unifying (i.e. to serve systematic, sustainable development within any organization at any scale). The FSSD has been shown to increase the value of any well thought-through concept or tool for sustainable development, and its unifying quality has also been empirically tested in case studies of numerous business organizations, municipalities, and cities around the world.

The FSSD builds on communication between five distinct levels (see Box 1.3.1).

Level 2 (defining success) is of founding importance for the other levels in strategic planning. If we don't know where we want to be we cannot be strategic, by definition, in our choices of actions and tools. A significant intellectual barrier with society's current unsustainable direction is that suggested solutions are too often initiated directly from the (i) systems level and trying to 'fix' problems here.

Box 1.3.1 The FSSD, a five-level framework

(i)   **The systems level**. The overall principle functioning of a system (in this case the biogeochemical cycles of the biosphere and the basic relationship of this system with the flows and practices of human society) is studied enough to arrive at a …

(ii) **Basic definition of success for any project** within the system (in this case sustainability) which in turn is mandatory to develop …

(iii) **Strategic guidelines**—in this case a systematic step-by-step approach to comply with the definition of success (e.g. back-casting), feeding the process of choosing the appropriate …

(iv) **Concrete actions**—that is, every concrete move in the transition towards sustainability should follow the strategic guidelines, which in turn require …

(v)   **Tools** that can systematically monitor the (iv) actions so that they are (iii) strategic to arrive at (ii) success in the (i) system.

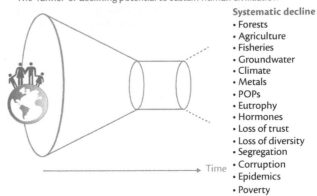

Sustainable development - A dynamic challenge

The 'funnel' of declining potential to sustain human civilization

Systematic decline
• Forests
• Agriculture
• Fisheries
• Groundwater
• Climate
• Metals
• POPs
• Eutrophy
• Hormones
• Loss of trust
• Loss of diversity
• Segregation
• Corruption
• Epidemics
• Poverty

Time

Fig. 1.3.1 Non-sustainable development can be visualized as entering deeper and deeper into a funnel, in which the margins for a healthy society become narrower and narrower as natural resources systematically decrease, while the demands of a growing population systematically increase. We lose more and more forests, cropland, purity, trust, and so on.
Reproduced courtesy of Karl-Henrik Robèrt.

As a result, the 'lens' of the second (ii) and the third (iii) levels are generally lacking. This often leads to narrow framing of an issue, typically solving one problem by inventing another. A striking example of this is how diesel was introduced as a technology in Europe to reduce CO_2 emissions in the 1990s, but without considering the whole picture, including health impact. It is now recognized as causing a considerable health burden due to its large emissions of particulate matter ($PM_{2.5}$ and PM_{10}) and oxides of nitrogen (NO_x). To avoid this kind of common pitfall, we need to achieve a competence of 'Planning in Complex Systems' comprising all levels, as described in the framework above.

One: the systems level

Human society is comprised of many interrelated pieces that are essential to scientifically understand for getting an overview of the natural underpinning of our existence. Examples are the solar-driven cycles in nature, the relationships among the species, and the exchange of resources and waste between society and ecosystem. Science describes the underlying functional processes of this system and informs us of its status. The latter is, from a sustainability perspective, today characterized by an increasing number of destructive impacts that implies a severe and dynamic challenge: the potential of the system to sustain civilization is gradually declining (see Fig. 1.3.1).

Metaphorically, it can be described as if we are systematically moving deeper into a funnel of declining potential for living prosperous and healthy lives. Here we can identify the clash between the large systems perspective of unsustainability, and our knowledge of individual impacts. From a systems perspective, we can logically conclude that the overall societal course will end in disaster unless we correct the underlying systemic errors, even though system complexities do not allow us to foresee the exact details of the disaster. This means that, in order to avoid disaster, we must prepare ourselves for making decisions out of a principled understanding of the situation, rather than to continue to react solely to

impacts. With this change of perception, many other things change too. This is not the least with regard to a very often missed aspect of sustainable development, the self-benefit, or 'business-case', thereof (Finster and Hernke, 2014). The funnel metaphor comes in very handy when this has to be explained (Holmberg and Robèrt, 2000).

What will happen to resource costs in the funnel of declining resources? What will happen to waste management costs as we keep producing more? Insurance costs for those who contribute relatively more to the problem?

And, perhaps most importantly, what will happen to opportunity costs for those who fail to understand how human needs will evolve further ahead in the funnel? Sustainability is about survival—for nature and people—and survival arguments are very convincing in the end. For those who do not foresee how 'markets' will evolve further ahead in the funnel, very expensive 'fire fighting' will be the option. And vice versa—companies like Electrolux foresaw, before competitors, what would happen to the inherently unsustainable use of Freon (chloroflourocarbons or CFCs) in refrigerators. They applied the FSSD and gradually developed sustainable options. In relation to competitors, who waited until CFCs were forbidden by law and consequently hit the walls of the funnel, Electrolux had relatively much lower costs (McNall *et al.*, 2011).

Understanding the funnel and learning how to move step-wise to its opening, rather than into its wall, will provide an opportunity for gradually turning to the leading competitive advantage—survival issues are very convincing in the end. Unfortunately, many leaders' lack of a sufficiently broad systems perspective on the unsustainability problem is linked to a flawed societal discourse (see Fig. 1.3.2).

The flawed cylinder paradigm

This paradigm considers all social and ecological harms from societal activities as 'costs' for the economic welfare we enjoy: 'The trees are not so green (e.g. drought), the bees are not so happy (e.g. pesticides), and those in poverty face overwhelming adversity, but in

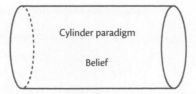

Cylinder paradigm

Belief

Funnel paradigm

Reality

Sustainability is an unrealistic dream. Programmes, audits, and life cycle assessments should focus on impacts, which are the known, isolated, transient, inevitable costs of our welfare. If stakeholders prove enough harm, ethics justify remedies that cost less than utility gained, but only in step with international agreements. Beyond-compliance action increases costs and reduces competitiveness.

Sustainability strategically corrects, at lowest cost, system errors driving destruction of conditions for welfare. Success principles address interconnections of impacts, even those not yet known, by focusing on their basic causes. Role models create competitive advantages and momentum for international agreements by combining ethics and self-benefit via alignment with the way the world actually functions.

Fig. 1.3.2 Cylinder versus funnel paradigms.

return society is quite successful.' So we need to balance the good with the bad. It is as if nature and the liberties and opportunities of less fortunate people are relatively compressed, but the 'cylinder' metaphor says nothing about the progressive decline of the overall potential to sustain civilization.

Reality: a funnel paradigm

Problems resulting from unsustainability are not just a series of negative but absorbable impacts, but more fundamentally, underlying systemic errors of societal design that will make problems worse and worse until, in the end, it will be impossible for society to sustain itself. Fixing problems one by one at the level of the 'leaf' is not a solution (e.g. banning dangerous substances such as DDT and CFCs only once their negative impacts are fully understood). Until the systemic errors are identified and eradicated at the 'trunk and branch' levels, the very conditions for survival and prosperity will continue to decline.

A further consideration is the vicious cycle between social and ecological impacts. Social systems, that constrain people's capacity to meet their needs, reduce their participation and their investment in those systems. A leadership incapable of seeing the larger picture of ecological sustainability, reduces trust even more among people at a time when we direly need trusting and collaborative relationships to correct looming ecological problems. And we have ample evidence how much a decline of trust in the social system costs, as we experience the walls of the funnel through any of the costs related to failures to avoid destruction of ecosystems in time. They are completely intuitive things such as costs related to transactions (when there is a general lack of trust, more lawyers are needed), lower grades of loyalty to communities and organizations, higher levels of sick leaves, lower creativity and productivity, and poor performance in talent wars since intelligent people look for jobs with meaning.

The broad systems perspective of sustainability does not mean an idealistic situation without adverse effects. It means that things at least do not get any worse, which is the main attribute of sustainability. We can also go further to be restorative, for example by making gardens from deserts, cleaning polluted lakes, and restoring a meaningful sense of safety and community.

Two: the success level

In soccer, success is achieved when one team gets the ball more times into the opponent's goal than vice versa. In chess, the principle of checkmate determines success. In the game of 'sustainable

development in the biosphere', success is defined through four basic socioecological principles[1]. Those are derived from the basic mechanisms of the gradually increasing destruction pictured by the funnel. What are those mechanisms? If we knew, we could turn those mechanisms to basic sustainability principles by equipping them with a 'not'. Or, in design terms, presenting the sustainability principles as exclusion criteria for redesign. Within the FSSD the mechanisms were deduced by asking: 'How can the myriad of increasing problems be clustered into a few basic mechanisms of destruction'? (see Box 1.3.2).

The fourth principle with its five subcategories, presented below, is a new version outlined in a recent doctorate (Missimer, 2013). This level of systems thinking is perhaps the most essential, yet least exploited, aspect of scientific responsibility in decision-making—to define basic conditions and constraints relevant to all desired outcomes.

Answers to the reverse question—by what principle ways could we destroy the biosphere and society's ability to sustain human society?—made it possible to address problems upstream in cause-and-effect chains where basic principle errors of societal design trigger the myriad of negative impacts that later occur downstream. Correcting errors at the upstream systems level creates comprehension to deal with current problems, and avoids new problems that are looming in the future. At this level of first approximation where

---

Box 1.3.2 The four basic sustainability principles

In a sustainable society, nature is not subject to systematically increasing:

1. concentrations of substances extracted from the Earth's crust

2. concentrations of substances produced by society

3. degradation by physical means

and

4. in that society people are not subject to structural obstacles to ...

- health
- influence
- competence
- impartiality
- meaning-making

complexity is minimized, it is possible to design the problems out of the system without knowing exactly what disasters will arise from not doing so.

The myriad of negative impacts related to ecological unsustainability can be categorized into three separate mechanisms by which we destroy the ability of the sun-driven biosphere's biogeochemical cycles to sustain society:

1. A systematic increase in concentration of elements that are net-introduced into the biosphere from mining (e.g. heavy metals and petroleum used in dissipative ways leading to increased concentrations of contaminants in soils and climate change from increasing CO_2 in the atmosphere).

2. A systematic increase in concentration of matter that is produced within the biosphere (such as very large emissions of naturally occurring substances, e.g. NO_X, or even minimal leakages of persistent compounds foreign to nature like CFCs).

3. A systematic destruction by physical means (e.g. overfishing, and draining of water tables).

These three mechanisms frame ecological sustainability, implying a set of restrictions within which sustainable societal activities must be incorporated. The fourth, social sustainability principle, is derived by understanding the basic mechanism for eroding of trust, the key element of a functional social system. It has been shown that trust erodes from various modes of power abuse. When we do not trust people in power, trust does not only erode towards our leaders. When we don't trust them, there is a strong risk for corruption and segregation to follow. Or in other words, there is a clear tendency for trust also eroding interindividually. In a socially sustainable society or community, power is not abused, which can occur along five different dimensions (see Box 1.3.2).

As a first step for an organization or society to implement sustainability planning, the basic sustainability principles can be translated into objectives that are relevant to each individual organization. For an organization, family, business, municipality, public institution, or government that does not want to be part of the unsustainability problem, an inverse phrasing of the basic unsustainability mechanisms define the objective of sustainability:

When we are sustainable, we have

1. eliminated our contribution to systematic increases in concentrations of substances from the Earth's crust …

2. as follows in accordance with Box 1.3.2: the four basic sustainability principles.

Each individual organization must draw its own conclusions from these basic principles regarding problems, solutions, and goals. It opens up a greater awareness to realize the full scope of current activities from a sustainability perspective. This allows us to not only tackle existing problems, but also to make sure that the proposed solutions accord with sustainability principles upfront, which avoids increasing problems now and in the future.

Three: the strategic level

This level describes the strategic guidelines for achieving success in the system. In soccer, one of the strategic guidelines to succeed is to spread out and pass the ball around, as opposed to everyone running after the ball at the same time. In terms of sustainable development, this level involves: i) a step-by-step approach towards the four basic principles for sustainability by allowing; ii) each step to be a platform for the next, while; iii) at the same time ensuring that each step is advantageous so that the process does not come to a halt due to a lack of resources (money, natural resources, time, and so on).

Backcasting

It follows from the description of the five levels of 'Planning in Complex Systems' that a strategy requires a clear idea of where we want to be. For example, in playing chess, it is very difficult to foresee exactly how the game will play out. Only one thing is known for certain—that victory must comply with the principles of checkmate. Even if we cannot look into the future, we can still play the 'sustainable development' game by 'backcasting' from a principle definition of sustainability. Once we understand the basic principles of any particular 'winning', we can pragmatically begin making moves that are as economizing as possible—that is, money or chess-pieces or any other resources—while at the same time creating flexible platforms to arrive at the basic principles of sustainability. Each time reality (or an opponent) makes another move, the situation is reassessed in real time with the same basic principles of success guiding the continuation of the game moment by moment.

The core concept in backcasting is to proceed from desired outcomes and thereafter plan backward in time, asking 'what can we do now to get there?' The variant of backcasting proposed here is not backcasting from successful scenarios, that is, simplified images of the future (Robinson, 1990), but backcasting from principles for success (i.e. this way of 'playing the sustainability game' is more like chess than laying puzzles) (Holmberg and Robèrt, 2000; Ny et al., 2006). Because many potential solutions will be compatible with the principles for sustainability, people can brainstorm various approaches to sustainability. Afterwards, organizations can prioritize various measures to create flexible platforms for further investments in the direction of principle success, while also realizing organizational benefits.

When people suggest an investment or policy, the question is not solely snapshot evaluations of whether the benefits outweigh the means. The term strategy implies a perspective on trade-offs guided by questioning what options will provide the best rational platform for future moves towards success, while striking a good balance between pace of progress and income. Planning for global health this way is process-orientated, exciting, and relevant. And it adds an essential element, that of 'enlightened self-interest'.

It is on this third level we put the precautionary principle. When we know the basic principles of sustainability, we can expand the meaning of the precautionary principle. CFCs, for instance, could have been avoided upfront since they by definition violate the second principle.

Forecasting

Forecasting is derived from forecasts of previous and current trends into the future. This planning approach dreams of a future that is similar to today, minus some problems we wish to solve. But simply correcting a range of current problems does not describe progress. When the tree trunk and branches are not correct, no makeshift solutions in the foliage will help in the long run.

Dreborg (1996) prescribes backcasting, not forecasting, when the relevant system is very complex, and when breaking with trends is called for. For example, if the current high price of bio-fuel, the low taxation of fossil fuels, and politicization of climate change are responsible for the torpor in phasing out fossil fuels, then forecasting cannot resolve the problem. Forecasting views a switch to renewable fuels as unrealistic until the prices are competitive, tantamount to not exercising until one is fit.

A systematic process (ABCD) to help people jointly apply the principles for backcasting has been developed and utilized by an increasing number of businesses, corporations, municipalities, cities, and in academia for systematic co-creation of sustainable futures (see Ny *et al.*, 2006; Robèrt *et al.*, 2013).

A. First, participants discuss the principles, and what they imply as boundary conditions for any vision or joint venture they may dream of.

B. Next, current challenges and strengths are assessed, referring to the desirable sustainable objective or vision.

C. In a similar fashion, possible solutions complying with the objective and its sustainability principles are listed.

D. A step-wise transition plan is set in motion, where early actions and investments are prioritized to strike the balance between income and pace towards the objective. At this step, when the gap between today and the desirable future is on the table, tools for decision support and monitoring of the transition are also selected/designed, which brings us to level 5 of the FSSD, the tools level.

Four: the actions level

This level comprises what tangibly occurs in practice. This level should not be confused with the strategic level (level 3) or the success level (level 2) but often is. Renewable energy is often inaccurately described as a principle of sustainability. Switching to renewable energy may be aligned with sustainability principles and something we might opt to do. But if done incorrectly (e.g. widespread deforestation by excessive biofuels production, or utilizing corn as biofuels such that food prices increase), we would conflict with the basic sustainability principles 3 and 4, respectively. Confusing what we do (level 4) with the principles of how to do it (level 3) or why we do it (level 2), risks solving one problem while creating another.

How to put the *sustainability principles* into practice

Though the basic sustainability principles are not prescriptive (they are just objective descriptions of the constraints for sustainability), and though individual organizations must seek their own solutions, some overall conclusions can be drawn to guide concrete actions.

◆ SC1: Substitute certain minerals that are scarce in nature with others that are more abundant, using all mined materials efficiently, and systematically reducing dependence on fossil fuels.

◆ SC2: Systematically substitute certain persistent and unnatural compounds with ones that are normally abundant or break down more easily in nature, and using all substances produced by society efficiently.

◆ SC3: Draw resources only from well-managed ecosystems, systematically pursuing the most productive and efficient use both of those resources and land, and exercising caution in all kinds of modification of nature (e.g. overharvesting and introductions).

◆ SC4–8: Avoid all practices, now or in the future, which restrict people's opportunities to health, influence, competence, meaning, and impartiality.

Five: the tools level

At this level we describe the different tools that can help us foster: (4) actions to be (3) strategic to arrive at (2) success in the (1) system.

Tools ensure that actions (level 4) accord with strategic principles (level 3) to improve the likelihood of achieving success (level 2) in the system (level 1). It may be tools for analyses (e.g. life cycle assessments following sustainability-related impacts of a practice from sourcing through production, use, and end-use), decision support (e.g. modelling and simulation of sustainable solutions within the constraints set by the sustainability principles), measurement (e.g. indicators; an organization might track its progress by eliminating persistent compounds that are foreign to nature, or removing the concrete barriers to people's trust outlined under the fourth sustainability principle), or reporting/auditing and communication (e.g. management systems). To make effective use of existing tools, it is essential that they are put in the context of the above outlined strategy. This means putting the gap between now and sustainability with its challenges and opportunities on the table, design the overall strategic plan to bridge that gap, and only now select and design the tools that will be needed (Robèrt *et al.*, 2002).

Global health and sustainability from a systems perspective

Causal relationships between specific environmental aspects and disease, and an overall systems perspective, are inseparably interlinked. Below are concrete examples regarding each of the basic sustainability principles and global public health.

Sustainability principle I

Societal flows of certain elements that are introduced from mining and drilling are multiples higher than nature's own flows, such as from volcanos and weathering (Azar *et al.*, 1996), and many of those elements are systematically increasing in concentration in biota, approaching unknown ecotoxic thresholds (e.g. silver, copper, lead, and chromium).

Burning fossil fuels extracted from Earth's crust has driven atmospheric CO_2 to levels not seen in millions of years. How will climate change, inevitably happening as a consequence of further fossil CO_2 increases in the atmosphere, affect ecosystems as we know them? What will happen to climate zones in relation to the agriculture zones civilization has created? How will this influence our food production capacity? How will increased acidity in the oceans, from further CO_2 increases there, affect the marine ecosystems? What will a future society look like that doesn't allow systematic net-increases in the biosphere of flows of matter from the Earth's crust?

This will not happen if we only talk about the evidence for this or that health impact from more and more silver or CO_2 injected into the biosphere. The exact future of these effects cannot be foreseen due to complexity. We can only state for sure that continuous use of fossil fuels or dissipative use of heavy metals violates the first system condition and is inherently unsustainable. As long as society allows a myriad of mined materials to increase in the biosphere, the risks to global health increase systematically. Questions based in principles for sustainability would lead to a vision of completely new energy systems and flows of metals, a phase-out of certain metals from large-scale use, and substitution with other materials that are easier, cheaper, and safer to use within the constraints set by the first system condition.

Sustainability principle II

What will a future society look like that doesn't allow any matter that is produced by society to systematically increase in the biosphere?

This will not happen if we only talk about the evidence for a particular health impact limiting concentrations to certain thresholds and then try to design our policies accordingly. For example, NOx are series of nitrogen compounds that are produced in combustion and incineration and contribute significantly to asthma, cancer, acidity, and eutrophication. No matter where the exact ecotoxic thresholds are, it is safe to say that it is not sustainable to systematically trespass the assimilation capacity of the biogeochemical cycles. The same is true about certain compounds that are foreign to nature and relatively persistent, since the 'allowable' emissions within sustainability constraints are then much smaller (e.g. dioxins, CFCs, and polychlorobiphenyl (PCB) with others looming on the horizon). In this way, we can avoid significant problems in the future—endocrine disruption from a great number of plastic additives, unknown effects from bromine organic antiflammables in our blood, and systematic increase of antibiotic resistant strains of microbes from accumulation of antibiotics in biota, and so on.

The conclusion is simple: if we are heading for sustainability, we cannot chase all chemicals one by one as they exceed their respective toxic and ecotoxic thresholds followed by a long lead-time until we have proven the effect epidemiologically. We need to draw the principle conclusions and ask the right questions so that no chemicals, per societal design, will systematically increase in the biosphere. Further, that no chemicals that are relatively persistent and foreign to nature, are used outside of very tight technical loops. If such compounds leak out and exceed their respective ecotoxic thresholds, they will hang around for long time periods after phase-out of use, and continue to exert negative affects (e.g. CFCs and endocrine disruptors).

Sustainability principle III

What will a future society look like that doesn't allow more and more encroachment on natural systems by physical means and the subsequent depletion of ecological services they provide to sustain human health? How can we live our lives in prosperity without exploiting more and more pristine areas for oil, or destroying more and more biotopes through strip-mining?

An overall systems error leads us to systematically encroach more and more on ecosystems through strip-mining, overfishing, clear-cutting, paving over fertile land, and systematically drawing down water tables for irrigation. We need to ask ourselves about future potentials for not violating the principle, and then make systematic moves in that direction. The challenge of this third system condition is increased by interplay with the first. Once we stop 'cheating' by use of stored energy (fossil and nuclear), which costs us in terms of ecosystem purity, a real consideration for spatial planning becomes paramount. Sustainable farming, forestry, fisheries, harvesting of materials, and capturing of primary energy (sun energy,

tidal waters, geothermal, and so on) are extensive industries whose collective space requirement must match the biosphere's ongoing capacity to provision. Cropland for instance, that does not rely on (i) large amounts of fossil fuels for machinery and for the production of phosphate and nitrogen fertilizers, (ii) pesticides, and (iii) irrigation systems that make water tables decline, must be managed at a landscape scale to simultaneously produce enough food and ecosystem services. The success of such systems also requires that we pay farmers fairly for the labour required for such a profound transition towards sustainable farming, which brings us to the social principle.

Sustainability principle IV

What will a future society look like that doesn't allow a systematic undermining of people's trust, anywhere in the world?

This will not happen if we only talk about the proofs for this or that health impact from insufficient management of climate change, or if we get bogged down on the detail level when it comes to determining the possible link between an unfair global distribution of energy and other resources on the one hand, and underlying factors leading to war and terrorism on the other. Concretely, this implies that we address the following questions regarding the use of power and governance: What does a future look like where the use of political power in no way creates barriers to:

1. People's health (this principle is closely related to human rights, e.g. asking questions about incomes to live from, dangers at work-places, and so on).

2. Influence (learning and responding to what people think, e.g. asking questions about staff interviews, fairness of polls, quality of general elections, and so on).

3. Competence (regarding possibilities for people to learn, develop, and grow, e.g. asking questions about learning programmes, schools, work-training, and so on).

4. Meaning (regarding clear and worthy endeavours and joint ventures, e.g. asking questions about dignified missions, whether leaders are trustworthily aligned with such missions, and so on).

5. Impartiality (respecting the universalism principle and treating all people equitably, e.g. asking questions about distribution of gender, skin colour and other diversity questions among leaders and boards, and so on).

Conclusion

To understand the need for basic principles of success in complex planning endeavours is not difficult. What is difficult, however, is to change mindsets in large paradigm shifts. The traditional ways of thinking and planning within the medical and public health fields have not taken basic sustainability principles for global health into account. Modern medicine and public health are accustomed to relying on epidemiology when causalities between environmental factors and morbidity are to be determined. When it comes to the basic flaws of societal design that are related to increasing impacts of unsustainability, this traditional paradigm is no longer sufficient. It sets out to fix a growing avalanche of disparate problems, instead of avoiding them by understanding the underlying mechanisms. We need to expand traditional thinking using systems-based science to see the broader picture, and then draw conclusions even before epidemiology can predict exactly how disasters may unfold in the future. It is essential that the medical and public health communities learn to include this perspective in their primary responsibilities, particularly a prevention-focus within medical training. Increasing global health problems from an unsustainably designed society is no less an essential responsibility of the health profession than it is of engineers, economists, policy makers, and others.

Note

1. In the communities of business and municipalities, those basic sustainability principles are referred to as The Natural Step System Conditions, named after the non-governmental organization (NGO), The Natural Step, that promotes them.

References

Azar, C., Holmberg, J., & Lindgren, K. (1996). Socio-ecological indicators for sustainability. *Ecol Econ*, 18 (2), 89–112.

Dreborg, K. H. (1996). Essence of backcasting. *Futures*, 28, 813–28.

Finster, M. P. & Hernke, Michael T. (2014). Benefits organizations pursue when seeking competitive advantage by improving environmental performance. *J Industrial Ecol*, 18, 652–62

Foster, K. R., Vecchia, P., & Repacholi, M. H. (2000). Science and the precautionary principle. *Science*, 288, 979–81.

Hileman, B. (1992). Industrial ecology route to slow global change proposed. *Chemical and Engineering News*, 70, 7–14.

Holmberg, J. & Robèrt, K.-H. (2000). Backcasting from non-overlapping sustainability principles—a framework for strategic planning. *Int J Sust Develop World Ecol*, 7, 291–308.

Kumar, R. & Kumar, A. (1997). Introduction to www.ISO14001.com. *Environmental Progress*, 16, F13–15.

McNall, S. G., Hershauer, J. C., & Basile, G. (2011). *The Business of Sustainability: Trends, Policies, Practices, and Stories of Success*. Santa Barbara, CA: ABC-CLIO, LLC.

Missimer, M. (2013). The social dimension of strategic sustainable development. Licentiate (Blekinge Institute of Technology).

Ny, H., MacDonald, J. P., Broman, G. I., & Robèrt, K.-H. (2006). Sustainability constraints as system boundaries: An approach to making life-cycle management strategic. *Journal of Industrial Ecology*, 10, 61–77.

Pandey, J. S., Khan, S., Joseph, V., & Singh, R. N. (2001). Development of a dynamic and predictive model for ecological footprinting (EF). *Journal of Environmental Systems*, 28, 279–91.

Postlethwaite, D. (1994). Development of Life Cycle Assessment (LCA): The role of SETAC (Society of Environmental Toxicology and Chemistry) and the 'Code of Practice'. *Environmental Science and Pollution Research*, 1, 54–5.

Robèrt, K.-H. (2000). Tools and concepts for sustainable development, how do they relate to a general framework for sustainable development, and to each other?. *Journal of Cleaner Production*, 8, 243–54.

Robèrt, K.-H., Broman, G. I., & Basile, G. (2013). Analyzing the concept of planetary boundaries from a strategic sustainability perspective: How does humanity avoid tipping the planet?. *Ecology and Society*, 18, 5.

Robèrt, K.-H., Schmidt-Bleek, B., Aloisi de Larderel, J., et al. (2002). Strategic sustainable development—selection, design and synergies of applied tools. *Journal of Cleaner Production*, 10, 195–296.

Robinson, J. B. (1990). Futures under glass: a recipe for people who hate to predict. *Futures*, 22, 820–42.

Young, M. D. (1995). Inter-generational equity, the precautionary principle and ecologically sustainable development. *Nature and Resources*, 31, 16–27.

The physiology of stress and stress recovery

Peter Wåhrborg, Panagiota Pervanidou, and George P. Chrousos

The history and philosophy of the stress concept

During the 1930s and 1940s, Hans Selye, a Hungarian-Canadian endocrinologist, first conceptualized the adaptive response of an organism to external or internal threats, as a process he called 'The General Adaptation Syndrome'. In 1956, he published the 'Stress of Life' (Selye, 1956) presenting the principal features of what he had originally termed the 'general adaptation syndrome', to which he also referred as the 'stress syndrome' or simply 'stress' (Jackson, 2012). *The Stress of Life* was his most influential publication of the relations between stress, health, and disease and his model remains the basis of our biopsychosocial understanding of stress today (Pervanidou and Chrousos, 2007).

Before Selye, Walter Cannon attributed the neuroendocrine response to an injury and the release of catecholamines, as part of the 'fight or flight reaction'. Selye was the first to describe the crucial role of the pituitary and the adrenal cortex in the physiology of the stress response and he termed the external or internal force causing stress, the 'stressor'. Another important contribution was the distinction between positive 'eustress' and negative 'distress' (Lazarus, 1966; Selye, 1974).

Selye, however, did not only describe the neuroendocrine processes involved in stress reactions, but also diseases related to stress, such as cardiovascular and inflammatory disorders and peptic ulcer (Szabo, 1998). Furthermore, Selye reflected on the philosophical aspects of stress research: individuals possessed a certain amount of 'adaptation energy' that was gradually consumed by the 'wear and tear of life', leading to physiological ageing and death (Selye, 1956). A longer and healthier life could be achieved by protecting 'adaptation energy' by 'living wisely in accordance to natural laws'. Selye argued that the study of nature would allow people to 'derive philosophical lessons': similarly to 'biological harmony achieved by intracellular altruism (the biological rules governing cells and organs)', social harmony and human satisfaction could be enhanced by 'interpersonal altruism' (Selye, 1974; Jackson, 2012).

Homeostasis and stress physiology

Stress is defined as the state of threatened homeostasis, the complex equilibrium that all living organisms try to maintain (Chrousos and Gold, 1992). Homeostasis is normally challenged by everyday external or internal forces, the stressors. The nature, intensity, and duration of stressors, as well as the timing of exposure and the perception of stress are important in stress reactions. When a stressor exceeds a certain threshold, the adaptive homeostatic systems of the organism are compensatory activated, in an innate stereotypic response, to regulate homeostasis and protect the organism during acute stress. These adaptive alterations take place both in the central nervous system (CNS) and the periphery and include facilitation of neural pathways that promote arousal and vigilance, and, simultaneously, inhibition of pathways related to eating, growth, and reproduction (Chrousos, 2009). Additional adaptive changes include increased oxygenation of the brain, heart, and skeletal muscles, all essential organs participating in the acute stress response (Chrousos, 2009).

The stress reaction is mainly coordinated by the stress system, consisting of central and peripheral mediators that will be described in the following. Homeostatic mechanisms exert their effects in a U-shaped curve, where, healthy homeostasis, or eustasis, is achieved in the middle of the curve, and suboptimal effects may occur on either side of the curve leading to a state of dyshomeostasis, also called allostasis or cacostasis, which may have damaging effects on the short- and long-term health of the individual (Chrousos and Gold, 1998; Chrousos, 2009).

The activation of the stress system is followed either by return to basal homeostasis (eustasis) or by a state of maladaptive response (inadequate or excessive), and the organism falls into cacostasis. In a third possibility, the organism gains from the experience, and a new, improved homeostatic capacity (hyperstasis) is attained (Fig. 1.4.1) (Chrousos, 2009).

Perception and inception of the stress reaction

The brain is the integrative centre for coordinating the behavioural and neuroendocrine response to challenges, some of which qualify as 'stressors'. The evolutionary modern mammalian part of the brain, once described as the neocortex (MacLean, 1990), is certainly involved, but also a number of other cortical structures are important actors in the perception and interpretation of potential stressors. The most important of these structures are

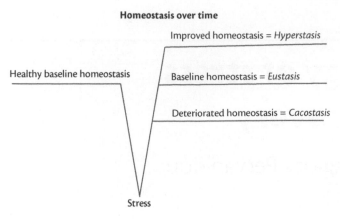

Fig. 1.4.1 Following a stressful situation, during which baseline homeostasis is disturbed and the adaptive response is activated, homeostasis is usually successfully regained (eustasis). However, two other states are possible: (i) the individual survives at the expense of the well-being of the individual (allostasis or cacostasis); or (ii) the organism 'learns' and gains from the experience, and a new, improved homeostasis (hyperstasis) at the benefit of well-being is attained. Reproduced with permission from Chrousos GP, 'Stress in Early Life: A Developmental and Evolutionary Perspective,' pp. 29-40 in Hochberg Z, *Evo-Devo of Child Growth: Treatise on Child Growth and Human Evolution*, Wiley-Blackwell Company, Hoboken, NJ, USA, Copyright © 2012.

found in the border zone between the 'intellectual brain' (neo-cortex) and the 'emotional brain' (paleocortex). These interconnected structures are often described as the limbic system (Broca, 1878) and they are of utmost importance for functions like memory (hippocampus), emotions and emotional reactions (amygdala), and emotional control (cingulate gyrus and prefrontal cortex in the frontal lobes).

A significant role in the perception of stress and our reactions to the environment is played by the frontal lobes. During evolution, these important structures have developed an exclusive ability to anticipate threats, and in fact also 'create' them as such (i.e. by worrying about things). In the most frontal part of these lobes the prefrontal cortex is located. They are not only of importance for emotional control, but also for integration and evaluation of different stimuli. The prefrontal cortex plays a major role for the coordination and activation of behavioural as well as physiological reactions to perceived threats and are closely linked to structures in the limbic system.

However, the brain is not organized in strict hierarchical lines. A number of neural networks are involved in perception, and for the interpretation of and reaction to stimuli, in the outer as well as in the inner world (Le Doux, 2003). It is obvious that the human brain has developed to a very complex structure, where simple boundaries for different functions of the brain have to be constantly redefined. Despite this complexity, certain areas seem to have more a important impact on the diffuse reaction we call stress.

The most explicit, and the first visible reaction to a 'stressful' experience, is emotional adaptation. From an evolutionary point of view, the emerging behaviour is aimed at preparing for fight or flight. Hostility, irritation, frustration, and anger are common behaviours in this kind of situation. During exposure to long-term stress, the behaviour tends to be dominated by exhaustion, depressive symptoms, anxiety, and more pronounced cognitive difficulties (Währborg, 2009).

Amygdala—the conductor of the stress reaction

A crucial part of the limbic system is the almond-shaped amygdala nuclear complex with its 13 different grains individually enforcing different access paths with other parts of the brain. Amygdala deal with both 'incoming' and 'outgoing' nerve traffic. Incoming information is apprehended from the neocortex and the body via the hypothalamus and thalamus. This information is of decisive importance for its conduction of responses to the perceived situation, in the outer as well as in the inner world of the individual. The coordination is essential for our ability to react on different stimuli and to prepare for proper action that has to be taken in order to avoid or deal with different challenges in our lives.

From the central nuclei in the amygdala, neurons are distributed to different projection areas; for example, to the paraventricular nucleus in the hypothalamus (Herman *et al.*, 2005). The amygdala is therefore an important actor in setting different stress mediator systems in motion (see Le Doux, 1996 for an overview).

The amygdala and the prefrontal cortex are not only the executers of stress reactions, but they are also vulnerable victims to its consequences. The prefrontal cortex plays an important role in working memory and executive function and is also involved in extinction of learning. Both these regions are targets of stress hormones, and stress is known to precipitate and exacerbate mood disorders. In long-term depressive illness, the hippocampus and prefrontal cortex undergo atrophy, whereas the amygdala is hyperactive in anxiety and mood disorders and may undergo a biphasic change in structure, increasing in size in acute depression and shrinking in long-term depression. In animal models of acute and chronic stress, neurons in the hippocampus and prefrontal cortex respond to repeated stress by showing atrophy that leads to memory impairment, whereas neurons in the amygdala show a growth response that leads to increased anxiety and aggression. Yet, these are not necessarily 'damaged' and may be treatable (Vyas *et al.*, 2002; Roozendaal *et al.*, 2009).

The hippocampus, a vulnerable master of memory and an important stress regulator

Stress modulates the brain's function and can facilitate or even impair the memory process. Emotionally arousing experiences generally lead to stronger memories than more ordinary events, whereas high stress levels seem to interfere with the retrieval of previously acquired memories. As mentioned, the brain is not only an executer of stress reactions but also a target for its biological consequences.

The hippocampus, often called 'the gateway to our memory', was the first brain region (beside the hypothalamus) to be recognized as a target of glucocorticoids. Stress and stress hormones produce both adaptive and maladaptive effects on this brain region throughout the life course. It has been shown that early life events influence lifelong patterns of emotionality and stress responsiveness and alter the rate of brain and body ageing. The hippocampus, the amygdala, and the prefrontal cortex undergo stress-induced structural remodelling, which alters behavioural and physiological responses (for an overview, see McEwen, 2004 and 2005).

The hippocampal region is located in the medial temporal lobe of the brain and plays a central role for different memory functions. Learning capacity is mainly related to the anterior parts of the hippocampus formation, while recall is related to the posterior parts (Lepage et al., 1998; Schacter and Wagner, 1999). Interestingly, the hippocampus is also strongly involved in emotionally contextual memories (Eichenbaum et al., 1992; Le Doux, 1995; Pugh et al., 1997).

The hippocampal formation is not only an important structure for different kinds of learning and memory, but also for the control of autonomic and vegetative functions like adrenocorticotropin (ACTH) secretion via feedback regulation of the hypothalamic–pituitary–adrenal (HPA)-axis (Jacobson and Sapolsky, 1991). It was shown already in 1968 (McEwen et al., 1968) that hippocampal neurons express receptors for circulating adrenal steroids. Two different receptor types are present in hippocampal neurons, type I (mineralocorticoid) and type II (glucocorticoid). Excitatory amino acids, such as N-methyl-D-aspartate (NMDA) receptors, play important roles in the functional and structural changes produced in the hippocampus by steroid hormones.

There are two different forms of structural plasticity in the hippocampal formation which are affected by stress. Repeated stress in animals causes atrophy of dendrites in a specific region of the hippocampus. Both acute and chronic stress have further been shown to suppress neurogenesis, that is, development of 'new' granule neurons in the dentate gyrus (for extensive review, see McEwen, 1999). It has even been suggested that severe long-term stress, often described as burnout, is an exponent of stress-mediated decrease in adult neurogenesis. This can lead to a decreased ability to cope with stress through decreased hippocampal function, possibly involving a disturbed hippocampal regulation of the HPA axis (Eriksson and Wallin, 2004).

An interesting hypothesis proposes that decreased glucocorticoid production also might lead to psychopathologies. Haller and co-workers (2007) have shown that aggressiveness can be driven by chronic hypoarousal due to glucocorticoid deficit. This is a situation described and found also in post-traumatic stress disorder, depression, and in burnout patients. A possible theoretical link might be found to serotonergic transmission which seems to lose its impact on aggression. Also in certain prefrontal areas, neurons are weakly activated, whereas the central amygdala acquires important roles.

Mediators of stress

Based on genetic and epigenetic parameters, stress mediators regulate homeostasis and stress responses to acute or chronic threats. The HPA axis and the sympathetic nervous system (SNS) are the main components of the stress system; however, a variety of neurotransmitters, growth factors, and cytokines interact with the classic neuroendocrine hormones to maintain homeostasis.

The central mediators of the stress system include the hypothalamic paraventricular nucleus hormones corticotrophin-releasing hormone (CRH) and arginine-vasopressin (AVP), the arcuate nucleus proopiomelanocortin-derived peptides α-melanocyte–stimulating hormone (MSH), and β-endorphin, and the brainstem norepinephrine (NE) produced in the A1/A2 centres of the locus coeruleus (LC) and in the central nuclei of the SNS. Research has shown that the hypothalamic CRH-AVP and brainstem norepinephrine centres

of the stress system mutually innervate and stimulate each other (Chrousos, 1995; Chrousos and Gold, 1992).

In the periphery, the end-effectors of the HPA axis are the glucocorticoids and those of the sympathetic system are the catecholamines epinephrine (E) and norepinephrine (NE). Catecholamines stimulate interleukin (IL)-6 release by immune- and other peripheral cells via β-adrenergic receptors (Papanicolaou et al., 1998).

The targets of these stress mediators are brain structures and functions related to emotion and behaviour, as well as peripheral tissues related to metabolism, growth, reproduction, immunity, and cardiovascular function.

Stress-induced metabolic and cardiovascular actions include the increase of heart rate and arterial blood pressure, while increased glucocorticoids and catecholamines induce gluconeogenesis, glycogenolysis, lipolysis, and stimulation of hepatic glucose secretion.

Stress also affects the immune system, influencing innate and acquired immunity (Chrousos, 1995; Chrousos, 2000). Both the glucocorticoids and the catecholamines suppress the secretion of pro-inflammatory cytokines (tumour necrosis factor [TNF], IL-1, IL-6, IL-8 and IL-12) and affect traffic and function of leukocytes and accessory immune cells, whereas both hormone families induce a systemic switch from cellular to humoral immunity (Chrousos, 2009).

Effects of perceived stress and trauma—stress-related disorders

As previously described, the activation of the stress system by everyday stressors results in adaptive endocrine, metabolic, behavioural, and cardiovascular changes with the purpose to maintain homeostasis. However, the experience of intense or long-standing perceived stressors (e.g. accidents, natural disasters, violent attacks, terrorism, or witnessing traumas) can lead to excessive and prolonged activation of stress mediators or, in a subgroup of individuals, to chronic hypoactivation of the stress system, which is equivalent to a cacostatic state with a variety of psychologic and biological consequences (Pervanidou and Chrousos, 2010; Pervanidou and Chrousos, 2012a).

Stress can lead to both acute or chronic physical conditions and diseases in predisposed individuals (Chrousos and Kino, 2007). For instance, acute or long-standing stress can trigger allergic manifestations, such as asthma or eczema, gastrointestinal symptoms, such as pains or diarrhoea, and disturbances in arterial pressure. Furthermore, stress-related somatic manifestations often present in clusters and are chronic. The term 'functional somatic syndrome' (FSS) refers to a broad cluster of physical symptoms, such as fatigue, abdominal pain, musculoskeletal pain, and headache, which cannot be explained by modern medicine. Such symptoms are also named 'medically unexplained symptoms' (MUS) (Fischer et al., 2014)

Abnormalities in stress system mediators have been reported in behavioural and psychiatric disorders such as anxiety, depression, post-traumatic stress disorder, and eating disorders (Chrousos, 2009; Pervanidou and Chrousos, 2012b). Increased or decreased concentrations of CRH and peripheral stress mediators may be responsible for physical complications and increased morbidity in these populations.

The important role of stress physiology in the pathophysiology of mental health disorders is highlighted in the latest (2013) revision of the *Diagnostic and Statistical Manual for Mental Disorders* (DSM), where a new class appears, the 'trauma and stressor-related disorders', including acute stress disorder (ASD) and post-traumatic stress disorder, which were both previously classified as anxiety disorders (APA, 2013).

Post-traumatic stress disorder

Post-traumatic stress disorder (PTSD) represents the most typical mental disorder linked to chronic distress. Indeed, a large body of evidence supports the crucial role of the stress system in the pathophysiology of PTSD.

The concept of 'psychic trauma', as an individual's experience of a perceived life threat caused by an external life event is attributed to Sigmund Freud (Freud, 1973). Trauma is not simply an extreme form of stress, but psychological and physiologic aspects of both trauma and stress contribute to the understanding of PTSD, as an entity of behavioural, emotional, and physiologic responses to perceived stress.

The term PTSD describes a syndrome of distress that develops after exposure to traumas like witnessing death or threatened death, actual or threatened serious injury, actual or threatened sexual violence, and by direct exposure to or witnessing violence (APA, 2013).

The clustering of symptoms, according to DSM-5, includes intrusion, avoidance, negative alterations in cognition and mood, and alterations in arousal and negativity (APA, 2013).

PTSD has been associated with dysregulation of the stress system and more precisely with increased CRH centrally (Baker *et al.*, 1999) together with decreased cortisol and elevated catecholamines in the periphery (Yehuda *et al.*, 1994, Pervanidou and Chrousos, 2010).

In a prospective and longitudinal study in children and adolescents experiencing motor vehicle accidents, the natural history of neuroendocrine alterations in relation to the development and maintenance of PTSD were investigated (Pervanidou *et al.*, 2007a; 2007b). These children had no previous trauma exposure, nor current or past psychopathology. Thus, the effects of a single acute and quite common stressor in children from the community were studied. Thirty per cent (30%) of the children developed PTSD one month after the event and 15 maintained PTSD six months later.

Evening salivary cortisol and morning serum interleukin-6 in the aftermath of the trauma were both higher in children that later developed PTSD, whereas norepinephrine (NE) was normal. Children with PTSD exhibited gradually greater NE concentrations compared to those who experienced an accident, but did not develop PTSD. This study supports an initial elevation of cortisol in individuals exposed to a single acute stressor, followed by a gradual normalization of cortisol as time passes from the stressor, which might lead to decreased cortisol in the periphery, months or years after the traumatic exposure. At the same time, a progressive elevation of NE is noted in individuals that continue to exhibit PTSD symptoms. It seems that a longitudinal interaction of peripheral measures of the sympathetic systems and the HPA axis characterizes those that develop and maintain the disorder (Pervanidou, 2008).

Early life stress and trauma

The term 'early life stress' (ELF) refers to a broad spectrum of negative exposures during foetal life, childhood, and adolescence. Commonly studied early life stressors include: physical or sexual abuse, neglect, social deprivation, emotional maltreatment, poverty, war, school bullying, but also single stressors, such as natural catastrophes, accidents, terrorism, attacks, or witnessing violence. Evidence has shown that a significant percentage of the population has experienced emotional, physical, or sexual abuse in childhood, while less have experienced emotional and physical neglect. In total, two-thirds of a large epidemiological sample of adults reported at least one adverse childhood experience, whereas the presence of one stressful experience significantly increased the prevalence of having additional adverse childhood experiences (Dong *et al.*, 2004). Furthermore, extensive research has revealed a strong relation between early life stress and the development of psychiatric disorders, such as depression, anxiety, and PTSD, as well as a variety of physical health problems in adult life (Infrasca, 2003; Levitan *et al.*, 2003; Pervanidou and Chrousos, 2007; Brown *et al.*, 2009).

There is convincing evidence today that chronic or intense stress during childhood affects developing brain structures and functions, and programmes the brain to react with more anxiety to new stressors (Lupien *et al.*, 2009).

Indeed, and as discussed earlier in this chapter, animal studies have shown that chronically elevated stress mediators may lead to alterations in brain development through accelerated loss of neurons, delays in myelination, or abnormalities in developmentally appropriate synaptic pruning and/or decreased neurogenesis (Sapolsky, 2000; Huang *et al.*, 2001). Moreover, cortisol hypersecretion *in utero* alters neuronal development in areas rich in glucocorticoid receptors (GC) (Lauder, 1988). Thus, although cortisol exposure is essential for brain and HPA axis development, studies in animals indicate the substantial and permanent effects of increased stress mediators on brain morphology during prenatal and postnatal brain development.

Studies in humans also confirm the detrimental effects of early life stress in brain morphology. Studies using magnetic resonance imaging have suggested that adults having experienced early life stress have smaller hippocampal volumes compared to controls (Bremner, 2002; 2003).

A study in a large sample of adults without history of psychopathology revealed volumetric differences in brain structure in those with a history of childhood trauma, compared to those with minimal ELF. Reductions in brain volumes were apparent in the anterior cingulate cortex (ACC) and the caudate nucleus (Cohen *et al.*, 2006). A recent study revealed that the age of exposure is an important variable determining the effects of stress on brain morphology (Baker *et al.*, 2013). This study indicates that adolescence is also a vulnerable period for the effects of stress in the brain and that stress might act differently in specific time windows of brain development. This is also supported by evidence indicating diverse effects of stress during foetal life depending on sex, as sex-dependent factors have different organizational effects on foetal neural circuits. Indeed, females seem to have an increased susceptibility to affective problems, such as anxiety and depression, whereas males are more vulnerable to developmental disorders, such as autism spectrum disorders and attention deficit and hyperactivity disorders (ADHD) (Davis and Pfaff, 2014).

Positive and negative adaptations

Apart from the detrimental effects of traumatic experiences, especially childhood trauma on stress reactivity, stress can also affect resilience. Resilience can be defined as a positive personality characteristic that enhances individual adaptation. A high number of interindividual differences in stress responses predispose an individual's vulnerability or resilience to environmental challenges.

Genetic predisposition is an important factor in the cumulative stress hypothesis of vulnerability or resilience to stress-related mental disorders. According to this hypothesis, in a given context, the accumulation of traumatic stress experiences and the failure to cope with such experiences enhances vulnerability (McEwen, 1998). Another concept of cumulative stress exposure, the 'three hits hypothesis' (Daskalakis et al., 2013), suggests also the timing of exposures as a critical point in determining vulnerability or resilience: hit-1, is the genetic predisposition; hit-2 is the early life environment; and hit-3 is the late life environment.

As depicted in Figure 1.4.2, the acute stress reaction is associated with acute activation of stress mediators—hormones, cytokines, growth factors, and receptors, as well as with epigenetic changes and alterations in gene expression. Stress responses are also dependent on the stressor: acute stressors may act differently than chronic experiences. Moreover, convincing evidence supports that timing and intensity of the exposure are crucial variables determining short- and long-term stress-related alterations and conferring either an adaptive advantage or a risk for mental and physical disorders (Taylor, 2010). The sex and personality traits of the individual, as well as prior psychiatric symptoms and coping mechanisms are of importance (Daskalakis et al., 2013).

Previous trauma, especially during early life, has received considerable interest in interpreting stress system activity in the sequelae of a traumatic experience, but also in the cumulative stress hypothesis in relation to long-term consequences. According to the cumulative stress hypothesis, if the accumulation of adversities in the lifespan exceeds a certain threshold, at-risk individuals will develop some psychopathology (McEwen, 1998). However, other theories, such as the predictive adaptive responses (Gluckman et al., 2009) suggest that the neuroendocrine, metabolic, and cardiovascular plasticity associated with early life stress might promote positive adaptations when the individual is exposed to a new stressor, since adaptive changes 'predict' an adverse future environment (read more about the developmental origin of health and disease in Chapter 1.2). In this view, exposure to a challenging, though moderate stressor might promote active coping and resilience to future stress exposures (Daskalakis et al., 2013).

The physiology of stress recovery

In a number of recent clinical studies, stress recovery has been explored with physiological and biochemical measures of different kind. Apart from clinical status and diagnostic criteria, various techniques have been used, such as ECG-based methods (e.g. heart rate variability—to measure sympathetic and parasympathetic tone), neuroimaging techniques (e.g. functional MRI to detect deviances in visible cortex regions), haemodynamic measures (e.g. blood pressure and heart rate), coagulation measures (e.g. activated blood clotting time), and of course neuroendocrine measures (e.g. cortisol, norepinephrine, testosterone, and so on). This kind of study is often supplemented with psychometric instruments in order to capture depression, anxiety, well-being, personality, and degree of stress.

Despite the number of methods used to monitor stress, there is yet not one single method existing with the reliable capacity to distinguish long-term pathological stress from normal stress. An example illustrating this is the measurement of morning awakening

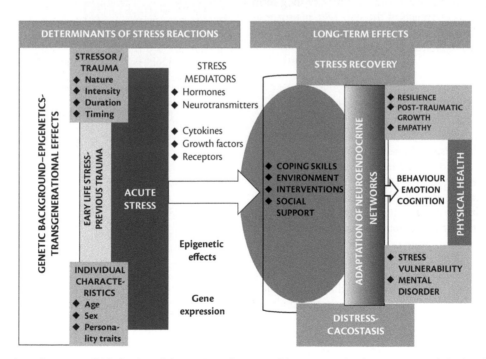

Fig. 1.4.2 Stress reactions, depending upon individual traits and characteristics, the nature of the stressor and early experiences might lead, in the long term, to either stress recovery or chronic distress. Acute reactions include the activation of stress mediators (hormones, growth factors, cytokines, neurotransmitters), epigenetic effects, and alterations in gene expression. Long-term positive or negative effects, through chronic adaptive changes in neuroendocrine networks, affect behaviour, emotion, and cognition, and the physical health of the individual. Positive adaptations might include increased resilience and empathy and post-traumatic growth. Negative adaptations include stress vulnerability and stress-related mental disorders.

cortisol levels. In patients defined as under long-term stress ('burn-out'), both increased (Grossi *et al.*, 2005), decreased (Pruessner *et al.*, 1999), and normal levels of cortisol (Mommersteeg *et al.*, 2006) have been reported in comparison with control groups. Since there is no single (patognomonic) physiological or biochemical marker to capture long-term stress in a reliable manner, there is neither any entirely acceptable method to evaluate spontaneous or therapy-induced recovery. It is indeed possible to feel well and being without cognitive difficulties and at the same time having an overload of measureable neuroendocrine activity.

Another difficulty in evaluating stress recovery involves the time courses of the behavioural, physiological, and biochemical processes. Most often the premorbid status is unknown for the researcher and it is also associated with difficulties to follow nervous, cardiovascular, and biochemical changes over time, especially if these are occurring at different times in the stressed individual, which most often also is the case. Since stress is such a broad concept and no general marker exists, the most fruitful design would be to break this wide concept down to variables that are possible to define and operationalize. In doing so, a number of interventions have been proven valuable. Pharmacological therapy has been shown to improve the regulation of neuroendocrine-autonomic systems as well as metabolism (Ljung *et al.*, 2001).

Physical activity has also been shown to improve neuroendocrine function and possibly protect the brain against the negative consequences of affective and stress-related disorders (Bjornebekk *et al.*, 2005; Jonsdottir 2006).

In addition, nature-assisted therapy has been proven to increase well-being and reduce the need for healthcare in patients with stress-related disorders (Annerstedt *et al.*, 2012; Annerstedt and Währborg, 2011).

All therapeutic efforts in the treatment of short- or long-term stress aim to reduce different aspects of the state (e.g. neuroendocrine responses, behaviour changes, and so on). A number of indirect measures can be used to indicate stress recovery.

Conclusion

Advances in neuroscience, endocrinology, molecular biology, genetics, and social sciences provide a new eco-bio-developmental framework for understanding the promotion of health and prevention of disease across the lifespan. Genetic predisposition, interacting with environmental factors and perceived positive or negative experiences, determine dynamic brain development and systems of neuroendocrine adaptation, affecting behaviour, cognition, learning, and physical health. In contrast to tolerable and mild stress, intense or chronic stress (also called toxic stress), especially in early life, has a critical role in disrupting neural networks in the brain and affecting other regulatory systems of the organism, increasing the risk for physical and mental disease.

Preventive societal interventions might include educational efforts, mainly focused on parents and school teachers, to increase awareness of the effects of stress in health and disease, and community investments on the development of services and environment to reduce sources of stress and to intervene, with collaborative works by mental health professionals and social workers, after adverse exposures. These prevention and intervention strategies might be more effective if applied to young age groups, in the form of early intervention programmes.

References

American Psychiatric Association (APA) (2013). *Diagnostic and Statistical Manual of Mental Disorders*, 5th edition. Arlington, VA: American Psychiatric Publishing.

Annerstedt, M. & Währborg, P. (2011). Nature-assisted therapy: systematic review of controlled and observational studies. *Scand J Public Health*, 39, 371–88.

Annerstedt, M., Ostergren, P. O., Björk, J., Grahn, P., Skärbäck, E., & Währborg, P. (2012). Green qualities in the neighbourhood and mental health—results from a longitudinal cohort study in Southern Sweden. *BMC Public Health*, 8, 12, 337.

Baker, D. G., West, S. A., Nicholson, W. E., *et al.* (1999). Serial CSF corticotropin-releasing hormone levels and adrenocortical activity in combat veterans with posttraumatic stress disorder. *Am J Psychiatry*, 156, 585–8.

Baker, L. M., Williams, L. M., Korgaonkar, M. S., Cohen, R. A., Heaps, J. M., & Paul, R. H. (2013). Impact of early vs. late childhood early life stress on brain morphometrics. *Brain Imaging Behav*, 7, 196–203.

Bjornebekk, A., Mathe, A. A., & Brene, S. (2005). The antidepressant effect of running is associated with increased hippocampal cell proliferation. *Int J Neuropsychopharmacol*, 8, 357–68.

Bremner, J. D. (2002). Neuroimaging studies in post-traumatic stress disorder. *Curr Psychiatry Rep*, 4, 254–63.

Bremner, J. D. (2003). Long-term effects of childhood abuse on brain and neurobiology. *Child Adolesc Psychiatr Clin N Am*, 12, 271–92.

Broca, P. (1878). Anatomie comparee des circonvolutions cerebrales: Le grand lobe limbique et la scissure limbique dans la serie des mammifères. *Revue d'Anthropologie*, 1, 385–498.

Brown, D. W., Anda, R. F., Tirmeier, H., *et al.* (2009). Adverse childhood experiences and the risk of premature mortality. *Am J Prev Med*, 37, 389–96.

Chrousos, G. P. (1995). The hypothalamic–pituitary– adrenal axis and immune-mediated inflammation. *N Engl J Med*, 332, 1351–62.

Chrousos, G. P. (2000). The stress response and immune function: clinical implications; the 1999 Novera H. Spector lecture. *Ann NY Acad Sci*, 917, 38–67.

Chrousos, G. P. (2009). Stress and disorders of the stress system. *Nat Rev Endocrinol*, 5, 374–81.

Chrousos, G. P. & Gold, P. W. (1992). The concepts of stress and stress system disorders. *J Am Med Assoc*, 267, 1244–52.

Chrousos, G. P. & Gold, P. W. (1998). A healthy body in a healthy mind and vice versa—the damaging power of "uncontrollable" stress. *J Clin Endocrinol Metab*, 83, 1842–5.

Chrousos, G. P. & Kino, T. (2007). Glucocorticoidaction networks and complex psychiatric and/or somatic disorders. *Stress*, 10, 213–9.

Cohen, R. A., Grieve, S., Hoth, K. F., *et al.* (2006). Early life stress and morphometry of the adult anterior cingulate cortex and caudate nuclei. *Biol Psychiatry*, 59, 975–82.

Daskalakis, N. P., Bagot, R. C., Parker, K. J., Vinkers, C. H., & De Kloet, E. R. (2013). The three-hit concept of vulnerability and resilience: toward understanding adaptation to early-life adversity outcome. *Psychoneuroendocrinology* 38, 1858–73.

Davis, E. P. & Pfaff, D. (2014). Sexually dimorphic responses to early adversity: Implications for affective problems and autism spectrum disorder. *Psychoneuroendocrinology*, 49, 11–25

Dong, M. X., Anda, R. F., Felitti, V. J., *et al.* (2004). The interrelatedness of multiple forms of childhood abuse, neglect, and household dysfunction. *Child Abuse Negl*, 28, 771–84.

Eichenbaum, H., Otto, T., & Cohen, N. J. (1992). The hippocampus—what does it do? *Behav Neural Biol*, 57, 2–3.

Eriksson, P. & Wallin, L. (2004). Functional consequences of stress-related suppression of adult hippocampal neurogenesis—a novel hypothesis on the neurobiology of burnout. *Acta Neurol Scand*, 110, 275–80.

Fischer, S., Lemmer, G., Gollwitzer, M., & Nater, U. M. (2014). Stress and resilience in functional somatic syndromes--a structural equation modeling approach. *PLoS One*, 9, e111214.

Freud, S. (1973). Fixation to traumas-the unconscious. In: Strachey, J. (Trans.). *Introductory lectures on psychoanalysis.* New York, NY: Penguin Books.

Gluckman, P. D., Hanson, M. A,. Buklijas, T., Low, F. M., & Beedle, A. S. (2009). Epigenetic mechanisms that underpin metabolic and cardiovascular diseases. *Nat Rev Endocrinol*, 5, 401–8.

Grossi, G., Perski, A., Ekstedt, M., Johansson, T., Lindström, M., & Holm, K. (2005). The morning salivary cortisol response in burnout. *J Psychosom Res*, 59, 103–111.

Haller, J., Halasz, J., Mikics, M., Toth, M., & Barsy, B. (2007). *Hyper- and hypoarousal in the control of aggressiveness: The role of glucocorticoids.* 2nd World Conference of Stress, August 23–26, Budapest, Hungary.

Herman, J. P., Ostrander, M. M., Mueller, N. K., & Figueiredo, H. (2005). Limbic system mechanisms of stress regulation: hypothalamo-pituitary-adrenocortical axis. *Prog Neuropsychopharmacol Biol Psychiatry*, 29, 1201–13.

Huang, W. L., Harper, C. G., Evans, S. F., Newnham, J. P., & Dunlop, S. A. (2001). Repeated prenatal corticosteroid administration delays myelination of the corpus callosum in fetal sheep. *Int J Dev Neurosci*, 19, 415–25.

Infrasca, R. (2003). Childhood adversities and adult depression: an experimental study on childhood depressogenic markers. *J Affect Disord*, 76, 103–11.

Jackson, M. (2012). The pursuit of happiness: The social and scientific origins of Hans Selye's natural philosophy of life. History of the Human Sciences, 25, 13–29.

Jacobson, L. & Sapolsky, R. (1991). The role of the hippocampus in feedback regulation of the hypothalamic-pituitary-adreocortical axsis. *Endocr Rev*, 12, 118–34.

Jonsdottir, I. (2006). Stress, exercise and consequences for memory function and affective disorders. *Helix Review series, Neurology and Cognitive Neuroscience*, 1, 1–5.

Lauder, J. M. (1988). Neurotransmitters as morphogens. *Prog Brain Res*, 73, 365–87.

Lazarus, R. S. (1966). *Psychological Stress and the Coping Process.* London, UK: McGraw-Hill Book Co.

Le Doux, J. E. (1995). In search of an emotional system in the brain: leaping from fear to emotion and consciousness. In: Gazzaniga, M. (ed.) *The Cognitive Neurosciences*, pp. 1049–61. Cambridge, MA: MIT Press.

Le Doux, J. E. (1996). *The Emotional Brain: The Mysterious Underpinnings of Emotional Life.* New York, NY: Simon and Schuster.

Le Doux, J. E. (2003). *Synaptic Self.* New York, NY: Penguin Books.

Lepage, M., Habib, R., & Tulving, E. (1998). Hippocampal PET activation of memory encoding and retrieval: the HIPER model. *Hippocampus*, 8, 313–22.

Levitan, R. D., Rector, N. A., Sheldon, T., & Goering, P. (2003). Childhood adversity associated with major depression and/or anxiety disorders in a community sample of Ontario: issues of co-morbidity and specificity. *Depress Anxiety*, 17, 34–42.

Ljung, T., Ahlberg, A. C., Holm, G., *et al.* (2001). Treatment of abdominally obese men with a serotonin reuptake inhibitor: a pilot study. *J Intern Med*, 250, 219–24.

Lupien, S. J., McEwen, B. S., Gunnar, M. R., & Heim, C. (2009). Effects of stress throughout the lifespan on the brain, behaviour and cognition. *Nat Rev Neurosci*, 10, 434–45.

MacLean, P D. (1990). *The Triune Brain in Evolution: Role in Paleocerebral Functions.* New York, NY: Plenum Press.

McEwen, B. S. (1998). Stress, adaptation, and disease. Allostasis and allostatic load. *Ann N Y Acad Sci*, 840, 33–44.

McEwen, B. S. (1999). Stress and hippocampal plasticity. *Ann Rev Neurosci*, 22, 105–22.

McEwen, B. S. (2004). *The End of Stress As We Know It.* Washington, DC: Joseph Henry Press.

McEwen, B. (2005). Protective and damaging effects of stress mediators. *N Engl J Med*, 338, 171–9.

McEwen, B. S., Weiss, J., & Schwartz, L. (1968). Selective retention of corticosterone by limbic structures in rat brain. *Nature*, 220, 911–12.

Mommersteeg, P. M., Heijnen, C. J., Verbraak, M. J., & van Doornen, L. J. (2006). Clinical burnout is not reflected in the cortisol awakening response, the day-curve or the response to a low dose dexamethasone suppression test. *Psychoneuroendocrinology*, 31, 216–25.

Papanicolaou, D. A., Wilder, R. L., Manolagas, S. C., & Chrousos, G. P. (1998). The pathophysiologic roles of interleukin-6 in humans. *Ann Intern Med*, 128, 127–37.

Pervanidou, P. (2008). Biology of post-traumatic stress disorder in childhood and adolescence. *J Neuroendocrinol*, 20, 632–8.

Pervanidou, P. & Chrousos, G. P. (2007). Post-traumatic stress disorder in children and adolescents: from Sigmund Freud's "trauma" to psychopathology and the (dys) metabolic syndrome. *Horm Metab Res*, 39, 413–9.

Pervanidou, P. & Chrousos, G. P. (2010). Neuroendocrinology of post-traumatic stress disorder. *Prog Brain Res*, 182, 149–60.

Pervanidou, P. & Chrousos, G. P. (2012a). Posttraumatic stress disorder in children and adolescents: neuroendocrine perspectives. *Sci Signal*, 5, pt6.

Pervanidou, P. & Chrousos, G. P. (2012b). Metabolic consequences of stress during childhood and adolescence. *Metabolism*, 61, 611–19.

Pervanidou, P., Kolaitis, G., Charitaki, S., *et al.* (2007a). Elevated morning serum interleukin (IL)-6 or evening salivary cortisol concentrations predict posttraumatic stress disorder in children and adolescents six months after a motor vehicle accident. *Psychoneuroendocrinology*, 32, 991–9.

Pervanidou, P., Kolaitis, G., Charitaki, S., & Chrousos, G. (2007b). The natural history of neuroendocrine changes in pediatric posttraumatic stress disorder after motor vehicle accidents: Progressive divergence of noradrenaline and cortisol concentrations over time. *Biological Psychiatry*, 62, 1095–110.

Pruessner, J. C., Hellhammer, D. H., & Kirschbaum, C. (1999). Burn out, perceived stress, and cortisol responses to awakening. *Psychosom Med*, 61, 197–204.

Pugh, C. R., Tremblay, D., Fleshner, M., & Rudy, J. W. (1997). A selective role for corticosterone in contextual-fear conditioning. *Behav Neurosci* 111:503–511.

Roozendaal, B., McEwen, B. S., & Chattarji, S. (2009). Stress, memory and the amygdala. *Nat Rev Neurosci*, 10, 423–33.

Sapolsky, R. M. (2000). Glucocorticoids and hippocampal atrophy in neuropsychiatric disorders. *Arch Gen Psychiatry*, 57, 925–35.

Schacter, D. & Wagner, A. (1999). Medial temporal lobe activations in fMRI and PET studies of episodic encoding and retrieval. *Hippocampus*, 9, 7–24.

Selye, H. (1956). *The Stress of Life.* New York, NY: McGraw-Hill.

Selye, H. (1974). *Stress Without Distress.* New York, NY: Harper and Row.

Szabo, S. (1998). Hans Selye and the development of the stress concept. Special reference to gastroduodenal ulcerogenesis *Ann NY Acad Sci*, 851, 19–27.

Taylor, S. E. (2010). Mechanisms linking early life stress to adult health outcomes. *Proc Natl Acad Sci, U S A*, 107, 8507–12.

Vyas, A., Mitra, R., Shankaranarayana Rao, B. S., & Chattarji, S. (2002). Chronic stress induces contrasting patterns of dendritic remodeling in hippocampal and amygdaloid neurons. *J Neurosci*, 1, 6810–18.

Währborg, P. (2009). *Stress och den nya ohälsan [Stress and ill health].* Stockholm, Sweden: NaturandKultur.

Yehuda, R., Teicher, M. H., Levengood, R. A., Trestman, R. L., & Siever L J. (1994). Circadian regulation of basal cortisol levels in posttraumatic stress disorder. *Ann N Y Acad Sci*, 746, 378–80.

CHAPTER 1.5

Unifying mechanisms: nature deficiency, chronic stress, and inflammation

William Bird, Elissa Epel, Jeannette R. Ickovics, and Matilda van den Bosch

Stress, inflammation, and disease

Chronic stress, in combination with contemporary unhealthy life-styles, which may be directly or indirectly associated with disconnection from nature, can lead to direct behavioural changes such as increased calorie intake, inactivity, excess alcohol intake, and smoking, as well as chronic inflammation through these behaviours and mediating biological factors. These factors include an increase in visceral fat, changes in gut microbiota, mitochondrial damage, and telomere shortening. The interactions between chronic inflammation, mitochondrial damage, and behavioural change all contribute to the rising prevalence of non-communicable diseases, such as diabetes, dementia, depression, and cardiovascular disease, as well as premature ageing and disability. Relating this scenario to exposure to nature, it is worth considering that disconnection from nature may lead to chronic stress and subsequent disease through several mechanisms (see e.g. Chapters 1.4. and 3.2). Thus, by reconnecting or increasing interactions with nature, it may possible to help prevent from the link between chronic stress and development of chronic disease.

In this chapter we will present the biological fundaments of chronic stress, how it develops, and how those biological processes can be a precursors of chronic inflammation and disease. Within this context, we will discuss the biochemical damage to the cells' metabolism and genetic material, by chronic stress and its consequences (Fig. 1.5.1).

Chronic stress

As discussed in Chapter 1.4, stress reactions can be explained in terms of stressors, resilience, and coping mechanisms. The balance between these factors determines the outcome and potential disease development related to acute and chronic stress. A poor response to current stressors (e.g. as seen in people with reduced resilience), leads to chronic stress (or toxic stress) in which negative effects of stress lead to yet more stress and as a consequence depression and anxiety. Resilience depends on a person coping with the current level of stress, instead of developing an 'allostatic overload' (see Chapter 1.4). Apart from genetic predisposition, resilience can

be affected by several variables (Fig. 1.5.1, PATHWAY A), such as past trauma and current unresolved stressors, loneliness, financial worries, unsupportive relationships, poor environments, lack of autonomy, or worries at work (Shonkoff et al., 2012).

A past and current connection to nature, and other life quality factors, seem to enhance resilience and increase the ability to cope with stressors (Fig. 1.5.1, PATHWAY B) and may therefore reduce the risk of developing chronic stress (Wells, 2012). See also Chapter 8.1 for a discussion on the reduced resilience to social stress in urban populations as compared to rural.

Chronic inflammation

Chronic low-grade inflammation is the result of the immune system failing to switch off and instead continues to generate pro-inflammatory cytokines, such as tumour necrosis factor-α (TNF-α), interleukin (IL)-6, IL-1β, IL-18, and C-reactive protein (CRP). Cytokines are small proteins that work as signals between the cells, mainly as immunomodulating agents.

Chronic inflammation has a few characteristics distinguishing it from acute inflammation. It is organ systemic (affects the whole body), of lower magnitude than acute stress, not time limited, and has no apparent, specific stimulus. In comparison to the acute stress reactions, which causes time-limited inflammatory responses, chronic pro-inflammatory activity can last for weeks, months, or even years (Straub, 2012).

Most non-communicable diseases (NCDs) can also be classified as chronic inflammatory diseases or at least associated with systemic inflammation (e.g. type 2 diabetes, cardiovascular disease, obesity, and common mental disorders). Inflammatory bowel diseases are also considered as chronic inflammatory diseases. These are a major cause of mortality and morbidity all over the world, having a significant impact on disability and performance over the life course.

A state of low-grade inflammation has been called the 'cause of causes' (Pruimboom et al., 2015) since it remains the fundamental common factor underlying these diseases, most of which were rare 200 years ago. Despite substantial investments by healthcare organizations around the world, their prevalence continues to rise, with

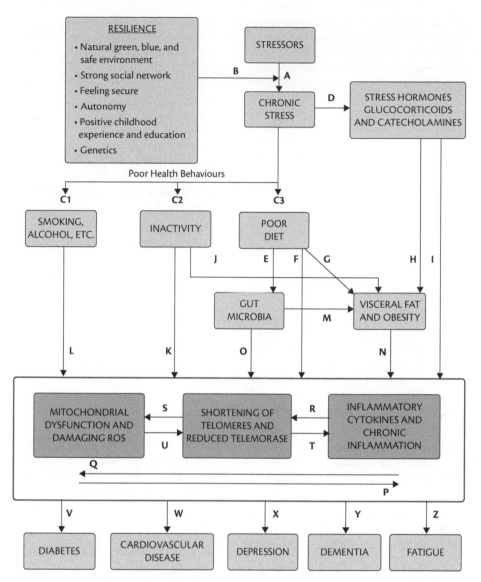

Fig. 1.5.1 This diagram demonstrates the pathways that lead away from a green natural environment, and/or other factors that decrease resilience, to the final cell damage, inflammation, premature ageing, and disease. Each pathway has a letter that is referred to in the text. The complex interactions between inflammation, oxidative stress, and telomere shortening have been grouped together to help simplify the interrelated mechanisms. However, some areas such as inactivity can increase oxidative stress and develop inflammation and shorten telomeres, both collectively and independently.

the most rapid rate in low- and middle-income countries. This represents a 'mismatch' between our evolutionarily developed adaptive responses to stressors and today's societies, demands, and lifestyles (Gluckman and Bergstrom, 2011; Gluckman *et al.*, 2005). Here we address the cause of the causes—chronic stress, which can precede and precipitate inflammation.

How chronic stress leads to chronic inflammation

A cascade of mechanisms turns chronic stress into chronic inflammation. Chronic stress leads to a continual activation of the hypothalamic pituitary adrenal (HPA) axis. This results in raised levels of glucocorticoids (e.g. cortisol) and catecholamines that eventually lead to glucocorticoid resistance, oxidative damage, and a prolonged pro-inflammatory state (Fig. 1.5.1, PATHWAY D). While glucocorticoids have a strong anti-inflammatory effect in the acute

stress phase, the same hormones lead to chronic inflammation with prolonged secretion (Tian *et al.*, 2014). At the early stage, stress downregulates pro-inflammatory cytokines, while simultaneously upregulating anti-inflammatory cytokines, creating an anti-inflammatory environment. However, with sustained stress, the HPA-axis reaches a state of 'fatigue' with downregulation of glucocorticoid receptor expression and thus glucocorticoid resistance (Cohen *et al.*, 2012). In combination with an increased release of pro-inflammatory cytokines, the initially anti-inflammatory response turns into a pro-inflammatory state. There are two types of glucocorticoid receptor GR alpha and GR beta. GR beta is inactive and competes with GR alpha receptors. Pro-inflammatory cytokines increase the expression of GR beta receptors leading to increasing insulin resistance, a reduced anti-inflammatory state, and increased pro-inflammatory state (Fig. 1.5.1, PATHWAY I) Carvalho *et al.* (2014). The release of IL-1, IL-6, and TNF-alpha further enhances the chronic inflammatory response.

A review by Rohleder (2014) proposes that catecholamine release during chronic stress redistributes immune cells into the circulation and activates the intracellular inflammatory signalling pathway. These pro-inflammatory responses seem to be exaggerated in populations living under socioeconomically deprived conditions (Krueger *et al.*, 2011), demonstrating the impact of social and physical environments in chronic disease development.

Finally, chronic stress tends to encourage unhealthy behaviours (Fig. 1.5.1, PATHWAY C), such as inactivity (*C2*), poor diet (*C3*), smoking, drinking, and poor sleeping habits (*C1*), which all contribute to the pro-inflammatory state. This can, in turn, lead to further increase in stress. These behavioural pathways are explained below.

Chronic stress, inactivity, and inflammation

Chronic stress can increase the risk of sedentary behaviour (Mouchacca *et al.*, 2013). Inactivity, in turn, leads to a chronic inflammatory state through three mechanisms (Fig. 1.5.1, PATHWAY K).

1. First, muscle contraction during physical activity releases over 100-fold levels of anti-inflammatory myokines, which subsequently stimulate production and release of other anti-inflammatory molecules, such as lysozyme and lactoferrin, by the immune system (Pedersen, 2011). Thus, exercise leads to a reduction of post-prandial inflammation (MacEneaney *et al.*, 2009). By remaining inactive, the rise in inflammation after a meal remains unchecked.

2. Secondly, inactivity favours the relative rise in visceral fat (Fig. 1.5.1, PATHWAY J), which is a powerful generator of pro-inflammatory cytokines (Smith *et al.*, 2013) (Fig. 1.5.1, PATHWAY N).

3. Lastly, inactivity leads to an increase in oxidative stress due to the charged mitochondria releasing reactive oxidative species (ROS, or free radicals), which damages the DNA of mitochondria. This, in turn, creates more ROS damage and subsequent inflammation. The high levels of ROS and inflammation in turn can damage telomeres. Bouts of exercise instead provide a controlled release of ROS that reduces damage in the long term (Bo *et al.*, 2013). A constantly active person is therefore set into a protective, low inflammatory state.

Chronic stress, poor diet, and inflammation

Chronic stress leads to two major changes associated with diet, outlined below (Epel *et al.*, 2001).

1. **Altering the number and diversity of the gut microbiota and increasing the permeability of the intestine.** There are between 10^{13} and 10^{14} microbes in the human gut, which work in symbiosis and are essential to immune function, nutrient processing, and also the development of the central nervous system (Gill *et al.*, 2006). Chronic stress has, mostly in animal studies, been linked to reduced diversity and amount of microbes in the gut (Watanabe *et al.*, 2016). This leads to a reduced resilience to stress. Interestingly, this negative effect can be reversed by ingestion of probiotics, returning the gut to normal (Zareie *et al.*, 2006). In addition, sensory neurons in the myenteric plexus of the gastrointestinal tract link straight to the vagal nerve (Stakenborg *et al.*, 2013). In germ-free guts, these neurons

are less excitable. This provides a possible mechanism as to how the microbes can affect the brain in what is termed the gut-brain axis (Hoban *et al.*, 2016, Kennedy *et al.*, 2016) (Fig. 1.5.1, PATHWAYS E and O).

Chronic stress also increases the gut permeability (Fig. 1.5.1, PATHWAY F) leading to leakage of Gram-negative bacteria outside the gastrointestinal tract, which triggers an inflammatory response reaction (Gareau *et al.*, 2008). The effects can also turn into a negative loop with an 'inflammatory gut' creating inflammation in the brain, resulting in enhanced stress reactions and increased risk of anxiety and depression and poor coping mechanisms, thus creating further chronic stress (Lucas *et al.*, 2014).

2. **Change of diet preference towards more palatable food with higher levels of fat.** It has been shown that, compared to a healthy diet, highly palatable foods increase levels of the appetite-stimulating hormone ghrelin, reducing the feeling of satiety and fuelling a further and unnecessary calorie intake, increasing the likelihood of obesity (Buss *et al.*, 2014) (Fig. 1.5.1, PATHWAY G).

The increase in fat and sugar and low consumption of fruit and vegetables, combined with an increase in stress hormones, can reduce the diversity of the gut microbiota and negatively affect the balance between beneficial (e.g. bacteroides) and harmful bacteria (e.g. *Clostridium*). Together, this stimulates an inflammatory process (Bailey *et al.*, 2011).

Chronic stress, obesity, and inflammation

Obese individuals with chronic stress have a higher ratio of visceral fat compared to subcutaneous fat (Marniemi *et al.*, 2002) (Fig. 1.5.1, PATHWAY H). One possible reason for this is that adipocytes in subcutaneous and visceral fat respond differently to chronic stress. Fat stemming from subcutaneous reserves is removed and transported to provide energy to the brain, whereas in visceral fat stress leads to macrophage invasion and the release of TNF, which alters glucose transport and favours further visceral fat accumulation (Peters and McEwen, 2015). The amount of macrophage infiltration in adipose tissue, which releases pro-inflammatory cytokines, is strongly associated with metabolic syndrome (Aschbacher *et al.*, 2014). The increasing size of adipocytes is associated with increased inflammation and insulin resistance (Acosta *et al.*, 2016).

Chronic stress, addictive behaviours, and inflammation

Chronic stress seems to promote addictive behaviours, such as smoking (Pomerleau and Pomerleau, 1991), drug use (Sinha, 2008), and excessive drinking of alcohol (Brady and Sonne, 1999) (Fig. 1.5.1, PATHWAY C1). All of these activities promote inflammatory markers and lead to a state of chronic inflammation (Fig. 1.5.1, PATHWAY L).

Chronic stress, poor sleep, and inflammation

Chronic stress is generally associated with poor sleep quality (Åkerstedt, 2006). Although the evidence is somewhat inconsistent, there seem to a positive association between sleep deprivation and pro-inflammatory activity, especially in combination with increased visceral fat (Prather *et al.*, 2014).

Inflammation and disease

We have now discussed how acute stress can evolve into chronic stress, if no opportunities for recovery are given, and how this can manifest itself in a state of chronic inflammation. How is this displayed in terms of actual health outcomes and disease burden? As previously mentioned, chronic inflammation is associated with a wide range of diseases, which will be presented in more detail here.

Inflammation and depression

There is strong evidence that clinical depression is associated with chronic inflammation (Allison and Ditor, 2014; Tansey and Lee, 2015) (Fig. 1.5.1, PATHWAY X). The pro-inflammatory cytokines in the peripheral blood pass the blood–brain barrier and alter the metabolic processes of certain neurotransmitters, such as serotonin and dopamine (Dunn *et al.*, 1999). The pro-inflammatory cytokines also activate corticotropine-releasing hormone (CRH) and upregulate adrenocorticotropic hormone (ACTH) and cortisol. There is considerable evidence that the overexpression of CRH is a key link between chronic stress and depression (Owens and Nemeroff, 1991; Chang *et al.*, 2015).

It is important to note that remission of clinical depression is accompanied by a normalization of inflammatory markers (Hannestad *et al.*, 2011), while lack of treatment or treatment response is associated with persistently elevated levels of inflammatory markers (Strawbridge *et al.*, 2015).

Inflammation and dementia

Chronic inflammation is one of the central pathological features of dementia (Prokop *et al.*, 2013) (Fig. 1.5.1, PATHWAY Y). Inflammatory markers are present in mild cognitive impairment cases that eventually progress to Alzheimer's disease (Olsson *et al.*, 2013). Chronic stress is known to augment neuroinflammatory process in the cortex through increased levels of glucocorticoids. Metabolic syndrome is a significant risk factor for the development of dementia, but some studies suggest that this association is only held in combination with elevated serum pro-inflammatory markers, suggesting that inflammation can be a mediating factor (Yaffe *et al.*, 2004).

Inflammation and diabetes

Diabetes is thought to be, at least partly, an inflammatory disease with overproduction of IL-6, TNF-alpha, and IL-1 (Van Greevenbroek *et al.*, 2013) (Fig. 1.5.1, PATHWAY V). Dandona *et al.* (2004) demonstrated that TNF-alpha can induce insulin resistance, whereas lack of TNF-alpha reduces insulin resistance. Insulin itself is a pro-inflammatory factor and beta cells of the pancreas, which secrete insulin, can potentially be disrupted by the pro-inflammatory cytokines (Perreault and Marette, 2001). However, a recent study has shown that sudden onset of obesity causes oxidation damage of the insulin-regulated glucose transporter type 4 (GLUT4), which probably results in insulin resistance even before inflammation starts (Boden *et al.*, 2015).

Inflammation and cardiovascular disease

Cardiovascular disease is associated with high levels of IL-1, IL-6, and TNF-alpha (Frostegård, 2013) (Fig. 1.5.1, PATHWAY W). These cytokines contribute to the formation of atherosclerotic plaques and cardiac irritability. The plaques start with a fatty streak which is an accumulation of lipid laden cells, macrophages, and T-cells beneath the endothelium of the vascular wall (Hansson, 2005). The activated macrophages induce a release of inflammatory cytokines and free radicals, which cause inflammation, tissue damage, and furthers the plaque formation.

Intracellular changes and disease

Apart from the relation between chronic stress, inflammation, and disease, intracellular changes to the cells' DNA and mitochondria are key to understanding the full impact that chronic stress and unhealthy lifestyles have on our health.

Mitochondria

The energy-producing mitochondria are central components in the cell biology of health and disease. In our evolutionary past, eukaryotic cells engulfed primitive mitochondria-like bacteria, resulting in an organism with an energy-producing advantage that has evolved to the mitochondria in all contemporary eukaryotic organisms. Mitochondria provide energy by converting adenosine diphosphate (ADP) to adenosine triphosphate (ATP) through the citric acid cycle (or Krebs cycle). ROS are created as a normal consequence of this metabolic process and are usually balanced by antioxidants. However when this balance is disturbed, the ROS levels increase, which can damage the cells' DNA and reduce the effectiveness of the mitochondria. This imbalance is called oxidative stress.

Oxidative stress is strongly associated with the following;

1. Physical inactivity and high calorie intake (Fig. 1.5.1, PATHWAY K and N)

2. Stress and the presence of cortisol (Fig. 1.5.1, PATHWAY I)

3. Underlying chronic inflammation (Fig. 1.5.1, PATHWAY Q)

4. Short telomeres (Fig. 1.5.1, PATHWAY S)

Physical inactivity and high calorie intake

James and colleagues (James *et al.*, 2012) describe that when the body is sedentary there is a low ATP demand, leading to a high proton motive force (electrochemical gradient), a low respiration rate (that leads to excess oxygen), and increased mitochondrial superoxide formation. Therefore inactivity leads to an excessive and damaging supply of ROS. The overconsumption of calories provides a surplus of electrons to the respiratory chain, further increasing the number of ROS, and thus initiating a vicious circle (Fig. 1.5.1, PATHWAYS F&N).

Stress and cortisol

Animal studies have shown that brief administration of high-dose cortisol improves mitochondrial function and has neuroprotective effects, whereas long-term high-dose cortisol administration dramatically decreases mitochondrial function and promotes cell death (Du *et al.*, 2009). Moreover, at low concentrations, reactive oxygen and lipid species activate cytoprotective pathways that increase antioxidants (Gutierrez *et al.*, 2006). Aschbacher *et al.* (2013) found that participants who had an increase in anticipatory stress had increased oxidative damage compared to controls. This suggests that stress hormones, such as cortisol, exacerbate the oxidative damage due to increased ROS.

Chronic inflammation

Deviation from the mitochondrial biochemical status quo triggers activation of the inflammatory response. Inflammation strongly influences the production of ROS, but ROS can also help trigger widespread chronic inflammation. Boden *et al.* (2015) found that after a very high calorie ingestion over two days, the initial change was the presence of oxidative damage. This was followed by inflammation and subsequent insulin resistance, indicating that oxidative damage is one of the first changes to take place in the aetiology of inflammation.

Telomere shortening

Telomere shortness can also trigger dysfunction in the mitochondria. Through a well-mapped out signalling pathway, short telomeres send out signals about damage to the mitochondria. As a result, the mitochondria become impaired, resulting in increased levels of ROS (Sahin *et al.*, 2011). The following section 'Telomeres and health' will outline the function of telomeres and how they can be harmed by chronic stress and unhealthy environments (Park *et al.*, 2015; Schaakxs *et al.*, 2016).

Telomeres and health

Recent research points to the crucial roles of telomeres and telomerase in cellular ageing and potentially in disease (Lindqvist *et al.*, 2015; Reynolds, 2016). Telomeres are DNA–protein complexes that cap and protect the chromosomal ends, promoting chromosomal stability. When cells divide, the telomere is not fully replicated, leading to telomere shortening with every replication. *In vitro*, when telomeres shorten sufficiently, the cell is arrested into senescence. In people, telomeres shorten with age in all replicating somatic cells that have been studied, including fibroblasts and leukocytes. Thus, telomere length can serve as a biomarker of a cell's biological (versus chronological) 'age', or its potential for further cell division.

Telomere length defines how much a cell or tissue has the potential to proliferate and stay healthy over years. When the telomeres are too short, there is limited ability to replenish the tissue. When measured in blood, it represents level of senescence in the immune system.

Telomere length is a biomarker related to cardiometabolic risk and cardiovascular disease (Haycock *et al.*, 2014), mental disorders (Colpo *et al.*, 2015, Czepielewski *et al.*, 2016), and diabetes (Willeit *et al.*, 2014). Telomere length is also related to modifiable health determinants, such as healthy behaviours (Puterman and Epel, 2012). Thus, telomere length may offer clues about which aspects of our physical and social environments appear to be 'getting under our skin', associated with accelerated cellular ageing.

Telomere length shortness is associated with chronic stress exposure, including the stress of impoverished urban environments. In contrast, exposure to greenery can reduce stress, and could theoretically slow telomere attrition. Here we take a closer look at these links.

Telomeres and stress

Several studies and reviews show that severe stress during childhood, or chronic or perceived stress during adulthood, is associated with telomere shortness (Price *et al.*, 2013; Starkweather *et al.*, 2014; Schutte and Malouff, 2014). The exact pathways are not fully explicated, but it is likely that the excessive stress hormones, inflammation, and oxidative stress associated with severe distress may be part of the systemic milieu that dampens the enzyme telomerase and promotes telomere shortening (Epel, 2009).

Telomere maintenance and environmental factors

Differences in socioeconomic status are mirrored in health inequalities and living under disadvantaged conditions results in adverse health outcomes (Marmot, 2005). Some of these adverse effects seem to be mitigated by access to greenery in the neighbourhoods (Mitchell and Popham, 2008; Mitchell *et al.*, 2015) and the stress-reducing effects of greenery (see Chapter 3.2) appear to be particularly pronounced among vulnerable populations (Roe *et al.*, 2013; Ward Thompson *et al.*, 2012). (Read more about health inequalities and the relation to natural environments in Chapter 6.3.)

A few studies have examined associations between telomere length and urban environments, all suggesting a link between telomere length and socioenvironmental disorder (Park *et al.*, 2015). One study examined the relation between neighbourhood environment and salivary telomere length of 99 children living in New Orleans (Theall *et al.*, 2013). The children's parents rated the level of disorder in the neighbourhood environment with indicators like presence of litter, broken glass, and vacant buildings. Both the level of poverty and the level of neighbourhood disorder were associated with shorter telomere length.

A larger study assessed the relationship between telomere length among adults and neighbourhood environment (Needham *et al.*, 2014). The researchers examined neighbourhood socioeconomic status, as defined by census track data of factors such as mean income, occupational level, wealth, and type of housing. They also conducted a fine grain analysis of aspects of the social environment based on mean ratings of three subscales: aesthetic quality (litter, noise, and attractiveness); social cohesion (perception of neighbours' trustworthiness, willingness to help, and value sharing); and safety (whether they felt safe walking in their neighbourhood and level of violence). The strongest indicator of telomere length was social environment. Those living in the neighbourhoods with the worst perceived social environments had telomeres that appeared shorter by the equivalent of eight years of natural telomeric shortening as compared to those living in the best social environments. In another study of the same cohort, deprived neighbourhood environments were associated with shorter sleep (DeSantis *et al.*, 2013). A recent study (Olafsdottir *et al.*, 2016) of 60 adults tested the difference between five months of (i) 'green exercise', (ii) indoor gym-based exercise, or (iii) no exercise programme. Telomere length increased in both exercise groups, but not in the control group. However, telomerase activity decreased in the gym group, but not in the green exercise. Green exercise thus seemed to be associated with better cell ageing profiles, as compared to indoor gym-based or no exercise.

Lastly, one study examined telomere length in over 900 elderly men living in Hong Kong, and compared types of neighbourhoods, including level of greenness (Woo *et al.*, 2009). They compared densely populated urban areas with a district outside of the city which borders a river and has many parks. In adjusted models, it was found that those in the urban areas were much less likely to have long telomeres. While other factors could be responsible for the association, this may suggest a certain protective role of nature (see Box 1.5.1).

Box 1.5.1 Pathways to understanding the association between parks and recreational facilities with multiple health outcomes—empirically testing a conceptual model

In an article, published 2014 in *Annual Review of Public Health*, Terry Hartig and his colleagues propose a conceptual model describing the associations between nature and health via multiple and diverse pathways: air quality, physical activity, social cohesion, and stress (Hartig *et al.*, 2014). They suggest that because the associations between nature and health are complex, multiple pathways are likely to be engaged simultaneously. These pathways emphasize different aspects of nature as a physical environment, a setting for individual and social behaviour, and a human experience. Together, they may impact an array of health outcomes.

The objective of the here-presented study is to examine the direct and indirect effects of nature on health and factors that may mediate this association, by empirically testing the model articulated in the review by Hartig and colleagues. We test the overall model and examine direct and indirect effects of access to parks on four health outcomes—body mass index, number of chronic conditions, self-rated health, and depressive symptoms—via the hypothesized mediators: air quality, physical activity, social cohesion, and stress. The data come from a community health assessment (N = 1307) in the greater New Haven, Connecticut region, US, representative of the population.

The definition of 'nature' was based on perceived access to parks and other recreational facilities as vital community resources.

Model testing

Structural equation modelling was used to test the direct and indirect associations between variables specified in the conceptual model linking nature to health. The final, trimmed structural equation model is presented in Figure 1.5.2.

To address the issue of self-selection bias, where healthier (or wealthier) people might choose to live in areas with greater park access, we tested the reverse models: health outcomes leading to park access, with the specified mediators and controlling for participant age, sex, race/ethnicity, income, and length of residency. The data did not fit the reverse model as well as the original model (χ^2 (28) = 468.37, p = 0.000; RMSEA = 0.121, CI = 0.112–0.131; CFI = 0.451), providing support for the original conceptual model as specified by Hartig and colleagues.

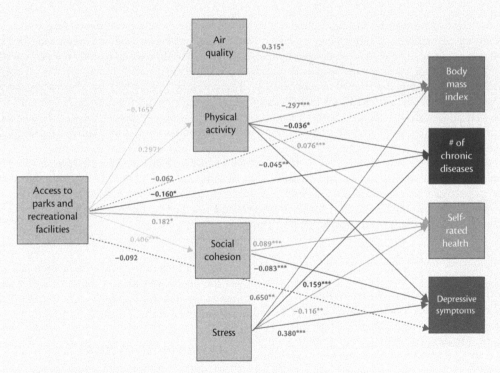

$^\dagger p$ <0.10, *p<0.05, **p<0.01, ***p<0.001
Note: All potential mediators and health outcomes were regressed on five control variables: age, race/ethnicity, gender, income, and length of residency

Fig. 1.5.2 Structural equation model results with beta coefficients.

Source: data from Terry Hartig *et al.*, 'Nature and Health', *Annual Review of Public Health*, Volume 35, pp. 207-228, Copyright © 2014 by Annual Reviews, DOI: 10.1146/annurev-publhealth-032013-182443.

(continued)

Box 1.5.1 (Continued)

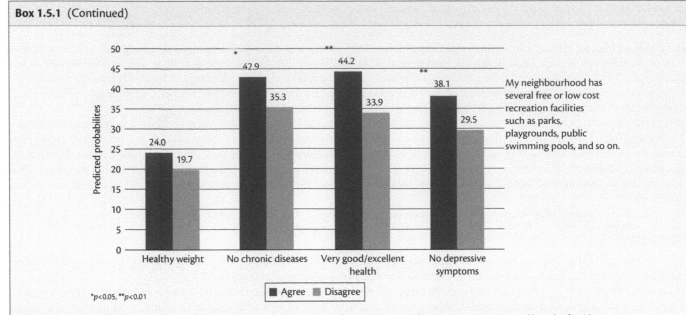

Fig. 1.5.3 Predicted probabilities of health outcomes by park access, adjusted for age, sex, race/ethnicity, income, region, and length of residency.
Source: data from Terry Hartig *et al.*, 'Nature and Health,' Annual Review of Public Health, Volume 35, pp. 207-228, Copyright © 2014 by Annual Reviews, DOI: 10.1146/ annurev-publhealth-032013-182443.

Discussion

The findings support our hypotheses and the conceptual model linking nature to health via several important mediators. Access to parks and other outdoor recreational facilities were associated with all the health outcomes we measured—body mass index, number of chronic diseases, self-rated health, and depressive symptoms (Fig. 1.5.3)—directly and/or via the proposed pathways. Physical activity was the most important mediator between park access and all measured health outcomes. Social cohesion, though only related to self-rated health (a strong predictor of overall health) (Idler and Benyamini, 1997) and depressive symptoms, was a strong and significant correlate along these pathways. Air quality was retained in the overall model, though was only associated with body mass index. Stress was significantly associated with all health outcomes; however, after controlling for socioeconomic and demographic characteristics, it was not associated with park access and thus not considered as mediating the association between nature and health in this study.

  This study represents a relatively large sample (>1300 people) across 13 cities and towns diverse in level of urbanization and community design. All analyses were controlled for age, sex, race/ethnicity, income, and length of residency. Although evidence demonstrates that more deprived populations have less access to usable and safe green space, urban planners have argued that socioeconomic position itself does not independently affect use of green space if readily available to residents. Thus, urban greening can positively impact the health of all residents, regardless of individual socioeconomic resources.

Conclusion

The described intricate links between environment, stress, inflammation, and molecular mechanisms open the floor for an innovative research agenda. Recently established research programmes investigate, for example, how telomere length, and other biomarkers, change with exposure to greenery over time. With the use of technology for ambulatory monitoring of behaviour and well-being, and increasing ease of biomarker sampling in field studies, we are getting closer to providing biological explanations to existing theories around the links between nature and health, years before chronic disease develops. From this perspective, the early cause of the triggers for disease, chronic stress and its mediators—chronic inflammation, mitochondrial damage, and telomere length—may prove to be central factors for improving our knowledge and understanding. Combined with existing epidemiological evidence around the positive health outcomes related to nature (described in the following chapters of the book), this kind of biochemical evidence could contribute to establishing a firm evidence base in the intriguing field of nature and health.

Acknowledgements

The authors would like to acknowledge the contributions of Kate Gilstad-Hayden, Julia Anderson, Spencer Meyer, Colleen Murphy-Dunning, Amy Carroll-Scott, and Bradford Gentry (all at Yale University at the time the work was completed) for their contributions to conceptual and empirical work on the 'pathways' between nature and health, along with Mark Abraham (DataHaven, Inc.) for his contributions and provision of the data. The research was supported, in part, by the Berkeley Conferences and the Center for Business and the Environment at the Yale School of Forestry and Environmental Studies, Centers for Disease Control and

Prevention, and the Patrick and Catherine Weldon Donaghue Medical Research Foundation.

References

Acosta, J. R., Douagi, I., Andersson, D. P., et al. (2016). Increased fat cell size: a major phenotype of subcutaneous white adipose tissue in non-obese individuals with type 2 diabetes. *Diabetologia*, 59, 560–70.

Åkerstedt, T. (2006). Psychosocial stress and impaired sleep. *Scand J Work Environ Health*, 32, 493–501.

Allison, D. J. & Ditor, D. S. (2014). The common inflammatory etiology of depression and cognitive impairment: A therapeutic target. *Journal of Neuroinflammation*, 11.

Aschbacher, K., Kornfeld, S., Picard, M., et al. (2014). Chronic stress increases vulnerability to diet-related abdominal fat, oxidative stress, and metabolic risk. *Psychoneuroendocrinology*, 46, 14–22.

Aschbacher, K., O'Donovan, A., Wolkowitz, O. M., Dhabhar, F. S., Su, Y., & Epel, E. (2013). Good stress, bad stress and oxidative stress: insights from anticipatory cortisol reactivity. *Psychoneuroendocrinology*, 38, 1698–1708.

Bailey, M. T., Dowd, S. E., Galley, J. D., Hufnagle, A. R., Allen, R. G., & Lyte, M. (2011). Exposure to a social stressor alters the structure of the intestinal microbiota: implications for stressor-induced immunomodulation. *Brain Behav Immun*, 25, 397–407.

Bo, H., Jiang, N., Ji, L. L., & Zhang, Y. (2013). Mitochondrial redox metabolism in aging: Effect of exercise interventions. *J Sport Health Sci*, 2, 67–74.

Boden, G., Homko, C., Barrero, C. A., et al. (2015). Excessive caloric intake acutely causes oxidative stress, GLUT4 carbonylation, and insulin resistance in healthy men. *Sci Translat Med*, 7, 304re7.

Brady, K. T. & Sonne, S. C. (1999). The role of stress in alcohol use, alcoholism treatment, and relapse. *Alcohol Res Health*, 23, 263–71.

Buss, J., Havel, P. J., Epel, E., Lin, J., Blackburn, E., & Daubenmier, J. (2014). Associations of ghrelin with eating behaviors, stress, metabolic factors, and telomere length among overweight and obese women: preliminary evidence of attenuated ghrelin effects in obesity? *Appetite*, 76, 84–94.

Carvalho, L. A., Bergink, V., Sumaski, L., et al. (2014). Inflammatory activation is associated with a reduced glucocorticoid receptor alpha/beta expression ratio in monocytes of inpatients with melancholic major depressive disorder. *Transl Psychiatry*, 4, e344.

Chang, H. S., Won, E., Lee, H. Y., Ham, B. J., & Lee, M. S. (2015). Association analysis for corticotropin releasing hormone polymorphisms with the risk of major depressive disorder and the response to antidepressants. *Behav Brain Res*, 292, 116–24.

Cohen, S., Janicki-Deverts, D., Doyle, W. J., et al. (2012). Chronic stress, glucocorticoid receptor resistance, inflammation, and disease risk. *Proc Natl Acad Sci U S A*, 109, 5995–9.

Colpo, G. D., Leffa, D. D., Köhler, C. A., Kapczinski, F., Quevedo, J., & Carvalho, A. F. (2015). Is bipolar disorder associated with accelerating aging? A meta-analysis of telomere length studies. *J Affective Disord*, 186, 241–8.

Czepielewski, L. S., Massuda, R., Panizzutti, B., et al. (2016). Telomere length in subjects with schizophrenia, their unaffected siblings and healthy controls: Evidence of accelerated aging. *Schizophr Res*, 174, 39–42.

Dandona, P., Aljada, A., & Bandyopadhyay, A. (2004). Inflammation: the link between insulin resistance, obesity and diabetes. *Trends Immunol*, 25, 4–7.

DeSantis, A. S., Roux, A. V. D., Moore, K., et al. (2013). Associations of neighborhood characteristics with sleep timing and quality: the Multi-Ethnic Study of Atherosclerosis. *Sleep*, 36, 1543.

Du, J., Wang, Y., Hunter, R., Wei, Y., Blumenthal, R., Falke, C., Khairova, R., Zhou, R., Yuan, P., Machado-Vieira, R. and McEwen, B. S. (2009). Dynamic regulation of mitochondrial function by glucocorticoids. *Proceedings of the National Academy of Sciences*, 106(9), 3543–8.

Dunn, A. J., Wang, J., & Ando, T. (1999). Effects of cytokines on cerebral neurotransmission. *Cytokines, Stress, and Depression*, 461, 117–27.

Epel, E., Lapidus, R., McEwen, B., & Brownell, K. (2001). Stress may add bite to appetite in women: a laboratory study of stress-induced cortisol and eating behavior. *Psychoneuroendocrinology*, 26, 37–49.

Epel, E. S. (2009). Psychological and metabolic stress: a recipe for accelerated cellular aging. *Hormones (Athens)*, 8, 7–22.

Frostegård, J. (2013). Immunity, atherosclerosis and cardiovascular disease. *BMC Med*, 11, 117.

Gareau, M. G., Silva, M. A., & Perdue, M. H. (2008). Pathophysiological mechanisms of stress-induced intestinal damage. *Curr Mol Med*, 8, 274–81.

Gill, S. R., Pop, M., Deboy, R. T., et al. (2006). Metagenomic analysis of the human distal gut microbiome. *Science*, 312, 1355–9.

Gluckman, P. & Bergstrom, C. (2011). Evolutionary biology within medicine: A perspective of growing value. *BMJ (Online)*, 343, d7671.

Gluckman, P. D., Hanson, M. A., & Spencer, H. G. (2005). Predictive adaptive responses and human evolution. *Trends Ecol Evol*, 20, 527–33.

Gutierrez, J., Ballinger, S. W., Darley-Usmar, V. M., & Landar, A. (2006). Free radicals, mitochondria, and oxidized lipids: the emerging role in signal transduction in vascular cells. *Circ Res*, 99, 924–32.

Hannestad, J., Dellagioia, N., & Bloch, M. (2011). The effect of antidepressant medication treatment on serum levels of inflammatory cytokines: a meta-analysis. *Neuropsychopharmacology*, 36, 2452–9.

Hansson, G. K. (2005). Inflammation, atherosclerosis, and coronary artery disease. *N Engl J Med*, 352, 1685–95.

Hartig, T., Mitchell, R., De Vries, S., & Frumkin, H. (2014). Nature and health. *Ann Rev Public Health*, 35, 207–28.

Haycock, P. C., Heydon, E. E., Kaptoge, S., Butterworth, A. S., Thompson, A., & Willeit, P. (2014). Leucocyte telomere length and risk of cardiovascular disease: systematic review and meta-analysis.

Hoban, A. E., Moloney, R. D., Golubeva, A. V., et al. (2016). Behavioural and neurochemical consequences of chronic gut microbiota depletion during adulthood in the rat. *Neuroscience*, 339, 463–77.

Idler, E. L. & Benyamini, Y. (1997). Self-rated health and mortality: A review of twenty-seven community studies. *J Health Soc Behav*, 38, 21–37.

James, A. M., Collins, Y., Logan, A., & Murphy, M. P. (2012). Mitochondrial oxidative stress and the metabolic syndrome. *Trends Endocrinol Metab*, 23, 429–34.

Kennedy, P. J., Murphy, A. B., Cryan, J. F., Ross, P. R., Dinan, T. G., & Stanton, C. (2016). Microbiome in brain function and mental health. *Trends Food Sci Technol*, 57, 289–301.

Krueger, P. M., Saint Onge, J. M., & Chang, V. W. (2011). Race/ethnic differences in adult mortality: the role of perceived stress and health behaviors. *Soc Sci & Med*, 73, 1312–22.

Lindqvist, D., Epel, E. S., Mellon, S. H., et al. (2015). Psychiatric disorders and leukocyte telomere length: Underlying mechanisms linking mental illness with cellular aging. *Neurosci Biobehav Rev*, 55, 333–64.

Lucas, M., Chocano-Bedoya, P., Shulze, M. B., et al. (2014). Inflammatory dietary pattern and risk of depression among women. *Brain Behav Immun*, 36, 46–53.

MacEneaney, O. J., Harrison, M., O'Gorman, D. J., Pankratieva, E. V., O'Connor, P. L. & Moyna, N. M. (2009). Effect of prior exercise on postprandial lipemia and markers of inflammation and endothelial activation in normal weight and overweight adolescent boys. *Eur J Appl Physiol*, 106, 721–9.

Marmot, M. (2005). Social determinants of health inequalities. *Lancet*, 365, 1099–104.

Marniemi, J., Kronholm, E., Aunola, S., et al. (2002). Visceral fat and psychosocial stress in identical twins discordant for obesity. *J Int Med*, 251, 35–43.

Mitchell, R. & Popham, F. (2008). Effect of exposure to natural environment on health inequalities: an observational population study. *Lancet*, 372, 1655–60.

Mitchell, R. J., Richardson, E. A., Shortt, N. K., & Pearce, J. R. (2015). Neighborhood environments and socioeconomic inequalities in mental well-being. *Am J Prev Med*, 49, 80–4.

Mouchacca, J., Abbott, G. R., & Ball, K. (2013). Associations between psychological stress, eating, physical activity, sedentary behaviours and body weight among women: a longitudinal study. *BMC Public Health*, 13, 828.

Needham, B. L., Carroll, J. E., Roux, A. V. D., Fitzpatrick, A. L., Moore, K., & Seeman, T. E. (2014). Neighborhood characteristics and leukocyte telomere length: The Multi-Ethnic Study of Atherosclerosis. *Health & Place*, 28, 167–72.

Olafsdottir, G., Cloke, P., Epel, E., et al. (2016). Green exercise is associated with better cell ageing profiles. *Eur J Public Health*, 26(Suppl 1), ckw165.021.

Olsson, B., Hertze, J., Lautner, R., et al. (2013). Microglial markers are elevated in the prodromal phase of Alzheimer's disease and vascular dementia. *J Alzheimers Dis*, 33, 45–53.

Owens, M. J. & Nemeroff, C. B. (1991). Physiology and pharmacology of corticotropin-releasing factor. *Pharmacol Rev*, 43, 425–73.

Park, M., Verhoeven, J. E., Cuijpers, P., Reynolds, C. F. III, & Penninx, B. W. J. H. (2015). Where you live may make you old: The association between perceived poor neighborhood quality and leukocyte telomere length. *PLoS One*, 10, e0128460.

Pedersen, B. K. (2011). Muscles and their myokines. *J Exp Biol*, 214, 337–46.

Perreault, M. & Marette, A. (2001). Targeted disruption of inducible nitric oxide synthase protects against obesity-linked insulin resistance in muscle. *Nature Med*, 7, 1138–43.

Peters, A. & McEwen, B. S. (2015). Stress habituation, body shape and cardiovascular mortality. *Neurosci Biobehav Rev*, 56, 139–50.

Pomerleau, O. F. & Pomerleau, C. S. (1991). Research on stress and smoking: progress and problems. *Br J Addict*, 86, 599–603.

Prather, A. A., Puterman, E., Epel, E. S., & Dhabhar, F. S. (2014). Poor sleep quality potentiates stress-induced cytokine reactivity in postmenopausal women with high visceral abdominal adiposity. *Brain Behav Immun*, 35, 155–62.

Price, L. H., Kao, H.-T., Burgers, D. E., Carpenter, L. L., & Tyrka, A. R. (2013). Telomeres and early-life stress: an overview. *Biol Psychiatry*, 73, 15–23.

Prokop, S., Miller, K. R., & Heppner, F. L. (2013). Microglia actions in Alzheimer's disease. *Acta Neuropathol*, 126, 461–77.

Pruimboom, L., Raison, C. L., & Muskiet, F. A. (2015). Physical activity protects the human brain against metabolic stress induced by a postprandial and chronic inflammation. *Behav Neurol*, 2015, 569869.

Puterman, E. & Epel, E. (2012). An intricate dance: life experience, multisystem resiliency, and rate of telomere decline throughout the lifespan. *Soc Personal Psychol Compass*, 6, 807–25.

Reynolds, C. F. III (2016). Telomere attrition: A window into common mental disorders and cellular aging. *Am J Psychiatry*, 173, 556–8.

Roe, J., Thompson, C., Aspinall, P., et al. (2013). Green space and stress: Evidence from cortisol measures in deprived urban communities. *Int J Environ Res Public Health*, 10, 4086–103.

Rohleder, N. (2014). Stimulation of Systemic Low-Grade Inflammation by Psychosocial Stress. *Psychosom Med*, 76, 181–9.

Sahin, E., Colla, S., Liesa, M., et al. (2011). Telomere dysfunction induces metabolic and mitochondrial compromise. *Nature*, 470, 359–65.

Schaakxs, R., Wielaard, I., Verhoeven, J. E., Beekman, A. T. F., Penninx, B. W., & Comijs, H. C. (2016). Early and recent psychosocial stress and telomere length in older adults. *Int Psychogeriatr*, 28, 405–13.

Schutte, N. S. & Malouff, J. M. (2014). The relationship between perceived stress and telomere length: A meta-analysis. *Stress Health*, 32, 313–19.

Shonkoff, J. P., Garner, A. S., Siegel, B. S., et al. (2012). The lifelong effects of early childhood adversity and toxic stress. *Pediatrics*, 129, e232–46.

Sinha, R. (2008). Chronic stress, drug use, and vulnerability to addiction. *Ann N Y Acad Sci*, 1141, 105–30.

Smith, H., Storti, K., Arena, V., et al. (2013). Associations between accelerometer-derived physical activity and regional adiposity in young men and women. *Obesity*, 21, 1299–305.

Stakenborg, N., Di Giovangiulio, M., Boeckxstaens, G. E., & Matteoli, G. (2013). The versatile role of the vagus nerve in the gastrointestinal tract. *EMJ Gastroenterol*, 1, 106–14.

Starkweather, A. R., Alhaeeri, A. A., Montpetit, A., et al. (2014). An integrative review of factors associated with telomere length and implications for biobehavioral research. *Nurs Res*, 63, 36.

Straub, R. H. (2012). Evolutionary medicine and chronic inflammatory state—known and new concepts in pathophysiology. *J Mol Med*, 90, 523–34.

Strawbridge, R., Arnone, D., Danese, A., Papadopoulos, A., Herane Vives, A., & Cleare, A. J. (2015). Inflammation and clinical response to treatment in depression: A meta-analysis. *Eur Neuropsychopharmacol*, 25, 1532–43.

Tansey, M. G. & Lee, J. K. (2015). Inflammation in nervous system disorders. *Neuroscience*, 302, 1.

Theall, K. P., Brett, Z. H., Shirtcliff, E. A., Dunn, E. C., & Drury, S. S. (2013). Neighborhood disorder and telomeres: Connecting children's exposure to community level stress and cellular response. *Soc Sci & Med*, 85, 50–8.

Tian, R., Hou, G., Li, D., & Yuan, T.-F. (2014). A possible change process of inflammatory cytokines in the prolonged chronic stress and its ultimate implications for health. *ScientificWorldJournal*, 2014, 780616.

Van Greevenbroek, M., Schalkwijk, C., & Stehouwer, C. (2013). Obesity-associated low-grade inflammation in type 2 diabetes mellitus: causes and consequences. *Neth J Med*, 71, 174–87.

Ward Thompson, C., Roe, J., Aspinall, P., Mitchell, R., Clow, A., & Miller, D. (2012). More green space is linked to less stress in deprived communities: Evidence from salivary cortisol patterns. *Landscape Urban Planning*, 105, 221–9.

Watanabe, Y., Arase, S., Nagaoka, N., Kawai, M., & Matsumoto, S. (2016). Chronic psychological stress disrupted the composition of the murine colonic microbiota and accelerated a murine model of inflammatory bowel disease. *PLoS One*, 11, e0150559.

Wells, N. M. (2012). The role of nature in children's resilience: cognitive and social processes. In: Tidball, G. G. & Krasny, M. E. (eds) *Greening in the Red Zone*. Dordrecht, the Netherlands: Springer.

Willeit, P., Raschenberger, J., Heydon, E. E., et al. (2014). Leucocyte telomere length and risk of type 2 diabetes mellitus: new prospective cohort study and literature-based meta-analysis. *PLoS One*, 9, e112483.

Woo, J., Tang, N., Suen, E., Leung, J., & Wong, M. (2009). Green space, psychological restoration, and telomere length. *Lancet*, 373, 299–300.

Yaffe, K., Kanaya, A., Lindquist, K., et al. (2004). The metabolic syndrome, inflammation, and risk of cognitive decline. *JAMA*, 292, 2237–42.

Zareie, M., Johnson-Henry, K., Jury, J., et al. (2006). Probiotics prevent bacterial translocation and improve intestinal barrier function in rats following chronic psychological stress. *Gut*, 55, 1553–60.

SECTION 2

How nature can affect health—theories and mechanisms

CHAPTER 2.1

Environmental psychology

Agnes E. van den Berg and Henk Staats

Environmental psychology in a health context

This chapter aims to give an overview of theories relevant to understanding positive impacts of nature on health. Most of these theories originate in the field of environmental psychology. Environmental psychology is a social science discipline concerned with the interplay between individuals and their physical environment (Steg *et al.*, 2012). The discipline has been recognized as a field of psychology since the late 1960s and is therefore a relatively young scientific area (Proshansky *et al.*, 1970).

As an applied science, environmental psychology has adapted and changed over time to address questions arising from the social and political context of the time. In the early years, when societies were facing the post-war challenges of providing decent housing and facilities for the general public, environmental psychology was primarily devoted to studying human interactions with the built environment, for example homes, offices, hospitals, and schools. In this period, natural environments were mostly investigated in the context of leisure and tourism, with a special interest in the assessment of visual quality or scenic beauty (Shafer and Mietz, 1969). The natural environment gained a more central focus in the 1990s, when it became clear that increasing urbanization and industrialization were rapidly taking their toll on nature and landscape, and thus on the quality of people's living environment. In response to these developments, modern environmental psychology now takes an active interest in studying people's interactions with natural environments in relation to their health and well-being. In particular, the restorative or stress-relieving functions of contact with nature have become a major topic for research and theorizing (Van den Berg *et al.*, 2007).

Our review of theories in this chapter follows the historical developments in the field of environmental psychology. The first sections give an overview of classic theories on environmental aesthetics, followed by a discussion of research and theorizing on restorative environments and the health benefits of nature. We then explore recent advances in environmental psychology, including theories on the basic visual processes that may underlie the restorative effects of natural environment experiences.

Environmental aesthetics and landscape preferences

The experience of beauty is an important dimension of people-environment interactions. In general, people will derive less benefit from contact with a setting if they experience it as aesthetically unpleasant. From this perspective, theories on environmental aesthetics and landscape preferences provide an important backdrop for understanding which environments are benign for human health and well-being. In this section, we give an overview of several influential theoretical frameworks: arousal theory, prospect-refuge theory, and information processing theory. What these theories have in common is that they assume a biological or evolutionary basis for aesthetics and environmental preferences.

Arousal theory

Daniel Berlyne (1924–1976) made important contributions to a number of areas in experimental psychology. Professor Berlyne was a motivational theorist who wanted to understand why people display curiosity and explore their environment. He developed a general theory on aesthetic pleasure and the properties of physical stimuli that optimize the aesthetic experience (Berlyne, 1960; 1971).

Stated simply, this theory postulates that people prefer stimuli which help them reach and maintain an optimal level of arousal (arousal being the general level of activation or excitement). The stimuli that bring about an optimal level of arousal typically contain a mixture of arousal-increasing properties (e.g. complexity, novelty, and ambiguity), and arousal-decreasing properties (e.g. familiarity and patterning). Such stimuli are much preferred, because they afford a pleasurable rise or 'boost' in arousal while at the same time ensuring that the arousal will stay in the intermediate range, or can be returned quickly to a comfortable level should it rise too high.

Berlyne's arousal theory provides a psychobiological underpinning of the age-old aesthetic principle of 'unity-in-variety', or order imposed on complexity, a principle that was already known to the early Greek philosophers and is still popular among architects and designers (Hekkert, 2006). Although the theory was originally developed to explain people's reactions to art, its relevance to environmental preferences has been widely acknowledged. In particular, Joachim (Jack) Wohlwill (1928–1987), one of the founding fathers of environmental psychology, underlined the relevance of Berlyne's work to understanding people's responses to nature and landscape. Among other things, Wohlwill noted that visual attributes of natural environments tend to converge to produce a desirable, intermediate level of complexity, characterized by 'irregular lines and curvilinear lines and edges, continuous gradations of shape and colour, and irregular, rough textures' (Wohlwill, 1983).

Prospect-refuge theory

British geographer Jay Appleton (1919–2015) stressed the evolutionary advantages of landscape views that simultaneously afford prospect (wide, open views from which approaching predators could be seen) and refuge (protected settings that prevent the viewer from being seen or that protect the viewer's back) (1975). Landscapes that offer both prospect and refuge allowed our ancestors to 'see without being seen', which would have enabled them to safely explore and gather information and food while out of sight of predators. Environmental preferences are therefore, according to Appleton, directly linked with the potential of an environment or 'habitat' to satisfy a biologic drive.

Appleton (1975) illustrated his theory, which has been aptly named 'hide and seek aesthetics', mainly through an analysis of landscape paintings, poetry, and park designs. He concluded that prospect-refuge symbolism, as indicated by sign-stimuli like panoramas and shelters, is omnipresent in landscape art and design, and thus seems to represent a universal value. However, the few studies that have empirically verified the theory have often found ambiguous results, especially with respect to refuge (Stamps, 2008). It therefore seems wise to maintain some caution in assuming the utility of the theory.

Information processing theory

The scholarly work of Stephen and Rachel Kaplan, both professors at the University of Michigan, has profoundly influenced the field of human-environment studies. In 1989, the Kaplans published their influential book *The Experience of Nature*, in which they offer a research-based analysis of the vital psychological role that nature plays in people's lives. The Kaplans developed an information processing theory on landscape preferences that it is grounded in cognitive psychology (Kaplan and Kaplan, 1989; Kaplan, 1987). However, the theory also builds on evolutionary assumptions and predicts a preference for natural settings that impose order over complexity. Information processing theory assumes that selection pressures during human evolution in natural environments would have favoured a cognitive ability to quickly detect conditions for survival by gaining knowledge of the environment. More specifically, Kaplan and Kaplan (1989) predict that humans have acquired a positive response to four basic informational characteristics, two of which (coherence and legibility) help one understand the environment, and the other two (complexity and mystery) encourage its exploration.

Empirical research has shown that especially mystery is a powerful predictor of landscape preference (Kaplan *et al.*, 1989b). Mystery is the promise that more information could be gained by moving deeper into the setting, as indicated by, for example, a trail disappearing, a bend in a road, meandering streams, or a view that is partially blocked by a hill. However, like arousal theory and prospect-refuge theory, information processing theory assumes that informational characteristics must act in combination for an optimal aesthetic experience. A scene must have sufficient complexity and mystery to invite the individual to gather more information, but these characteristics must be based on enough coherence and legibility to keep the scene from becoming too overwhelming (Kaplan *et al.*, 1998, see also Fig. 2.1.1).

Variations: group differences

Consistent with evolutionary theories, empirical research has shown a high degree of consensus in landscape preferences (Tveit *et al.*, 2012). However, there also exist important variations between groups and subcultures, which relate primarily to the preferred balance between nature and human influences (Konijnendijk and Van den Berg, 2012). These variations between groups and subcultures

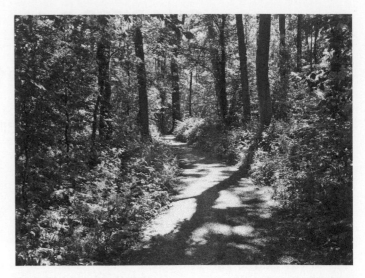

Fig. 2.1.1 A winding path adds mystery to a landscape. It makes you want to find out what is behind the bend.
Photograph reproduced courtesy of Carlo Konings, Copyright © Carlo Konings 2016.

may at least partly reflect differences in the relative strength of understanding (or refuge) and exploration (or prospect) needs (Kaplan & Kaplan, 1989). For example, the need for understanding an environment may become more salient when other aspects of one's life are temporarily or chronically less orderly and controlled, resulting in a higher preference for settings with a high degree of coherence and legibility (Koole and Van den Berg, 2005).

These insights are also relevant to people's health responses. When designing natural environments for vulnerable populations with a high need for understanding, like older people or hospital patients with acute health problems, it may be better to keep to simple designs without too much complexity or ambiguity. More information about healthy and biophilic design can be found in Chapter 8.3, 'Nature in buildings and health design'.

Psychological restoration: classic theories

A main finding of research on environmental preferences is that natural environments elicit more positive responses than built environments (Wohlwill, 1983). This finding has stimulated environmental psychologists to go beyond aesthetics and formulate theories on the beneficial, restorative functions that people derive from interacting with nature. In this section we discuss two theories, Stress Reduction Theory (SRT) and Attention Restoration Theory (ART), which have become leading theoretical frameworks for research on restorative environments.

Stress Reduction Theory

Roger Ulrich is a professor of architecture who is renowned for his research on evidence-based design of healthcare environments. In 1983, he first published his psycho-evolutionary theory on aesthetic and affective responses to natural landscapes (Ulrich, 1983), which is more commonly known as Stress Reduction Theory (SRT, Ulrich *et al.*, 1991) The theory assumes that certain environmental features and patterns elicit rapid, affective reactions (i.e. like/dislike) which occur without conscious processing. These affective reactions very quickly initiate physiological mobilization and subsequent adaptive or survival-enhancing behaviour. The environmental features or 'preferenda' that may automatically elicit positive affective reactions include the presence of natural content like vegetation and water, gross structure (e.g. symmetries), depth and spatial cues, smooth texture, a deflected vista, and the absence of threats.

What makes Ulrich's approach stand out from previously discussed evolutionary theories is that it explicitly acknowledges restoration as an adaptive need that provides a 'breather from stress', perhaps partly to restore energy to sustain behaviours to exploit food, water, or other advantages of the area (Ulrich et al., 1991). SRT makes a number of testable predictions about the restorative response. For example, it is stated that restorative influences of unthreatening natural scenes following a stressor should be evident in a shift towards a more positively toned emotional state, and in decreased levels of physiological arousal. It is also predicted that such restoration should occur fairly quickly (i.e. often within minutes rather than hours, depending on the intensity of the stress response). Furthermore, SRT maintains that 'modern humans might have a biologically prepared readiness to quickly and readily acquire restorative responses with respect to many unthreatening natural settings, but have no such preparedness for most urban or built contents and configurations' (Ulrich et al., 1991). Thus, the theory explicitly assigns a restorative advantage to natural environments over built environments.

Experiments guided by SRT have confirmed that viewing natural settings can provide more effective restoration from acute stress than viewing built scenes, as indicated by, for example, a stronger reduction in muscle tension, skin conduction, blood pressure, and heart rate, and more positive changes in self-reported affect (Laumann et al., 2003;Van den Berg et al., 2003). These restorative responses occur very quickly, usually within the first minutes after the start of exposure to nature. A prediction that has not been empirically confirmed is, however, that restorative responses are moderated by adaptive and aesthetically important features, such as a deflected vista or presence of water. Indeed, one of the first experiments (Ulrich et al., 1991) already showed that natural scenes with water were not more effective in providing restoration from stress than natural scenes without water. In general, research suggests

that nearly all kinds of nature are about equally restorative, apart from scenes that induce perceptions of danger, like unstructured, enclosed woods (Gatersleben and Andrews, 2013).

Attention Restoration Theory

While doing research among participants of wilderness programmes and members of gardening groups, Kaplan and Kaplan (1989) were struck by the general and universal positive value and meaning of nature to people. Or, in their own words (Kaplan & Kaplan, 1989): 'Trees and water, flowers and green things, the sense that the plants grow and that they will always be there—these indeed seem to be as close to universals as one can find.' The universal positive value of nature stimulated Kaplan and Kaplan to formulate a new theory on restorative experiences with nature, to complement and extend their theory on landscape preferences. Thus, Attention Restoration Theory (ART; Kaplan et al., 1989a; Kaplan, 1995) has become the most influential theory on benefits of nature for health and well-being.

While SRT considers restoration as an affect-driven process, ART emphasizes the importance of cognitive mechanisms, referring to those as 'directed attention' and 'fascination'. A core assumption of ART is that people only have a limited capacity to direct their attention to something that is not in itself captivating. The mechanism necessary to focus on things that require cognitive effort, called the central executive function, becomes depleted with prolonged or intensive use according to the theory (Kaplan and Berman, 2010). Depletion of the central executive function could result in something called mental (or attentional) fatigue. Entering a situation that does not require cognitive efforts ('directed attention') permits a fatigued person to rest and replenish the central executive function.

ART identifies four qualities of environmental experiences that would help restore mental fatigue: *being away* from daily hassles and obligations; a sense of *extent* or connectedness; *fascination* or the capacity of an environment to automatically and effortlessly draw attention; and a *compatibility* between the individual's inclinations and the characteristics of the environment (see Fig. 2.1.2). Of these four qualities, fascination is thought to play a key role by

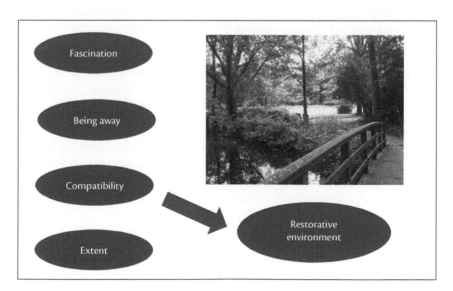

Fig. 2.1.2 The four components of Attention Restoration Theory.
Photograph reproduced courtesy of Carlo Konings, Copyright © Carlo Konings 2016.

Box 2.1.1   Hard and soft fascination

Attention Restoration Theory makes a distinction between two types of fascination or involuntary attention (Herzog *et al.*, 1997; Kaplan, 1995):

♦ Hard fascination occurs when events or activities grab attention so fully that it is hard to think about anything else. Examples include watching sport, playing violent computer games, or visiting a nightclub.

♦ Soft fascination is a more moderate form of involuntary attention that leaves room for thought and self-reflection. Soft fascination seems to be especially, but not exclusively, evoked by natural events that are pleasant to watch, like sunsets, the play of light on foliage, a butterfly flapping its wings, or the motion of the leaves in a breeze.

While soft fascination is suggested to be highly supportive of restoration from mental fatigue and stress, hard fascination would provide only very limited space and time for reflection or recovery.

Source: data from Herzog TR *et al.*, Reflection and attentional recovery as distinctive benefits of restorative environments,' *Journal of Environmental Psychology*, Volume 17, Issue 2, pp. 165-170, Copyright ©1997 Academic Press; and Kaplan S, 'The restorative benefits of nature: Toward an integrative framework,' *Journal of Environmental Psychology*, Volume 15, Issue 3, pp. 169-182, Copyright © 1995, published by Elsevier Ltd.

alleviating demands on the central executive function, with the other three enhancing or sustaining fascination (see Box 2.1.1). Because a combination of these four qualities is more commonly found in natural environments than in most built settings, natural environments tend to be more effective in countering mental fatigue. However, some built environments, like museums or monasteries, could also be conducive to restoration, albeit mainly for selective groups (Staats, 2012).

ART posits that there are four successive and progressive stages of restoration (Kaplan and Kaplan, 1989). The first stage consists of the 'clearing the head' function, which frees the mind from residual clutter. The second stage is recharging directed attention capacity. The cognitive quiet and reduced 'internal noise' gained in these initial stages of restoration prepare the person to enter the third stage of restoration, during which one can more clearly hear unbidden thoughts or matters on one's mind. The final and deepest stage involves 'reflections on one's life, on one's priorities and possibilities, on one's actions and one's goals' (Kaplan and Kaplan, 1989). It should be mentioned, however, that the claims made regarding this sequence of restorative stages have not been critically examined through empirical research.

ART provides useful insights in what happens during a single restorative experience. However, one such experience will of itself do little to promote lasting good health and well-being. In recognition of this fact, ART has highlighted the importance of cumulative effects of repeated restorative experiences with nature in the living environment. For example, Rachel Kaplan (2001, Kaplan, 1993) has discussed the cumulative value of 'micro-restorative experiences' afforded by a window view onto trees and other natural features from the home or the workplace. Consistent with this line of

reasoning, many studies have reported particularly strong relationships between green space in the living environment and public health and well-being (Groenewegen *et al.*, 2012; see also Section 3 'Public health impact by nature contact—pathways to health promotion and disease prevention' in this book).

Integration of theories

Although at first glance SRT and ART seem to offer competing theoretical perspectives, it has been argued that the theories complement, rather than speak against, each other. For example, Terry Hartig, an influential scholar who has from the outset been at the forefront of restorative environment research, has pointed out that psychophysiological stress and mental fatigue often occur independently of each other (Hartig *et al.*, 1991). Which theory is most predictive of the restoration process thus depends largely on the restorative needs of the person. If a person suffers from acute stress as indicated by elevated arousal and negative affect, exposure to nature would bring about quick psychophysiological recovery. If a person suffers from mental fatigue due to prolonged engagement in cognitively demanding activities, exposure to nature would initiate the more time-consuming process of attentional restoration. And should stress and mental fatigue coincide, which often is the case, the two theories may jointly predict the different dimensions and phases of a restorative process.

Attempts have also been made to link theories on environmental preferences with theories on restorative experiences. In particular, Henk Staats and colleagues (Hartig and Staats, 2006; Staats *et al.*, 2010) have shown that people who are in need of restoration, or imagine themselves to be so, express greater preferences for a walk in a forest or a park, over a walk in a built environment. Preferences for walking also correlated positively with ratings of the likelihood of experiencing attentional recovery during the walk. These findings have been interpreted as an indication that common preference for natural over urban environments is, at least in part, driven by the greater (perceived) restorative potential of natural environments (Van den Berg *et al.*, 2003).

Advances in environmental psychology

The area of environmental psychology has inspired much discussion and new theorizing. In this section we discuss several theoretical advancements in research on restorative environments and the health benefits of nature. Some of these have considered the basic neural mechanisms and visuospatial processes that lie behind the 'automatic affective response' and 'soft fascination'. Others have proposed alternative pathways to the restorative and health-promoting effects of nature.

Visuospatial mechanisms underlying restorative responses to nature

A common assumption of SRT and ART is that restorative responses to nature are driven by a bottom-up mechanism that is triggered by visual information. SRT proposes that there is an automatic affective response to viewing natural content based on millions of years of evolution; ART holds that natural scenes elicit soft fascination by automatically capturing attention without requiring any effort. However, both theories fall short in defining the basic neural mechanisms and visuospatial processes that lie behind the 'automatic affective response' and 'soft fascination'. Several theoretical propositions have been advanced to try and find this missing piece of the puzzle.

The Perceptual Fluency Account (PFA, Joye, 2007; Joye and Van den Berg, 2011) proposes that natural scenes evoke more positive affect and capture attention more easily than built scenes, because the visual information contained in natural scenes is processed more fluently or easily than the visual information contained in built scenes. Specifically, PFA suggests that fluent processing of natural scenes is triggered by fractal patterns that are ubiquitous in nature, but mostly absent in built environments. See Chapter 2.5, 'Biological mechanisms and neurophysiological responses to sensory impact from nature' for further insights in this topic.

A related approach, referred to as Reward Restoration Theory (RRT, Valtchanov, 2013), has linked restorative responses to the activation of reward pathways in ventral areas of the brain. These pathways are thought to be activated by mid-to-high spatial frequencies (or wavelengths) that are common to non-threatening nature scenes. Notably, mid-to-high spatial frequencies are also common to fractals, making this account highly compatible with the PFA. The predictions made by RRT are supported by a number of experiments which have demonstrated positive links between mid-to-high spatial frequencies and various measures of restoration like blink-rates, number of fixations, self-reported stress and pleasantness (Valtchanov, 2013).

Connectedness to nature

A recent theoretical approach has argued that people derive a sense of meaning and emotional well-being from being connected to the natural world (Mayer and Frantz, 2004; Schultz, 2002). This approach draws on three lines of theorizing. First, in mainstream social psychology, the need to belong to human groups and to feel like a valued member of a community has been highlighted as a basic human need (Baumeister and Leary, 1995). Second, ecologists and ecopsychologists have proposed that a sense of belonging to the broader natural community is a prerequisite for environmental protection and human well-being (Roszak et al., 1995). Third, the biophilia hypothesis (Kellert and Wilson, 1993) argues that people have a biologically based need to affiliate with and feel connected to the broader natural world.

Within this approach, several instruments have been developed to measure how connected an individual feels to nature, including the connectedness to nature scale (Mayer and Frantz, 2004), the nature relatedness scale (Nisbet and Zelenski, 2013), and the inclusion of self in nature scale (Schultz, 2002). Studies that have used these measures have shown that individuals who are highly connected to nature report higher well-being (e.g. Howell et al., 2011). In addition, it has been found that a visit to nature can strengthen people's connectedness to nature (Schultz and Tabanico, 2007). Read more about these theories and their implications in Chapter 2.6, 'The role of nature and environment in behavioural medicine'.

Learned associations and positive beliefs

Finally, we want to draw attention to an alternative explanation of restorative effects of nature in terms of learned associations. This explanation is basically a logical argument that has been referred to as the 'cognitive perspective' (Valtchanov, 2013). The cognitive perspective has no formal citation, but is often brought up as an alternative explanation for the positive effects of nature by both scholars and non-scholars alike. The argument states that, during the lifespan, modern city dwellers experience natural and built environments in different contexts, which may shape their beliefs about the restorative and healthy effects of nature. Natural environments may be experienced while on holiday, during leisure time, and when spending time with family and friends, whereas built environments are mostly experienced while at work, doing chores, and generally in more stressful circumstances. To some extent these learned associations, including environment, behaviour, and social context, may affect beliefs about the health-related characteristics of these physical environments.

Consistent with these notions, surveys in different countries have shown that the majority of the population believes that being around nature will relieve stress. For example, 95% of the Dutch population agrees with the statement that visiting nature is a useful way of relieving stress (Van den Berg et al., 2007). Thus, there exist pervasive beliefs on restorative and healthy effects of nature which may influence the way individuals respond to natural and built scenes. This explanation may be especially relevant to studies in which participants are asked to rate environments on the perceived likelihood of restoration as an alternative to assessing actual changes in restorative functioning. Such ratings are guided by beliefs, and may or may not be representative of the actual restorative potential of an environment at a given moment for a specific individual. However, they usually will give a fair approximation, because most people have experienced these outcomes on multiple occasions. Indeed, the present literature provides multiple examples of congruence between people's ratings of the restoration likelihood of natural versus built settings and outcomes of objective measures of attention and/or physiology while walking in or viewing these settings (Hartig, 2011). Moreover, positive beliefs about nature may also lead to real and measurable improvements in mental and physical health and well-being, even if they are unrealistic or illusory (Taylor et al., 2000).

Conclusion

After more than 30 years of theorizing and experimentation, we have come to understand more about the drivers of people's positive and health-promoting responses to natural environments. In this chapter, we have not covered all available theories on human–nature interactions comprehensively, but instead have focused on those that are most relevant to understanding the benefits of nature for public health. It is clear from the work presented that much progress has been made, but the expectation remains that theorizing in this area can be enhanced, extended, and deepened. Among other things, this can be achieved by making connections with relevant domains of mainstream psychology, such as work and organizational psychology where stress is a major research topic, and research on emotion regulation, which has increasingly looked at environmental strategies. Much also remains to be done to inform organizations and authorities responsible for health promotion to make realistic assessments of what nature-based interventions can and cannot do and what would be cost-efficient or not. Part of this task involves explaining how different mechanisms or 'active ingredients' of 'nature as medicine' may be combined for optimal health promotion. These theoretical developments may inform and benefit many people as they seek better health and quality of life through contact with nature in their everyday living environment.

References

Appleton, J. (1975). *The Experience of Landscape*. New York, NY: John Wiley and Sons.

Baumeister, R. F. & Leary, M. R. (1995). The need to belong: desire for interpersonal attachments as a fundamental human motivation. *Psychol Bull*, 117, 497.

Berlyne, D. E. (1960). *Conflict, Arousal, and Curiosity*. New York, NY, McGraw-Hill.

Berlyne, D. E. (1971). *Aesthetics and Psychobiology*, East Norwalk, CT: Appleton-Century-Crofts.

Gatersleben, B. & Andrews, M. (2013). When walking in nature is not restorative—The role of prospect and refuge. *Health Place*, 20, 91–101.

Groenewegen, P. P., Van den Berg, A. E., Maas, J., Verheij, R. A., & De Vries, S. (2012). Is a green residential environment better for health? If so, why? *Ann Assoc Am Geogr*, 102, 996–1003.

Hartig, T. (2011). Issues in restorative environments research: Matters of measurement. In: Fernández-Ramírez, B., Hidalgo-Villodres, C., Salvador-Ferrer, C. M., & Martos, M., M. J. (eds) *Psicología Ambiental 2011: Entre los estudios urbanos y el análisis de la sostenibilidad. Proceedings of the 11th Conference on Environmental Psychology in Spain*. Almería, Spain: University of Almería & the Spanish Association of Environmental Psychology.

Hartig, T., Mang, M., & Evans, G. W. (1991). Restorative effects of natural-environment experiences. *Environ Behav*, 23, 3–26.

Hartig, T. & Staats, H. (2006). The need for psychological restoration as a determinant of environmental preferences. *J Environ Psychol*, 26, 215–226.

Hekkert, P. (2006). Design aesthetics: principles of pleasure in design. *Psychol Sci*, 48, 157.

Herzog, T. R., Black, A. M., Fountaine, K. A., & Knotts, D. J. (1997). Reflection and attentional recovery as distinctive benefits of restorative environments. *J Environ Psychol*, 17, 165–70.

Howell, A. J., Dopko, R. L., Passmore, H.-A., & Buro, K. (2011). Nature connectedness: Associations with well-being and mindfulness. *Pers Indiv Differ*, 51, 166–71.

Joye, Y. (2007). Architectural Lessons From Environmental Psychology: The Case of Biophilic Architecture. *Rev Gen Psychol*, 11, 305–28.

Joye, Y. & Van den Berg, A. E. (2011). Is love for green in our genes? A critical analysis of evolutionary assumptions in restorative environments research. *Urban Forestry & Urban Greening*, 10, 261–8.

Kaplan, R. (1993). The role of nature in the context of the workplace. *Landscape and Urban Planning*, 26, 193–201.

Kaplan, R. (2001). The nature of the view from home—Psychological benefits. *Environ Behav*, 33, 507–42.

Kaplan, R. & Kaplan, S. (1989). *The Experience of Nature: A Psychological Perspective*. New York, NY: Cambridge University Press.

Kaplan, R., Kaplan, S., & Brown, T. (1989a). Environmental preference a comparison of four domains of predictors. *Environ Behav*, 21, 509–30.

Kaplan, R., Kaplan, S., & Brown, T. (1989b). Environmental preference: a comparison of four domains of predictors. *Environ Behav*, 21, 509–30.

Kaplan, R., Kaplan, S., & Ryan, R. (1998). *With People in Mind: Design and Management of Everyday Nature*. Washington, DC: Island Press.

Kaplan, S. (1987). Aesthetics, affect, and cognition: environmental preference from an evolutionary perspective. *Environ Behav*, 19, 3–32.

Kaplan, S. (1995). The restorative benefits of nature: Toward an integrative framework. *J Environ Psychol*, 15, 169–82.

Kaplan, S. & Berman, M. G. (2010). Directed attention as a common resource for executive functioning and self-regulation. *Perspect Psychol Sci*, 5, 43–57.

Kellert, S. R. & Wilson, E. O. (1993). *The Biophilia Hypothesis*. Washington, DC: Island Press.

Konijnendijk, C. C. & Van den Berg, A. E. (2012). Ambivalence toward nature and natural landscapes. In: Steg, E. M., Van den Berg, A. E.,

De Groot, J. I. M. (eds) *Environmental Psychology: An Introduction*. London, UK: Wiley-Blackwell.

Koole, S. L. & Van den Berg, A. E. (2005). Lost in the wilderness: Terror management, action orientation, and nature evaluation. *J Pers Soc Psychol*, 88(6), 1014–28.

Laumann, K., Garling, T., & Stormark, K. (2003). Selective attention and heart rate responses to natural and urban environments. *J Environ Psychol*, 23, 125–34.

Mayer, F. S. & Frantz, C. M. (2004). The connectedness to nature scale: A measure of individuals' feeling in community with nature. *J Environ Psychol*, 24, 503–15.

Nisbet, E. K. & Zelenski, J. M. (2013). The NR-6: a new brief measure of nature relatedness. *Front Psychol*, 4, 813.

Proshansky, H. M., Ittelson, W. H., & Rivlin, L. G. (1970). *Environmental Psychology: People and Their Physical Settings*. New York, NY: Holt, Rinehart & Winston.

Roszak, T. E., Gomes, M. E., & Kanner, A. D. (1995). *Ecopsychology: Restoring the Earth, Healing the Mind*, San Francisco, CA: Sierra Club Books.

Schultz, P. W. (2002). Inclusion with nature: The psychology of human-nature relations. In: Schmuck, P. & Schultz, P. W. (eds) *Psychology of Sustainable Development*. New York, NY: Springer.

Schultz, P. W. & Tabanico, J. (2007). Self, identity, and the natural environment: Exploring implicit connections with nature. *J Appl Soc Psychol*, 37, 1219–47.

Shafer, E. L. & Mietz, J. (1969). Aesthetic and emotional experience rate high with Northwest wilderness hikers. *Environ Behav*, 1, 187–197.

Staats, H. (2012). Restorative environments. In: Clayton, D. (ed.) *The Oxford handbook of environmental and conservation psychology*, pp. 445-458. Oxford, UK: Oxford University Press.

Staats, H., Van Gemerden, E., & Hartig, T. (2010). Preference for restorative situations: Interactive effects of attentional state, activity-in-environment, and social context. *Leisure Sciences*, 32, 401–17.

Stamps, A. E. (2008). Some findings on prospect and refuge: I. *Percept Mot Skills*, 106, 147–62.

Steg, L., Van den Berg, A. E., & De Groot, J. I. M. (2012). *Environmental Psychology: An Introduction*. London, UK: Wiley-Blackwell.

Taylor, S. E., Kemeny, M. E., Reed, G. M., Bower, J. E., & Gruenewald, T. L. (2000). Psychological resources, positive illusions, and health. *Am Psychol*, 55, 99.

Tveit, M. S., Sang, Å. O., & Hägerhäll, C. M. (2012). Scenic beauty: Visual landscape assessment and human landscape perception. In: Steg, E. M., Van Den Berg, A. E., & De Groot, J. I. M. (eds) *Environmental Psychology: An Introduction*. London, UK: Wiley-Blackwell.

Ulrich, R. S. (1983). Aesthetic and affective response to natural environment. In: Altman, I. & Wohlwill, J. F. (eds) *Human Behavior and Environment: Advances in Theory and Research, Volume 6*. New York, NY: Plenum Press.

Ulrich, R. S., Simons, R. F., Losito, B. D., Fiorito, E., Miles, M. A., & Zelson, M. (1991). Stress recovery during exposure to natural and urban environments. *J Environ Psychol*, 11, 201–30.

Valtchanov, D. (2013). *Exploring the Restorative Effects of Nature: Testing a Proposed Visuospatial Theory*. Dissertation, University of Waterloo.

Van den Berg, A. E., Hartig, T., & Staats, H. (2007). Preference for nature in urbanized societies: Stress, restoration, and the pursuit of sustainability. *J Soc Issues*, 63, 79–96.

Van den Berg, A. E., Koole, S. L., & Van Der Wulp, N. Y. (2003). Environmental preference and restoration: (How) are they related? *J Environ Psychol*, 23, 135–146.

Wohlwill, J. F. (1983). The concept of nature: A psychologist's view. In: Altman, I. & Wohlwill, J. F. (eds) *Behavior and the Natural Environment: Advances in Theory and Research, Volume 6*. New York, NY: Plenum.

CHAPTER 2.2

Therapeutic landscapes, restorative environments, place attachment, and well-being

Mardie Townsend, Claire Henderson-Wilson, Haywantee Ramkissoon, and Rona Weerasuriya

Nature and well-being

Despite health interventions and other factors contributing to reduced morbidity and mortality and increased life expectancies in much of the developed world, increasing rates of depression and other mental illnesses seem to indicate declining overall well-being. This view is supported by the definition of well-being from the US Centers for Disease Control (2013): 'Well-being is a valid population outcome measure beyond morbidity, mortality, and economic status that tells us how people perceive their life is going from their own perspective.' In the face of declining well-being, there has been over recent years an increasing recognition of the importance of contact with nature—a view which was pervasive (though at times tacit) in pre-industrial societal structures.

This chapter introduces the concepts of therapeutic landscapes, restorative environments, and place attachment and their relationships with well-being. It briefly outlines the relevance of perceptual psychology and ecopsychology for exploring explanations of people's landscape preferences and the ways in which landscapes underpin a sense of coherence in people's lives. It goes on to examine place-related challenges to health and well-being, including the changes over recent decades which have necessitated this renewed focus on therapeutic landscapes and restorative environment. The chapter then illustrates these ideas through case studies.

Key concepts

Therapeutic landscapes

Therapeutic landscapes have a long history, with evidence dating back to 406 BC highlighting nature-based approaches to treating illness (Huelat, 2003). Between the eleventh and fourteenth centuries, the predominant European source of care for the sick was monasteries, which often featured therapeutic gardens (Gerlach-Spriggs et al., 1998). The concept of 'therapeutic landscapes' has been subject to significant discussion and debate over recent decades, with cultural geographer Wilbert Gesler (1993) providing the foundations for much of this by exploring the 'environmental, individual, and societal factors that come together in the healing process in both traditional and non-traditional landscapes'. Gesler (1996) went on to note that: 'A therapeutic landscape arises when physical and built environments, social conditions and human perceptions combine to produce an atmosphere which is conducive to healing.' While Gesler's definition does not incorporate specific reference to human intention, it can be argued that in the current context the distinction between 'therapeutic landscapes' and 'restorative environments' revolves around human intention (i.e. the inclusion of a specific therapeutic goal, or set of goals in the former versus the absence of any formal therapeutic goals in the latter).

Restorative environments

The notion of 'restorative environments' is based on Attention Restoration Theory, or ART for short (Kaplan and Kaplan, 1989), which holds that 'intensive or prolonged use of directed attention, the kind that requires effort, leads to the fatigue of the mechanisms that serve it' (Herzog et al., 2003). Restorative environments are deemed to be those settings that, through escape from pressures, restful occupation of the mind, moderate or 'quiet fascination' (Kaplan, 1995), and compatibility with an individual's inclinations, the recovery of effective functioning is fostered. Read more about ART and other theories around nature and health in Chapter 2.1, 'Environmental psychology'.

Place attachment

The bonds developed between people and places are often referred to by environmental psychologists as 'place attachment' (Ramkissoon et al., 2012; Davenport and Anderson, 2005). Underpinning such attachment is people's 'sense of place', defined by Curtis and Rees Jones (1998) as 'the meaning, intention, felt value and significance that individuals or groups give to particular places'. Over time, different characterizations of the relationships between the various place-related concepts have been put forward. For example, whereas Rogan et al. (2005) see 'sense of place' as an overarching concept, under which sit 'place identity' (the cognitive dimension) and 'place attachment' (the emotive dimension), Ramkissoon et al. (2012) present a conceptual framework with place attachment as an overarching construct comprised of four subdimensions—place dependence, place identity, place affect, and place social bonding. They posit that these subdimensions of place attachment are individually and collectively associated with pro-environmental behavioural intentions, constructs, and psychological well-being (expressed as satisfaction with the environmental settings). There is a substantial body of evidence to support a link between engagement with the natural environment and pro-environmental behaviour which, in turn, contributes to the ongoing availability of natural settings for restorative purposes. For example, Ramkissoon et al. (2013a; 2013b) explore how visitors' attachment to a national park (an attitude) influences their intentions to engage in park-specific pro-environmental behaviours that can help protect and sustain the park's resources and environment. This may in turn lead to a sense of connectedness with nature, resulting in positive effects on psychological well-being (Kamitsis and Francis, 2013).

The relevance of perceptual psychology and ecopsychology

But what is it that determines the attitudes, values, and understandings outlined in the definitions above, and what disciplines can we use to shed light on such concepts? Knez and Thorsson (2008) draw on *perceptual psychology* (a subset of cognitive psychology) to highlight the fact that experience and culture influence the ways in which we perceive people, events, and places, and thus affect our attitudes and behaviours towards them. In 2009, Thomas Doherty, the founding Chief Editor of the journal *Ecopsychology* noted that people's emotional connection with the natural environment is important. He argued that ecopcyschology is rooted in environmental and conservation psychology, and draws from several studies on the relationship between humans and nature, and its restorative effects, which promotes public health and well-being (Frumkin and Jackson, 2014).

Context

It can be argued that in 2015 there is a multiplicity of external factors underpinning humans' need for therapeutic landscapes and restorative environments. These challenges to health and well-being (all of which are either place-related or have place-related flow-on effects) include: increasing urbanization and urban densification; technological developments; economic changes; and sociocultural changes.

Increasing urbanization and urban densification

This is a summary of nature–health-related issues of urbanization. For more reading on urban health and other aspects of urbanization, see Section 8 'The nature of the city'.

In recent decades, as the world's population has expanded, there has been a rapid increase in 'urbanization'—'change in size, density, and heterogeneity of cities' (Vlahov and Galea, 2002). The health and well-being implications of global urbanization are likely to include: communicable diseases related to inadequate sanitation, sewerage and waste disposal systems; transport-related injury and accidents; respiratory problems and cancers related to biological, chemical, and physical pollution of air, water, and land; non-communicable diseases related to physical inactivity or substance abuse; and creation of slums and social isolation (Baum,

2008; Butterworth, 2000; Cyril et al., 2013; Friel, 2010; Galea and Vlahov, 2005).

Specific physical aspects of urban environments which have been found to impact on residents' health and well-being include: density of developments; the mix of land uses; the scale and connectivity of street networks; the aesthetic qualities of the environment; and the availability of green spaces (Baur et al., 2013; Dannenberg et al., 2003; Galea and Vlahov, 2005). Social aspects of the urban environment have also been found to impact on residents' health and well-being. For example, social isolation can be experienced by urban residents as the density and diversity of their neighbourhood increases, yet public spaces for residents to gather, interact, and form relationships may be inadequate (Baur et al., 2013).

The importance of the preservation of natural environments and provision of natural areas within cities which could be 'restorative' was highlighted by famous American urban planner Frederick Law Olmsted in 1865. He stated that natural scenery 'employs the mind without fatigue and yet exercises it; tranquilizes it and yet enlivens it; and thus, through the influence of the mind over the body, gives the effect of refreshing rest and reinvigoration to the whole system' (Olmsted, 1865, cited in Kaplan, 1995). Given the increasing rate of urbanization, the need for restorative environments is even greater in twenty-first century urban living than it was in the context in which Olmsted was speaking.

Economic changes

Compounding (and, to a degree, reflecting) these land-use management and technological changes are economic changes. Recent evidence from Australia indicates that housing is becoming increasingly unaffordable in our major cities. The ratio of housing costs to annual income doubled between the 1960s and the beginning of the twenty-first century (Yates, 2007) and house prices are continuing to escalate in many major cities. This has implications for time-use, necessitating a growing proportion of households where both parents are involved in the paid workforce (Qu, 2008) and, consequently, the likelihood of diminished time available for non-work related activities, like being outdoors for recreation. This link is borne out in the academic literature which generally notes a correlation between increased hours of workforce participation and decreased total and leisure-time physical activity (Vandelanotte et al., 2015). Moreover, Japanese research has also demonstrated a link between greater levels of time devoted to work and lower levels of pro-environmental behaviour (Matsumoto et al., 2014), further contributing to a disconnect between humans and nature and impaired environments.

Sociocultural changes

Associated with these changes in urban environments, technologies, and economic circumstances are changes which might be grouped under the title of 'sociocultural changes'. Francis and colleagues (2012a) note that among these recent sociocultural changes are changing perceptions of neighbourhood safety and a declining sense of community. These changes are, to some extent at least (but not exclusively), influenced by the changes outlined above.

Given the complexity and the apparent enormity of these urban developmental, technological, economic, and sociocultural changes, the limited extent to which the therapeutic or restorative potential of outdoor spaces is capitalized on in modern society comes as no surprise (Francis et al., 2012a). Yet, as the following section indicates, there is growing evidence to affirm this potential, and there are strategies which could be adopted to increase the take-up of these benefits.

Evidence: case studies from Australia illustrating the links between therapeutic landscapes, restorative environments, place attachment, and well-being

Case study 1: park visitors' pro-environmental behaviour and its links to psychological well-being

A study undertaken by Ramkissoon and colleagues in 2011 used data from 452 visitors to the Dandenong Ranges National Park, Victoria, Australia. Located 35 km east of Melbourne, the park is a convenient recreational spot offering a variety of outdoor activities including picnicking, bushwalking, photography, nature study, birdwatching, car touring, cycling, and horse riding. The study used questionnaires administered face-to-face to investigate the relationship between place attachment, visitors' levels of satisfaction, and their pro-environmental behaviour.

The path relationships between the different constructs were tested using structural equation modelling, a robust statistical tool (Nunkoo *et al.*, 2013) used in social sciences. Ramkissoon *et al.* (2013a) established and confirmed the validity of place attachment as a second-order factor comprising the four subconstructs of dependence, identity, affect, and social bonding. Place attachment was found to have a significant and positive influence on the pro-environmental behavioural intentions of park visitors. An examination of the relationship between visitors' place attachment and their well-being captured by their levels of place satisfaction (e.g. I am happy visiting this national park) revealed that the former had a positive and significant influence on the latter.

In further analysis of the data by Ramkissoon and Mavondo (2014), pro-environmental behaviour was shown to mediate the relationship between place affect and visitors' satisfaction levels. This implies that visitors with more experience in natural settings have stronger levels of place affect, which may enhance their psychological well-being as compared with those with lesser experience. The largest statistically significant mediating effect of visitors' pro-environmental behaviour in Ramkissoon and Mavondo's (2014) analysis was on the relationship between visitors' levels of place identity and their satisfaction with the park. These findings suggest that maintaining a place's distinctiveness and uniqueness through identification of the self with the natural environment may lead to high levels of well-being. Pro-environmental behaviour in nature-based settings can be encouraged by providing visitors with descriptions of important species of plants and their role in the environment, and emphasizing the importance of conservation and preservation of biodiversity (Ramkissoon and Mavondo, 2014).

Read more about pro-environmental behaviour and nature connectedness in Chapter 2.6 'The role of nature and environment in behavioural medicine'.

Case study 2: 'Feel Blue, Touch Green'

The 'Feel Blue, Touch Green' project was undertaken in 2005/6 by a team from Deakin University in collaboration with Barwon Health, Parks Victoria, and Surf Coast Shire, and funded by Alcoa World Alumina Australia through the People and Parks Foundation. The small pilot project involving 10 participants explored the potential of nature-based activities in a restorative setting for promoting well-being among people suffering from depression, anxiety, and related social isolation.

Anglesea Heath, located approximately 100 km to the south-west of Melbourne, provided a restorative setting for engaging participants in supported nature-based activities with Angair (the Anglesea and Airey's Inlet Society for Protection of Flora and Fauna). Participants were referred by local medical practitioners and support workers, and each participant committed to undertake at least 10 hours of supported hands-on nature-based activities over a period of six weeks. Through observation, surveys based on validated scales, and qualitative interviews with participants, the well-being effects of the project were evaluated.

According to the Emotional State Scale (ESS), which was used pre- and post-activities, participants experienced positive emotional change across all activities. These positive results in terms of the ESS were borne out in the in-depth interviews, where participants highlighted a range of positive impacts arising from the programme:

- developing skills, taking risks and confronting challenges;
- improving mental health, confidence, and sense of self-worth;
- positive cognitive changes, and stress and anxiety management;
- managing depression and depressed mood;
- improving physical health;
- building social connections; and
- improving the natural environment.

The participants reported distinct mental health and healing benefits from the ecological nature of the activities, in addition to reporting benefits from meeting environmental challenges, with an associated sense of gratification. But the restorative nature of the environment in which the activities took place was particularly highlighted in the face-to-face interviews. One participant commented: 'I need natural environments to maintain [my mental] health. I've had it with support groups and counsellors' (Weerasuriya, 2016).

The engagement in nature-based activities also promoted positive topics of conversation between participants, such as talking about nature instead of worries, and this was associated with positive cognitive changes. 'It takes the tension and focus away from myself … [and I] forget reality … This [natural environment] grabs you' (Weerasuriya, 2016).

Accompanying the positive cognitive changes from focus on self to focus on ecology were cognitive changes from anxiety to calmness. As the following quote from one participant indicates, the cognitive changes associated with becoming calm may have been associated, in part, with the 'pleasant' stimuli offered in natural environments: 'In the bush there are not a lot of intrusive noises such as electronic sounds and beeping trucks. The natural sounds are pleasant while the mechanical sounds are irritating' (Weerasuriya, 2016). This quote highlights the importance of restorative environments in the context of the modern technologically mediated world described by this participant. While this project focused on people with mental health issues, there is reason to believe that the restorative nature of such settings would have benefits for a much wider sector of the population, given the population-densified, time-pressured, and technologically mediated and rapidly changing sociocultural lives of twenty-first century citizens.

Case study 3: exploring the health and well-being experiences of staff, patients, and visitors who accessed hospital gardens in Australia

The current body of evidence which continues to grow indicates multiple health and well-being benefits from passive viewing and directly accessing nature within healthcare settings (Cooper Marcus and Barnes, 1995; Davis, 2011; Detweiler *et al.*, 2008; Ulrich, 1984). Undertaken between 2012 and 2014, this phenomenological study explored the experiences of hospital staff, patients, and visitors accessing gardens at three hospitals in the inner northern suburbs of Melbourne, Australia: Austin Hospital, Royal Talbot Rehabilitation Centre, and the Heidelberg Repatriation Hospital (Fig. 2.2.1).

It should be noted that, at the present time, it is only the garden at the Royal Talbot Rehabilitation Centre which is used 'therapeutically' (i.e. having specific therapeutic goals associated with its use), whereas the other (newer) hospital gardens at Austin Hospital and the Repatriation Hospital are currently being used more as restorative environments.

Purposive and snowball sampling techniques were employed for recruiting all 72 participants. Given the lack of research exploring the benefits of therapeutic landscapes for acquired brain injury (ABI) patients, these patients were specifically targeted during recruitment. Additionally, staff with limited access to the gardens were interviewed at baseline and later following relocation to a new ward, where more direct access to an indoor courtyard garden was provided. Face-to-face semi-structured interviews were conducted, together with the photo elicitation technique (Epstein *et al.*, 2006; Harper 2002), which was used to trigger reflection and gather richer data. The longitudinal sample comprised 14 nursing staff, bringing the total number of interviews conducted to 86.

The key findings indicated the qualities of the garden setting which afforded restoration, relaxation, and holistic healing. Being drawn into and immersed in a setting, which allowed for experiencing a sense of escape, a connection to the 'larger world', a sense of being comforted and protected, in a space which was welcoming and safe led to the experience of relaxation, rejuvenation, and an improved mood. Dealing with and regulating confronting emotions common to all the participants was reportedly made easier in

a setting which afforded these experiences. The appreciation for the connections to a 'larger world' depicting normality and the associated sense of peace afforded in the gardens is illustrated in a comment by a visitor who noted, 'I can sit here with my brother and I can have a conversation and we can hear the birds chirping and there's a sense of peace … this is connected with the real world …' (Weerasuriya, 2016).

This sense of connection to normality was seen to be enhanced particularly by the therapeutic use of the garden at the Royal Talbot Rehabilitation Centre, where patients engage in potting plants and tending the garden as part of the rehabilitation process.

One ABI patient commented: 'It's nice to know you can go out and work and help out. It's good fun.' And a visitor to the ABI Unit commented: 'I felt really excited to tell Mxxx's dad that this place was so beautiful and that the garden was here and that perhaps Mxxx would have the possibility to work in the garden; it was really, yeah it felt like, it gave us a point of hope I suppose and purpose, which I think is crucial for recovery' (Weerasuriya, 2016).

Similarly, the restorative effects of the garden reported by staff members were highlighted by a nurse who stated, 'When working in a stressful situation and when you come out and see the garden, you relax and you forget your pain and sorrows and your tiredness' (Weerasuriya, 2016). Two additional themes indicated the gardens facilitated connecting with 'living energy' and 'people'. Connections to living energy were mainly facilitated through experiencing the seasons and observing regeneration, as well as through the elements, water features, and other ornamental features placed throughout the garden. Users appreciated this experience in the context of dealing with illness, tragedy, and at times despair, as noted by a visitor: 'When you come here to the Talbot, you can go from that medical, institutional environment, straight out into a garden that is beautiful… It takes you away from that medical model, into a … sense of being a part of life again, as opposed to being a part of illness' (Weerasuriya, 2016). While observing the seasons and regeneration instilled hope, acceptance, provided perspective on life, and acknowledged the passing of time, the elements and ornaments both visually and symbolically connected to 'life' and to its positive energy.

The third theme was the connection to 'people'. Garden access both visually and directly promoted dialogue and socialization, afforded a certain degree of refuge and quiet time in private, allowed cloistered conversations in a setting which was more homelike and familiar, and offered a play space for children.

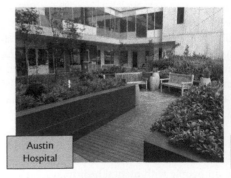
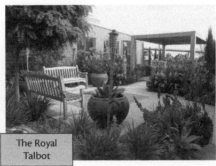
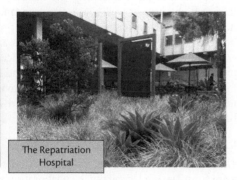

Austin Hospital

The Royal Talbot

The Repatriation Hospital

Fig. 2.2.1 The hospital gardens at Austin Health campuses, Victoria, Australia.
Photographs Copyright © Steven Wells.

Analysis of the data collected from the staff followed longitudinally, indicated that the frequency of garden access improved, when closer, more direct access was provided. Further, level of job satisfaction, perception of work environment, and perception of efficiency at work improved following relocation. While the concept of 'recommending the hospital as a workplace' was not perceived to be directly related to garden access, a number of users felt the improved quality of access would enhance their recommendation. However, it is important to note that these findings are likely to be somewhat impacted by the brand new ward environment that staff experienced following relocation.

The provision of a hospital garden has a plethora of implications at a population, ecosystem, and city planning level. The health and well-being benefits to users and consequent improvements to psychophysiological well-being and healing in a hospital context, a deeper connection with nature than otherwise observed among city dwellers, significant impacts on ecological and conservation efforts, and sustainable growth at an urbanization level is implied by these findings. The consequences of access to hospital gardens spreads far and wide across these domains.

Conclusion

In the context of societies and communities increasingly disconnected from the natural environment, societies in which technology impinges on every moment, in which mental illness is on the rise, and in which sociocultural changes are occurring at a rate beyond many humans' capacity to adapt, these case studies highlight the efficacy of reconnection with place. They highlight the restorative nature of natural environments and the potential for much greater intentional inclusion of therapeutic landscapes in treatment plans and programmes. But they also highlight the lack of awareness and understanding, in the community at large and in the healthcare community in particular, of these potentialities.

References

Baum, F. (2008). *The New Public Health*, 3rd edition. South Melbourne, Victoria: Oxford University Press.

Baur, J. W. R., Gómez, E., & Tynon, J. F. (2013). Urban Nature Parks and Neighborhood Social Health in Portland, Oregan. *JPRA*, 31, 23–44.

Butterworth, I. (2000). The relationship between the built environment and wellbeing: a literature review. Report prepared for the Victorian Health Promotion Foundation, Melbourne, Australia. Available at: https://www.vichealth.vic.gov.au/~/media/.../built_environment. ashx (accessed 17 December 2012) [Online].

Centers for Disease Control and Prevention (2013). *Health-Related Quality of Life (HRQOL): Well-Being Concepts*. Available at: http://www.cdc.gov/hrqol/wellbeing.htm#three (accessed 1 May 2015) [Online].

Cooper Marcus, C. & Barnes, M. (1995). *Gardens in Health Care Facilities: Uses, Therapeutic Benefits, and Design Recommendations*. Martinez, CA: The Center of Health Design.

Curtis, S. & Rees Jones, I. (1998). Is there a place for geography in the analysis of health inequality?. *Sociology of health & illness*, 20(5), 645–672.

Cyril, S., Oldroyd, J., & Renzaho, A. (2013). Urbanisation, urbanicity, and health: a systematic review of the reliability and validity of urbanicity scales. *BMC Public Health*, 13, 513–24.

Dannenberg, A. L., Jackson, R. J., Frumkin, H., *et al.* (2003). The impact of community design and land-use choices on public health: A scientific research agenda. *Am J Public Health*, 93, 1500–8.

Davenport, M. A. & Anderson, D. H. (2005). Getting from sense of place to place-based management: An interpretive investigation of place meanings and perceptions of landscape change. *Society & Natural Resources*, 18, 625–41.

Davis, B. E. (2011). Rooftop hospital gardens for physical therapy: a post-occupancy evaluation. *HERD*, 4, 14–43.

Detweiler, M., Murphy, P., Myers, L. & Kim, K. (2008). Does a wander garden influence inappropriate behaviors in dementia residents? *Am J Alzheimers Dis Other Demen*, 23, 31–45.

Doherty, T. J. (2009). A peer reviewed journal for ecopsychology. Editorial. *Ecopsychology*, 1, 1–7.

Epstein, I., Stevens, B., McKeever, P., & Baruchel, S. (2006). Photo elicitation interview (PEI): Using photos to elicit children's perspectives. *IJQM*, 5, 1–9.

Francis, J., Giles-Corti, B., Wood, L., & Knuiman, M. (2012a). Creating sense of community: The role of public space. *J Environ Psychol*, 32, 401–9.

Friel, S. (2010). Climate change, food insecurity and chronic diseases: sustainable and healthy policy opportunities for Australia. *NSW Public Health Bull*, 21, 129–33.

Frumkin, H. & Jackson, R. (2014). Ecopsychology and Public Health. *Ecopsychology*, 6, 131–3.

Galea, S. & Vlahov, D. (2005). Urban health: evidence, challenges, and directions. *Annu Rev Public Health*, 26, 341–65.

Gerlach-Spriggs, N., Kaufman, R. E., & Warner, S. B. Jr. (1998). *Restorative Gardens: The Healing Landscape*. New Haven, CT: Yale University Press,

Gesler, W. M. (1993). Therapeutic landscapes: medical issues in the light of the new cultural geography. *Soc Sci Med*, 34, 735–46.

Gesler, W. M. (1996). Lourdes: healing in a place of pilgrimage. *Health Place*, 2, 95–105.

Harper, D. (2002). Talking about pictures: a case for photo elicitation. *Visual Studies*, 17, 13–26.

Herzog, T. R., Maguire, C. P., & Nebel, M. B. (2003). Assessing the restorative components of environments. *J Environ Psychol*, 23, 159–70.

Huelat, B. J. (2003). *Healing Environments: Design For the Body, Mind and Spirit*. Arlington, VA: MEDEZYN in collaboration with PEECAPRESS.

Kamitsis, I. & Francis, A. (2013). Spirituality mediates the relationship between engagement with nature and psychological wellbeing. *J Environ Psychol*, 36, 136–43.

Kaplan, S. (1995). The restorative benefits of nature: towards an integrative framework. *J Environ Psychol*, 15, 169–82.

Kaplan, R. & Kaplan, S. (1989), *The Experience of Nature: A Psychological Perspective*. New York, NY: Cambridge University Press.

Knez, I. & Thorsson, S. (2008). Thermal, emotional and perceptual evaluations of a park: Cross-cultural and environmental attitude comparisons. *Building and Environment*, 43, 1483–90.

Matsumoto, T., Hiroyuki, A., & Tatsuya, H. (2014). Effects of olfactory stimulation from the fragrance of the Japanese citrus fruit yuzu (Citrus junos Sieb. ex Tanaka) on mood states and salivary chromogranin A as an endocrinologic stress marker. J Alt Complement Med, 20, 500–6.

Misra, S. & Stokols, D. (2012). Psychological and health outcomes of perceived information overload. *Environ Behav*, 44, 737–59.

Nunkoo, R., Ramkissoon, H., & Gursoy, D. (2013). Use of structural equation modeling in tourism research: past, present, and future. *J Travel Res*, 52, 759–71.

Olmsted, F. L. (1865). The value and care of parks. In: *Report to the Congress of the State of California (Reprinted in Landscape Architecture)*. 17, 20–23.

Qu, L. (2008). Work and family balance. *Family Matters*, 80, 6–8.

Ramkissoon, H. & Mavondo, F. (2014). Pro-environmental behaviour: the link between place attachment and place satisfaction. *Tourism Analysis* 19, 673–88.

Ramkissoon, H., Smith, L. G. D., & Weiler, B. (2013a). Testing the dimensionality of place attachment and its relationships with place satisfaction and pro-environmental behaviours: A structural equation modelling approach. *Tour Manage*, 36, 552–66.

Ramkissoon, H., Smith, L. G. D., & Weiler, B. (2013b). Relationship between place attachment, place satisfaction, and pro-environmental behaviour in an Australian national park. *J Sust Tour*, 21, 434–57.

Ramkissoon, H., Weiler, W. & Smith, L. (2012). Place attachment and pro-environmental behaviour in national parks: the development of a conceptual framework. *J Sust Tour*, 20, 257–76.

Rogan, R., O'Connor, M., & Horwitz, P. (2005). Nowhere to hide: Awareness and perceptions of environmental change, and their influence on relationships with place. *J Environ Psychol*, 25, 147–58.

Ulrich, R. (1984). View from a window may influence recovery from surgery. *Science*, 224, 420–1.

Väistö, J., Eloranta, A-M., Viitasalo, A., *et al.* (2014). Physical activity and sedentary behaviour in relation to cardiometabolic risk in children: cross-sectional findings from the Physical Activity and Nutrition in Children (PANIC) Study. *Int J Behav Nutr Phys Act*, 11, 55.

Vandelanotte, C., Short, C., Rockloff, M., *et al.* (2015). How do different occupational factors influence total, occupational, and leisure-time physical activity? *J Phys Act Health*, 12, 200–7.

Vlahov, D. & Galea, S. (2002). Urbanization, urbanicity, and health. *J Urban Health*, 79, S1–S12.

Weerasuriya, R. (2016), The health and wellbeing experiences accessing nature in gardens within a healthcare setting. Unpublished PhD thesis, Deakin University.

Yates, J. (2007), *Affordability and access to home ownership: past, present and future?*, National Research Venture 3: Housing affordability for lower income Australians, Research Report No. 10. Sydney, Australia: Australian Housing and Urban Research Institute.

CHAPTER 2.3

Microbes, the immune system, and the health benefits of exposure to the natural environment

Graham Rook

Nature, health, and microbial diversity

Living close to the natural rural or coastal environment, often denoted 'green' or 'blue' space, respectively, increases subjective feelings of well-being and reduces overall mortality, cardiovascular disease, and depressive symptoms (Maas *et al.*, 2006; Mitchell and Popham, 2008; Wheeler *et al.*, 2012). The beneficial effects are particularly prominent in individuals of low socioeconomic status (Maas *et al.*, 2006; Mitchell and Popham, 2008). It is often assumed that the mechanism is psychological, but the data supporting this view have often lacked the controls that would enable the reader to distinguish between an effect specific to green space, and a non-specific effect of relaxation. Moreover, the immediate relaxing effects of the natural environment might not be relevant to long-term health benefits (Rook, 2013). There are also new data suggesting that exercise, although clearly beneficial in its own right, does not entirely explain the health benefits of green space (Maas *et al.*, 2008; Lachowycz and Jones, 2013) See Chapter 3.1. Other benefits might include exposure to the sun and social interactions. Thus, the reasons for the health benefits of exposure to the natural environment are not clear and are probably numerous as discussed in this book.

This chapter sets out an alternative (or additional) explanation. We now understand that human physiology requires exposure to the natural environment because it is a crucial source of microbial biodiversity. This microbial biodiversity is necessary for the development of many organ systems and for much of our metabolism, and crucially, in the context of this chapter, it is essential for the development and regulation of the immune system.

Failure of regulation of the immune system has consequences for a wide range of chronic inflammatory disorders that are increasing in high-income countries, particularly in urban settings. Failing immunoregulation also impacts on psychiatric diseases and stress resilience (Rook *et al.*, 2014a).

Humans as ecosystems

We are not individuals (Gilbert *et al.*, 2012). A human is an ecosystem, in which there are more microbial cells than human cells, and

at least 300-fold more microbial genes than human genes (O'Hara and Shanahan, 2006). Similarly, much of 'our' metabolism, assessed from metabolites in the blood, is in fact microbial (Wikoff *et al.*, 2009). Many of these symbiotic organisms reside in the various microbiotas (microbe populations), particularly the gut microbiota which may contain 10^{14} bacteria and *archaea* (single-celled prokaryotes that despite a superficial resemblance to bacteria, represent a distinct domain of life), and an even larger number of viruses. Moreover, signals from these microbiotas are also involved in development of mammalian organ systems, including gut, immune system, bone, and brain (reviewed in McFall-Ngai *et al.*, 2013). For example, neither the brain nor the hypothalamo-pituitary-adrenal axis can develop normally in germ-free animals (Heijtz *et al.*, 2011; Sudo *et al.*, 2004).

But the primary concern of this chapter is the immune system. The complex adaptive immune system of the vertebrates probably evolved in order to cope with the dual tasks of 'farming' the microbiota, while simultaneously protecting the ecosystem from pathogens (McFall-Ngai, 2007). At birth, the immune system is like a computer with hardware (anatomical structures) and software (genetically encoded programs), but few data. The system has some 'knowledge' of self, which it acquires in the thymus gland (Klein *et al.*, 2014), and minimal knowledge of the outside world transferred via the mother *in utero*. But after birth, the immune system needs to be educated with data derived from the microbial environment.

There are at least four reasons for this requirement (Fig. 2.3.1). First, microbial signals are needed to drive development and expansion of the lymphoid system. Secondly, exposure to a broad biodiversity of organisms builds up memory of diverse molecular structures that accelerates subsequent rapid recognition of novel dangerous organisms (Su *et al.*, 2013, Naik *et al.*, 2012). (This works because all life forms share fundamental molecular building blocks (McFall-Ngai *et al.*, 2013).) Thirdly, microbial components such as peptidoglycans and lipopolysaccharide (LPS) taken in from the gut maintain background activation of the innate immune system (Clarke *et al.*, 2010). Finally, and most important in the present context, microbial inputs drive expansion of the regulatory pathways

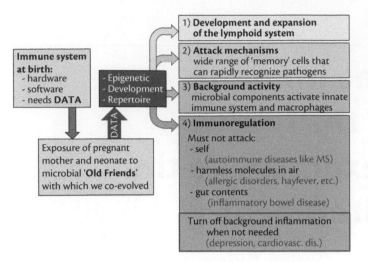

Fig. 2.3.1 Education of the immune system. At birth the immune system lacks data. Exposures to the microbiota of the mother and other people, organisms from the natural environment, and organisms with which we co-evolved (collectively designated 'old friends'), are required to expand the effector mechanisms of the immune system, provide a level of background activation, and above all, to set up the regulatory branches of the immune system. Adequate background levels of regulatory T-cells, dendritic cells, and other regulatory mechanisms are required to maintain suppression of responses to 'forbidden targets' involved in chronic inflammatory disorders, and to switch off inflammation completely when the danger is eliminated, so that pro-inflammatory mediators do not continue to circulate. Failure of immunoregulation, as indicated within rectangle 4, predisposes to many disorders that are increasing in modern urban environments.

Adapted with permission from Graham A. Rook, 'Regulation of the immune system by biodiversity from the natural environment: An ecosystem service essential to health,' *Proceedings of the National Academy of Sciences of the United States of America* (PNAS), Volume 110, Number 46, pp. 18360–18367, Copyright © 2013 PNAS.

that control the immune system and prevent it from attacking inappropriate targets (such as self, gut contents, or harmless allergens), and also shut it down when inflammation is not required.

Which organisms?

Which organisms are involved in driving the immunoregulatory circuits that are the concern of this chapter? Humans evolved as small hunter-gatherer groups colonized by the various microbiotas described in the previous section ('Humans as ecosystems'), which they obtained from their mothers and other family members. They were also exposed to microorganisms from the natural environment, some of which would have been able to establish themselves within the microbiotas (Mulder *et al.*, 2009). Finally, there were certain 'old' infections that established lifelong carrier states or subclinical infections, which were able to survive within small hunter-gatherer groups. Ancestral forms of tuberculosis, *Helicobacter pylori* (Matricardi *et al.*, 2000; Koloski *et al.*, 2008), gut helminths, and blood nematodes all fall into this category. Analysis of their phylogenetic trees and comparison with the human phylogenetic tree reveal how the old infections co-evolved and spread over the globe with human populations (Wolfe *et al.*, 2007; Comas *et al.*, 2013; Linz *et al.*, 2007).

These three categories of organism were constantly present, and had to be tolerated, and thus co-evolved roles in setting up immunoregulatory pathways. For example, blood nematodes are

powerfully immunoregulatory factors, and relatively harmless if tolerated, but aggressive immune responses that attempt (unsuccessfully) to eliminate them destroy the lymphatic system and result in elephantiasis (Babu *et al.*, 2006).

These three categories of immunoregulatory 'old friends' (microbiotas, old infections, and organisms from the natural environment) are depleted from the modern high-income urban environment by a whole range of mechanisms that are discussed below, and illustrated in Figure 2.3.2.

In sharp contrast, citizens of modern cities are exposed to more of the 'crowd infections' which evolved after human populations had expanded following the Neolithic revolution, and urbanization commenced. Crowd infections such as measles either kill the host or induce solid immunity, so they could not have survived in isolated Palaeolithic hunter-gatherer groups (Wolfe *et al.*, 2007; Black, 1966). As anticipated, therefore, epidemiological studies show that the 'crowd infections' do not drive immunoregulation, and do not protect from the chronic inflammatory disorders that are increasing in developed high-income countries (Benn *et al.*, 2004; Dunder *et al.*, 2007; Bremner *et al.*, 2008). The crowd infections are common, and increasingly so, in high-income urban communities, while modern air travel and population growth increase the threat from new crowd infections, such as avian influenza viruses.

Immunoregulatory mechanisms

Immunoregulation by the three categories of organisms (Fig. 2.3.2), collectively known as the 'old friends', has been reviewed in detail elsewhere (Rook, 2010; Rook *et al.*, 2013), but briefly, they can be shown to block or treat a wide range of chronic inflammatory disorders in animal models (Osada and Kanazawa, 2010). Although many more mechanisms remain to be revealed, several of them secrete molecules that expand regulatory T-cell (Treg) populations (Round *et al.*, 2011; Atarashi *et al.*, 2011; Grainger *et al.*, 2010), or cause dendritic cells to drive Treg rather than inflammatory effector cells (Smits *et al.*, 2005; Correale and Farez, 2013).

Unidentified organisms from the natural environment implicated in experiments with piglets also appeared to decrease gut inflammation and block inappropriate immune responses to a novel food by increasing Treg numbers (Mulder *et al.*, 2011; Lewis *et al.*, 2012). Expansion of Treg populations is notably driven by *Bacteroides fragilis*, and by two clusters of the genus *Clostridium* that are commonly found in the gut microbiota (Round *et al.*, 2011; Atarashi *et al.*, 2011).

An active immunoregulatory polysaccharide has been isolated from *B. fragilis* (Round *et al.*, 2011), as has an anti-inflammatory component of a filarial nematode. In fact, progress is being made towards developing novel drugs based on analogues of this material (Rzepecka *et al.*, 2014).

There is a possibility that immunoregulation-inducing probiotics can be used to substitute for some of these microbes, though the regulatory climate needs to be tightened so that when an immunoregulatory effect is required, strains with that specific property are used. Such strains are being identified (Poutahidis *et al.*, 2014b), but studies in humans are at a very early stage. *Lactobacillus plantarum* taken orally is able to induce changes in gene expression in the human duodenum that correlate with induction of tolerance (van Baarlen *et al.*, 2009).

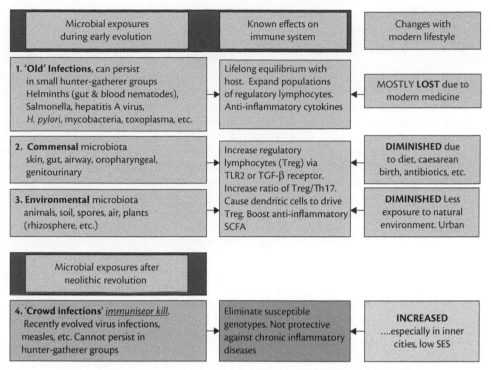

Fig. 2.3.2 Microbial 'old friends'. Humans co-evolved with the 'old infections' that could persist in isolated hunter-gatherer groups as lifelong carrier states or subclinical infections. This required activation of immunoregulatory mechanisms to avoid incapacitating the host and to limit potentially fatal immunopathology. Organisms from the natural environment (soil, animals, and so on) were abundantly present, as were the commensal microbiotas. These also had to be tolerated and drove immunoregulatory mechanisms. When human communities increased in size after the Neolithic revolution, 'crowd' infections were able to evolve, such as the childhood virus infections and influenza. These usually kill or immunize so could not persist in small hunter-gatherer groups, but can become endemic in large populations. Modern urban life reduces contact with the three categories of 'old friends' for the reasons indicated in the figure, but *increases* exposure to the crowd infections. This is particularly true of urban people of low socioeconomic status who have little opportunity for rural holidays or secondary homes.

(Treg = regulatory T-cell, TLR2 = toll-like receptor 2, TGF-β = transforming growth factor beta, SCFA = short chain fatty acid, SES = socioeconomic status.)

Adapted from Graham A. Rook *et al.*, 'What Does Immunology Have To Do With Brain Development and Neuropsychiatric Disorders,' *Brain Research*, Volume 1617, pp. 47–62, Copyright © 0006-8993/& 2014 The Authors. Published by Elsevier B.V. This is an open access article under the CC BY license (http://creativecommons.org/licenses/by/3.0/).

Although the emphasis of research has been the gut microbiota, it is clear that the microbiotas of the skin and lungs also have unique immunoregulatory roles (Whitlock and Feelisch, 2009; Naik *et al.*, 2012; Gollwitzer *et al.*, 2014).

Failed regulation of the immune system and chronic inflammation

Modern medicine deprives us of the old infections, while caesarean sections, failure to breast feed, antibiotics, and the modern lifestyle reduce exchange of human microbiota (Fig. 2.3.2). The maternal microbiota is an essential part of the infant's inheritance and many mechanisms have evolved to promote the transfer from mother to child. For example, neither the placenta nor breast milk is sterile (Aagaard *et al.*, 2014; Latuga *et al.*, 2014), and both play a role in transferring the microbiota, as obviously does birth via the female genital tract. Human behaviour tends to exacerbate the problem. For example babies are healthier if, rather than sterilizing the pacifier (dummy) after it has fallen on the floor, mothers simply suck it clean and replace it in the infant's mouth (Hesselmar *et al.*, 2013).

Transfer of skin microbiota is also compromised by modern life. Triclosan (an antibacterial and antifungal agent added to many contemporary soaps, shampoos, deodorants, toothpastes, mouthwashes, and cleaning materials) and alkylbenzene sulphonate

detergents are extremely toxic to ammonia-oxidizing bacteria that might have colonized the skin in hunter-gatherer times (Whitlock and Feelisch, 2009). Meanwhile, we live in air-conditioned buildings with little exposure to organisms from the natural environment.

When the microbial inputs fail, regulation of the immune system is impaired, and the risks of several types of inflammatory disorder increase. The high-income countries, particularly urban centres within those countries, have been undergoing explosive increases in the incidences of disorders that are at least partly attributable to failure of immunoregulation (Bach, 2002; Rook *et al.*, 2014b).

Autoimmune disease, inflammatory bowel disease, and allergies

The chronic inflammatory disorders that are increasing in high-income urban settings include autoimmune disorders such as multiple sclerosis and type 1 diabetes, which involve inappropriate immune responses to self-components (Fleming, 2013). Similarly, there are dramatic increases in allergic disorders due to unnecessary immune responses to harmless allergens in air or food (Eder *et al.*, 2006).

Inflammatory bowel diseases, mainly due to damaging immune responses to the gut microbiota also increase, and patients' microbiota show reduced biodiversity (Rehman *et al.*, 2010). The same is probably true for skin disorders (Zeeuwen *et al.*, 2013). There is an abnormal microbiota and reduced diversity on skin subject to eczema, with a tendency to return to greater diversity following effective treatment (Kong *et al.*, 2012), and similar findings in psoriasis (Fahlen *et al.*, 2012).

Obesity, metabolic syndrome, and type 2 diabetes

The gut microbiota of lean and obese human individuals differ, and can transfer the tendency to leanness or adiposity to germ-free mice maintained on a standard diet (Turnbaugh *et al.*, 2006). Obesity is associated with microbiota of reduced biodiversity (Turnbaugh *et al.*, 2009). The mechanisms by which microbiota influence adiposity have been reviewed elsewhere (Karlsson *et al.*, 2013).

In an animal model, the adipogenic and pro-inflammatory effects of the Western fast food diet can be opposed by a probiotic (*Lactobacillus reuteri*) via a pathway that depends on the simultaneous presence of a normal gut microbiota, and is mediated by Treg (Poutahidis *et al.*, 2013).

Cancers associated with poorly regulated inflammation

The incidence of a number of cancers also increases in high-income urbanized settings. These include colorectal, breast, prostate, classical Hodgkin's lymphoma (HL), and acute lymphatic leukaemia of childhood (ALL) (Rook and Dalgleish, 2011; von Hertzen *et al.*, 2011). The epidemiology of these cancers is strikingly similar to that of the chronic inflammatory disorders (Greaves, 2006; Rastogi *et al.*, 2008). The probable explanation is that inflammation can enhance mutation (Colotta *et al.*, 2009) and also releases growth factors and angiogenic factors that enhance growth, vascularization, and metastasis (Porta *et al.*, 2009). Interestingly, nonsteroidal anti-inflammatory agents, including aspirin and specific cycloxygenase-2 (COX-2) inhibitors such as celecoxib, reduce the risk of developing colon and breast cancer and reduce the mortality caused by them (Cuzick *et al.*, 2009), although the known side effects (which include gastrointestinal bleeding) limit their use. Protection from such cancers can be demonstrated in animal models where immunoregulation-inducing organisms can oppose or even treat neoplasia (Erdman *et al.*, 2010; Lakritz *et al.*, 2013; Poutahidis *et al.*, 2014a).

Chronic background inflammation manifested as raised C-reactive protein

When no inflammation is required, the immune system should become quiescent, and C-reactive protein (CRP), a good biomarker of background inflammatory activity, should fall to almost zero. This is seen in low-income developing country settings, where episodes of infection lead to high CRP levels, but when the infection is cleared the immunoregulatory mechanisms switch inflammation off completely (McDade, 2012). This is in sharp contrast to the situation in the urbanized high-income settings, where the major classes of chronic inflammatory disorder have increased. Here, even in people with no apparent reason for an inflammatory response, there is often a permanently raised CRP demonstrable in longitudinal studies, indicating a failure to suppress inflammation when it is no longer required (McDade, 2012). This type of chronic failure to regulate background inflammation is dangerous and correlates with subsequent cardiovascular disease and depression (Gimeno *et al.*, 2009; Valkanova *et al.*, 2013; Rietzschel and De Buyzere, 2012).

Depression and reduced stress resilience

It is estimated that depression will become among the major causes of human disability by 2030 (Mathers and Loncar, 2006). Chronically raised levels of inflammatory mediators are routinely associated with risk of depression in high-income countries (Valkanova *et al.*, 2013; Gimeno *et al.*, 2009; Rook *et al.*, 2014b). For example, children with raised interleukin-6 (IL-6) at nine years of age are more likely to suffer from depression when aged 18 years (Khandaker *et al.*, 2014). Some of the mechanisms that link chronic low-level inflammation to depression have been reviewed elsewhere (Miller *et al.*, 2013).

It should be noted that clinical administration of the pro-inflammatory cytokine interferon-alpha (IFN-α) to treat some cancers or viral hepatitis, commonly causes depression as a side effect (Raison *et al.*, 2009). Thus decreasing exposure to microbial biodiversity, by reducing the efficiency of immunoregulatory circuits, is likely to be contributing to the increases in depression and reduced stress resilience in high-income settings (Rook *et al.*, 2013). Meanwhile, a carefully controlled experiment using functional magnetic resonance imaging (fMRI) has demonstrated that administering a fermented milk product to women can alter the brain areas responding to an emotional stimulus (Tillisch *et al.*, 2013). We do not yet know if this was an immunoregulatory effect, or some other manifestation of the gut–brain axis, but it clearly opens the door to more research.

Human microbiota and the natural environment

To what extent are reduced microbe-driven education of the immune system's regulatory pathways and reduced biodiversity of human microbiota a consequence of changes in the biodiversity of the environment in which we live, or of our exposure to it? Humans and other mammals obtain much of their microbiota from their mothers during delivery (Dominguez-Bello *et al.*, 2010), and via the milk (which is not sterile), and from family members (Jost *et al.*, 2013). However, most animal species, probably all of them, obtain a major component of their microbiota by ingesting soil (Troyer, 1984; Mulder *et al.*, 2011), and consumption of soil (geophagy) by human infants is almost certainly an evolutionary relic of this.

The gut microbiota of US citizens is different from that of Amerindian hunter-gatherers, and strikingly less biodiverse (Yatsunenko *et al.*, 2012). Although the reasons for these differences are not formally identified, evidence from studies of the effects of contact with farms, animals, and green spaces suggest that humans acquire important microbial biodiversity from the environment (Fig. 2.3.3).

Health benefits of exposure to farms

Exposure of the pregnant mother or infant to the farming environment protects the child against allergic disorders and juvenile forms of inflammatory bowel disease (Riedler *et al.*, 2001, Radon *et al.*, 2007). This protection appears to be attributable to airborne microbial biodiversity assayed in children's bedrooms (Ege *et al.*, 2011). Similarly, mere proximity to agricultural land rather than

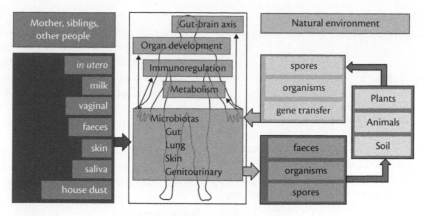

Fig. 2.3.3 Humans, microbiotas, and the natural environment. The microbiotas are provided mostly by the mother, starting *in utero* (the foetus may not be entirely sterile) but then via the vaginal microbiota and breastfeeding (breast milk is not sterile), and transfer from faeces, skin, saliva (kissing), and so on. These microbiotas play essential roles in organ development, metabolism, the gut–brain axis, and immunoregulation. But the ecosystem that constitutes a human is also constantly exchanging organisms, genes, and spores with the natural environment. The main text outlines the evidence that spores, microbes, and horizontal gene transfer of microbial genetic material acquired via contact with green space and animals are important for health.

to urban agglomerations increased the biodiversity of skin microbiota, reduced atopic sensitization, and increased release by blood cells of IL-10, an anti-inflammatory mediator (Hanski *et al.*, 2012). There is considerable overlap between bacterial communities that colonize the child, and those found in the dust in a child's home (Konya *et al.*, 2014).

Animals and dogs

Some of the relevant microbiota come from animals. Contact with cows and pigs in the perinatal period protects against allergic disorders (Riedler *et al.*, 2001; Sozanska *et al.*, 2013). Contact with dogs, with which humans have co-evolved for many millennia (Axelsson *et al.*, 2013; Thalmann *et al.*, 2013), also protects from allergic disorders (Ownby *et al.*, 2002; Aichbhaumik *et al.*, 2008). People share their microbiota via dogs (Song *et al.*, 2013), which greatly increase the microbial biodiversity of the home (Fujimura *et al.*, 2010; Dunn *et al.*, 2013).

In a developing country, the presence of animal faeces in the home correlated with better ability to control background inflammation (CRP levels) in adulthood (McDade *et al.*, 2012), and in Russian Karelia (where the prevalence of childhood atopy is 4-fold lower, and type 1 diabetes is 6-fold lower than in Finnish Karelia), house dust contained a 7-fold higher number of clones of animal-associated species than was present in Finnish Karelian house dust (Pakarinen *et al.*, 2008).

Interestingly, when mice were gavaged with house dust from homes with dogs, there was significant restructuring of the lower gut microbiota and this was accompanied by attenuation of allergic responses to cockroach allergen (Fujimura *et al.*, 2014).

The natural environment

Particularly relevant experiments have been performed with piglets, showing that when maintained with the sow in a field they developed a characteristic gut microbiota rich in *Firmicutes*, particularly *Lactobacilli*. On the other hand, similar piglets maintained with the sow on the same diet, but in a clean indoor environment developed a gut microbiota that was deficient in *Firmicutes*, and biopsies of the gut epithelium revealed increased expression of inflammatory

genes such as type 1 interferon and Major Histocompatibility Complex class I (Mulder *et al.*, 2009). Moreover, the piglets deprived of environmental exposure had reduced numbers of regulatory T-cells (Treg) and a predisposition to making antibody following introduction of a novel food (Lewis *et al.*, 2012). This represents an elegant model of the way that human babies are reared in high-income settings with minimal contact with environmental biodiversity, and parallels the rising incidence of food allergies and other immunoregulatory abnormalities in such babies.

In a mouse model of allergy, it was noted recently that appropriate bacterial colonization of the airways during the first weeks of life could block their tendency to develop allergic response when exposed to potential allergens (Gollwitzer *et al.*, 2014).

A recent human study monitored the faecal microbiota in volunteers who consumed diets consisting entirely of animal-derived materials, or entirely of plant matter. It was noticed that the microbiota began to contain food-associated bacteria and fungi, and that many of these microbes remained viable after passing through the digestive tract and appeared to be metabolically active there (David *et al.*, 2014).

Spores

About one-third of the bacteria in the gut microbiota are spore-forming, and spores are readily demonstrable in human faeces (Hong *et al.*, 2009). Spores are remarkably resistant, and can remain viable for thousands, possibly millions of years (reviewed in Nicholson, 2002).

It has been calculated that many billions of tons of animal and human faeces are generated every year; therefore, faeces-derived spores accumulate in the natural environment and might constitute a resource that can be called upon when different metabolic requirements arise, perhaps as a result of a change of diet (David *et al.*, 2014).

Moreover, there are also spore-forming bacteria such as *Bacillus spp.* that are usually considered to be soil organisms, but which can germinate and replicate in the human gut (Hong *et al.*, 2009, discussed and referenced in Rook *et al.*, 2014b). We do not currently know how much of the human microbiota is derived from the microbial environment, but it seems likely that at least some of it comes from spores that constitute a major reservoir of microbial genetic diversity.

Horizontal gene transfer

In addition to exchange of whole organisms and spores with animals and the natural environment, we need to consider horizontal gene transfer (HGT) (Smillie *et al.*, 2011). HGT refers to the transfer of genetic material (DNA or RNA) from one organism to another by mechanisms distinct from the vertical transfer of conventional reproduction. For example, genetic material from one organism may be taken up and expressed by another, even by a different species. In some cases specialized bacterial structures, bacteriophages, or plasmids are involved in this transfer of genetic material.

HGT is common between bacteria, particularly those that are adapted for residence in the gut, and recent work has revealed the existence of a global network of HGT between members of the human microbiota, even between phylogenetically very divergent bacteria separated by billions of years of evolution. Examples include the horizontal transfer of genetic material encoding antibiotic resistance genes from soil microbes (Forsberg *et al.*, 2012). Similarly, consumption of seaweed by the Japanese induces horizontal transfer to their microbiota from the environmental microbes of genes that enable the catabolism of novel seaweed-associated carbohydrates (Hehemann *et al.*, 2012). Thus, the adaptability of the human microbiota depends upon appropriate contact with potential sources of genetic innovation and diversity, and might therefore be threatened by loss of biodiversity in the gene reservoir of environmental microbes.

Conclusion

The extraordinary dietary and environmental flexibility of humans is at least partly attributable to the fact that the natural environment is a reservoir of genetic potential. It is a resource that provides humans with genetic and metabolic flexibility, and it also provides essential data inputs to the immune system. Even when environmental microbiota do not colonize permanently, they can still modulate the immune system, as discussed elsewhere (Rook, 2013).

The massive recent progress in techniques for sequencing and identifying microorganisms has led to increased understanding of the composition-crucial roles of the various commensal microbiotas, particularly the organisms in the gut. However, the current methods fail to identify many of the organisms present, often because they have not been previously recorded. Even when species-level identification is achieved, this is not usually sufficient to ascertain whether the organism is the same *strain* as that found in the natural environment (this might require epigenetic studies), and organisms present only as spores are often neglected entirely. However, essentially all animals gain some of their microbiota from the environment, and a mass of circumstantial and correlative evidence suggests that the same is true for humans.

During the next few years we will learn a lot more about the nature and extent of the interchange of organisms and genes between the environmental and the human microbiotas. The story will be complex; we already know that the benefits of proximity to green space can depend on the precise location (Fuertes *et al.*, 2014). Humans evolved as a grassland species, which might provide

some clues in the future. Meanwhile, in addition to psychological factors, sunlight, and exercise, we can already make a strong case for the view that much of the beneficial effect of green space is attributable to contact with microbial biodiversity. Therefore we need to think about how to restore human interactions with green space. The chronic inflammatory disorders (often denoted 'non-communicable diseases' or NCDs) are a major and increasing scourge of modern urban life, particularly among people of low socioeconomic status.

The understanding that lack of appropriate microbial exposures can deregulate the immune system provides powerful new medical reasons for finding ways to incorporate green space in the design of cities.

References

Aagaard, K., Ma, J., Antony, K. M., *et al.* (2014). The placenta harbors a unique microbiome. *Sci Transl Med*, 6, 237ra65.

Aichbhaumik, N., Zoratti, E. M., Strickler, R., *et al.* (2008). Prenatal exposure to household pets influences fetal immunoglobulin E production. *Clin Exp Allergy*, 38, 1787–94.

Atarashi, K., Tanoue, T., Shima, T., *et al.* (2011). Induction of colonic regulatory t cells by indigenous clostridium species. *Science*, 331, 337–41.

Axelsson, E., Ratnakumar, A., Arendt, M. L., *et al.* (2013). The genomic signature of dog domestication reveals adaptation to a starch-rich diet. *Nature*, 495, 360–4.

Babu, S., Blauvelt, C. P., Kumaraswami, V., *et al.* (2006). Regulatory networks induced by live parasites impair both Th1 and Th2 pathways in patent lymphatic filariasis: implications for parasite persistence. *J Immunol*, 176, 3248–56.

Bach, J. F. (2002). The effect of infections on susceptibility to autoimmune and allergic diseases. *N Engl J Med*, 347, 911–20.

Benn, C. S., Melbye, M., Wohlfahrt, J., *et al.* (2004). Cohort study of sibling effect, infectious diseases, and risk of atopic dermatitis during first 18 months of life. *Brit Med J*, 328, 1223–8.

Black, F. L. (1966). Measles endemicity in insular populations: critical community size and its evolutionary implication. *J Theor Biol*, 11, 207–11.

Bremner, S. A., Carey, I. M., Dewilde, S., *et al.* (2008). Infections presenting for clinical care in early life and later risk of hay fever in two UK birth cohorts. *Allergy*, 63, 274–83.

Clarke, T. B., Davis, K. M., Lysenko, E. S., *et al.* (2010). Recognition of peptidoglycan from the microbiota by Nod1 enhances systemic innate immunity. *Nature Medicine*, 16, 228–31.

Colotta, F., Allavena, P., Sica, A., *et al.* (2009). Cancer-related inflammation, the seventh hallmark of cancer: links to genetic instability. *Carcinogenesis*, 30, 1073–81.

Comas, I., Coscolla, M., Luo, T., *et al.* (2013). Out-of-Africa migration and Neolithic coexpansion of Mycobacterium tuberculosis with modern humans. *Nat Genet*, 45, 1176–82.

Correale, J. & Farez, M. F. (2013). Parasite infections in multiple sclerosis modulate immune responses through a retinoic acid-dependent pathway. *Journal of Immunology*, 191, 3827–37.

Cuzick, J., Otto, F., Baron, J. A., *et al.* (2009). Aspirin and non-steroidal anti-inflammatory drugs for cancer prevention: an international consensus statement. *Lancet Oncol*, 10, 501–7.

David, L. A., Maurice, C. F., Carmody, R. N., *et al.* (2014). Diet rapidly and reproducibly alters the human gut microbiome. *Nature*, 505, 559–63.

Dominguez-Bello, M. G., Costello, E. K., Contreras, M., *et al.* (2010). Delivery mode shapes the acquisition and structure of the initial microbiota across multiple body habitats in newborns. *Proc Natl Acad Sci U S A*, 107, 11971–5.

Dunder, T., Tapiainen, T., Pokka, T., *et al.* (2007). Infections in child day care centers and later development of asthma, allergic rhinitis, and atopic dermatitis: prospective follow-up survey 12 years after controlled randomized hygiene intervention. *Arch Pediatr Adolesc Med*, 161, 972–7.

Dunn, R. R., Fierer, N., Henley, J. B., et al. (2013). Home life: factors structuring the bacterial diversity found within and between homes. *PLoS ONE*, 8, e64133.

Eder, W., Ege, M. J. and Von Mutius, E. (2006). The asthma epidemic. *N Engl J Med*, 355, 2226–35.

Ege, M. J., Mayer, M., Normand, A. C., et al. (2011). Exposure to environmental microorganisms and childhood asthma. *N Engl J Med*, 364, 701–9.

Erdman, S. E., Rao, V. P., Olipitz, W., et al. (2010). Unifying roles for regulatory T cells and inflammation in cancer. *Int J Cancer*, 126, 1651–65.

Fahlen, A., Engstrand, L., Baker, B. S., et al. (2012). Comparison of bacterial microbiota in skin biopsies from normal and psoriatic skin. *Arch Dermatol Res*, 304, 15–22.

Fleming, J. O. (2013). Helminth therapy and multiple sclerosis. *Int J Parasitol*, 43, 259–74.

Forsberg, K. J., Reyes, A., Wang, B., et al. (2012). The shared antibiotic resistome of soil bacteria and human pathogens. *Science*, 337, 1107–11.

Fuertes, E., Markevych, I., Von Berg, A., et al. (2014). Greenness and allergies: evidence of differential associations in two areas in Germany. *J Epidemiol Community Health*, 68, 787–90.

Fujimura, K. E., Demoor, T., Rauch, M., et al. (2014). House dust exposure mediates gut microbiome Lactobacillus enrichment and airway immune defense against allergens and virus infection. *Proc Natl Acad Sci U S A*, 111, 805–10.

Fujimura, K. E., Johnson, C. C., Ownby, D. R., et al. (2010). Man's best friend? The effect of pet ownership on house dust microbial communities. *J Allergy Clin Immunol*, 126, 410–12, 412 e1–3.

Gilbert, S. F., Sapp, J. and Tauber, A. I. (2012). A symbiotic view of life: we have never been individuals. *Q Rev Biol*, 87, 325–41.

Gimeno, D., Kivimaki, M., Brunner, E. J., et al. (2009). Associations of C-reactive protein and interleukin-6 with cognitive symptoms of depression: 12-year follow-up of the Whitehall II study. *Psychol Med*, 39, 413–23.

Gollwitzer, E. S., Saglani, S., Trompette, A., et al. (2014). Lung microbiota promotes tolerance to allergens in neonates via PD-L1. *Nat Med*, 20, 642–7.

Grainger, J. R., Smith, K. A., Hewitson, J. P., et al. (2010). Helminth secretions induce de novo T cell Foxp3 expression and regulatory function through the TGF-beta pathway. *J Exp Med*, 207, 2331–41.

Greaves, M. (2006). Infection, immune responses and the aetiology of childhood leukaemia. *Nat Rev Cancer*, 6, 193–203.

Hanski, I., Von Hertzen, L., Fyhrquist, N., et al. (2012). Environmental biodiversity, human microbiota, and allergy are interrelated. *Proc Natl Acad Sci U S A*, 109, 8334–9.

Hehemann, J. H., Kelly, A. G., Pudlo, N. A., et al. (2012). Bacteria of the human gut microbiome catabolize red seaweed glycans with carbohydrate-active enzyme updates from extrinsic microbes. *Proc Natl Acad Sci U S A*, 109, 19786–91.

Heijtz, R. D., Wang, S., Anuar, F., et al. (2011). Normal gut microbiota modulates brain development and behavior. *Proc Natl Acad Sci U S A*, 108, 3047–52.

Hesselmar, B., Sjoberg, F., Saalman, R., et al. (2013). Pacifier Cleaning Practices and Risk of Allergy Development. *Pediatrics*, 131, e1829–37.

Hong, H. A., Khaneja, R., Tam, N. M., et al. (2009). Bacillus subtilis isolated from the human gastrointestinal tract. *Res Microbiol*, 160, 134–43.

Jost, T., Lacroix, C., Braegger, C. P., et al. (2013). Vertical mother-neonate transfer of maternal gut bacteria via breastfeeding. *Environ Microbiol*, 16, 2891–904.

Karlsson, F., Tremaroli, V., Nielsen, J., et al. (2013). Assessing the human gut microbiota in metabolic diseases. *Diabetes*, 62, 3341–9.

Khandaker, G. M., Pearson, R. M., Zammit, S., et al. (2014). Association of serum interleukin 6 and c-reactive protein in childhood with depression and psychosis in young adult life: a population-based longitudinal study. *JAMA Psychiatry*, 71, 1121–8.

Klein, L., Kyewski, B., Allen, P. M., et al. (2014). Positive and negative selection of the T cell repertoire: what thymocytes see (and don't see). *Nat Rev Immunol*, 14, 377–91.

Koloski, N. A., Bret, L. and Radford-Smith, G. (2008). Hygiene hypothesis in inflammatory bowel disease: a critical review of the literature. *World J Gastroenterol*, 14, 165–73.

Kong, H. H., Oh, J., Deming, C., et al. (2012). Temporal shifts in the skin microbiome associated with disease flares and treatment in children with atopic dermatitis. *Genome Res*, 22, 850–9.

Konya, T., Koster, B., Maughan, H., et al. (2014). Associations between bacterial communities of house dust and infant gut. *Environ Res*, 131, 25–30.

Lachowycz, K. & Jones, A. P. (2013). Towards a better understanding of the relationship between greenspace and health: Development of a theoretical framework. *Landscape and Urban Planning*, 118, 62–9.

Lakritz, J. R., Poutahidis, T., Levkovich, T., et al. (2013). Beneficial bacteria stimulate host immune cells to counteract dietary and genetic predisposition to mammary cancer in mice. *Int J Cancer*, 135, 529–40.

Latuga, M. S., Stuebe, A. & Seed, P. C. (2014). A review of the source and function of microbiota in breast milk. *Semin Reprod Med*, 32, 68–73.

Lewis, M. C., Inman, C. F., Patel, D., et al. (2012). Direct experimental evidence that early-life farm environment influences regulation of immune responses. *Pediatr Allergy Immunol*, 23, 265–9.

Linz, B., Balloux, F., Moodley, Y., et al. (2007). An African origin for the intimate association between humans and Helicobacter pylori. *Nature*, 445, 915–18.

Maas, J., Verheij, R. A., Groenewegen, P. P., et al. (2006). Green space, urbanity, and health: how strong is the relation? *J Epidemiol Community Health*, 60, 587–92.

Maas, J., Verheij, R. A., Spreeuwenberg, P., et al. (2008). Physical activity as a possible mechanism behind the relationship between green space and health: a multilevel analysis. *BMC Public Health*, 8, 206.

Mathers, C. D. and Loncar, D. (2006). Projections of global mortality and burden of disease from 2002 to 2030. *PLoS Med*, 3, e442.

Matricardi, P. M., Rosmini, F., Riondino, S., et al. (2000). Exposure to foodborne and orofecal microbes versus airborne viruses in relation to atopy and allergic asthma; epidemiological study. *Brit Med J*, 320, 412–17.

McDade, T. W. (2012). Early environments and the ecology of inflammation. *Proc Natl Acad Sci U S A*, 109 (Suppl 2), 17281–8.

McDade, T. W., Tallman, P. S., Madimenos, F. C., et al. (2012). Analysis of variability of high sensitivity C-reactive protein in lowland ecuador reveals no evidence of chronic low-grade inflammation. *Am J Hum Biol*, 24, 675–81.

McFall-Ngai, M. (2007). Adaptive immunity: care for the community. *Nature*, 445, 153.

McFall-Ngai, M., Hadfield, M. G., Bosch, T. C., et al. (2013). Animals in a bacterial world, a new imperative for the life sciences. *Proc Natl Acad Sci U S A*, 110, 3229–36.

Miller, A. H., Haroon, E., Raison, C. L., et al. (2013). Cytokine targets in the brain: impact on neurotransmitters and neurocircuits. *Depress Anxiety*, 30, 297–306.

Mitchell, R. & Popham, F. (2008). Effect of exposure to natural environment on health inequalities: an observational population study. *Lancet*, 372, 1655–60.

Mulder, I. E., Schmidt, B., Lewis, M., et al. (2011). Restricting microbial exposure in early life negates the immune benefits associated with gut colonization in environments of high microbial diversity. *PLoS One*, 6, e28279.

Mulder, I. E., Schmidt, B., Stokes, C. R., et al. (2009). Environmentally-acquired bacteria influence microbial diversity and natural innate immune responses at gut surfaces. *BMC Biol*, 7, 79.

Naik, S., Bouladoux, N., Wilhelm, C., et al. (2012). Compartmentalized control of skin immunity by resident commensals. *Science*, 337, 1115–19.

Nicholson, W. L. (2002). Roles of Bacillus endospores in the environment. *Cell Mol Life Sci*, 59, 410–16.

O'Hara, A. M. & Shanahan, F. (2006). The gut flora as a forgotten organ. *EMBO Rep*, 7, 688–93.

Osada, Y. and Kanazawa, T. (2010). Parasitic helminths: new weapons against immunological disorders. *J Biomed Biotechnol*, 2010, 743–58.

Ownby, D. R., Johnson, C. C., & Peterson, E. L. (2002). Exposure to dogs and cats in the first year of life and risk of allergic sensitization at 6 to 7 years of age. *JAMA*, 288, 963–72.

Pakarinen, J., Hyvarinen, A., Salkinoja-Salonen, M., *et al.* (2008). Predominance of Gram-positive bacteria in house dust in the low-allergy risk Russian Karelia. *Environ Microbiol*, 10, 3317–25.

Porta, C., Larghi, P., Rimoldi, M., *et al.* (2009). Cellular and molecular pathways linking inflammation and cancer. *Immunobiology*, 214, 761–77.

Poutahidis, T., Kleinewietfeld, M., & Erdman, S. E. (2014a). Gut Microbiota and the Paradox of Cancer Immunotherapy. *Front Immunol*, 5, 157.

Poutahidis, T., Kleinewietfeld, M., Smillie, C., *et al.* (2013). Microbial reprogramming inhibits Western diet-associated obesity. *PLoS One*, 8, e68596.

Poutahidis, T., Springer, A., Levkovich, T., *et al.* (2014b). Probiotic microbes sustain youthful serum testosterone levels and testicular size in aging mice. *PLoS One*, 9, e84877.

Radon, K., Windstetter, D., Poluda, A. L., *et al.* (2007). Contact with farm animals in early life and juvenile inflammatory bowel disease: a case-control study. *Pediatrics*, 120, 354–61.

Raison, C. L., Borisov, A. S., Majer, M., *et al.* (2009). Activation of central nervous system inflammatory pathways by interferon-alpha: relationship to monoamines and depression. *Biol Psychiatry*, 65, 296–303.

Rastogi, T., Devesa, S., Mangtani, P., *et al.* (2008). Cancer incidence rates among South Asians in four geographic regions: India, Singapore, UK and US. *Int J Epidemiol*, 37, 147–60.

Rehman, A., Lepage, P., Nolte, A., *et al.* (2010). Transcriptional activity of the dominant gut mucosal microbiota in chronic inflammatory bowel disease patients. *J Med Microbiol*, 59, 1114–22.

Riedler, J., Braun-Fahrlander, C., Eder, W., *et al.* (2001). Exposure to farming in early life and development of asthma and allergy: a cross-sectional survey. *Lancet*, 358, 1129–33.

Rietzschel, E. & De Buyzere, M. (2012). High-sensitive C-reactive protein: universal prognostic and causative biomarker in heart disease? *Biomark Med*, 6, 19–34.

Rook, G. A. W. (2010). 99th Dahlem conference on infection, inflammation and chronic inflammatory disorders: Darwinian medicine and the 'hygiene' or 'old friends' hypothesis. *Clin Exp Immunol*, 160, 70–9.

Rook, G. A. W. (2013). Regulation of the immune system by biodiversity from the natural environment: An ecosystem service essential to health. *Proc Natl Acad Sci U S A*, 110, 18360–7.

Rook, G. A. W. & Dalgleish, A. (2011). Infection, immunoregulation and cancer. *Immunol Rev*, 240, 141–59.

Rook, G. A. W., Lowry, C. A., & Raison, C. L. (2013). Microbial Old Friends, immunoregulation and stress resilience. *Evol Med Public Health*, 2013, 46–64.

Rook, G. A. W., Lowry, C. A., & Raison, C. L. (2014a). Hygiene and other early childhood influences on the subsequent function of the immune system. *Brain Res*, 1617, 47–62.

Rook, G. A. W., Raison, C. L., & Lowry, C. A. (2014b). Microbial 'Old Friends', immunoregulation and socio-economic status. *Clin Exp Immunol*, 177, 1–12.

Round, J. L., Lee, S. M., Li, J., *et al.* (2011). The Toll-like receptor 2 pathway establishes colonization by a commensal of the human microbiota. *Science*, 332, 974–7.

Rzepecka, J., Coates, M. L., Saggar, M., *et al.* (2014). Small molecule analogues of the immunomodulatory parasitic helminth product ES-62 have anti-allergy properties. *Int J Parasitol*, 44, 669–74.

Smillie, C. S., Smith, M. B., Friedman, J., *et al.* (2011). Ecology drives a global network of gene exchange connecting the human microbiome. *Nature*, 480, 241–4.

Smits, H. H., Engering, A., Van Der Kleij, D., *et al.* (2005). Selective probiotic bacteria induce IL-10-producing regulatory T cells in vitro by modulating dendritic cell function through dendritic cell-specific intercellular adhesion molecule 3-grabbing nonintegrin. *J Allergy Clin Immunol*, 115, 1260–7.

Song, S. J., Lauber, C., Costello, E. K., *et al.* (2013). Cohabiting family members share microbiota with one another and with their dogs. *Elife*, 2, e00458.

Sozanska, B., Blaszczyk, M., Pearce, N., *et al.* (2013). Atopy and allergic respiratory disease in rural Poland before and after accession to the European Union. *J Allergy Clin Immunol*, 133, 1347–53.

Su, L. F., Kidd, B. A., Han, A., *et al.* (2013). Virus-specific CD4(+) memory-phenotype T cells are abundant in unexposed adults. *Immunity*, 38, 373–83.

Sudo, N., Chida, Y., Aiba, Y., *et al.* (2004). Postnatal microbial colonization programs the hypothalamic-pituitary-adrenal system for stress response in mice. *J Physiol*, 558, 263–75.

Thalmann, O., Shapiro, B., Cui, P., *et al.* (2013). Complete mitochondrial genomes of ancient canids suggest a European origin of domestic dogs. *Science*, 342, 871–4.

Tillisch, K., Labus, J., Kilpatrick, L., *et al.* (2013). Consumption of fermented milk product with probiotic modulates brain activity. *Gastroenterology*, 144, 1394–401, 1401 e1–4.

Troyer, K. (1984). Behavioral acquisition of the hindgut fermentation system by hatchling Iguana iguana. *Behav Ecol Sociobiol*, 14, 189–93.

Turnbaugh, P. J., Hamady, M., Yatsunenko, T., *et al.* (2009). A core gut microbiome in obese and lean twins. *Nature*, 457, 480–4.

Turnbaugh, P. J., Ley, R. E., Mahowald, M. A., *et al.* (2006). An obesity-associated gut microbiome with increased capacity for energy harvest. *Nature*, 444, 1027–31.

Valkanova, V., Ebmeier, K. P., & Allan, C. L. (2013). CRP, IL-6 and depression: a systematic review and meta-analysis of longitudinal studies. *J Affect Disord*, 150, 736–44.

van Baarlen, P., Troost, F. J., Van Hemert, S., *et al.* (2009). Differential NF-kappaB pathways induction by Lactobacillus plantarum in the duodenum of healthy humans correlating with immune tolerance. *Proc Natl Acad Sci U S A*, 106, 2371–6.

von Hertzen, L. C., Joensuu, H., & Haahtela, T. (2011). Microbial deprivation, inflammation and cancer. *Cancer Metastasis Rev*, 30, 211–23.

Wheeler, B. W., White, M., Stahl-Timmins, W., *et al.* (2012). Does living by the coast improve health and wellbeing? *Health Place*, 18, 1198–201.

Whitlock, D. R. & Feelisch, M. (2009). Soil bacteria, nitrite, and the skin. In: Rook, G. A. W. (ed.) *The Hygiene Hypothesis and Darwinian Medicine*. Basel, Switzerland: Birkhäuser.

Wikoff, W. R., Anfora, A. T., Liu, J., *et al.* (2009). Metabolomics analysis reveals large effects of gut microflora on mammalian blood metabolites. *Proc Natl Acad Sci U S A*, 106, 3698–703.

Wolfe, N. D., Dunavan, C. P., & Diamond, J. (2007). Origins of major human infectious diseases. *Nature*, 447, 279–83.

Yatsunenko, T., Rey, F. E., Manary, M. J., *et al.* (2012). Human gut microbiome viewed across age and geography. *Nature*, 486, 222–7.

Zeeuwen, P. L., Kleerebezem, M., Timmerman, H. M., *et al.* (2013). Microbiome and skin diseases. *Curr Opin Allergy Clin Immunol*, 13, 514–20.

CHAPTER 2.4

Environmental enrichment: neurophysiological responses and consequences for health

Heidi Janssen, Julie Bernhardt, Frederick R. Walker, Neil J. Spratt, Michael Pollack, Anthony J. Hannan, and Michael Nilsson

Environmental effects on disease and rehabilitation

Evidence from animal models of disease and clinical research suggests that the environment in which an individual either recovers from an acute illness, or undertakes rehabilitation for a significant brain injury, has the potential to have a significant effect on their outcome. This chapter will present current theories and evidence concerning the causal mechanisms hypothesized to be related to the favourable effects associated with health environments which enable access to stimulating and natural environments, with a particular focus on environmental enrichment. The chapter will discuss the effect of the surrounding environment in animal models of disease and brain injury, the evidence in humans supporting the benefits of environments that include multisensory stimulation and nature, and proposed mechanisms linked to the favourable outcomes observed when recovering in these stimulating environments.

Environmental enrichment in animal models

Origins

The positive and negative effects of the environment on a healthy, diseased, and more recently a degenerating neurological system, are now being seriously considered by clinicians and hospital administrators. In 1947, neuropsychologist Donald Hebb was the first to scientifically demonstrate that exposure to an enriched environment is advantageous for the mammalian brain, resulting in improvements in both motor and cognitive function. Hebb took rats from his laboratory housed in small cages with only food, nesting, and water, home to roam free in his relatively more enriched family home. When returned to the laboratory for testing, compared with those remaining in the laboratory cages, those taken home showed significant improvements in learning and memory (Hebb, 1947).

Hebb's work led to the development of a scientific model of environmental enrichment (EE) (Rosenzweig et al., 1962). Models of EE have been used in a large body of work to better understand what role both the surrounding environment (i.e. our surroundings) and our experience within it has on the developing, healthy, disease-affected, and injured brain.

EE, as it has primarily been used in research, does not include exposure to 'nature' (i.e. natural environments which incorporate sunlight, flora, changing temperatures, smells, and other sensory stimuli). Nature offers in-built complex and ever changing stimulation in which we humans as animals have evolved. Nature provides novel stimulation which has demanded a need for a process which facilitates and allows adaptation (e.g. to changing weather, vegetation, or risk of predators).

Environments which are stimulating by their novelty and complexity, as explained hereafter, appear to be important in building resilience and enabling us as a species to thrive. Hence, these experimental models of EE provide us with the opportunity to explore the importance of environmental stimulation on maintaining healthy brain function, augmenting recovery after brain injury and, to a lesser degree, to understand how our surroundings, while unwell, contribute to our overall health. Drawing on this research, it is possible to hypothesize that natural environments may be considered as inherently enriched, and therefore potentially containing similar qualities and restorative effects as traditionally used enriched environments.

Definition

In animal studies, EE describes conditions which, relative to deprived (e.g. social isolation, with one animal per cage) or standard (e.g. basic bedding and nesting materials only, with two or more animals per cage) conditions, provide greater multisensory stimulation (i.e. sensorimotor or cognitive stimulation and socialization) (Nithianantharajah and Hannan, 2006). Compared to deprived or standard conditions (see Fig. 2.4.1), enriched environments usually involve larger cages which are filled with objects and toys which are frequently changed and/or rearranged and often also include

(a)

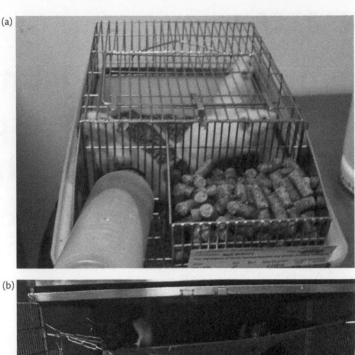

(b)

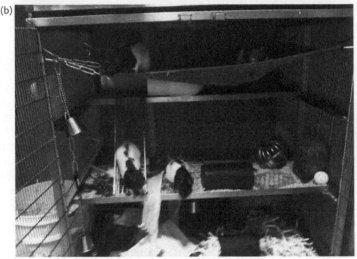

Fig. 2.4.1 Standard versus enriched environment housing in animal models. (a) Standard housing; and (b) enriched environment housing.
Reproduced courtesy of Spratt and Nilsson-Walker Laboratories.

a greater number of animals per cage ('social enrichment') (see Fig. 2.4.1b). Animals in an enriched environment are free (i.e. not forced) to voluntarily explore and engage in challenge-free interaction with each other and the cage contents (Sale *et al.*, 2009).

Sensorimotor (or sensory and physical) stimulation in an animal model of enrichment is provided via the cage contents. This may include such items as novel inanimate objects (balls and toys), horizontal boards, ladders, chains, tunnels, and ropes, thus providing increased environmental complexity. Additional voluntary 'exercise' is available due to the increased space available in the significantly larger enriched cages, and in some cases through the presence of running wheels (Nithianantharajah and Hannan, 2006). Cognitive stimulation is provided within the enriched cage through (i) the novelty of the cage contents (i.e. toys and objects not familiar to laboratory animals) and (ii) frequent removal and addition and/or rearrangement of cage contents. This enhanced environmental novelty requires enriched animals to formulate and continually update spatial maps associated with their surrounds (Nithianantharajah and Hannan, 2006). Remodelling of the cage also provides multisensory stimulation through the changing

smells, tastes, and textures. Although not commonly employed, cognitive stimulation has also been encouraged in EE models where access to food, treats or water is dependent on successful completion of mazes or tunnels within the enriched cage (Knieling *et al.*, 2009). Social stimulation is provided by increasing the number of animals per cage (Nithianantharajah and Hannan, 2006).

Effects of exposure to environmental enrichment and proposed underlying mechanisms

Healthy models

EE has been found to have a range of beneficial effects on the behaviour of healthy laboratory mice and rats (van Praag *et al.*, 2000; Nithianantharajah and Hannan, 2006). Healthy animals exposed to enriched environments generally demonstrate less anxiety, better spatial and non-spatial memory, higher levels of activity, greater exploratory behaviour, and better stimulus discrimination (Alwis and Rajan, 2014).

The neuroanatomical changes underlying these behavioural changes induced by EE in healthy laboratory rodents are many. One important change is an increase in volume of specific brain areas (e.g. neocortical regions and hippocampus). Exposure to EE results in an increase in the number and size of neurons, dendritic length and branching, and dendritic spine density. These changes are thought to contribute to the increased volume of specific brain regions. Change in dendritic morphology is accompanied by an increase in the number of synapses and synaptic connections. Specifically, hippocampal neurogenesis and neuronal survival is enhanced in enriched animals compared to animals in relatively non-enriched (standard) housing conditions (Fabel et al., 2009).

A large number of molecular changes also occur in several different brain regions following exposure to enrichment. Specifically, the brains of animals in an enriched environment show an increase in neurotrophic factors, such as brain-derived neurotrophic factor (BDNF) and nerve growth factor (NGF) and in neurotransmitters (e.g. serotonin, acetycholine, and noradrenaline), which are all important in promoting neuroplasticity. Molecular mediators of glutamatergic excitatory neurotransmission also change in brains of enriched animals. Extracellular glutamate and expression of AMPA and NMDA receptors all increase within the hippocampus (Alwis and Rajan, 2014). Lastly, EE has been shown to alter the phenotype of microglia from neurotoxic to phagocytic, reducing neuroinflammation and increasing neuroprotection (Jurgens and Johnson, 2012).

Models of neurological injury and disease and neurodegeneration

Structural changes occurring in the injured brain of enriched animals after experimental stroke are related to the process of cortical re-organization (Nilsson and Pekny, 2007). These changes within the neural circuitry are considered instrumental in the recovery of function (Nudo, 2006). Similar to healthy animals, stroke-affected animals exposed to an enriched environment have a greater number of dendritic spines, normalized astrocyte-neuron ratios, and an increase in the level of neurotrophic factors (e.g. BDNF) (Nithianantharajah and Hannan, 2006). Additionally, behavioural effects including significant improvements in sensorimotor function and a trend towards better learning are observed (Janssen et al., 2010). Similarly, use of EE in animal models of traumatic brain injury (TBI) shows reduced brain lesions, increased neuronal survival, and less neuronal degeneration in the affected cortex. This is also accompanied by better recovery of sensorimotor and cognitive function (Nithianantharajah and Hannan, 2006). These benefits are also observed in models of spinal cord injury (SCI): animals housed in enriched conditions are significantly more active and outperform animals housed in standard conditions, both (i) with and (ii) without daily forelimb and locomotor training, on a variety of neurological and functional tests (Starkey et al., 2014).

EE has been shown to delay the onset and progression of Huntington's disease (HD) in mice expressing a human HD transgene (van Dellen et al., 2000; Spires et al., 2004), augments learning and memory in transgenic mouse models of Alzheimer's disease (Nithianantharajah and Hannan, 2006) and enhances motor recovery in models of Parkinson's disease (Jadavji et al., 2006).

Additionally, EE has been shown to have beneficial effects in many models of psychiatric disorders. For example: schizophrenia (McOmish et al., 2008), post-traumatic stress disorder (Hendriksen et al., 2010), and depression (Schloesser et al., 2010). Finally, exposure to EE can reduce drug use vulnerability (and addiction) (Stairs and Bardo, 2009) and there is emerging evidence that it may play a role in inhibiting cancer growth (Cao et al., 2010) and alleviate symptoms of chronic pain (Vachon et al., 2013). We refer readers to Nithianantharajah and Hannan (2006) and Fox, Merali and Harrison (2006) for a more detailed review of EE in these and other disease models (Nithianantharajah and Hannan, 2006; Fox et al., 2006).

Proposed underlying mechanisms of effects

Exactly how EE induces this variety of beneficial effects remains unclear. It is likely to be a result of a combination of several characteristics specific to these models. One popular hypothesis is that higher levels of brain activation, a result of the multisensory stimulation and greater activity experienced by the animal, triggers the molecular cascades outlined previously, which are important for neuronal function and neuroplasticity (Fox et al., 2006; Azar et al., 2012). Specifically, one proposed mechanism is that a shift in the excitatory-inhibitory balance of the brain to one of greater excitation contributes to this experience-dependent plasticity (Alwis and Rajan, 2014). At behavioural and cognitive levels, EE can involve repeated exposure to mild stressors, and having positive and adaptive responses to such stressors may enable the development of coping strategies which build resilience, preparing the occupant for future stress. This 'stress inoculation' theory can help explain the positive effects observed in experimental models of several psychiatric conditions (Crofton et al., 2015). Refer to Alwis and Rajan (2014) and Crofton et al. (2015) for a more in-depth discussion on the proposed mechanisms (Alwis and Rajan, 2014; Crofton et al., 2015).

How do stressors within our environment affect our health?

There is evidence supporting the harmful effects of too much stress on our health in both animal models and human studies (Golbidi et al., 2015; Lagraauw et al., 2015). This and the favourable effects observed in models of EE illustrates the need to understand the role that repeated exposures to stress (or little relief from repeated stressors) may play in influencing our health within hospital and institutional care settings.

Humans have evolved in the presence of fluctuating environmental demands and have required moment-by-moment physiological changes that compensate for these varying conditions. Some of these challenges are routine (e.g. temperature fluctuation) while others can be intense, unpredictable, and life-threatening (e.g. predatory attack). While the presence of these challenges in human life has long been appreciated, it was only in the middle of the last century when it was recognized that the body may have developed a specific response mechanism to assist in meeting these challenges. Specifically, Hans Seyle proposed that the body could engage a relatively stereotypical physiological response to assist in the rapid reorientation of an organism's cognitive and physiological systems to deal with the impending challenge (Day, 2005). This mechanism has come to be known as the stress response. Read in detail about stress physiology in Chapter 1.4 'The physiology of stress and stress recovery'.

Researchers have come to differentiate between the event that causes a response in the body, and the body's actual response to it. Specifically, it is now accepted that a stressor is any stimulus (real or imagined) that substantially threatens the homeostatic balance that exists within the body, while the stress response is the reaction of the body aimed at re-establishing homeostatic balance (Day, 2005). More recently, this concept has been further extended to consider that events are stressors only if they are (i) uncontrollable and/or (ii) unpredictable and (iii) considered to be salient (Koolhaas et al., 2011; Day and Walker, 2007).

While this definition of a stressor is useful theoretically, it is also helpful to place this definition within the context of actual life events. In this respect, actual or imminent unemployment, poverty, medical illness or disability, and loss, are all frequently experienced stressors (Hammen, 2005). The intensity of these stressors can be significantly moderated by the individual's personality, coping strategies, and level of social support (Hammen, 2005).

From a biological perspective, once an event has been determined to be a stressor, the stress response is initiated. This involves significant changes in the release of a variety of molecules into the bloodstream. Of these, the most well characterized is cortisol, released from the adrenal cortex, and catecholamines, released via activation of the sympathetic nervous system (SNS) (Ulrich-Lai and Herman, 2009). These two systems work in a hand-in-hand manner, with the catecholamines acting to provide near instantaneous changes required for dealing with a challenge, and the slower acting effects of cortisol working to mobilize the body's resources for more sustained action (Ulrich-Lai and Herman, 2009).

From an evolutionary standpoint, the benefit of a biological mechanism that can rapidly provide the body with sufficient resources to deal with serious and immediate challenges appears obvious. Problems, however, can arise when the stress response is repeatedly engaged or inadequately terminated. With respect to humans, it is now well established that stress, and in particular chronic stress, is a major risk factor for a variety of diseases, including diabetes, cardiovascular diseases (including stroke), depression, autoimmune diseases, and cancer (Bercovich et al., 2014; Keinan-Boker et al., 2015; Stojanovich and Marisavljevich, 2008). Read more about stress in relation to disease in Chapter 1.4, 'The physiology of stress and stress recovery'.

In response to the very well-recognized ability of chronic stress to complicate disease processes, a variety of strategies have been deployed. While greater emphasis has been placed overall on the development of pharmacological interventions, promising environmental manipulations have also been canvassed. Of this latter class, EE has been the most intensively studied. While a detailed account of these many studies is beyond the scope of the current chapter, many studies across the course of two decades have consistently identified the ability of EE to significantly modulate stress-induced surges in circulating corticosterone (Fox et al., 2006), although the mechanism remains unclear.

Enriched environments and their role in optimizing health environments for humans

With an ageing population comes an increase in demand for health services and hence increasing need for cost-effective outcomes from the health system. Manipulating the environment to augment recovery from acute medical and more permanent and disabling neurological injury is an attractive means by which to compensate for mismatch between the availability of health resources and this growing demand. Despite favour with the concept among clinicians and the experimental evidence outlined here, a comparable human model of EE has yet to be proven effective within the clinical setting. Translation of EE into such settings is difficult for many reasons; one of which is that hospital environments and their occupants are inherently more complex than laboratory cages and the animals they house. For example, patient safety, dose of enrichment and patient personal preference for enrichment must be considered to ensure successful translation.

What is environmental enrichment for patients within a hospital environment?

As in animal models, EE for humans involves conditions in which the occupants of an environment are exposed to more multisensory stimulation; the provision of greater sensory (i.e. visual, tactile, and olfactory stimulation), physical, cognitive, and social activity. As described earlier, EE is a relative term, comparing the multisensory stimulation provided in one environment to that of another comparable environment (or, in most situations, the environment prior to applying the enrichment). One way of 'enriching' a hospital environment or applying EE within a hospital space (i.e. a hospital ward) is by adding in or providing greater access to both passive and active forms of novel and enjoyable stimulation.

Passive stimulation (i.e. passive EE) encompasses that which is added into the environment but which is not dependent on the occupant (patient) actively engaging or interacting with it. Exposure to a passive enrichment strategy may exert effects on the occupant at a subconscious level; it may result in emotional, psychological, and/or physiological responses which the occupant has very little control over. They may or may not be aware of their response to the stimulation. For example, aromas, noises, and sunlight are forms of enrichment that do not require the patient to consciously acknowledge or interact with them. The patient may consciously observe a (i) change in or (ii) distinguishing feature within their surrounding environment, but not necessarily interact with it.

Active stimulation (i.e. active EE) requires the occupant (patient) to engage or interact with the environment and/or the contents and people within it. Specifically, active EE entices the occupant to engage in activity by providing opportunities to be more physically active (e.g. exercise or move more), cognitively active (e.g. problem solve or strategize, such as when playing games), and/or socially active (e.g. interact more with people within their environment).

There are many strategies of EE which incorporate both passive and active stimulation. Cultural enrichment activities are one such example; partnered dancing, music or group singing, and gardening. These examples involve simultaneous movement (physical activity), memory and pattern recognition (cognitive activity), and socialization (social activity). They also have the added layer of stimulation of other sensory systems via touch, sound, and smell.

The challenge for translation of an enriched environment into the clinical setting is that what one person finds 'stimulating', another may not. Personalities, personal experience, and preference for and motivation to be engaged in certain types of activities varies greatly between individuals. There is also variability in the patient's ability to interact and/or communicate. Some generalizations are however possible. Recent qualitative research regarding patient preferences during their hospital stay indicates that being active, being stimulated (i.e. not bored), and having control and input into their rehabilitation is important (Luker *et al.*, 2015). Similar sentiments have been conveyed by surgical patients who identified having positive distraction, control of their immediate environment and an opportunity for socialization as priorities (Devlin *et al.*, 2016).

Although we are yet to fully understand the mechanisms by which EE exerts the cellular and functional effects observed in animal models, there is gathering evidence that it is advantageous for humans to live a more enriched life. In particular, greater exposure to multisensory stimulation and participation in physical, cognitive, and social activities is associated with delaying the onset of cognitive decline of those at risk and cognitive decline in those with dementia (Nithianantharajah and Hannan, 2011; Ruthirakuhan *et al.*, 2012). This highlights the potential advantages of creating health environments that provide interesting and engaging environments which promote activity and multisensory stimulation (i.e. passive and active sensory, physical, cognitive, and social stimulation). Providing a range of opportunities to allow patients a degree of control over their surroundings (patient choice) also appears to be important. Exposure to mild stressors in the form of sensory stimulation, novel activities, and social interactions in a controlled and supported environment may help build resilience and develop the coping mechanisms required for the future.

Evidence indicating exposure to multisensory stimulation contributes to better health outcomes

Removing people from deprived environments is important. Relocating institutionalized children and adults from impoverished environments to ones with better access to social and leisure stimulation, education, and better nutrition has contributed to significant improvements in levels of arousal and attention (Raine *et al.*, 2001) and in behaviour and cognitive function (Vogel *et al.*, 1968). Similarly, providing those with dementia with greater stimulation and in particular socialization (i.e. through better communication with staff and family and friends) in institutionalized care improves behaviour and reduces agitation (Livingston *et al.*, 2014).

Interest in applying EE within rehabilitation hospitals is growing, driven by the emerging evidence for the benefits of multisensory situation in animal models of disease and the knowledge that patients spend large amounts of their non-therapy time being inactive and alone (Janssen *et al.*, 2014a). Human equivalent models of EE for the purposes of providing multisensory stimulation have been developed with preliminary results, indicating that such models facilitate patient activity (Janssen *et al.*, 2014b) and potentially even contribute to a reduction in stress and better recovery (Khan *et al.*, 2016).

Enrichment through the use of cultural activities (i.e. dancing, art, and so on) and access to nature (i.e. sunlight, views, garden spaces) has also been incorporated into typical rehabilitation and institutional settings. In addition to efficacy in humans, dosage and timing of multisensory stimulation following acute injury or disease onset has yet to be determined. The amount and time to commencement of multisensory stimulation is likely to be different, dependent on the stage of recovery, neurological impairments and needs certain patient populations. For example, differing amounts

of certain social and sensory stimulation within the surrounding environment can 'trigger' seizure activity (of varying severity) in individuals with epilepsy (Shraiky *et al.*, 2012).

Cultural activities as enrichment improves mood and reduces the stress associated with hospital admission and institutionalization

Recovering in hospital environments in which patients feel disempowered and disconnected from the world outside (of the hospital) may contribute to the development of mood disorders. Patients experiencing low mood and/or in a state of great distress (i.e. high stress) are less likely to engage actively in rehabilitation, preventing them from achieving optimal functional recovery (Turner, 2012). Similarly, disengaged residents in institutional care living in unstimulating environments are equally at risk of deteriorating further or developing psychological disorders, losing motivation, and the ability to be independent and enjoy a good quality of life. Multisensory cultural enrichment activities implemented in these environments offer a gateway through which occupants can engage with their surroundings and normalize their hospital experience, or in the case of institutional care, engage in behaviours typical of similarly aged people living in the community. Unsurprisingly, cultural enrichment which incorporates a mixture of active and passive stimulation is enjoyed and felt to be worthwhile by most patients, residents, and staff (Drahota *et al.*, 2012; Luker *et al.*, 2015; Guzman-Garcia *et al.*, 2013).

There are behavioural and physiological benefits to including these cultural enrichment activities when used with people living with dementia. Music listening activities used with dementia patients in institutionalized care has been shown to reduce: agitation (Sung *et al.*, 2010), anxiety (Ueda *et al.*, 2013), and physically and verbally aggressive behaviour (Chang *et al.*, 2010). Similar effects have been seen when used with people who are acutely confused or have dementia, but are also acutely unwell in the hospital setting (Helmes and Wiancko, 2006). In particular, individualized or preferred music listening (and/or that known to be enjoyed by the person in earlier years) evokes memories associated with positive feelings, which soothe and prevent or alleviate agitation (Gerdner, 1997). Evidence-based guidelines have been developed concerning the use of music as a means to evoke memories and improve behaviour and the well-being of people living with dementia (Gerdner, 2013) with programmes such as 'Music & Memory' in place at numerous dementia care institutions throughout Australia, the Netherlands, and the United States (Music & Memory).

Dance and music are advantageous for recovery from cancer and surgery and when used with people undergoing neurological rehabilitation. Music movement therapy has been shown to be effective when used with women receiving breast cancer radiotherapy in reducing perceived stress and pain (Ho *et al.*, 2016). Listening to self-selected music postoperatively has been shown to reduce pain, systolic blood pressure, heart rate, and anxiety (Vetter *et al.*, 2015). Similar effects and reduced stress have been observed in patients recovering from a recent myocardial infarct (Laursen *et al.*, 2014). Dance during inpatient rehabilitation for stroke is beneficial for facilitating socialization and balance (Demers and McKinley, 2015). Self-selected music listening daily for an hour, commenced very early after stroke, has been shown to contribute to improvements in focused attention, verbal memory, and better mood two months post-event (Sarkamo *et al.*, 2008).

Creative arts (i.e. painting and literature) as active enrichment can also improve the capacity of health environments to heal. For example, stroke survivors given access to arts during a hospital stay experienced less anxiety and depression (Ali *et al.*, 2014), with the opportunity to express their emotions and engage in greater social activity (Reynolds, 2012). Art therapy, and art groups in particular, are used frequently as active enrichment for people with mental health disorders, but the evidence regarding the benefits on health outcomes has yet to be confirmed (Uttley *et al.*, 2015).

Our understanding of how engaging in multisensory stimulating enrichment cultural activities contributes to the effects outlined above is still relatively poor. More importantly, the effects this has at a physiological, and particularly for music, at a neurological level, and how these effects alter healing and health, is yet to be fully understood. Most cultural activities added into these health environments appear to be able to exert an effect on mood, often reducing stress and/or anxiety. Read more about cultural enrichment and the relation to natural enrichment in health interventions in Chapter 4.3 'Similarities, disparities, and synergies with other complex interventions—stress as a common pathway'.

EE in animal models of disease reduces stress. As observed in animals, providing patients with access to multisensory stimulation (i.e. active and passive EE) within their hospital environment or their permanent aged care residence, may in fact be very advantageous for healthy brain function and in particular for maximizing recovery following injury to the central nervous system. Increasing stimulation is, however, not always appropriate. For example, when emerging from a post-traumatic brain injury coma, tactile and visual stimulation is minimized so as to reduce patient agitation (Williams *et al.*, 1990).

Exposure to aspects of nature contributes to improved health outcomes

Nature, through its inherent complex visual, tactile, and olfactory stimulation, along with the memories and emotions it evokes, offers both passive and active environmental stimulation within a traditionally sterile clinical health setting. The inclusion and use of gardens within a healthcare environment is the most commonly used strategy to provide patients and residents with access to nature. Gardens within hospitals and institutionalized care can have therapeutic benefits by reducing stress, relieving physical symptoms, and improving a person's sense of well-being (Cooper Marcus and Barnes, 1999). Similarly to EE, gardens incorporate both (i) passive stimulation or passive experience of nature, and (ii) active stimulation or experience of nature by providing a space for interaction via horticultural/garden therapy and/or a space for physical rehabilitation (Cooper Marcus and Barnes, 1999). The specific effects of nature, as a potentially enriched environment, is covered in several sections and chapters of this book.

Architecture in health and institutional care environments

Given our deep understanding of the influence of the physical environment on behaviour in animal models, it is somewhat surprising that it is only recently that researchers in human health and disease have turned their attention to the physical or built environment in which healthcare is provided. Medical research has for many years focused primarily on the search for 'evidence-based interventions' to improve human health, with little consideration of the potential impact of the built environment on health behaviours and outcomes.

Historically, consumers of care, or the health providers themselves, have had limited ability to influence the design of new hospitals or health facilities. Building design has predominantly been in the purview of the architects, building managers, and the funders, driven largely by regulatory standards and economic constraints. Perhaps this inability to influence architecture and building design explains why health researchers have not invested much time or energy in the study of the built environment to date. Or perhaps we have simply always believed that the care we provide is the dominant driver of health outcomes, and the built environment has little role in 'wellness' or in recovery from illness.

With the advent of the 'evidence-based architecture' movement, attitudes are slowly shifting. Increased engagement of stakeholder groups in the design of healthcare spaces is changing the way we design both buildings and the services delivered within them. While it remains common for health providers to be presented with new building plans, or even a new building, as a 'fait accompli', increasingly the principles of co-design are being applied, with greater lead time allowing for meaningful stakeholder consultation. An increasing commitment to patient-centred care in much of the Western world appears to be driving greater consideration of what patients want in their built environments. Higher demands by patients and families in conjunction with the mounting experimental, and to a lesser degree clinical, evidence in support for more 'enriched environments' is influencing design.

For example, single-bed rooms are becoming increasingly common in new hospital design. There is evidence from small controlled clinical trials or strong associations in clinical studies that suggest that being cared for in a single-bed room reduces hospital-acquired infections, noise, improves sleep quality, perceived privacy, and supports family and staff interactions (Ulrich *et al.*, 2010). However, recent debate on this topic highlights that not one size fits all, and that in the United Kingdom, at least, some patients show a strong preference for multibed rooms, which they argue increases socialization and reduces isolation and boredom (Pennington and Isles, 2013). It is likely that one size does not fit all, and that in some cases the potential negative effects of a single-bed room may outweigh the potential positive effects. There is evidence in animal models of stroke that animals housed with many other conspecifics (and can therefore at least see, smell, and touch another animals) have significantly better recovery and less stress than those housed individually without any access to other animals (Venna *et al.*, 2014; Verma *et al.*, 2014). The importance of designing health environments which enable multisensory stimulation and space for rest and restoration is becoming a focus of those involved in building and managing hospitals and aged care institutions.

Conclusion

Environmental enrichment, through multisensory stimulation in models of healthy, diseased, and brain-injured animals, contributes to anatomical, morphological, and molecular changes within the brain. Beyond these cellular changes, EE also drives significant behavioural and cognitive changes. While much remains to be discovered about the specific pathways through which EE induces these changes, brain excitation and stress inoculation are likely to play a role.

Extending beyond the pre-clinical domain, it appears that EE in the form of multisensory stimulation for humans residing in health environments and institutionalized care is warranted and is likely to be advantageous for their recovery and sense of well-being. Incorporating nature and novel and engaging cultural activities as strategies to enrich the environment can provide greater opportunities for patients and residents to experience both passive and active stimulation.

Larger-scale implementation of EE in clinical domains requires further research. Firstly, to understand the mechanism by which multimodal stimulation, including passive and active engagement with nature, exerts effects on people with an injured or diseased brain. It is critical to deduce what are the minimum set of features that constitute EE, so that interventions can be modularized and deployed in a cost-effective and clinically efficient manner. Equally as important is identifying the key elements necessary to ensure successful implementation of EE for the purpose of improving patient (and resident) health outcomes and quality of life. Finally, the largest challenge will be in ensuring the sensory, physical, cognitive, and social stimulation, and the built and natural environment that facilitate and support them, address the needs at both individual and group levels in a cost-effective and sustainable manner.

References

Ali, K., Gammidge, T., & Waller, D. (2014). Fight like a ferret: a novel approach of using art therapy to reduce anxiety in stroke patients undergoing hospital rehabilitation. *Med Humanit*, 40, 56–60.

Alwis, D. S. & Rajan, R. (2014). Environmental enrichment and the sensory brain: the role of enrichment in remediating brain injury. *Front Syst Neurosci*, 8, 156.

Azar, T. A., Sharp, J. L., & Lawson, D. M. (2012). Effects of cage enrichment on heart rate, blood pressure, and activity of female Sprague-Dawley and spontaneously hypertensive rats at rest and after acute challenges. *J Am Assoc Lab Anim Sci*, 51, 339–44.

Bercovich, E., Keinan-Boker, L., & Shasha, S. M. (2014). Long-term health effects in adults born during the Holocaust. *Isr Med Assoc J*, 16, 203–7.

Cao, L., Liu, X., Lin, E. J., et al. (2010). Environmental and genetic activation of a brain-adipocyte BDNF/leptin axis causes cancer remission and inhibition. *Cell*, 142, 52–64.

Chang, F. Y., Huang, H. C., Lin, K. C., & Lin, L. C. (2010). The effect of a music programme during lunchtime on the problem behaviour of the older residents with dementia at an institution in Taiwan. *J Clin Nurs*, 19, 939–48.

Cooper Marcus, C. & Barnes, M. (1999). *Healing Gardens: Therapeutic Benefits and Design Recommendations*. New York, NY: Wiley.

Crofton, E. J., Zhang, Y., & Green, T. A. (2015). Inoculation stress hypothesis of environmental enrichment. *Neurosci Biobehav Rev*, 49, 19–31.

Day, T. A. (2005). Defining stress as a prelude to mapping its neurocircuitry: no help from allostasis. *Prog Neuropsychopharmacol Biol Psychiatry*, 29, 1195–1200.

Day, T. A. & Walker, F. R. (2007). More appraisal please: a commentary on Pfaff et al. (2007) 'Relations between mechanisms of CNS arousal and mechanisms of stress'. *Stress*, 10, 311–13; discussion 314–15.

Demers, M. & McKinley, P. (2015). Feasibility of delivering a dance intervention for subacute stroke in a rehabilitation hospital setting. *Int J Environ Res Public Health*, 12, 3120–32.

Devlin, A. S., Andrade, C. C., & Carvalho, D. (2016). Qualities of inpatient hospital rooms: patients' perspectives. *HERD*, 9, 190–211.

Drahota, A., Ward, D., Mackenzie, H., Stores, R., Higgins, B., Gal, D., & Dean, T. P. (2012). Sensory environment on health-related outcomes of hospital patients. *Cochrane Database Syst Rev*, 3, CD005315.

Fabel, K., Wolf, S. A., Ehninger, D., Babu, H., Leal-Galicia, P., & Kempermann, G. (2009). Additive effects of physical exercise and environmental enrichment on adult hippocampal neurogenesis in mice. *Front Neurosci*, 3, 50.

Fox, C., Merali, Z., & Harrison, C. (2006). Therapeutic and protective effect of environmental enrichment against psychogenic and neurogenic stress. *Behav Brain Res*, 175, 1–8.

Gerdner, L. (1997). An individualized music intervention for agitation. *J Am Psychiatr Nurses Assoc*, 3, 177–84.

Gerdner, L. (2013). *Evidence Based Guideline: Individualised Music for Persons with Dementia*, 5th edition. Standford, CA: Stanford University School of Medicine.

Golbidi, S., Frisbee, J. C., & Laher, I. (2015). Chronic stress impacts the cardiovascular system: animal models and clinical outcomes. *Am J Physiol Heart Circ Physiol*, 308, H1476–98.

Guzman-Garcia, A., Hughes, J. C., James, I. A., & Rochester, L. (2013). Dancing as a psychosocial intervention in care homes: a systematic review of the literature. *Int J Geriatr Psychiatry*, 28, 914–24.

Hammen, C. (2005). Stress and depression. *Annu Rev Clin Psychol*, 1, 293–319.

Hebb, D. O. (1947). The effects of early experience on problem solving at maturity. *Am Psychol*, 2, 306–7.

Helmes, E. & Wiancko, D. C. (2006). Effects of music in reducing disruptive behavior in a general hospital. *J Am Psychiatr Nurses Assoc*, 12, 37–44.

Hendriksen, H., Prins, J., Olivier, B., & Oosting, R. S. (2010). Environmental enrichment induces behavioral recovery and enhanced hippocampal cell proliferation in an antidepressant-resistant animal model for PTSD. *PLoS One*, 5, e11943.

Ho, R. T., Fong, T. C., Cheung, I. K., Yip, P. S., & Luk, M. Y. (2016). Effects of a short-term dance movement therapy program on symptoms and stress in patients with breast cancer undergoing radiotherapy: a randomized, controlled, single-blind trial. *J Pain Symptom Manage*, 51, 824–31.

Jadavji, N. M., Kolb, B., & Metz, G. A. (2006). Enriched environment improves motor function in intact and unilateral dopamine-depleted rats. *Neuroscience*, 140, 1127–38.

Janssen, H., Ada, L., Bernhardt, J., et al. (2014a). Physical, cognitive and social activity levels of stroke patients undergoing rehabilitation within a mixed rehabilitation unit. *Clin Rehabil*, 28, 91–101.

Janssen, H., Ada, L., Bernhardt, J., et al. (2014b). An enriched environment increases activity in stroke patients undergoing rehabilitation in a mixed rehabilitation unit: a pilot non-randomized controlled trial. *Disabil Rehabil*, 36, 255–62.

Janssen, H., Bernhardt, J., Collier, J. M., et al. (2010). An enriched environment improves sensorimotor function post-ischemic stroke. *Neurorehabil Neural Repair*, 24, 802–13.

Jurgens, H. A. & Johnson, R. W. (2012). Environmental enrichment attenuates hippocampal neuroinflammation and improves cognitive function during influenza infection. *Brain Behav Immun*, 26, 1006–16.

Keinan-Boker, L., Shasha-Lavsky, H., Eilat-Zanani, S., Edri-Shur, A., & Shasha, S. M. (2015). Chronic health conditions in Jewish Holocaust survivors born during World War II. *Isr Med Assoc J*, 17, 206–12.

Khan, F., Amatya, B., Elmalik, A., et al. (2016). An enriched environmental programme during inpatient neuro-rehabilitation: A randomized controlled trial. *J Rehabil Med*, 48, 417–25.

Knieling, M., Metz, G. A., Antonow-Schlorke, I., & Witte, O. W. (2009). Enriched environment promotes efficiency of compensatory movements after cerebral ischemia in rats. *Neuroscience*, 163, 759–69.

Koolhaas, J. M., Bartolomucci, A., Buwalda, B., et al. (2011). Stress revisited: a critical evaluation of the stress concept. *Neurosci Biobehav Rev*, 35, 1291–1301.

Lagraauw, H. M., Kuiper, J., & Bot, I. (2015). Acute and chronic psychological stress as risk factors for cardiovascular disease: Insights gained from epidemiological, clinical and experimental studies. *Brain Behav Immun*, 50, 18–30.

Laursen, J., Danielsen, A., & Rosenberg, J. (2014). Effects of environmental design on patient outcome: a systematic review. *HERD*, 7, 108–19.

Livingston, G., Kelly, L., Lewis-Holmes, E., *et al.* (2014). Non-pharmacological interventions for agitation in dementia: systematic review of randomised controlled trials. *Br J Psychiatry*, 205, 436–42.

Luker, J., Lynch, E., Bernhardsson, S., Bennett, L., & Bernhardt, J. (2015). Stroke survivors' experiences of physical rehabilitation: a systematic review of qualitative studies. *Arch Phys Med Rehabil*, 96, 1698–708 e10.

McOmish, C. E., Burrows, E., Howard, M., *et al.* (2008). Phospholipase C-beta1 knockout mice exhibit endophenotypes modeling schizophrenia which are rescued by environmental enrichment and clozapine administration. *Mol Psychiatry*, 13, 661–72.

Music & Memory. *Music & Memory* [Online]. Available at: http://musicandmemory.org (accessed 2016) [Online].

Nilsson, M. & Pekny, M. (2007). Enriched environment and astrocytes in central nervous system regeneration. *J Rehabil Med*, 39, 345–52.

Nithianantharajah, J. & Hannan, A. J. (2006). Enriched environments, experience-dependent plasticity and disorders of the nervous system. *Nat Rev Neurosci*, 7, 697–709.

Nithianantharajah, J. & Hannan, A. J. (2011). Mechanisms mediating brain and cognitive reserve: experience-dependent neuroprotection and functional compensation in animal models of neurodegenerative diseases. *Prog Neuropsychopharmacol Biol Psychiatry*, 35, 331–9.

Nudo. R. J. (2006). Plasticity. *NeuroRx*, 3, 420–7.

Pennington, H. & Isles, C. (2013). Should hospitals provide all patients with single rooms? *BMJ*, 347, f5695.

Raine, A., Venables, P. H., Cyril-Dalais, P. H., Mellingen, K., Reynolds, C., & Mednick, S. A. (2001). Early education and health enrichment at age 3–5 years is associated with increased autonomic and central nervous system arousal and orienting at age 11 years: Evidence from the Mauritius Child Health Project. *Psychophysiology*, 38, 254–66.

Reynolds, F. (2012). Art therapy after stroke: Evidence and a need for further research. *Arts Psychother*, 39, 239–44.

Rosenzweig, M. R., Krech, D., Bennett, E. L., & Diamond, M. C. (1962). Effects of environmental complexity and training on brain chemistry and anatomy: a replication and extension. *J Comp Physiol Psychol*, 55, 429–37.

Ruthirakuhan, M., Luedke, A. C., Tam, A., Goel, A., Kurji, A., & Garcia, A. (2012). Use of physical and intellectual activities and socialization in the management of cognitive decline of aging and in dementia: a review. *J Aging Res*, 2012, 384875.

Sale, A., Berardi, N., & Maffei, L. (2009). Enrich the environment to empower the brain. *Trends Neurosci*, 32, 233–9.

Sarkamo, T., Tervaniemi, M., Laitinen, S., *et al.* (2008). Music listening enhances cognitive recovery and mood after middle cerebral artery stroke. *Brain*, 131, 866–76.

Schloesser, R. J., Lehmann, M., Martinowich, K., Manji, H. K., & Herkenham, M. (2010). Environmental enrichment requires adult neurogenesis to facilitate the recovery from psychosocial stress. *Mol Psychiatry*, 15, 1152–63.

Shraiky, J., Schoonover, J., Sirven, J., & Helepololei, L. (2012). Sensory-based design & epilepsy: Analyzing effects of design innovations on patient treatment and recovery. *Enquiry: A Journal for Architectural Research*, 9.

Spires, T. L., Grote, H. E., Varshney, N. K., *et al.* (2004). Environmental enrichment rescues protein deficits in a mouse model of Huntington's disease, indicating a possible disease mechanism. *J Neurosci*, 24, 2270–6.

Stairs, D. J. & Bardo, M. T. (2009). Neurobehavioral effects of environmental enrichment and drug abuse vulnerability. *Pharmacol Biochem Behav*, 92, 377–82.

Starkey, M. L., Bleul, C., Kasper, H., *et al.* (2014). High-impact, self-motivated training within an enriched environment with single animal tracking dose-dependently promotes motor skill acquisition and functional recovery. *Neurorehabil Neural Repair*, 28, 594–605.

Stojanovich, L. & Marisavljevich, D. (2008). Stress as a trigger of autoimmune disease. *Autoimmun Rev*, 7, 209–13.

Sung, H. C., Chang, A. M., & Lee, W. L. (2010). A preferred music listening intervention to reduce anxiety in older adults with dementia in nursing homes. *J Clin Nurs*, 19, 1056–64.

Turner, J. (2012). Environmental factors of hospitalisation which contribute to post-stroke depression during rehabilitation for over 65 year olds. *JARNA*, 15, 11–15 5p.

Ueda, T., Suzukamo, Y., Sato, M., & Izumi, S. (2013). Effects of music therapy on behavioral and psychological symptoms of dementia: a systematic review and meta-analysis. *Ageing Res Rev*, 12, 628–41.

Ulrich-Lai, Y. M. & Herman, J. P. (2009). Neural regulation of endocrine and autonomic stress responses. *Nat Rev Neurosci*, 10, 397–409.

Ulrich, R. S., Berry, L. L., Quan, X., & Parish, J. T. (2010). A conceptual framework for the domain of evidence-based design. *HERD*, 4, 95–114.

Uttley, L., Stevenson, M., Scope, A., Rawdin, A., & Sutton, A. (2015). The clinical and cost effectiveness of group art therapy for people with non-psychotic mental health disorders: a systematic review and cost-effectiveness analysis. *BMC Psychiatry*, 15, 151.

Vachon, P., Millecamps, M., Low, L., *et al.* (2013). Alleviation of chronic neuropathic pain by environmental enrichment in mice well after the establishment of chronic pain. *Behav Brain Funct*, 9, 22.

van Dellen, A., Blakemore, C., Deacon, R., York, D., & Hannan, A. J. (2000). Delaying the onset of Huntington's in mice. *Nature*, 404, 721–2.

van Praag, H., Kempermann, G., & Gage, F. H. (2000). Neural consequences of environmental enrichment. *Nat Rev Neurosci*, 1, 191–8.

Venna, V. R., Xu, Y., Doran, S. J., Patrizz, A., & McCullough, L. D. (2014). Social interaction plays a critical role in neurogenesis and recovery after stroke. *Transl Psychiatry*, 4, e351.

Verma, R., Friedler, B. D., Harris, N. M., & McCullough, L. D. (2014). Pair housing reverses post-stroke depressive behavior in mice. *Behav Brain Res*, 269, 155–63.

Vetter, D., Barth, J., Uyulmaz, S., *et al.* (2015). Effects of art on surgical patients: a systematic review and meta-analysis. *Ann Surg*, 262, 704–13.

Williams, L. M., Morton, G. A., & Patrick, C. H. (1990). The Emory cubicle bed: an alternative to restraints for agitated traumatically brain injured clients. *Rehabil Nurs*, 15, 30–3.

Vogel, W., Kun, K. J., & Meshorer, E. (1968). Changes in adaptive behavior in institutionalized retardates in response to environmental enrichment or deprivation. *J Consult Clin Psychol*, 32, 76–82.

Biological mechanisms and neurophysiological responses to sensory impact from nature

Caroline Hägerhäll, Richard Taylor, Gunnar Cerwén, Greg Watts, Matilda van den Bosch, Daniel Press, and Steven Minta

Searching for the mechanisms

An increasing number of epidemiological studies demonstrate correlation and even causal relation between access to nature and improved health. However, before we can define the strength of evidence for this relation we need a better understanding of the biomechanistic explanations and what physiological reactions account for positive health effects of nature. Given the dynamics and complexity of natural environments such research is complicated, as randomized control studies are rarely plausible to pursue. Most experimental studies in the field have concerned visual input and often in very general terms from, for example photos, films, or window views. Nevertheless, some attempts have been done to study more specifically defined elements of the visual input and to monitor physiological responses to also other sensory input from nature, including smell and sound.

This chapter will outline the current understanding of human physiological responses to specific visual stimuli, sounds, and smells of nature, including mechanistic theories and biological explanations. The chapter also includes reports on recent studies using advanced neurophysiological monitoring for determining the impact of nature sensory input.

Viewing the patterns of nature

Defining what we see in nature

Most studies on the visual qualities of nature apply a broad and relatively vague definition of nature. Furthermore, there have been few attempts to investigate biological mechanisms of the visual uniqueness of nature and why viewing nature, as compared to another kind of environment, may be particularly beneficial to health. In this section we will present empirical research and discuss an explanation that is beginning to gain support, namely that the psychophysiological effects can be attributed partly to the fractal properties of the patterns found in nature (Hägerhäll, 2005; Joye and Van Den Berg, 2011).

A fractal object features patterns that recur on finer and finer scales, building shapes of immense complexity. Figure 2.5.1 shows two common examples. The branches of a tree are fractal—the patterns created by the fine-scale twigs match the coarse-scale patterns created by the thick branches. The swirling pattern within a nautilus shell is also fractal. In this second case, the rate of shrinkage is set by the golden ratio, serving as a hint to the aesthetic qualities of fractals.

Fractals are abundant in nature (Mandelbrot, 1982), but can also be found in the man-made world, for example in art (Taylor *et al.*, 1999), architecture (Bovill, 1995), landscape design (Van Tonder *et al.*, 2002), and archaeology (Brown *et al.*, 2005).

An important parameter for quantifying a fractal pattern's visual complexity is the fractal dimension, D. D describes how the patterns occurring at different magnifications combine to building the resulting fractal shape. A fractal's D-value lies between 1 and 2. By increasing the amount of fine structure in the fractal mix of repeating patterns, the D-value moves closer to 2. Thus, for fractals described by a low D-value, the small content of fine structure builds a very smooth, sparse shape. However, for fractals with a D-value closer to two, the larger content of fine structure builds a shape full of intricate, detailed structure (Taylor and Sprott, 2008).

Psychophysiological responses to visual fractal patterns

Over the past 15 years, pioneering research has built a body of consistent results showing that experiencing fractals is not only aesthetically pleasing, but also has the capacity to affect human physiology, with for example a potential to lower stress. It has been proposed that fractal patterns are easier to process than artificial shapes, and that this perceptual fluency results in positive affect, stress reduction, and attention restoration (Joye and Van Den Berg, 2011).

Empirical data is emerging that supports this theoretical claim. For instance, when the observer is engaged in free viewing of visual stimuli, their eye movements trace out a fractal trajectory quantified by mid-range D-values (Taylor *et al.*, 2011). Since mid-range

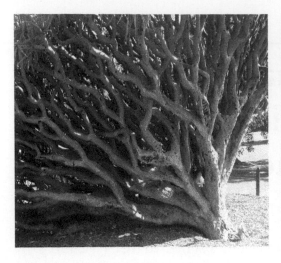
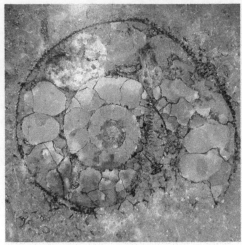
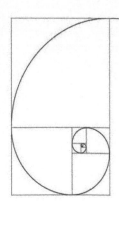

Fig. 2.5.1 Examples of fractal patterns observed in nature. The branches of a tree (left) and the swirling pattern within a nautilus shell (middle) repeat at increasingly fine size scales. The schematic on the right shows how the golden ratio sets the rate of shrinkage of the shell pattern.
Reproduced courtesy of Richard Taylor.

fractals are dominant in nature, it is plausible that the human visual system has evolved to more efficiently recognize and process these prevalent patterns. Another explanation declares that the observer has an evolved familiarity with mid-range D-fractals due to repeated exposure, an idea that draws support from functional magnetic resonance imaging (fMRI) studies showing that fractals induce activity in the regions of the brain associated with long-term memory (Taylor *et al.*, 2011).

Empirical research on natural fractals is still very limited. The authors of this chapter-section are pioneers in the field and in the following, a few of our studies are presented.

Perception studies of nature's fractal silhouettes

The starting point of our initial empirical work focused on photographs of scenery and natural phenomena, from which visually salient contours of landscape scenes were extracted. In particular, the silhouette outline between the sky and landscape was extracted from photographs. The results from these behavioural studies showed that people's preferences were higher for silhouettes of landscapes with mid-range D-values (Hägerhäll *et al.*, 2004; Hägerhäll, 2005). Furthermore, silhouettes with a D-value of 1.3 were rated as the most natural in appearance. Taken together, these results indicate that people prefer the most natural-looking fractals—those with a visual complexity that is neither too low nor too high.

However, using landscape photographs reduces the possibility of obtaining high D-silhouettes (approaching D = 2), since the amount of visual detail in the pattern is limited by the distance to the horizon and by photographic resolution limits. Furthermore, contours from real landscapes are often recognizable and may evoke subjective associations that can bias the preference judgements. To overcome these limitations, our follow-up studies moved away from fractal silhouettes extracted from photographs and instead used computer constructed, artificial fractal silhouettes.

Electroencephalogram responses to artificial fractal silhouettes

Using highly controlled sets of computer-generated fractal images (Fig. 2.5.2), we hypothesized that the preferences for mid D-fractals expressed in the perception studies would be mirrored in specific

effects on human neurophysiology. This idea was fuelled by earlier studies from the 1980s and 1990s, which highlighted preference for nature over built environments. In addition, neurophysiological measurements, such as from an electroencephalogram (EEG), found that natural environments featuring vegetation and water generated increased alpha response (Ulrich, 1981), an indicator of a wakefully relaxed state (Laufs *et al.*, 2003). Building on our hypothesis, we set out to investigate if a wakefully relaxed state could be

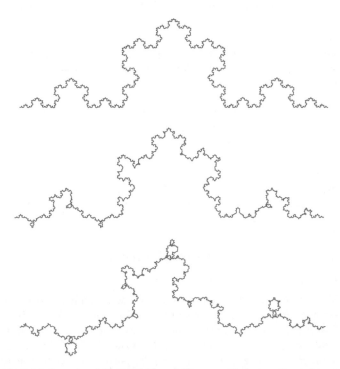

Fig. 2.5.2 Examples of the artificial fractal silhouettes. The bottom image shows an example of a natural-looking silhouette employed in the study of section 2. The top image shows an exact fractal silhouette used in the studies in section 3. The middle image shows a silhouette transitioning between the two.
Reproduced courtesy of Richard Taylor.

induced by mid-range D-fractals, using the computer-generated images of landscape silhouettes with different D-values.

Subjects were exposed to four silhouettes with D-values of 1.14, 1.32, 1.51, and 1.70. Each stimulus was shown for 60 seconds and interspaced with a neutral grey image for 30 seconds. EEG was continuously recorded. Our results revealed a significant difference in alpha response measured in the frontal area of the brain, with the highest response occurring for the silhouette with a D-value of 1.32. Hence the EEG data suggest that the positive effects of mid-range fractals extend beyond perceptual to physiological effects (Taylor *et al.*, 2011).

Natural aesthetics hypothesis, exact to statistical fractals

Fractals can serve a fascinating dual role in our visual surroundings—providing both a stimulus that evokes active interest and processing, and a stimulus that provides a visual background allowing for inward attention and restoration. Not all fractals are equal in this regard, however, and there seems to be a difference between the types of fractals we find in nature and those which are man-made.

Many man-made fractals are referred to as 'exact' because the patterns at different magnifications are exact replications of each other (Fig. 2.5.2, top image). In contrast, nature's patterns mix randomness into this fractal repetition and the patterns do not repeat exactly at different magnifications. Instead, only the statistical qualities of these natural 'statistical' fractals repeat. Consequently, the patterns at different magnifications appear similar to each other, rather than exact replications (Fig. 2.5.2, bottom image).

Computers have the capacity to generate both exact fractals and statistical fractals associated with nature. Yet most studies have been based on statistical fractals. Hence it was not known if the preferences and relaxation effects are induced by fractal geometry in general or specifically by the natural form of fractal. Hypothesizing that human responses are driven by the natural fractals, in the latest study (Hägerhäll *et al.*, 2015) we created and tested fractals of the same D-value that gradually evolved from an exact to a statistical fractal. Using a traditional fractal, the Koch curve, to generate our fractal silhouettes, we produced a set of nine curves with three different D-values (1.1, 1.3, and 1.5), which all evolved from exact to statistical in three steps. As in the previous study, we used continuous EEG recordings and an exposure time of 60 seconds for each image.

The results confirmed that responses to the two types of fractals differ, and that the natural form of fractals to a higher extent induces a relaxed state. Alpha response increased significantly as the fractal evolved from exact to statistical, and this was the case for all regions of the brain measured (the electrode positions used were F3F4, P3P4, and T5T6). The randomness that is integrated with the scaling properties in nature's statistical fractals seems to add to their visual qualities. The extra variation of the pattern may be particularly important for keeping the observer engaged in the stimulus over time. If the purpose of a pattern is to induce relaxation and attention restoration, then a pattern that holds attention, yet stays predictable and allows inward attention, would be preferable. Mid-range statistical fractals seem to offer this visual balance between predictability and unpredictability, and also between order and disorder.

The aesthetics of exact fractals

Therefore, it appears that statistical fractals offer a unique visual experience, one that triggers the aesthetic preference and relaxation associated with viewing nature's scenery. What of exact fractals? Although they follow the same generic scaling behaviour as their natural counterparts, our results indicate that this is not enough to trigger the favourable physiological impacts such as relaxation and attention restoration. What remains to be explored is the aesthetic qualities of exact fractals. Will they trigger the same preference for mid D-values as revealed by our previous studies on statistical fractals?

To date, only one minor study (Pickover, 1995) has considered the aesthetics of exact fractals. This study concentrated on relatively simple patterns formed by repeating squares and revealed a preference for high complexity patterns of D = 1.7. Perhaps the 'cleaner' visual experience generated by the exact repetition of patterns allows the viewer to accommodate a greater tolerance for complexity—so shifting preference to higher D-values, compared to the preferred mid D-values for statistical fractals? If so, it seems likely that the preferred D-value for exact fractals will not be universal, but will vary across different types of exact fractal pattern depending on their specific visual qualities. For example, the golden ratio (celebrated across art and nature for its ability to generate aesthetic patterns) can be used to create exact fractals with different D-values—demonstrating that aesthetic quality is not tied to one unique D-value.

The way forward

Our studies so far have concentrated on visual stimuli displayed on computer monitors. The next logical step is to extend these simple stimuli to make them more realistic to the viewer. Indeed, our studies of the relationship between exact and statistical fractals can be viewed as an example of moving towards a more realistic and well-defined representation of nature. The exact fractals are a simplified, 'cleaner' form of the fractals found in nature. Our studies highlighted the power of moving to the more realistic statistical fractals—these fractals induce higher levels of alpha responses than their artificial equivalents. Perhaps further positive responses will be achieved by making the fractal stimuli even more realistic replicas of nature? One approach to move further would be to use virtual reality techniques to sample subjects' responses as they walk through three-dimensional environments in which they are surrounded by fractal scenery. Will this heighten their aesthetic and physiological experiences? Will these experiences also be heightened by integrating the fractal visual experiences with tactile, olfactory, and sonic stimuli? Along these lines, the following sections present research on the sounds and smells of nature.

Soundscape

The experience of everyday sounds in the environment has been given increased attention in recent years. Whereas research has dealt primarily with the mapping of negative effects of noise, we are also beginning to understand the potential benefits inherent in the sonic environment, such as the role of nature sounds in recuperation from stress. The following section provides an introduction to sound and the concept of soundscape. The focus will then shift to sounds of nature and their known effects on human health and well-being. The section covers potential applications in environmental design, as well as healthcare.

Research on soundscape was first initiated in the 1960s. One of the pioneers was the Canadian composer Murray Schafer, who

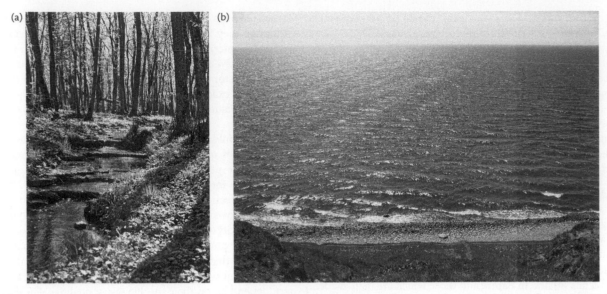

Fig. 2.5.3 Nature communicates with all senses, including sound. The sounds of nature, such as (a) streaming water, (b) waves of the sea, the twittering of birds, and rustling vegetation are generally perceived of as positive, and can have positive effects on health.
Images reproduced courtesy of Gunnar Cerwén.

applied his knowledge from the musical world to study everyday sounds. Drawing on artistic work by John Cage, Schafer (1994) uses an orchestra as a metaphor to describe the soundscape; thus underlining the inherent experiential qualities. In Schafer's orchestra, we are all musicians, as we are not only listening, but also creating sounds.

Soundscape is a broad concept. It has been used to describe anything from field recordings and sound art to musical compositions. The term is often used where there is a need to emphasize experiential and/or contextual qualities of sound.

For our purposes, we use soundscape to refer to the experience of everyday sounds or, as it was recently defined by the International Organization for Standardization (ISO), an 'acoustic environment as perceived or experienced and/or understood by a person or people, in context' (ISO, 2014). Following on from this definition, soundscape includes potential positive as well as negative effects of sound.

The nature of sound

Any sound is a result of a vibration caused by an activity. Sounds are therefore, by definition, good storytellers—they tell us what is happening around us. Through interactions between auditory and limbic systems of the brain, sound is linked to our emotions, positive as well as negative (Kraus and Canlon, 2012). This is well-known and utilized in many areas of society, including film-making, marketing, and music production.

While our vision is limited to approximately 180 degrees, we can hear sounds from any direction, including those behind us. In contrast to light, sound waves have a good ability to travel through walls and around corners. We can close our eyes, but we have no corresponding mechanism to close our ears—we are always immersed in sound.

This may be one of the reasons why the sonic environment often is taken for granted. Even though we are influenced by sounds, the experience tends to happen unconsciously. As an example, we can consider a humming fan that becomes noticeable only after it

has been turned off. Awareness of sound comes, instead, when we really like it—such as with our favourite music—or when we really cannot stand them, as is the case with extremely loud or jarring sounds.

Nevertheless, whether consciously or unconsciously, sound influences our health and well-being. Exposure to noise, especially for extended periods of time, has been shown to have negative effects on health including hearing disorders, cardiovascular disease, hypertension, and sleep disturbance (Basner et al., 2014). According to calculations by the World Health Organization, WHO (2011), the disease burden from noise pollution in Europe is between 1.0–1.6 million disability-adjusted life years (DALYs) annually.

Sound preference

Sound influences our appreciation of the environment. Although previous research on environmental appreciation has tended to focus on visual aspects, a growing number of preference studies based on different combinations of pictures and/or environmental sounds have pointed to the impact of sound (Preis et al., 2015). Among other things, it has been shown that congruence between visual and auditory stimuli can have a positive effect on preference, but more research is needed in order to fully understand the underlying mechanisms (see also Box 2.5.1).

In general, we tend to have a preference for sounds from nature (see Fig. 2.5.3), but dislike technological sounds (e.g. traffic), while sounds from human beings are somewhere in between (Nilsson and Berglund, 2006). Such categorical preferences vary depending on particular cues such as type of sound, physical qualities of the sound, the subject's mood, situation, previous experience, cultural identity, and present expectations of the environment. Furthermore, in real life, sounds are seldom found in isolation, but are mixed and have different intensities and come from different directions. The experience of the everyday sound environment is thus a complex phenomenon.

Box 2.5.1 A scientific study using fMRI to examine responses to tranquil and non-tranquil environments with nature sound as a potential mediator

Tranquillity is a positive psychological outcome that is often desired by visitors to parks and open spaces in the countryside (Department for Environment Food and Rural Affairs, 2001). It is known that tranquil environments are associated with natural surrounding and quiet and restful soundscapes. As a result, a tranquillity prediction tool has been developed which has the potential to assist in the design of tranquil spaces. This utilizes not only the average man-made noise level, but also the percentage of natural features in the scene (Pheasant *et al.*, 2008). By quantifying these two factors it becomes readily apparent that high man-made noise levels combined with little vegetation results in a low tranquillity score, while conversely a low noise level and high natural content results in high scores.

These studies reinforce the notion that multisensory processes are at work in the perceptual processes occurring in the brain and that both auditory and visual information need to be fully taken into account.

To further understand this interaction a series of studies including the use of functional magnetic resonance imaging (fMRI) have been carried out at the University of Sheffield (Hunter *et al.*, 2010). The paradigm adopted for the fMRI scans involved exposing participants to both tranquil and non-tranquil scenes, but using the same audio input so that the effects of the visual modulation on perception of tranquillity could be isolated. Fortunately, it had been previously recognized that the sounds produced by waves breaking on a shallow sandy beach (considered tranquil) are perceived to be similar to that experienced at a few hundred metres from a motorway site (non-tranquil). Both are characterized by a constant roar. A logarithmically averaged spectrum was derived from these two similar sound source spectra and used to shape broadband sound for use as the audio signal during the fMRI scans. It was demonstrated that using a beach and motorway scene with this same average sound spectrum would be construed as tranquil and non-tranquil respectively by the majority of participants (Watts *et al.*, 2009).

It is likely that the connected state of the auditory cortex is more important than its activation *per se* in determining the overall perceptual experience, including cognitive and affective aspects relevant to tranquillity. In the current fMRI study, participants were exposed to video clips with the visually distinct scenes as discussed above (beach scenes vs. motorway scenes) with the expectation that they would be experienced as tranquil and non-tranquil environments, even though the auditory input was identical for both sets of scenes. This allowed examination of visually induced changes in the auditory cortex's connections with other brain regions. Of particular interest were the supposed connections between the auditory cortex and medial prefrontal cortex, which has been implicated in a number of functions that relate to the experience of mental states including self-reflection (Johnson *et al.*, 2002) and empathy for others (Farrow *et al.*, 2001).

At each time point during scanning, participants were presented with short 3.5 s video clips of either a tranquil beach scene or a non-tranquil motorway scene, or a fixation cross. Each scene or cross was played concurrently with the same environmentally plausible broadband sound or in silence.

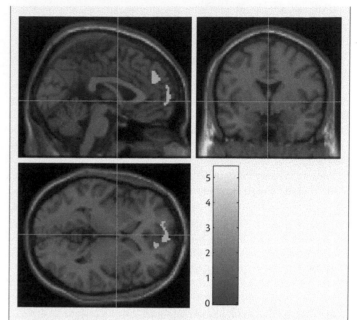

Fig. 2.5.4 Regions showing significantly enhanced connection with the auditory cortex under the tranquil (beach) condition compared with the non-tranquil (motorway) condition.
Adapted from Watts GR *et al.*, 'The use of fMRI techniques to investigate the perception of tranquillity,' Proceedings of Inter-Noise Conference, Ottawa, Canada, Copyright © 2009, with permission of the authors.

This approach amounts to a probe of effective connectivity and in this case identifies brain areas that receive significantly enhanced contribution from the auditory cortex under the tranquil visual condition compared with the non-tranquil visual condition.

Two foci in the medial prefrontal cortex demonstrated significantly enhanced connectivity (correlation) with the auditory cortex in the tranquil (beach) condition compared with the non-tranquil (motorway) condition as can be seen in Figure 2.5.4 ($p < 0.001$). No regions exhibited significantly greater connection with the auditory cortex in the non-tranquil condition than the tranquil condition.

It was concluded that responses in the medial prefrontal cortex are linked directly to activity in the auditory cortex under tranquil conditions, but not under non-tranquil conditions. This difference may be interpreted as greater engagement with tranquil environments and, in contrast, an apparent rejection of non-tranquil places. Such results are a first step in developing the fMRI technique for use in the design and improvement of tranquil spaces for amenity areas and in the development of appropriate restorative environments to aid recovery from illness and the improvement of well-being. In addition, the results of these studies further our understanding of how exposure to natural surroundings of sufficient quality, in terms of both visual and auditory input, can produce positive health outcomes.

The sound of nature

To say something general about the sound of nature is a difficult task; the variation and richness is vast. Sound sources in nature are innumerable, ranging from sounds of air, water, earth, and fire through to the sound of birds, insects, fish, and mammals.

If we consider some of the basic experiential variables in sound, such as loudness, timbre, pitch, and rhythm, we also find great variation. The sounds of nature include extremes—such as the powerful broadband sound of a waterfall or a stormy ocean—all the way to the barely audible pip of a newly hatched chick.

Similarly, rhythms of nature can be found on different scales and kinds; among frogs and birds, in breaking waves, or in the uneven pattern of the wind that passes through the forest canopy. It has been suggested that there is a relationship between the rhythmic qualities of ocean waves and well-being (Schafer, 1994; see also Box 2.5.1).

Sounds of nature vary in different regions, seasons, and situations. Forests come alive in springtime, when the birds are chirping, and the new leaves rustle in the wind. All forests have their individual character depending on the composition of plants and animals (c.f. biotopes). Biotopes thus relate to the sonic environment, a fact which led Hedfors (2003) to introduce the term *sonotope*.

A sonotope can be designed by changing the prerequisites for species composition. This can be accomplished, for example, by providing water and shrubberies to attract birds, or planting trees that rustle in the wind, like aspen. Such considerations have a direct influence on the qualities of the sonotope, and our appreciation of the environment. It has, for example, been shown that the types and combinations of bird species may have an impact on appreciation as well as stress recovery (Ratcliffe *et al.*, 2013, Hedblom *et al.*, 2014). Sonotopes have an impact, not only on humans, but also on the wildlife that resides in them as the animals' habitats can be disturbed by noise.

The sound of nature is a useful quality to consider in environmental design, also in urban contexts. The sound of water has, for example, been used as a design feature, not only for the quality it offers in itself, but also because of its ability to mask out or reduce the impact of unwanted sounds, like road noise (Cerwén, 2016). Covering a range of popular sound sources—like chirping birds, a brook, a rolling ocean, or the sound of a breeze in a tree—sounds of nature are generally perceived of as pleasant (Axelsson *et al.*, 2010), and may have the ability to influence mood (Benfield *et al.*, 2014).

Sounds of nature may also have a positive effect on health. Alvarsson *et al.* (2010) found that the recovery from a psychological stressor was faster when subjects were presented with nature sounds (sounds of a fountain and tweeting birds at 50 dB) compared to when presented with three different kinds of noises (40–80 dB). Similar findings were discovered by Annerstedt *et al.* (2013), where subjects recovered from stress more efficiently (as measured by cortisol and heart rate variability, HRV) through exposure to virtual nature (including nature sounds), while this was not the case in the control group exposed to an ordinary indoor setting or virtual nature without sound. Medvedev *et al.* (2015) recently reported a similar study in which subjects that were exposed to a stress task listened to five different sonic conditions during recovery (ocean, traffic, birdsong silence, and construction). No significant effects were found between sonic conditions and recovery (as measured by skin conductance level, SCL, and HRV). However, a significant relationship was found between recovery (SCL and HRV) and sounds that were not perceived as eventful (most typically ocean sound and birdsong). It was also found that sounds that subjects perceived of as pleasant (most typically birdsong, ocean sound, and music) produced lower skin conductance levels when at rest.

Sound of nature in healthcare

One of the earlier research studies in the area was conducted by Diette *et al.* (2003), demonstrating reduced pain experience during bronchoscopy by nature sounds. In another study, Saadatmand *et al.* (2013) investigated the effect of nature sound on stress reduction during mechanical ventilation. Data was collected using the Faces Anxiety Scale and Richmond Agitation Sedation Scale. The results indicated positive health effects, such as reduced blood pressure and reduced anxiety levels. Aghaie *et al.* (2014) found similar results in a study on the effects of nature-based sounds during the weaning of mechanical ventilation in coronary artery patients.

Experience from research on patients under anaesthesia show significant effects of nature sound exposure, such as decreased biomarkers for stress (salivary amylase) (Arai *et al.*, 2008). A randomized double-blind controlled study also showed effects in terms of blunted haemodynamic changes upon emergence from general anaesthesia and increased acceptability of the anaesthesia experience (Tsuchiya *et al.*, 2003).

Results from research thus far indicate that there is a connection between nature sounds and health-related outcomes, but we lack knowledge of effect variation depending on, for example, type of sound, physical characteristics of sound (such as sound pressure, level, and rhythm), individual nature connectedness, interacting sensory exposure, or population group. This calls for more studies exploring causality and interdependent factors.

An increased understanding of the role of nature sounds in relation to potential stress reduction and positive health effects could lead to improved environmental design and public health. However, it is important to remember that sound is always experienced in a context. While the study of one sensory input can reveal certain effects, it needs to be considered together with other cues in the environment in order to give as full an understanding as possible.

Smell, nature, and well-being

The research on associations between natural odours and health is very limited. This section will outline existing knowledge and discuss the impact of olfactory input. It will provide an insight to potential pathways between the smell of nature and health.

Smell and perception in an evolutionary context

Most of the ancestors to modern humans depended on olfaction for finding food, assessing its quality, and avoiding ingestion of harmful substances (Sell, 2014). Because olfaction is so important to survival, it became an important factor in the neural evolution of nearly all mammals.

The human threshold for sensing some odours is impressively low—the earthy scent of geosmin (a type of actinobacteria typically occurring after rain has fallen on the ground after a dry spell) can be detected at concentrations under 10 parts per trillion (Jiang *et al.*, 2007)—and it is estimated that humans can detect a number of scents ranging from a conservative 5,000 (Gerkin and Castro, 2015) to a theoretical upper limit of 1 trillion (Bushdid *et al.*, 2014).

However, as anyone familiar with canine tracking capabilities knows, non-human mammals are better than we are at distinguishing odours and parsing differences in concentrations.

Neurologically, decoding and using olfactory messages succeeds more in species that devote more cortical support to olfaction. Despite their reliance on vision, it would be inaccurate to say that primates have poor olfactory capacities (Yeshurun and Sobel, 2010). Instead, the ways in which olfaction is employed by primates may be more evolved than most species (Schaal and Porter, 1991).

Human olfaction relies on very old neural architecture, in what is sometimes called the 'reptilian or smell' brain. These primitive processes and connections have a direct limbic pathway, which has allowed humans to quickly catalogue compounds and events. These rapid assays of the world allow us to immediately determine, without a prior stop for reasoning and reflection, whether something is edible or dangerous.

Through olfaction, in contrast with the other senses, we directly sample the chemical composition of objects and our surroundings. Olfactory neurons lie only three synapses from the cerebral cortex. Odours are thus assayed directly from ambient air, with a first, coarse check for pattern recognition by the olfactory bulb and cortex. Through another short circuit, olfactory neurons provide major inputs to the limbic system, a critical locus of emotional stimulus and response.

Recalling stimuli by smell versus sight

We can easily and faithfully recall visual stimuli, and communicate these to others along with our feelings about them, but smell-based replay is effectively impossible and hard to communicate. When olfactory stimuli are present, emotions are triggered and we can readily call up memories, but the imagination is useless for replaying smell experiences. Vision thus provides highly reliable and communicable recall that can last a long time (low variance), but with highly variable and changeable emotional responses. Olfaction provides long-term signal strength with high emotional fidelity, but very low communicability.

Smell and culture

The sense of smell and the pervasive role of odour in people's lives have been neglected in histories and narratives, at least for Western cultures (Classen et al., 1994). What is clear is that as urban environments modernized, odour became a class issue. As Emmons (2014) put it ' … in the modern bourgeois world, the goal became a complete absence of scent, a deodorisation of both person and environment'. Smell seemingly became irrelevant to our sense of where we are; accordingly, we have relatively few examples of contemporary people who rely on olfaction to order the space around them.

Some native peoples, especially in non-urban environments, still use smell to recognize their territories; to distinguish group members from non-members; to make land-use decisions; and generally to choose between desirable and undesirable landscapes. Peoples from cultures all around the world rely on olfaction to convey the desirable qualities of their landscapes and for cues regarding the geological nature of their countries, as Yarde (2013) remarks in her study of the island of Dominica. In the mid-twentieth century, the anthropologist Gerardo Reichel-Dolmatoff (1985) documented how some of the tribes composing the eastern Tukanoan populations of the north-west Colombian Amazon used olfaction for communication, predation (what is proper to hunt) and territoriality. Read more about cultural factors related to experiences of nature in Chapter 6.4 ('Responses to nature from populations of varied cultural background').

Turning to the Global North, most members of the French wine industry and trade believe that their viticultural regions became organized into *appellations* and rankings according to the technocratic pursuit of efficiency and economic growth typical of French bureaucrats (Loubère, 1990). Vintners grudgingly accept that officially sanctioned differences between one *Grand Cru* (highly ranked) vineyard and its neighbouring parcel of much less distinction derive faithfully from a long history of trial and error, resulting inevitably in the best possible separation between wines with great reputations and wines considered ordinary. However, because wines are constantly sampled to make sure they meet quality norms, the rankings of the various *appellations* are ultimately mediated by *smell*. The sense modality acting as final arbiter between mediocre, good, and great vineyards (and consequently influencing land and wine prices) is olfaction.

Olfaction and nature

By relying so much on vision and language, have we limited our understanding of the natural world? What might we know about nature if we gave more importance to olfaction? Could we use olfaction instrumentally, say, to improve public and environmental health? Could we use olfaction to better understand our own health and to improve interactions with non-human life?

We continue this section exploring how olfaction can contribute to phenomenological, taxonomic, and health-based ways of interrogating and interacting with nature. We also discuss why it may be that scientific studies on odours and health are scarce and how we might change that paradigm.

Phenomenology

Olfactory inputs resist linguistic abstraction; in essence, we are not accustomed to paying close attention to (not to mention *believing*) any sort of cognition that is not represented symbolically (e.g. Batty, 2011).

Most of us have a soundtrack, a stream of words, in our mind that accompanies our mind's eye. We tend heavily towards accompanying all that we see, or replay in our memory, with language. But this is not typically the case with olfaction, because olfaction is a fundamentally different way of knowing. Olfactory cognition can—and does—happen quite well without language. As a consequence, we struggle to represent olfactory knowledge intersubjectively through symbols. In turn, what we cannot represent symbolically we treat as subjective and irreproducible, much as if olfactory data were evanescent intuitions, guesses, or impressions.

And yet, as hard as it is to name or describe discrete olfactory stimuli, our odour sensorium is superbly adapted to the task of retaining smell data for decades. Human olfaction powerfully demonstrates that our system of memory is often more stable than the laboured encoding we use every day with symbols used in, for example, math or language. This advantage in temporal stability invites us to contemplate how we might learn to encode different stimuli in different, non-linguistic ways.

Taxonomy

New uses for olfactory data can arise if we accept and amplify olfaction as a useful way of knowing.

If environmental scientists conducted olfactory sensory analyses on the same landscapes year after year, could they tell us something novel about different kinds of disturbances (e.g. climate change, floods, land conversion, pollution, or fire) and recoveries that we simply could not know otherwise? Drawing on the temporal advantages of olfaction, could such analyses offer some capacity to predict future stresses and thereby prevent potential diseases? Does a landscape harbouring disease vectors like mosquitos smell differently from one lacking them?

Olfaction and health

A growing body of literature establishes the importance of odours and odoriferous toxins for public health (see for example Nimmermark, 2004; Patel and Pinto, 2014). If practical field methods for olfactory assays can be developed (as suggested by Kern et al., 2014, with their Olfactory Function Field Exam, or OFFE), then using olfaction for regulatory purposes in public health-related aspects may not be so far off. Smeets and Dalton (2005) propose an information-processing model of chemosensory perception that combines odour perception with subjective experiences of irritancy, and suggest that the model could be used to set occupational exposure limits. Nuisance abatement standards could also be derived from better understanding olfaction and environmental quality (Nimmermark, 2004; Blanes-Vidal et al., 2014).

Some empirical data suggest that chemical compounds from forests and forest odours have a distinct impact on physiological processes, with potential impact on for example our immune system (Li, 2010). Much of this research is conducted within the concept of 'forest bathing' (Shinrin-yoku), which is presented in Chapter 5.1.

Given the strong and immediate connection between the olfactory sense and our emotions and memories, it is a plausible hypothesis that the specific odour of nature and its chemical compounds would have a specific health impact through neurophysiological or psychological influences.

For thousands of years humans have acquired sophisticated methods for mitigating toxins, formulating botanical remedies, and concocting healthful diets based on smell and flavour. It has only been in recent decades that science has begun to firmly establish the molecular and physiological mechanisms of olfaction and taste. The rapid progress has resulted in a proliferation of publications revealing the extraordinary complexity and interplay among olfactory–taste detection, behavioural responses, and somatic effects (e.g. Spence, 2015).

Our attraction or repulsion to chemicals is mediated primarily by two separate systems in nasal, ocular, and oral mucosae: the main olfactory and the trigeminal chemosensory. The modality of the trigeminal system is chemesthesis, which conveys the concept of chemical 'feel' for sensations that are neither odours nor tastes, but responses to volatile chemicals. These sensations are usually sharp or pungent, including prickling, piquancy, irritation, stinging, tingling, freshness, coolness, burning, and the like. Thus the trigeminal system responds to menthol, ammonia, acids, CO_2, and a myriad of other volatiles that elicit immediate behaviours of alertness, arousal, sharpness, or repugnance.

The extreme sensitivity of the trigeminal system serves to warn us against toxins, pathogens, and pollutants. For example, plants typically produce toxins to avoid being eaten. However, many such potentially noxious irritants may be harmless and even pleasant and beneficial in low concentrations, or when ameliorated by associated compounds or flavours within a plant—the basis of aromatherapy. In addition, at some low thresholds, a plant volatile may have medically therapeutic effects, or it may co-occur with other plant biochemicals having those effects. In the right ratios, humans are drawn to conjoined sensations, aromas, and flavours; for example, the volatiles in mint, cinnamon, mustard, chilli, and vanilla

Table 2.5.1 Examples of odours of nature and corresponding effects on cognitive capacity, stress, and mood

Odour	Cognitive performance	Stress	Mood
Lavender	**Improved concentration and computational accuracy and speed** (Sakamoto et al., 2005; Diego et al., 1998)	**Reduced stress and anxiety** (Toda & Morimoto, 2008; Lehrner et al., 2005)	**Increased relaxation** (Diego et al., 1998) **Improved mood** (Lehrner et al., 2005; Diego et al., 1998)
Peppermint	**Enhanced attention, alertness, arousal, memory, and task performance** (Moss et al., 2008; Barker et al., 2003)	**Increased eustress and reduced distress** (Toda & Morimoto, 2001)	
Rosemary	**Enhanced alertness and quality of memory** (Diego et al., 1998; Moss et al., 2003; Moss & Oliver, 2012)	**Reduced anxiety** (Diego et al., 1998)	**Stimulated and improved mood** (Sayorwan et al., 2012)
Citrus	**Improved scholastic performance** (Akpinar, 2005)	**Reduced stress and anxiety** (Matsumoto et al., 2013; Lehrner et al., 2005; Goes et al., 2012)	**Stimulated and improved mood** (Warrendburg, 2005; Lehrner et al., 2005)
Cypress		**Reduced blood pressure** (Chen et al., 2015)	**Relaxed and improved mood** (Ikei, Song, & Miyazaki, 2015; Chen et al., 2015)
Vanilla			**Relaxed and improved mood** (Warrenburg, 2005)

when diluted or added to food. Similarly, we can acquire a taste for wine and carbonated beverages that are mixes of volatiles and pleasant flavours. Volatiles are also readily absorbed from the air via the lungs and mucosa, without ingestion, and with the attraction and pleasure driven primarily by olfaction and chemesthesis.

A few research studies have demonstrated specific health-related effects from odours of plants, such as lavender, rosemary, citrus, and cypress (see Table 2.5.1).

According to a study by Glass and colleagues (2014), 'biophilic odours' (e.g. summer air) have been shown to evoke positive responses, such as improved mood and physical responses due to associative memory, while 'urban odours' (e.g. disinfectants) evoked negative responses.

From a planning and design perspective, it has been suggested to include natural scents in healthcare facilities in order to enhance well-being among patients. For example, odours of lavender or oranges may alleviate anxiety (Lehrner *et al.*, 2005), reduce agitation in patients with severe dementia (Perry and Perry, 2006), or lessen the demand for postoperative painkillers (Kim *et al.*, 2007). Olfactory stimuli may be of particular relevance for people with limited vision or hearing. However, using scents in healthcare facilities requires awareness of hyperreactivity or allergies, and it is important to use natural, hypoallergenic scents, controlled concentrations, and potentially containment to personal spaces.

More research will be needed to establish a causal chain between olfaction, affect (or even biophilia), and environmental management and sustainable health. Already, psychophysiological studies underscore the importance—for public health and quality of life—of pleasant olfactory environments, from infants (Coffield *et al.*, 2014) to adults (Nimmermark, 2004).

Conclusion

Altogether we can conclude that we still have a long way to go to elucidating the mechanisms behind humans' positive responses to nature exposure. However, from the research presented in this chapter, it is clear that specific features of nature provide certain sensory input to the brain with subsequent neurophysiological, physiological, and psychological responses. Such responses partly determine health impact and outcome. This means that independent of background, cultural context, or individual preferences, the objective sensory dimensions of nature may, on a general level, evoke bodily reactions with bearing for our health and well-being. This is a small, but central piece of knowledge, essential to explore further in order to provide better understanding and conclusive evidence on how nature influences human health.

References

Aghaie, B., Rejeh, N., Heravi-Karimooi, M., *et al.* (2014). Effect of nature-based sound therapy on agitation and anxiety in coronary artery bypass graft patients during the weaning of mechanical ventilation: A randomised clinical trial. *Int J Nurs Stud*, 51, 526–38.

Akpinar, B. (2005). The effects of olfactory stimuli on scholastic performance. *The Irish Journal of Education/Iris Eireannach an Oideachais*, 86–90.

Alvarsson, J. J., Wiens, S., & Nilsson, M. E. (2010). Stress recovery during exposure to nature sound and environmental noise. *Int J Environ Res Public Health*, 7, 1036–46.

Annerstedt, M., Jonsson, P., Wallergard, M., *et al.* (2013). Inducing physiological stress recovery with sounds of nature in a virtual reality forest—Results from a pilot study. *Physiol Behav*, 118, 240–50.

Arai, Y.-C., Ushida, T., Matsubara, T., *et al.* (2008). Intra-operative natural sound decreases salivary amylase activity of patients undergoing inguinal hernia repair under epidural anesthesia: 123. *Reg Anesth Pain Med*, 33, e234.

Axelsson, Ö., Nilsson, M. E., & Berglund, B. (2010). A principal components model of soundscape perception. *J Acoust Soc Am*, 128, 2836–46.

Basner, M., Babisch, W., Davis, A., *et al.* (2014). Auditory and non-auditory effects of noise on health. *Lancet*, 383, 1325–32.

Batty, C. 2011. Smelling lessons. *Philosophical Studies*, 153, 161–74.

Benfield, J. A., Taff, B. D., Newman, P., & Smyth, J. (2014). Natural sound facilitates mood recovery. *Ecopsychology*, 6, 183–8.

Blanes-Vidal, V., Bælum, J., Nadimi, E. S., Løfstrøm, P., & Christensen, L. P. (2014). Chronic exposure to odorous chemicals in residential areas and effects on human psychosocial health: Dose–response relationships. *Sci Total Environ*, 490, 545–54.

Bovill, C. (1995). *Fractal Geometry in Architecture and Design.* Berlin, Germany: Springer.

Brown, C. T., Witschey, W. R. T., & Liebovitch, L. S. (2005). The broken past: Fractals in archaeology. *J Arch Method Theory*, 12, 37–78.

Bushdid, C., Magnasco, M. O., Vosshall, L. B., & Keller, A. (2014). Humans Can Discriminate More than 1 Trillion Olfactory Stimuli. *Science*, 343, 1370–2.

Cerwén, G. (2016). Urban soundscapes: a quasi experiment in landscape architecture. *Landscape Research*. Available at: http://www.tandfonline.com/doi/abs/10.1080/01426397.2015.1117062?src=recsys&journalCode=clar20 [Online].

Chen, C.-J., Kumar, K., Chen, Y.-T., *et al.* (2015). Effect of hinoki and meniki essential oils on human autonomic nervous system activity and mood states. *Nat Prod Commun*, 10, 1305–8.

Classen, C., Howes, D. & Synnoy, A. (1994). *The Cultural History of Smell.* New York, NY: Routledge.

Coffield, C. N., Mayhew, E. M. Y., Haviland-Jones, J. M., & Walker-Andrews, A. S. (2014). Adding odor: Less distress and enhanced attention for 6-month-olds. *Infant Behav Dev*, 37, 155–61.

Department for Environment Food and Rural Affairs (2001). Survey of Public Attitudes to Quality of Life and the Environment. DEFRA, UK.

Diego, M. A., Jones, N. A., Field, T., *et al.* (1998). Aromatherapy positively affects mood, EEG patterns of alertness and math computations. *Int J Neurosci*, 96, 217–24.

Diette, G. B., Lechtzin, N., Haponik, E., Devrotes, A., & Rubin, H. R. (2003). Distraction therapy with nature sights and sounds reduces pain during flexible bronchoscopy: a complementary approach to routine analgesia. *Chest*, 123, 941–8.

Emmons, P. (2014). The place of odour in modern aerial urbanism. *J Archit*, 19, 202–15.

Farrow, T. F. D., Zheng, Y., Wilkinson, I. D., *et al.* (2001). Investigating the functional anatomy of empathy and forgiveness. *NeuroReport*, 12, 2433–8.

Gerkin, R. C., Castro, J. B. (2015). The number of olfactory stimuli that humans can discriminate is still unknown. *eLife*, 4, e08127.

Glass, S. T., Lingg, E., & Heuberger, E. (2014). Do ambient urban odors evoke basic emotions? *Applied Olfactory Cognition*, 158.

Goes, T. C., Antunes, F. D., Alves, P. B., & Teixeira-Silva, F. (2012). Effect of sweet orange aroma on experimental anxiety in humans. *J Altern Complement Med*, 18, 798–804.

Hägerhäll, C. M. (2005). Fractal dimension as a tool for defining and measuring naturalness. In: Martens, B. & Keul, A. G. (eds) *Designing Social Innovation—Planning, Building, Evaluating.* Cambridge, MA: Hogrefe & Huber.

Hägerhäll, C. M., Laike, T., Kuller, M., Marcheschi, E., Boydston, C., & Taylor, R. P. (2015). Human physiological benefits of viewing nature: eeg responses to exact and statistical fractal patterns. *Nonlinear Dynamics Psychol Life Sci*, 19, 1–12.

Hägerhäll, C. M., Purcell, T., & Taylor, R. (2004). Fractal dimension of landscape silhouette outlines as a predictor of landscape preference. *J Environ Psychol*, 24, 247–55.

Hedblom, M., Heyman, E., Antonsson, H., & Gunnarsson, B. (2014). Bird song diversity influences young people's appreciation of urban landscapes. *Urban For Urban Greening*, 13, 469–74.

Hedfors, P. (2003). *Site Soundscapes: Landscape Architecture in the Light of Sound.* (Doctoral Thesis) Dept. of Landscape Planning, SLU, Ultuna.

Hunter, M. D., Eickhoff, S. B., Pheasant, R. J., et al. (2010). The state of tranquility: Subjective perception is shaped by contextual modulation of auditory connectivity. *NeuroImage*, 53, 611–18.

International Organization for Standardization (ISO) (2014). ISO 12913-1:2014 Acoustics—Soundscape—Part 1: Definition and conceptual framework. Geneva, Switzerland: ISO.

Jiang, J., He, X., & Cane, D. E. (2007). Biosynthesis of the earthy odorant geosmin by a bifunctional Streptomyces coelicolor enzyme. *Nat Chem Biol*, 3, 711–15.

Johnson, S. C., Baxter, L. C., Wilder, L. S., Pipe, J. G., Heiserman, J. E., & Prigatano, G. P. (2002). Neural correlates of self-reflection. *Brain*, 125, 1808–14.

Joye, Y., & Van Den Berg, A. (2011). Is love for green in our genes? A critical analysis of evolutionary assumptions in restorative environments research. *Urban For Urban Greening*, 10, 261–8.

Kern, D. W., Wroblewski, K. E., Schumm, L. P., Pinto, J. M., & McClintock, M. K. (2014). Field survey measures of olfaction: The Olfactory Function Field Exam (OFFE). *Field Methods*, 26, 421–34.

Kim, J. T., Ren, C. J., Fielding, G. A., et al. (2007). Treatment with lavender aromatherapy in the post-anesthesia care unit reduces opioid requirements of morbidly obese patients undergoing laparoscopic adjustable gastric banding. *Obes Surg*, 17, 920–5.

Kraus, K. S. & Canlon, B. (2012). Neuronal connectivity and interactions between the auditory and limbic systems. Effects of noise and tinnitus. *Hear Res*, 288, 34–46.

Laufs, H., Krakow, K., Sterzer, P., et al. (2003). Electroencephalographic signatures of attentional and cognitive default modes in spontaneous brain activity fluctuations at rest. *Proc Natl Acad Sci U S A*, 100, 11053–8.

Lehrner, J., Marwinski, G., Lehr, S., Johren, P., & Deecke, L. (2005). Ambient odors of orange and lavender reduce anxiety and improve mood in a dental office. *Physiol Behav*, 86, 92–5.

Li, Q. (2010). Effect of forest bathing trips on human immune function. *Environ Health Prev Med*, 15, 9–17.

Loubère, L. A. (1990). *The Wine Revolution in France: The Twentieth Century.* Princeton, NJ: Princeton University Press.

Mandelbrot, B. B. (1982). *The Fractal Geometry of Nature.* San Francisco, CA: W. H. Freeman.

Matsumoto, T., Asakura, H., & Hayashi, T. (2014). Effects of olfactory stimulation from the fragrance of the Japanese citrus fruit yuzu (Citrus junos Sieb. ex Tanaka) on mood states and salivary chromogranin A as an endocrinologic stress marker. *J Altern Complement Med*, 20, 500–6.

Medvedev, O., Shepherd, D., & Hautus, M. J. (2015). The restorative potential of soundscapes: A physiological investigation. *Appl Acoustics*, 96, 20–6.

Moss, M., Cook, J., Wesnes, K., & Duckett, P. (2003). Aromas of rosemary and lavender essential oils differentially affect cognition and mood in healthy adults. *Int J Neurosci*, 113, 15–38.

Moss, M., Hewitt, S., Moss, L., & Wesnes, K. (2008). Modulation of cognitive performance and mood by aromas of peppermint and ylang-ylang. *Int J Neurosci*, 118, 59–77.

Nilsson, M. E. & Berglund, B. (2006). Soundscape quality in suburban green areas and city parks. *Acta Acustica United with Acustica*, 92, 903–11.

Nimmermark, S. (2004). Odour influence on well-being and health with specific focus on animal production emissions. *Ann Agric Environ Med*, 11, 163–73.

Patel, R. M. & Pinto, J. M. (2014). Olfaction: Anatomy, physiology, and disease. *Clin Anat*, 27, 54–60.

Perry, N. & Perry, E. (2006). Aromatherapy in the management of psychiatric disorders. *CNS Drugs*, 20, 257–80.

Pheasant, R., Horoshenkov, K., Watts, G., & Barrett, B. (2008). The acoustic and visual factors influencing the construction of tranquil space in urban and rural environments tranquil spaces-quiet places? *J Acoust Soc Am*, 123, 1446–57.

Pickover, C. (1995). *Keys to Infinity.* New York, NY: Wiley

Preis, A., Kociński, J., Hafke-Dys, H., & Wrzosek, M. (2015). Audio-visual interactions in environment assessment. *Sci Total Environ*, 523, 191–200.

Ratcliffe, E., Gatersleben, B., & Sowden, P. T. (2013). Bird sounds and their contributions to perceived attention restoration and stress recovery. *J Environ Psychol*, 36, 221–8.

Reichel-Dolmatoff, G. (1985). Tapir avoidance in the Colombian northwest Amazon. In: Urton, G. (ed.) *Animal Myths and Metaphors in South America.* Salt Lake City, UT: University of Utah Press.

Saadatmand, V., Rejeh, N., Heravi-Karimooi, M., et al. (2013). Effect of nature-based sounds' intervention on agitation, anxiety, and stress in patients under mechanical ventilator support: A randomised controlled trial. *Int J Nurs Stud*, 50, 895–904.

Sakamoto, R., Minoura, K., Usui, A., Ishizuka, Y., & Kanba, S. (2005). Effectiveness of aroma on work efficiency: lavender aroma during recesses prevents deterioration of work performance. *Chem Senses*, 30, 683–91.

Schaal, B., Porter, R. H. (1991). 'Microsmatic Humans' Revisited: The Generation and Perception of Chemical Signals. *Adv Study Behav*, 20, 135–99.

Schafer, R. M. (1994). *The Soundscape: Our Sonic Environment and the Tuning of the World.* Rochester, VT: Destiny Books.

Sell, C. S. (2014). *Chemistry and the Sense of Smell.* Hoboken, NJ: John Wiley & Sons.

Smeets, M. A. M. & Dalton, P. H. (2005). Evaluating the human response to chemicals: odor, irritation and non-sensory factors. *Environ Toxicol Pharmacol*, 19, 581–8.

Spence, C. (2015). Multisensory flavor perception. *Cell*, 161, 24–35.

Taylor, R. P., Micolich, A. P., & Jonas, D. (1999). Fractal analysis of Pollock's drip paintings. *Nature*, 399, 422.

Taylor, R. P., Spehar, B., Van Donkelaar, P., & Hägerhäll, C. M. 2011. Perceptual and physiological responses to Jackson Pollock's fractals. *Front Hum Neurosci*, 5, 60.

Taylor, R. P. & Sprott, J. C. (2008). Biophilic fractals and the visual journey of organic screen-savers. *Nonlinear Dynamics Psychol Life Sci*, 12, 117–29.

Toda, M. & Morimoto, K. (2008). Effect of lavender aroma on salivary endocrinological stress markers. *Arch Oral Biol*, 53, 964–8.

Toda, M. & Morimoto, K. (2011). Evaluation of effects of lavender and peppermint aromatherapy using sensitive salivary endocrinological stress markers. *Stress Health*, 27, 430–5.

Tsuchiya, M., Asada, A., Ryo, K., et al. (2003). Relaxing intraoperative natural sound blunts haemodynamic change at the emergence from propofol general anaesthesia and increases the acceptability of anaesthesia to the patient. *Acta Anaesthesiol Scand*, 47, 939–43.

Ulrich, R. S. 1(981). Natural versus urban scenes: some psychophysiological effects. *Environ Behav*, 13, 523–56.

van Tonder, G. J., Lyons, M. J., & Ejima, Y. (2002). Visual structure of a Japanese Zen garden. *Nature*, 419, 359–60.

Warrenburg, S. (2005). Effects of fragrance on emotions: moods and physiology. *Chem Senses*, 30, i248–9.

Watts, G. R., Hunter, M. D., Douglas, M., et al. (2009). The use of fMRI techniques to investigate the perception of tranquillity. 38th International Congress and Exposition on Noise Control Engineering 2009. INTER-NOISE 2009, 699–706.

World Health Organization (WHO) (2011). *Burden of disease from environmental noise: Quantification of healthy life years lost in Europe.* Bonn, Germany: The World Health Organization European Centre for Environment and Health.

Yarde, T. N. (2013). Sensing the natural in the Caribbean's nature island. *Senses Soc*, 8, 149–64.

Yeshurun, Y. & Sobel, N. (2010). An odor is not worth a thousand words: from multidimensional odors to unidimensional odor objects. *Ann Rev Psychol*, 61, 219–41.

CHAPTER 2.6

The role of nature and environment in behavioural medicine

Leonie Venhoeven, Danny Taufik, Linda Steg, Marino Bonaiuto, Mirilia Bonnes, Silvia Ariccio, Stefano De Dominicis, Massimiliano Scopelliti, Matilda van den Bosch, Paul Piff, Jia Wei Zhang, and Dacher Keltner

What is behavioural medicine?

The Society of Behavioural Medicine (www.sbm.org) defines behavioural medicine as an 'interdisciplinary field concerned with the development and integration of behavioural, psychosocial, and biomedical science knowledge and techniques relevant to the understanding of health and illness, and the application of this knowledge and these techniques to prevention, diagnosis, treatment, and rehabilitation'. From the perspective of behavioural medicine, many health problems are a result of undesirable behaviour and thus better health may be achieved by changing behaviour. Until now, behavioural medicine has mainly focused on behaviours with a direct impact on human health and well-being.

However, more recently, environmentally related behaviour, especially pro-environmental behaviour, has achieved attention as an indirect pathway to better health. Pro-environmental behaviour can be defined as the propensity to take actions and decisions with an ecologically sustainable impact and may result as a consequence of concerns regarding ecosystem destruction, climate change, and other harmful impacts of anthropogenic actions (Stern, 2000). Pro-environmental behaviour is related to decisions such as active transport (e.g. biking) instead of passive (e.g. car driving), recycling, or reduced red meat consumption. Several pathways are suggested for explaining a relation between pro-environmental behaviour and health. In the following, a few of these pathways are outlined. In addition, various potential mechanisms for inducing or changing environmentally related behaviours are discussed.

Connectedness to nature and the meaning of life

Being attached to natural environments and even having a feeling of connectedness to nature may provide an existential sense of well-being (Bonaiuto and Alves, 2012). As Stephen R. Kellert (1993) poses: 'Nature's diversity and healthy functioning are worthy of maintenance because they represent the best chance for people to experience a satisfying and meaningful existence.' Feeling connected to nature can induce many comforting emotions, such as positive affect, life satisfaction, happiness, feelings of vitality, and a sense of meaning and purpose in life (Passmore and Howell, 2014). These positive feelings may trigger pro-environmental behaviour in an individual—as we feel good by nature we want to protect it for our own well-being. If nature connectedness can promote positive feelings and behaviour, an important question to answer is how connectedness to nature can be achieved. Chapter 2.2 'Therapeutic landscapes, restorative environments, place attachment, and well-being' discusses the concept of place attachment and identity, which may be part of nature connectedness. It is also possible that living in more natural areas by default makes people more connected and familiar with nature. For example, people living in rural, natural settings may be more prone to act ecologically than people living in urban areas (Berenguer et al., 2005). Furthermore, spending time in nature can have an especially positive effect on pro-environmental behaviour when the experiences one has are pleasant, while the relationship might be less evident if activities performed in natural environments are unpleasant or part of common daily life (Collado et al., 2015).

Pro-environmental behaviour as a direct source of well-being

Several correlational studies suggest that engaging in pro-environmental behaviour may be a direct source of well-being. For instance, people who live in more ecologically sustainable ways are usually happier, and environmentally conscious consumption is related to well-being and life satisfaction in general (Brown and Kasser, 2005). An important theoretical question to answer, however, is why pro-environmental behaviour and well-being would be related.

Hedonic and eudaimonic well-being

In order to answer this question, it is important to consider the distinction between two types of well-being (Venhoeven *et al.*, 2013): hedonic and eudaimonic well-being. The former concept generally refers to feelings of *pleasure*, while the latter refers to feelings of *meaning*. Pleasure and meaning may be linked to pro-environmental behaviour in differing degrees. Acting pro-environmentally sometimes comes at a certain cost rather than providing pleasure. While cycling on a warm spring day for instance may be evaluated as very comfortable, taking a cold shower in winter is most probably not, in spite of knowing that you save energy. In fact, people may especially have the latter group of pro-environmental behaviours in mind, leading them to think acting pro-environmentally threatens well-being. Feelings of meaning (eudaimonic well-being), however, are at the core of pro-environmental behaviour. As acting pro-environmentally can benefit the quality of nature and the well-being of other people, it is regarded moral and thereby meaningful behaviour (Heberlein, 1972). Although environmentally friendly behaviour may induce discomfort on an individual level, it may at the same time be the perception of contributing to positive consequences for the environment that brings meaning and feelings of well-being for the individual.

Self-image

If the sense of meaning plays a role in explaining why acting in an environmentally friendly way feels good, the next question that arises is what leads meaning to have this effect. A possible answer to this question is that engagement in meaningful behaviour could induce well-being because this behaviour can *signal something positive about who you are*. One's self-image reflects a collection of components that together form a person's view of the self. One of the pillars on which people base their self-image is their own decisions and actions (Bem, 1972). How meaningful you perceive your behaviour to be may thereby affect how positive your self-image is: the more an activity involves eudaimonia (e.g. at a personal or social level), the more the person feels to have a correspondingly stronger personal or social identity (Mao *et al.*, 2016). If environmentally friendly behaviour is perceived to be meaningful, acting this way may boost your self-image, thereby eliciting positive emotions and well-being. In general, action and activities carried out in a place are a crucial component for person–environment relationships (Bonaiuto *et al.*, 2004). Furthermore, recent correlational data specifically show that there is a positive relation among the eudaimonia (measured as experience of 'flow', namely of being immersed in a place-related activity) experienced by a person while doing activities in a place one feels to belong to, and the place identity felt by the same person in relation to the very same place (coherently with the Eudaimonistic Identity Theory; Bonaiuto *et al.*, 2016).

The positive emotions that are elicited by 'meaningful behaviour' are also referred to as a 'warm glow'. 'Warm glow' (or 'helper's high') is a concept used to explain motivational factors behind non-selfish decisions and behaviours from an evolutionary perspective (Andreoni, 1990). By doing good to others (or the environment) your chances for survival increase, and the behaviour is therefore inherently enforced. There is also a biological fundament for this theory as the brain reacts on us 'doing good' by releasing 'feel good' neurotransmitters, like oxytocin (Moll *et al.*, 2006). The concept of 'warm glow' was first introduced in research on pro-social behaviour, such as altruism, but links are also drawn to pro-environmental behaviour (Taufik *et al.*, 2015).

Positive feelings affecting future behaviour

There are different perspectives on whether the good feeling induced by acting in an environmentally friendly manner in turn translates into future pro-environmental behaviour—thereby setting in motion a virtuous loop with continued societal and environmental benefits. The line of research that studies *moral licensing* suggests a good feeling would not necessarily initiate a chain of further good behaviours. As this literature argues, when the need to see yourself in a positive light is fulfilled by one good action, there is no immediate reason to engage in further good but costly behaviour. The process explaining this effect is referred to as moral balancing; people will stop performing moral actions once they 'have done enough' to reach their desired level of morality. Rather, engagement in moral behaviour can now lead to less moral behaviour on a later occasion (Tiefenbeck *et al.*, 2013). Some studies even suggest that moral licensing is more likely to occur when people receive a boost in their self-image (Khan and Dhar, 2006) especially if engagement in moral behaviour involves doing something unpleasant, like taking a cold shower, the desire to stay in a positive mood may outweigh the wish to behave morally.

Opposite to these arguments, however, stands the *broaden-and-build model* of positive emotions (Fredrickson, 2001). This model suggests that positive emotions broaden 'people's momentary thought-action repertoires'. More precisely, positive emotions allow people to become more creative, knowledgeable, resilient, socially integrated, and healthy over time—which can open the way for pro-environmental behaviour. As research indeed shows, doing good does not only feel good; people who feel good are also more likely to engage in good behaviour (Aknin *et al.*, 2012). A number of studies have demonstrated that a good feeling may lead people to engage in pro-environmental behaviour. Anticipating feelings of pride can encourage pro-environmental actions (Onwezen *et al.*, 2013). This line of reasoning would therefore suggest that the positive well-being effect of engagement in environmentally friendly behaviour does spark future pro-environmental behaviour, thereby bringing long-term benefits for society.

This knowledge is important for understanding measures to induce behavioural change. It has been found that environmental campaigns stressing moral motives to behave ecologically, for example to check one's tyre pressure (namely, because it helps to protect the environment), are more effective than those stressing financial motives (in the form of saving money). Seeing oneself as an ecologically sound person may create a more positive self-image than seeing oneself as a person driven by economical motives (Bolderdijk *et al.*, 2013).

Deliberate versus automatic decision-making

Whether the good feeling that pro-environmental actions elicit translates into future pro-environmental behaviour may, at least partly, depend on how conscious the pro-environmental behaviour was performed. Essentially, two kinds of processing in decision-making and behaviour are in function, often referred to as the 'dual system' (Chaiken and Trope, 1999). The first kind of processing is often defined as a 'reflective and conscious system' (Strack and Deutsch, 2004), which mainly depends on information processing and active elaborations (i.e. rational decisions). This processing system is controlled and deductive. The second kind of processing is defined as an 'impulsive, automatic system' (Strack and Deutsch, 2004). This system is uncontrolled, associative, and environmentally determined. From a neurobiological perspective, behavioural processing in relation to the external world is steered by the brain's mirror neuron system and the mentalizing system (Van Overwalle and Baetens, 2009). In particular, the mirror neuron system is believed to be activated automatically (Spunt and Lieberman, 2013).

Most of the literature within the field of environmental psychology has dealt with controlled, rational processes and antecedents that lead people to actively choose to behave in a pro-environmental manner (Harland *et al.*, 1999). Campaigns that try to influence pro-environmental behaviour via this rational route, however, are not always effective (Ockwell *et al.*, 2009). An explanation for this may be that a large proportion of our behaviour is the result of automatic, less conscious decision-making. Any external or internal stimulus induces reactions in the brain, resulting in particular behaviours that are often beyond our control of will. Depending on stimuli type, the brain reacts in different ways and our behaviour is subsequently directed in various ways. Apart from social stimuli (i.e. us reacting on other peoples' behaviour), environmental cues may induce reactions and guide our behaviour. For example, rat studies on 'enriched environments' show that stimulating environments with positive environmental cues increase levels of neurotrophic factors in the brain, making the rats more socially interactive (Sale *et al.*, 2009). Interestingly, certain experiences and stimuli in the environment do not only temporarily activate neurotrophic factors, but they actually change the structure and function of cerebral neurons as well, referred to as brain plasticity (Sale *et al.*, 2014). This would support the idea that using environmental cues to induce pro-environmental behaviour may lead to pro-environmental behaviour that is maintained over time. Read more about enriched environments in Chapter 2.4 'Environmental enrichment: Neurophysiological responses and consequences for health'.

Gaining understanding about how the automatic system influences environmental decision-making may be one way to potentially induce behaviour change towards a more sustainable lifestyle. For instance, one may use the set-up or the design of the environment (a concept which can relate and impact on the so-called 'choice architecture', namely the behavioural range a person has within a given spatial and temporal frame; Thaler and Sunstein, 2008) to stimulate or 'nudge' environmentally friendly choices. In other words, more or less disguised modifications of environmental features may be used to induce pro-environmental behaviour.

Most of the studies so far around these concepts have related to encouraging lifestyle behaviours to improve health (Hollands *et al.*, 2013). However, a recent study demonstrated that subtle environmental cues could induce 'mental shortcuts' that unconsciously influence decisions with beneficial consequences for the environment (Ölander and Thøgersen, 2014). There appear to be several ways through which pro-environmental choices can be promoted in a more or less automatic manner. Even mere exposure to nature can make people act more cooperatively (see Box 2.7.1) and increase the likelihood of pro-environmental actions (Zelenski *et al.*, 2015). As we know that nature has an automatic impact on our cognitive function and neurological processes (Bratman *et al.*, 2012), it is plausible that environmentally friendly behaviour may also be induced unconsciously.

Box 2.7.1 Pro-social behaviour and nature

Pro-social behaviour—inclinations to share, care, cooperate, and assist—is critical to the development and maintenance of strong social relationships and is also related to pro-environmental behaviour (Berenguer, 2010; Sevillano *et al.*, 2010). Pro-social behaviour can enable social ties that are reciprocal and mutually beneficial. Similarly to pro-environmental behaviour, pro-social behaviour can also incur many costs, and those who act pro-socially risk their sacrifices being unreciprocated or even exploited. How do individuals decide about where, when, and with whom to act in a pro-social fashion? Several lines of theorizing have focused on how social processes influence pro-social behaviour, positing that pro-sociality follows from rational cost-benefit analyses in which the individual takes stock of the person in need, the costs of helping, and the immediate or delayed rewards for the self to be derived from pro-social action (Keltner *et al.*, 2014).

Extending this framework and in parallel with understanding of automatically induced pro-environmental behaviour, emerging research in psychology suggests that pro-sociality can also arise from processes that are neither rational nor social. This work finds that pro-social behaviour can be influenced by people's relationship to the external natural environment. Research has documented a connection between experiences of nature and an enhanced orientation to others and social relationships. For instance, people who feel connected to nature report greater perspective taking (Mayer and Frantz, 2004), and people who perceive beauty in nature report more benevolence (Diessner *et al.*, 2013). In one experiment, people who saw images of nature, relative to images of urban scenes, endorsed greater communal aspirations (e.g. 'To have deep enduring relationships'). In a follow-up study, participants who completed the study in a lab with potted plants behaved more generously than participants in a room without plants (Weinstein *et al.*, 2009). A connection to nature, it would seem, can enhance social connections.

Other research was focused on two underlying processes that may help drive the effects of nature and the natural environment on human sociality: beauty and awe. It was found that exposure to natural beauty is a particularly significant driver of pro-social behaviour (Zhang *et al.*, 2014). In one study, participants were randomly assigned to watch a one-minute long slideshow that contained either 10 images of beautiful nature or 10 images of less beautiful nature. Participants then received 10 points (each of which would be equal to an additional five cent award at the end of the study) and were asked how many, if any, they wanted to allocate to an anonymous partner that they had been paired with in the study. Participants who had viewed images of beautiful nature gave away significantly more points than participants

(continued)

Box 2.7.1 (Continued)

in the less beautiful nature condition. In another study, participants who were exposed to more beautiful, as opposed to less beautiful nature offered more help to an experimenter by folding Japanese paper cranes for victims of a tsunami. Across studies it was also found that the effects of natural beauty on pro-social behaviour were driven by positive mood. In other words, participants who had been exposed to natural beauty felt better—they were happier—and their enhanced positivity drove their increased kindness towards others. This is another corresponding feature to the potential of 'warm glow' or other positive emotions driving pro-environmental behaviour.

In another focal area of research, the social consequences of awe—a cherished and transformative emotion that is deeply connected to experiences in nature—were examined (Shiota *et al.*, 2007). Awe arises via appraisals of stimuli that are vast, that transcend current frames of reference, and that require new schemata to accommodate what is being perceived. Although many stimuli can inspire awe, from beautiful buildings to elegant equations, the prototypical awe experience, at least in Western cultures, involves encounters with natural phenomena that are immense in size, scope, or complexity (e.g. panoramic vistas, the night sky, giant trees, waterfalls).

Studies have begun to document the influences of awe on sociality, effects that can be understood in terms of how awe directs attention to entities greater than oneself and triggers feelings that one's individual being is relatively less significant. In one study, participants primed to recall a past personal experience of awe reported perceptions of something greater than themselves, feeling smaller and less significant, and a sense that their attention was less focused on personal day-to-day concerns (Shiota *et al.*, 2007). In other research, eliciting awe via a nature video caused participants to feel more connected to others (Van Cappellen and Saroglou, 2012). Research found that experiences of awe can cause people to be more willing to forego self-interest in favour of others' welfare (Piff *et al.*, 2015). In one experiment, inducing awe via a five-minute video of scenic vistas, mountains, and canyons caused participants to share significantly more of a valued resource (lottery tickets for a cash prize) with a stranger, relative to participants who watched a video of nature that induced amusement or a neutral control video. In another experiment, participants were situated in a grove of towering eucalyptus trees and were asked to look up at the tall trees or to face the opposite direction and look up at a tall building (control) for 60 seconds; these experiences differed in the levels of awe they evoked. After 60 seconds had elapsed, participants' helping behaviour was assessed by observing and recording the number of pens they picked up to help an experimenter who had ostensibly dropped them by accident. Participants who stared up at trees gathered significantly more pens for the experimenter than participants in the control condition. It appears that even short-lived, fleeting experiences of awe in nature can have a meaningful impact on various types of pro-social judgements and behaviour. Moreover, across studies it was found that the effects of awe on pro-sociality were driven by self-reported feelings that the individual self and its interests were relatively diminished vis-à-vis something perceived to be more vast and powerful than oneself. In certain ways, then, experiences of awe towards nature may serve to shift people's focus away from the centre of their own individual worlds, towards the broader social context and their place within it.

The naturalist Jon Muir observed, ' ... in every walk with Nature one receives far more than he seeks' (Muir 1992), suggesting a psychological benefit to nature—an intuition many people share and that mounting evidence corroborates (Bratman *et al.*, 2012). Altogether perceptions of beauty, enhanced positive mood, and transformative experiences of awe are but a few of the myriad of benefits that arise from humans' relationship to nature, benefits that can extend beyond the individual to one's relationship partners, small groups, and social collectives.

Missing out on well-being by behaving automatically?

While automatic decision-making may be an interesting way to motivate engagement in pro-environmental behaviour, its consequences for the sense of well-being that people derive out of pro-environmental behaviour need to be studied in further detail. If people act in an environmentally friendly way following the process of automatic decision-making, they may not be fully aware of the fact they are doing something environmentally friendly and thus meaningful. Thereby, the good feeling that engagement in pro-environmental behaviour itself elicits may be lost. Furthermore, *making the choice* to engage in certain behaviour, rather than acting out of situational constraints or inputs, may particularly reveal something about who you are—not only to others, but also to yourself. Behaviour that is performed automatically may thus say less about an individual, than behaviour that is performed with deliberation. Pro-environmental behaviour performed via automatic decision-making may thus fail to boost the self-image of those people acting this way. Following this reasoning, it is likely that particularly those people who deliberately choose to act pro-environmentally will experience their behaviour to be meaningful and gain well-being from their actions (Evans and Jackson, 2008).

However, while automatically induced pro-environmental behaviour may possibly provide less individual well-being, on a broader public health level pro-environmental behaviour may have a much more general effect on health and well-being for populations across the world (Van den Bosch and Depledge, 2015). Moving beyond the individual perspective, pro-environmental behaviour should result in less environmental degradation and eventually also reduce the speed of climate change. It has been shown that environmentally aware households can substantially reduce carbon emissions, with little or no impact on general well-being (Dietz *et al.*, 2009). As worsened environmental conditions and climate change caused by anthropogenic impact are today among the major threats to human health, anything that hampers this process has the potential to improve public health in a long-term and global perspective. Thus, even if engagement in pro-environmental behaviour via the automatic route may not increase the well-being of the individual acting this way, it may eventually improve the health and well-being of the whole planet and its inhabitants.

Conclusion

We are at a point in time when behaviours related to nature and the environment are gaining increasing importance for public health.

Behavioural medicine must therefore expand to include human actions and decisions related to the environment. This would include aspects of how our behaviour affects the environment, but also how the natural environment affects our behaviour. Engagement in pro-environmental behaviour may bring health and well-being for different reasons. Behaving pro-environmentally can in itself feel good, since these actions are deemed meaningful and improve the self-image of those acting this way. In turn, the positive feelings that pro-environmental behaviour can set in motion a virtuous loop, stimulating future ecologically sound behaviour. Last, but not least, people's decisions and actions to fight climate change and improve our environment will eventually lead to healthier nature and living conditions, thereby protecting the health and well-being of everyone living on Earth now and in the future. Further evidence that environmental cues, and even natural environments themselves, could encourage automatic pro-environmental behaviour would be another argument for maintaining and developing natural environments and urban green spaces.

References

Aknin, L. B., Dunn, E. W., & Norton, M. I., (2012). Happiness runs in a circular motion: Evidence for a positive feedback loop between prosocial spending and happiness. *J Happiness Stud*, 13, 347–55.

Andreoni, J. (1990). Impure altruism and donations to public goods: A theory of warm-glow giving. *Econ J*, 100, 464–77.

Bem, D. J. (1972). Self-perception theory. In: Berkowitz, L. (ed.) *Advances in Experimental Social Psychology*, pp. 1–62. New York, NY: Academic Press.

Berenguer, J. (2010). The effect of empathy in environmental moral reasoning. *Environ Behav*, 42, 110–34.

Berenguer, J., Corraliza, J. A., & Martín, R. (2005). Rural-urban differences in environmental concern, attitudes, and actions. *Eur J Psychol Assess*, 21, 128–38.

Bolderdijk, J. W., Steg, L., Geller, E. S., Lehman, P. K., & Postmes, T. (2013). Comparing the effectiveness of monetary versus moral motives in environmental campaigning. *Nat Clim Chang*, 3, 413–16.

Bonaiuto, M. & Alves, S. (2012). Residential places and neighbourhoods: Toward healthy life, social integration, and reputable residence. In: Clayton, S. (ed.) *The Oxford Handbook of Environmental and Conservation Psychology*, pp. 221–47. Oxford, UK: Oxford University Press.

Bonaiuto, M., Bonnes, M., & Continisio, M. (2004). Neighborhood evaluation within a multi-place perspective on urban activities. *Environ Behav*, 36, 41–69.

Bonaiuto, M., Mao, Y., Roberts, S., et al. (2016). Optimal experience and optimal identity: Flow and the consolidation of place identity. *Front Psychol*, 7, 1654. eCollection 2016.

Bratman, G. N., Hamilton, J. P. & Daily, G. C. (2012). The impacts of nature experience on human cognitive function and mental health. *Ann N Y Acad Sci*, 1249, 118–36.

Brown, K. W. & Kasser, T. (2005). Are psychological and ecological well-being compatible? The role of values, mindfulness, and lifestyle. *Soc Indic Res*, 74, 349–68.

Chaiken, S. & Trope, Y. (1999). *Dual-Process Theories in Social Psychology*. New York, NY: Guilford Press.

Collado, S., Corraliza, J. A., Staats, H., & Ruiz, M. (2015). Effect of frequency and mode of contact with nature on children's self-reported ecological behaviors. *J Environ Psychol*, 41, 65–73.

Diessner, R., Iyer, R., Smith, M. M., & Haidt, J. (2013). Who engages with moral beauty?. *J Moral Educ*, 42, 139–63.

Dietz, T., Gardner, G. T., Gilligan, J., Stern, P. C. & Van Den Bergh, M. P. (2009). Household actions can provide a behavioral wedge to rapidly reduce US carbon emissions. *Proc Natl Acad Sci U S A*, 106, 18452–6.

Evans, D. & Jackson, T. (2008). *Sustainable Consumption: Perspectives from Social and Cultural Theory*. Guildford, UK: University of Surrey.

Fredrickson, B. L. (2001). The role of positive emotions in positive psychology: The broaden-and-build theory of positive emotions. *Am Psychol*, 56, 218–26.

Harland, P., Staats, H., & Wilke, H. A. M. (1999). Explaining proenvironmental intention and behavior by personal norms and the theory of planned behavior. *J Appl Soc Psychol*, 29, 2505–28.

Heberlein, T. A. (1972). The land ethic realized: Some social psychological explanations for changing environmental attitudes. *J Soc Issues*, 28, 79–87.

Hollands, G. J., Shemilt, I., Marteau, T. M., et al. (2013). Altering micro-environments to change population health behaviour: Towards an evidence base for choice architecture interventions. *BMC Public Health*, 13, 1218.

Kellert, S. R. (1993). The biological basis for human values of nature. In: Kellert, S. R. & Wilson, E. O. (eds) *The Biophilia Hypothesis*, pp. 42–69. Washington, DC: Island Press.

Keltner, D., Kogan, A., Piff, P. K., & Saturn, S. R. (2014). The sociocultural appraisals, values, and emotions (SAVE) framework of prosociality: Core processes from gene to meme. *Ann Rev Psychol*, 65, 425–460.

Khan, U. & Dhar, R. (2006). Licensing effect in consumer choice. *J Market Res*, 43, 259–66.

Mao, Y., Roberts, S., & Bonaiuto, M. (2016). Optimal experience and optimal identity: A multinational examination at the personal identity level. In: Harmat, L., Ørsted Andersen, F., Ullén, F., Wright, J., & Sadlo, G. (eds) *Flow Experience. Empirical Research and Applications*, pp. 289–308. Basel, Switzerland: Springer.

Mao, Y., Roberts, S., Pagliaro, S., Csikszentmihalyi, M., & Bonaiuto, M. (2016). Optimal experience and optimal identity: A multinational study of the associations between flow and social identity. *Front Psychol*, 7, 67.

Mayer, F. S. & Frantz, C. M. (2004). The connectedness to nature scale: A measure of individuals' feeling in community with nature. *J Environ Psychol*, 24, 503–15.

Moll, J., Krueger, F., Zahn, R., Pardini, M., De Oliveira-Souza, R., & Grafman, J. (2006). Human fronto-mesolimbic networks guide decisions about charitable donation. *Proc Natl Acad Sci U S A*, 103, 15623–8.

Muir, J. (1992). *The Eight Wilderness—Discovery Books*. United Kingdom: Diadem Books.

Ockwell, D., Whitmarsh, L., & O'Neill, S. (2009). Reorienting climate change communication for effective mitigation: Forcing people to be green or fostering grass-roots engagement?. *Sci Commun*, 30, 305–27.

Ölander, F. & Thøgersen, J. (2014). Informing versus nudging in environmental policy. *J Consum Policy*, 37, 341–56.

Onwezen, M. C., Antonides, G., & Bartels, J. (2013). The Norm Activation Model: An exploration of the functions of anticipated pride and guilt in pro-environmental behaviour. *J Econ Psychol*, 39, 141–53.

Passmore, H. & Howell, A. J. (2014). Nature involvement increases hedonic and eudaimonic well-being: A two-week experimental study. *Ecopsychology*, 6, 148–54.

Piff, P. K., Dietze, P., Feinberg, M., Stancato, D. M. & Keltner, D. (2015). Awe, the small self, and prosocial behavior. *J Pers Soc Psychol*, 108, 883–99.

Sale, A., Berardi, N., & Maffei, L. (2009). Enrich the environment to empower the brain. *Trends Neurosci*, 32, 233–9.

Sale, A., Berardi, N., & Maffei, L. (2014). Environment and brain plasticity: towards an endogenous pharmacotherapy. *Physiol Rev*, 94, 189–234.

Sevillano, V., Aragonés, J. I. & Schultz, P. W. (2010). Altruism and beyond: The motivational bases of pro-environmental behavior. In: Corral-Verdugo, V., Garcia-Caden, C. H., & Frias-Armenta, M. (eds). *Psychological Approaches to Sustainability: Current Trends in Theory, Research and Applications*, pp. 161–184. New York, NY:Nova Science Publishers.

Shiota, M. N., Keltner, D., & Mossman, A. (2007). The nature of awe: Elicitors, appraisals, and effects on self-concept. *Cogn Emot*, 21, 944–63.

Spunt, R. P. & Lieberman, M. D. (2013). The busy social brain: Evidence for automaticity and control in the neural systems supporting social cognition and action understanding. *Psychol Sci*, 24, 80–6.

Stern, P. C. (2000). New environmental theories: Toward a coherent theory of environmentally significant behavior. *J Soc Issues*, 56, 407–24.

Strack, F. & Deutsch, R. (2004). Reflective and impulsive determinants of social behavior. *Pers Soc Psychol Rev*, 8, 220–47.

Taufik, D., Bolderdijk, J. W. & Steg, L. (2015). Acting green elicits a literal 'warm-glow'. *Nat Clim Chang*, 5, 37–40.

Thaler, R. H. & Sunstein, C. R. (2008). *Nudge: Improving Decisions about Health, Wealth, and Happiness.* New Haven, CT: Yale University Press.

Tiefenbeck, V., Staake, T., Roth, K., & Sachs, O. (2013). For better or for worse? Empirical evidence of moral licensing in a behavioral energy conservation campaign. *Energy Policy*, 57, 160–71.

Van Cappellen, P. & Saroglou, V. (2012). Awe activates religious and spiritual feelings and behavioral intentions. *Psychology Religion Spirituality*, 4, 223–36.

Van Den Bosch, M. A. & Depledge, M. H. (2015). Healthy people with nature in mind. *BMC Public Health*, 15, 1232.

Van Overwalle, F. & Baetens, K. (2009). Understanding others' actions and goals by mirror and mentalizing systems: A meta-analysis. *NeuroImage*, 48, 564–84.

Venhoeven, L. A., Bolderdijk, J. W., & STEG, L. (2013). Explaining the paradox: How pro-environmental behaviour can both thwart and foster well-being. *Sustainability*, 5, 1372–386.

Weinstein, N., Przybylski, A. K., & Ryan, R. M. (2009). Can nature make us more caring? Effects of immersion in nature on intrinsic aspirations and generosity. *Pers Soc Psychol Bull*, 35, 1315–29.

Zelenski, J. M., Dopko, R. L. & Capaldi, C. A. (2015). Cooperation is in our nature: Nature exposure may promote cooperative and environmentally sustainable behavior. *J Environ Psychol*, 42, 24–31.

Zhang, J. W., Piff, P. K., Iyer, R., Koleva, S. & Keltner, D. (2014). An occasion for unselfing: Beautiful nature leads to prosociality. *J Environ Psychol*, 37, 61–72.

SECTION 3

Public health impact of nature contact— pathways to health promotion and disease prevention

CHAPTER 3.1

Promoting physical activity— reducing obesity and non-communicable diseases

Billie Giles-Corti, Fiona Bull, Hayley Christian, Mohammad Javad Koohsari, Takemi Sugiyama, and Paula Hooper

Planning for active living

'One generation plants the trees, and another gets the shade.'
Chinese Proverb

In the last two decades, there has been growing interest in the role of public open space in creating and enhancing health and well-being. This idea is not new: in the nineteenth century, public open space was seen as the 'lungs' of polluted industrial cities, and were developed to provide recreational opportunities and improve living conditions, particularly for the working classes living in squalid crowded housing (Sutton, 1971).

However, in the twenty-first century, renewed interest in public open space by the public health community has been sparked by its role in encouraging active living. Globally, the prevalence of non-communicable diseases (NCDs) is increasing, accounting for over 66% of all deaths annually (Lozano *et al.*, 2012). Leading NCDs (e.g. cardiovascular disease, diabetes, and some cancers) share common risk factors including obesity and physical inactivity. The way communities are planned—including the availability and quality of public open space—has an important role to play in reducing NCD risk behaviours. In this chapter, we overview the evidence of an association between physical activity and NCDs, then consider the role that public open space plays in encouraging active living across the life course from cradle to grave.

Why is physical activity important to health?

Undertaking regular physical activity is well established as promoting good health, preventing disease, and enhancing well-being. The ancient Greek physician, Hippocrates advised 'exercise in moderation' for good health, a statement now scientifically supported by the efforts of modern day study of the causes and prevention of disease. Since early pioneering work in the 1950s (Morris *et al.*, 1953), there has been a steadily growing body of scientific evidence documenting the extensive health-enhancing benefits of active living (Lee *et al.*, 2012; US Department of Health and Human Services, 2008; WHO, 2010).

Findings from a large number of epidemiological studies, many from Europe and North America but increasingly from other regions of the world, have measured the levels of physical activity in people and tracked health outcomes over time. These studies have established that the protective benefits of physical activity include a 30% reduced risk of ischaemic heart disease, a 27% reduced risk of diabetes, and a 21–25% reduced risk of breast cancer and colon cancer (WHO, 2010). In addition, regular physical activity lowers the risk of stroke and hypertension and is fundamental to maintaining a healthy energy balance and healthy body weight. Physical activity can reduce the development of the metabolic syndrome and is associated with favourable lipid profiles. For older adults, regular physical activity can maintain strength and functional abilities and prevent falls.

As noted, physical inactivity is now recognized as one of the four key behavioural risk factors of the leading NCDs, along with smoking, alcohol abuse, and unhealthy diet, three of which can lead to overweight and obesity. The World Health Organization (WHO) estimates that inactivity alone accounts for between 6–9% of NCDs and an estimated 3.2 million premature deaths annually, along with 32.1 million disability-adjusted life years, DALYs (2.1% of all global DALYs, a measure of diasability) (WHO, 2011). Physical inactivity is the fourth leading risk factor for global mortality after hypertension, tobacco, and high blood glucose levels (WHO, 2009; 2011), contributing to 15% more deaths than are attributed to obesity. A more recent estimate calculated that the impact of inactivity is possibly higher, suggesting that annually 5 million premature deaths could be prevented (Lee *et al.*, 2012). Furthermore, if adults met the recommended levels of activity life expectancy could be increased by 0.6 years (Lee *et al.*, 2012).

It is, however, not just physical health that benefits from regular exercise. There is a growing body of evidence that mental health and well-being can be improved and that physical activity is an effective therapeutic regime for depression and anxiety. More recent research has identified a potential protective effect against diseases such as Alzheimer's. The enjoyment of, and participation in, physical activities with other people can also provide and improve social connections, and through this gain health benefits which are important to health and well-being. It is clear that physical activity plays an extensive role in both maintaining good health and in the prevention and treatment of illness. In terms of multiple benefits of being physically active, the whole is considerably greater than the sum of the parts.

Indeed, the importance and breadth of benefits afforded by regular participation in physical activity was recognized by the United Nations in 2011 at its meeting to address the global concern regarding the rising burden of NCDs (UN, 2011). Noting that two out of every three premature deaths are due to NCDs, and that 80% of these occur in low- and middle-income countries, the UN Declaration provides a clear call to all countries (developed and developing) to increase efforts to promote participation in physical activity as part of a comprehensive response. The critical importance of reducing exposure to the core modifiable risk factors for NCDs was emphasized, and the subsequent Global Action Plan released by the WHO provides countries with a platform for action, as well as a global target of reducing the levels of inactivity by 10% by 2025 (WHO, 2013).

Importantly, both the UN and WHO have recognized that reducing NCDs and encouraging physical activity are not simply the responsibility of the health sector. Effective action requires a whole-of-government, whole-of-society approach. This highlights the important role played by sectors outside of health, and hence the importance of focusing on the potential contribution of well-designed and accessible public open space.

What is 'public open space' and how might it affect individual health and chronic disease?

Throughout this chapter, we refer to 'public open space'. This is defined as all land reserved for the provision of green space and natural environments that is freely accessible and intended for active or passive recreation (Edwards et al., 2013). Figure 3.1.1 defines the different categories of public open space that this might include: parks, natural environments (e.g. bushland, forests), school grounds, and residual green spaces.

Individuals and communities are affected by the quality and design of the settings in which they live, work, and play. Hence, there is growing recognition that the availability and design of public open space has an important role to play in community levels of physical activity (Kaczynski and Henderson, 2007). This reflects an 'ecological' model of active living (Sallis et al., 2006), as depicted in Figure 3.1.2. This model suggests that multiple factors influence the health and well-being of individuals. Notably, most of these factors—including the built environment—are outside of the health sector, illustrating a host of sectors influencing and creating the built environment that develops the conditions for good health. Broadly defined, the built environment refers to '… the physical environment that is constructed by human activity' (Saelens and Handy, 2008). Among other things, the built environment includes land use patterns, transportation systems, foot paths, and bike paths (Saelens and Handy, 2008), as well as public open space (Kaczynski and Henderson, 2007). Hence, optimizing health and well-being outcomes—including reducing risk factors for NCDs—requires the involvement of numerous disciplines and sectors responsible for designing and planning the built environment, including urban designers, planners, and

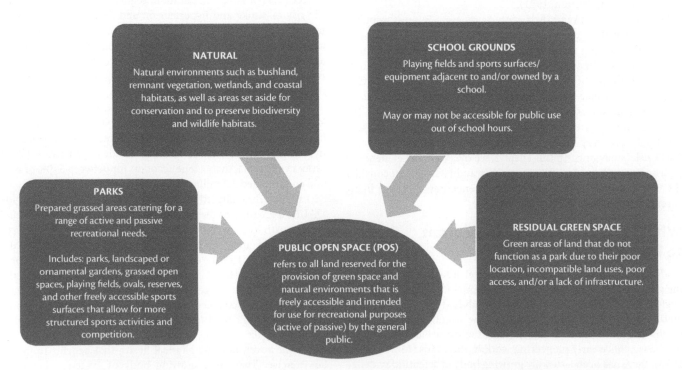

Fig. 3.1.1 Different types of public open spaces.

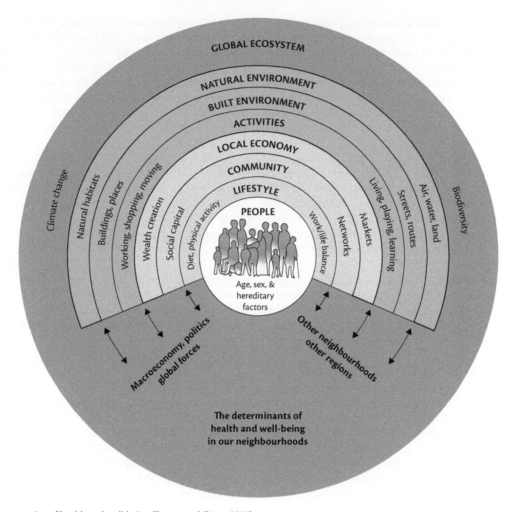

Fig. 3.1.2 Ecological perspective of health and well-being (Barton and Grant, 2006).
Reproduced with permission from Dahlgren G and Whitehead M, *Policies and Strategies to Promote Social Equity in Health*, Institute for Futures Studies, Stockholm, Sweden, Copyright © 1991.

landscape architects, as well as local government and the recreation sector. Importantly, public open space needs to be designed to cater for different user groups across the life course, as this will increase its use and in turn contribute to community levels of physical activity. In the sections that follow, we consider the evidence on the role of public open space in encouraging physical activity across the life course: from children through to older adults.

The importance of access to public open space for children and adolescents

Numerous health benefits are derived by children from access to public open space. Enhanced access is associated with increased physical activity (Babey *et al.*, 2008; Cohen *et al.*, 2006b; Coley *et al.*, 1997; Rodríguez *et al.*, 2012; Salmon and Timperio, 2007; Wheeler *et al.*, 2010; Giles-Corti *et al.*, 2009; Roemmich *et al.*, 2006) and decreased risk of overweight in children (Bell *et al.*, 2008; Coley *et al.*, 1997; Liu *et al.*, 2007; Potwarka *et al.*, 2008). Public open space is also important for child health and development because it facilitates different types of play—and in particular 'active play', which is an important source of physical activity for children (Brockman *et al.*, 2011).

Landscape features of public open space appear to influence physical fitness and motor development in young children. In quasi-experimental studies of 5–7 year olds, Fjørtoft showed that children who played in a natural landscape (i.e. forest), significantly increased their motor fitness, balance, and coordination compared with children who played only in traditional outdoor kindergarten playgrounds (Fjørtoft, 2004; Fjørtoft, 2001; Fjørtoft and Sageie, 2000). Young people exposed to nature also experience a wide range of cognitive, emotional, and social benefits. These topics and other impacts of nature on children's health are further elaborated on in Chapter 6.1. 'Children and nature'.

Importantly, children who spend more time outside are more physically active (Cleland *et al.*, 2008; Sallis *et al.*, 2000). There is strong empirical evidence that children's outdoor play and physical activity is positively associated with access to nature and public open space, including parks and playgrounds. For example, a US study of children aged 3–12 years found that levels of play in barren spaces were about half as much as play in spaces with trees and grass (Taylor *et al.*, 1998).

Moroever, the physical activity benefits associated with public open space appear to be greater for boys than girls. A recent Danish study used accelerometers and global positioning systems (GPS) to determine the proportion of time spent in moderate-vigorous physical activity in different settings. It found that compared with girls, boys spend a significantly larger proportion of their time doing moderate-to-vigorous physical activity in urban green space (24% vs. 17%) (Klinker *et al.*, 2014).

In addition, numerous studies have found that children are more likely to use parks closer to home (Cohen *et al.*, 2006a; Epstein *et al.*, 2006; Roemmich *et al.*, 2006). However, simply having access to nearby public open space may not be enough: park amenity is also important. An Australian study found that, regardless of age, gender, or socioeconomic status, children did not necessarily visit their closest park (Veitch *et al.*, 2006b). Instead they visited parks with better play equipment (Veitch *et al.*, 2008) and were less likely to use a park if it was perceived as boring and unchallenging (Veitch *et al.*, 2006b). Similarly, a study of adolescents living in a regional city found that adolescents—particularly boys—travelled further to use a public open space if it had amenities they enjoyed using, such as a skateboard ramp (Edwards *et al.*, 2015).

Thus, to facilitate children's play and physical activity in parks, public open space needs to be interesting and provide an element of risk. There is considerable evidence that nature-based features (i.e. trees, rocks, and water) in parks attract children and youth of all ages (Fjørtoft, 2001; Fjørtoft and Sageie, 2000; Lee and Christiansen, 1999; Loukaitou-Sideris and Stieglitz, 2002; Wood *et al.*, 2010); however, there are fewer studies examining other park attributes associated with levels of physical activity (Floyd *et al.*, 2011). One of the few studies to comprehensively examine the association between park attributes and youth physical activity found that out-of-school physical activity in adolescent girls was associated with access to local parks with walking paths, running tracks, playgrounds, basketball courts, and streetlights and floodlights (Cohen *et al.*, 2006b). Neighbourhood features surrounding a park can also either facilitate or discourage park visits by children. For example, the presence of high traffic volumes has been shown to decrease the likelihood of adolescent girls travelling to a park (Norman *et al.*, 2006) or park use by adolescents living in a regional city (Edwards *et al.*, 2013), while zebra crossings and traffic lights increase park accessibility for children (Timperio *et al.*, 2004).

Finally, a significant barrier to children's play and physical activity in parks is parental 'fear of strangers'. Parents are gatekeepers of children's behaviour. However, when the perceived risks of 'stranger danger' outweigh the real risks (Zubrick *et al.*, 2010), parents may negatively influence their children's opportunities for play and physical activity, particularly in public areas like neighbourhood parks. Read more about risk perception in Chapter 7.4. 'Risk and the perception of risk in interactions with nature'.

Only a handful of studies have investigated the influence of public open space interventions on child and adolescent physical activity levels, with mixed findings. An Australian study found no significant effects on children's park use or physical activity following a major upgrade to children's play areas (Bohn-Goldbaum *et al.*, 2013). In contrast, significant soccer and baseball playfield upgrades in two public parks significantly increased park use by children as well as the number of physically active visitors (regardless of ages), compared with the control park (Tester and Baker, 2009). Furthermore, a natural experiment of a playground upgrade found that compared with the control community, total physical activity increased for children with lower BMIs in the intervention community, but decreased for those with higher BMIs (Quigg

et al., 2011). Finally, safe transitional green spaces (e.g. green verge between the front fence and the footpath or road) between home and the wider neighbourhood are readily accessible play environments for children, yet little is known about their role in facilitating children's outdoor play and physical activity. In some countries, many of these 'near home' transitional green spaces have been lost over time, and are unlikely to be have been compensated for by the presence of neighbourhood parks and playgrounds (Foster *et al.*, 2011).

As cities urbanize and densify, the amount of private and public open space available for children's active play declines (Hall, 2010; Mccurdy *et al.*, 2010; Martin and Wood, 2012). This is worrying, as we have shown that time spent outdoors is associated with children's physical activity (Sallis *et al.*, 1993). If not carefully managed, reduced outdoor open space may result in a decline in children's play and physical activity with negative consequences for their overall health, weight status, and development. Hence, as cities become more compact (OECD, 2012), there is a need to carefully consider the needs for public open space for all population groups, but in particular the needs of children and young people who need public open space where they can be active and play.

Public open space and adults' physical activity

As with children, access to public open space confers numerous benefits to adults' mental and physical health. As disucssed in Chapter 3.2. 'Preventing stress and promoting mental health', access to public open space can be beneficial to mental health. By way of example, an Australian study found that the quality of public open space to be inversely associated with adults' psychosocial distress (Francis *et al.*, 2012), while a recent US study found higher neighbourhood greenness to be associated with lower symptomology for depression, anxiety, and stress among adults (Beyer *et al.*, 2014).

However, access to green space also appears to be protective of NCDs and their associated risk factors. For example, an Australian study found variability in greenness within neighbourhoods to be negatively associated with coronary heart disease and stroke in adults (Pereira *et al.*, 2012). Similarly, the amount and variability of greenness in a neighbourhood (Pereira *et al.*, 2013) as well as proximity to a large park (Rundle *et al.*, 2013) have been found to be negatively associated with weight status. In addition, a study in Denmark found the availability of green spaces within neighbourhoods to be inversely related to type 2 diabetes (Maas *et al.*, 2009).

Many of these positive effects of public open space on adults' health are likely to result from the opportunities provided for adults to be physically active. Public open space is a key neighbourhood setting for a variety of physical activities including walking and playing sports (Bedimo-Rung *et al.*, 2005; Kaczynski and Henderson, 2007). In the last decade, there have been a burgeoning number of studies of adults' physical activity examining different aspects of public open space including its proximity and features (Giles-Corti *et al.*, 2005a; Kaczynski *et al.*, 2008; Sugiyama *et al.*, 2010; Sallis *et al.*, 2016).

Most studies examining the proximity of public open space use the concept of 'shortest distance to', or the 'size of the nearest', public open space. Adults living closer to the nearest public open

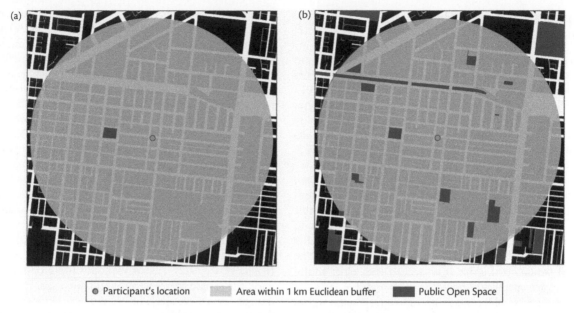

Fig. 3.1.3 Multiple sites of public opens space around participant's home versus single closest one: (a) single closest; (b) multiple.

space or whose closest public open space is larger tend to report more physical activity. For instance, an English study found that adults with shorter distances to formal parks were more likely to achieve recommended levels of physical activity (Coombes *et al.*, 2010). A Danish study also found the large size of the nearest urban green space to be positively associated with adults' physical activity undertaken within that setting (Schipperijn *et al.*, 2013). However, examining the impact of only a single public open space ignores the potential influence of other green and natural open spaces within the neighbourhood (Fig. 3.1.3). To address this issue, recent studies have analysed the impact of having multiple sites of public open space nearby on adults' physical activity. For example, a US study (Kaczynski *et al.*, 2009) found that the number and total area of parks within 1 km of residents' homes (but not the shortest distance to the closest park) played a significant role in increasing adults' park-related physical activity.

In addition to proximity, park attributes have been shown to be important in encouraging adults' physical activity. For instance, in the United States, Kaczynski *et al.* (Kaczynski *et al.*, 2008) found park features to be associated with adults' physical activity within parks, although no associations were found for distance to, and size of, parks. Among park attributes, the presence of trails were the most important correlate of physical activity. An Australian study however, showed that the presence of larger attractive public open space in a local area may encourage higher levels of walking regardless of the distance to such open space (Sugiyama *et al.*, 2010). Similarly, Foster *et al.* (2012) found public open space with more features, and safer parks with less disorder and more lighting were more likely to encourage recreational walking.

Nevertheless, a handful of studies have shown the proximity of public open space and their features to be unrelated to adults' physical activity. For example, a UK study of adults found access to green spaces was not associated with recreational walking (Foster *et al.*, 2009), while a Brazilian study found that distance to the nearest park was not associated with either adults' leisure-time physical activity or walking (Hino *et al.*, 2011). Similarly, a recent Australian

study found none of four public open space proximity measures to be associated with adults' walking to, or within, a public open space including distance to the nearest, total number, total area, or attractiveness of public open space (Koohsari *et al.*, 2013b). Finally, no association was observed between park use and perceived park safety among adults, unlike park size which was associated with park usage (Cohen *et al.*, 2010).

There appears to be several reasons for the mixed evidence related to the proximity and features of public open space and adults' levels of physical activity. First, the majority of previous studies used context-free measures of physical activity (Giles-Corti *et al.*, 2005b), such as the total physical activity independent of where it took place. This may include a substantial amount of physical activity undertaken outside one's neighbourhood (Troped *et al.*, 2010). Second, the inconsistencies may be caused by different studies using objective (e.g. geographic information systems) and perceived (e.g. surveys) measures of proximity and public open space features. Gebel and colleagues found that objective measures of the built environment do not necessarily reflect perceived measures (Gebel *et al.*, 2009). Hence, different findings may reflect measurement differences. Third, studies incorporating measures of the nearest public open space appear to assume that residents use their nearest public open space. However, the evidence suggests there is a wide range of factors that influence use, not least of which are its size and attributes. Hence, there may be a mismatch between the exposure measure (i.e. attributes of the nearest public open space) and the public open space actually used.

Last, most studies tend to ignore the characteristics of the built environment surrounding public open space (e.g. safety, aesthetics, walkability). These characteristics not only moderate the influence of proximity and public open space features on physical activity (Sugiyama *et al.*, 2014), but are also independently associated with adults' participation in physical activity. For example, providing more direct and lower speed streets around parks is associated with more park-related physical activity among adults (Kaczynski *et al.*, 2014).

Public open space and older adults' physical activity

Population ageing is taking place rapidly both in developed and developing countries: the number of older persons (aged 60 years or over) worldwide is expected to more than double between 2013 and 2050 (UN, 2013). There is now widespread agreement that many health problems of older life—including the onset of frailty and disability—could be postponed or delayed if older adults increased their levels of physical activity (Bishop, 1999; WHO, 1998; 2002).

Given the implications of population ageing on healthcare and ageing-related services, multisector initiatives are needed to support older adults' health, well-being, and independence. Accessible facilities for physical activity are important for older adults to maintain their levels of physical activity and functioning. Studies conducted in different geographical and cultural contexts show that access to local public open space is associated with older adults' physical activity, irrespective of how it is measured. For instance, in the United Kingdom, older men with more green space within 400 m of their residence were more likely to participate in regular physical activity (Gong et al., 2014); and in Hong Kong, it was found that the presence of parks within 400 m was associated with longer recreational walking in older Chinese adults (Cerin et al., 2013). Similarly, in the United States, local walking was associated with the density of green and open spaces within 800 m in older adults (Li et al., 2005b), while an Australian study found the percentage of green areas within 1 km of home was associated with walking and physical activity among adults over 45 years old (Astell-Burt et al., 2014). A Canadian study also found that the number and size of parks within 1 km of home were related to older adults' (55+ years) neighbourhood-based and park-based physical activity (Kaczynski et al., 2009). In a longitudinal study, older residents of neighbourhoods with access to recreational facilities, including parks, had lower rates of decline in walking over time (Li et al., 2005a). A review of qualitative studies also confirms that access to green spaces is a facilitator of older adults' physical activity (Moran et al., 2014). Together these quantitative and qualitative studies consistently show that local public open space is an important resource for older people, and vital for their participation in physical activity, particularly walking.

Nevertheless, there are a number of complexities to be considered. A Portuguese study found that proximity to the nearest park was unrelated to whether older residents engaged in leisure-time physical activity or not, yet among active male participants close park proximity was associated with longer duration of being active (Ribeiro et al., 2013). Conversely, a Japanese study found that access to proximate parks and green spaces (within 250, 500, and 1,000 m of home) was associated with the frequency of leisure-time physical activity, but not the duration of walking (Hanibuchi et al., 2011). These mixed findings seem to suggest there may be between-country differences in park distribution, and the way parks are used for physical activity by older residents. Moreover, the relationships between public open space attributes and physical activity in older adults may not be a simple linear association and moderation may be present. For example, a non-linear relationship has been identified between the amount of green space and walking, with older adults living in areas with medium density (4.5–8%) of park area having the highest likelihood of walking

more than one hour per week, compared with those living in areas with either lower (≤4.1%) or higher (8.1–35.2%) park density (Gomez et al., 2010). Thus, there may be an optimum amount of local public open space, beyond or below which public open space does not facilitate older people being more active. Furthermore, a prospective study has found an association between proximity to parks with a higher likelihood of maintaining or increasing walking in neighbourhoods in high but not low socioeconomic status (SES) neighbourhoods (Michael et al., 2010). The relationships between the availability of public open space and physical activity may vary by socioeconomic group. Moreover, in lower socioeconomic areas, the quality of public open space has been shown to be poorer (Crawford et al., 2008). Given that older adults tend to be more vulnerable and fearful, it may be that if public open space in lower income areas is of poor quality or not well maintained (Crawford et al., 2008; Mitchell and Popham, 2007), recreational walking may be lower, with detrimental impacts on mental health (Foster et al., 2012). Hence, without careful design and maintenance, the simple presence of public open space will not have the desired impact on levels of physical activity and the creation of health and well-being.

The contribution of green spaces to older adults' physical health is documented in a few studies. A Japanese study shows that older people who have walkable green spaces close to their residence tend to live longer (Takano et al., 2002). In Finland, the number of outdoor recreational facilities such as parks and green spaces within walking distance was shown to be associated with a decreased risk of developing walking difficulty (Eronen et al., 2014). This is important, given that functional decline is associated with falls, a major cause of death and disability in older adults (Todd and Skelton, 2004).

Most studies reviewed have focused on the availability of public open space (i.e. its presence, density, number, and proximity). Although public open space attributes such as amenities, activity facilities, vegetation, and maintenance are likely to be important, relatively little is known about which specific park features are relevant to older people's physical activity and park visits. Aesthetic aspects (pleasantness of open space and lack of nuisance) of local parks have been found to be related to older adults' recreational walking in a UK study (Sugiyama and Ward Thompson, 2008). A study examining older adults' preference for hypothetical parks with varying combinations of attributes has shown the relative importance of deterrents such as nuisances, vandalism, dog fouling, and heavy traffic en route, and of attractors such as cafes, toilets, vegetation, and things to watch (Aspinall et al., 2010). Although consistent with adult findings that the presence of disorder was negatively associated with recreational walking (Foster et al., 2012), this is an understudied area requiring further investigation in older adults.

Implications for policy and practice?

It is clear that public open space is an important setting to enhance the physical activities of residents in urban areas across the life course. The provision of public open space within towns and cities has long been an urban public policy concern and is determined by urban design and planning practices (Veal, 2012).

The evidence reviewed here suggests that the features of public open space that influence health and well-being outcomes vary depending on the user group or life stage (e.g. children, adolescents, adults, older adults). For example, different public open space amenities (e.g. local facilities and equipment) such as playgrounds are important for encouraging children's physical activity and independent play (Cohen et al., 2006b; Wood et al., 2010; Loukaitou-Sideris and Stieglitz, 2002; Fjørtoft, 2001; Lee and Christiansen, 1999; Fjørtoft and Sageie, 2000), while other types of amenity, facilities, and features within parks (e.g. toilets and seating) may encourage park use by older adults (Sugiyama and Ward Thompson, 2008). Even public open space proximity appears to be more meaningful for some user groups more than others. Notably, more vulnerable groups with less mobility, such as children and older adults, are more likely to use proximate public open space located within a short distance of their home (Gong et al., 2014; Cerin et al., 2013; Moran et al., 2014; Kaczynski et al., 2009). Public open space located further away may be less of a barrier for adolescents and adults. However, public open space with more amenities attracts specific user groups from afar, making proximity alone less important as the primary factor driving use, even in younger children (Veitch et al., 2006a; Veitch et al., 2008).

The evidence suggests that public open space with a variety of functions, characteristics, facilities, and amenities are important for encouraging use for different purposes (i.e. walking, playing sports, and relaxation) and by different population subgroups (i.e. children through to older adults). While the optimum mix of attributes is not clear, urban design and planning policies nevertheless therefore should ensure that neighbourhoods have a range of types of public open spaces available, which are accessible and conveniently located for use by the majority of residents. Importantly, public open space—particularly larger spaces—should cater for multiple user groups (e.g. a sporting field that can be used by recreational walkers and has a play area for children). However, recreational walkers are unlikely to be attracted to open flat sports fields, with unshaded, exposed boundary footpaths, and limited imaginative landscaping or vegetation, natural elements, or undulation. Rather, the accumulating evidence indicates that public open space that encourages active park use and walking has a range of features including the presence of footpaths, constructed or natural trails, trees, grass, natural settings, and water features, all of which are associated with active park use and walking within parks (Mccormack et al., 2010; Kaczynski et al., 2008). A number of studies have now found that parks with walking paths and trails were used more than those simply containing sports facilities (Reed et al., 2008; Giles-Corti et al., 2005a). Hence, with thoughtful (re-)design to include amenities for recreational walkers, sports fields (for example) could be optimized to make them an invaluable community resource catering for the needs of multiple user groups.

Increasingly, the provision of public open space is recognized as an 'environmental justice' issue to ensure the democratic provision of, and equitable access to, public open space in socially deprived and ethnically diverse neighbourhoods (Timperio et al., 2007). However, the evidence remains mixed (Badland et al., 2010), with some studies showing that public open space distribution disproportionately benefits more affluent communities.

To ensure equitable access, and provide opportunities for physical activity for everyone, public open space planning policies are required. Since the early to mid 1900s, common aspects of UK and US public open space planning policies (in some cases still used today) included the use of 'standards' and 'hierarchies' to guide the amount, types, spatial distribution, and accessibility of public open space throughout urban areas and neighbourhoods. Common standard-based approaches include: area-percentages (a specified percentage of land to be reserved for public open space); and catchment areas (specifications for various categories of public open space, typically based on size hierarchies) for maximum distances which residents should have to travel to gain access (Veal, 2012). Hierarchical standards have been deemed useful to analyse and categorize existing open space provision and to guide future provision or enhancement (Kellett and Rofe, 2009).

Veal (2012) notes that much of the international rationale on the provision of public open space and the development of provision standards appears to be premised in 'common sense' approaches (Kellett and Rofe, 2009) to quantify the space required for participation in recreational activity within reasonable distances of home, rather than being founded on empirical evidence (Wilkinson, 1985). One advantage of the standards is that they provide a legal basis for a defence of open space requirements demanded from developers (Kellett and Rofe, 2009) and give developers economic certainty in any calculation of profit from their development of land areas (Grose, 2009). Conversely, blanket standards are said to make it difficult for planners and environmental scientists to argue the case for more public open space, as developers feel they lose potential yield and profit (Grose, 2009). Importantly, however, internationally there appears to be few or no evidence-based approaches to developing planning standards for public open space provision (Veal, 2012) and clearly this is a gap in the literature. Importantly, the implementation of standards alone tends to ignore the quality of the public open space which, as evidenced by the review, is clearly an important determinant of use of public open space.

Hence, while the principles of setting open space standards and hierarchies have proved to be robust policy tools over a number of decades, current policy advice has shifted away from applying such prescriptive requirements given the range of development types, scales, and and densities. Needs-based assessment is increasingly being seen as preferable (Shiels, 1989; Veal, 2012) and may be more suitable than a standards-based approach to public open space provision.

Nevertheless, whether standards or needs-based assessment is adopted, the evidence presented in this review provides a persuasive argument that public open space is important infrastructure and there is a need to ensure equitable access to well-designed public open space that meets the needs of different people. The importance of including community participation in this process has been highlighted by the UK Commission for Architecture and the Built Environment (CABE Space, 2005), which noted that the nature, extent, and location of open space is best determined in consultation with existing and future residents taking into account the demographics of the local population.

Hence, in planning and designing public open space to support physical activity, it is imperative that local government, landscape architects, and urban designers ensure that the voices of all user groups are heard. This will ensure that the critical factors which encourage or discourage different groups from using public open space is considered in the (re)-design phase.

What evidence might help to advance the agenda of using green space to increase physical activity?

Generally there is consistent evidence that access to public open space is associated with physical activity across different age groups. However, with few exceptions, most research to date is cross-sectional. Longitudinal evidence is required to assess the causal relationships between access to public open space and physical activity patterns of residents. Findings from longitudinal studies are more scientifically robust and provide insights into strategies that might be effective to promote physical activity. For example, one longitudinal study of residents relocating to another neighbourhood found that those who gained access to different types of recreational destinations (e.g. a park, sports oval, or a beach) after relocating, increased their recreational walking by around 18 minutes per week for each different type of recreational destination gained (Giles-Corti et al., 2013). However, another longitudinal study of residents who remained in the same neighbourhood found the presence, proximity, and the size of the largest local public open space were associated with maintenance but not the uptake of walking over four years (Sugiyama et al., 2013). These results are important because they suggest a causal relationship between access to public open space and walking. However, they also suggest that the provision of public open space is necessary but insufficient alone to stimulate local walking; other strategies may be required to draw residents into local parks. Further prospective research, for example natural experiments (Veitch et al., 2014) that examine causal relationships between creating or upgrading public open space and physical activity patterns of nearby residents of different age groups, is warranted.

Second, methodological development is needed to more accurately measure physical activity in relation to public open space (as a destination, as a setting, and as a route). Currently, studies rely on self-report measures to identify public open space-related physical activities. Objective assessment using activity monitors is not totally suitable for this purpose, as they simply measure activity irrespective of context. GPS, which provides data on movement (speed) and location, can be a solution. There are already several studies that have employed GPS devices to identify physical activity undertaken in public open space (Dunton et al., 2014; Evenson et al., 2013). Further use of GPS is recommended to better understand issues the types of public open spaces used more by residents, how public open space can influence people's intention to walk through a route, and how far people of different age groups travel (and by what means) to use public open space and for what purpose. This technology is now readily used, and this research would simply provide another useful application.

Third, most existing studies examine linear associations between open space attributes and physical activity. However, as one study of older adults suggests (Gomez et al., 2010), open space attributes may have an optimal level that would best serve residents' physical activity. Examining the shape of associations (rather than magnitude) and identifying 'thresholds' for public open space characteristics are an important next step. For example, there is evidence that proximity to larger public open space is associated with more walking in adults (Sugiyama et al., 2010; Giles-Corti et al., 2005a). Future research could consider how close and how large open space needs to be to facilitate physical activity, the optimal level of park attributes (e.g. walking paths, trees, play equipment) required to increase physical activity; and how these differ by user groups (children through to older adults). Findings on thresholds will provide more practical, evidence-based information that can assist in planning and decision-making (Koohsari et al., 2013a). Moreover, identifying the combination of attributes that optimize levels of physical activity across the life course would increase the efficiency of this valuable community infrastructure.

In this regard, there is a growing interest in the cost-effectiveness of built environment interventions and this is a fourth area of future research (Gunn et al., 2014). For example, there appears to be no published research examining the cost-effectiveness of creating or upgrading public open space. Using tools developed in health economics that translate physical activities such as walking and cycling into financial terms (Kahlmeier et al., 2014), it may be possible to estimate the possible economic benefit of providing public open space, including various park attributes. Policy decisions are often made based on the balance between cost and benefit. Determining the co-benefits associated with public open space could assist policy makers to make informed decisions with this important investment.

Finally, research is needed to understand the value that people place on public open space, particularly those living in higher density housing. As cities urbanize and densities increase, there is likely to be a greater demand for public open space, particularly in higher density areas. There is already some evidence that apartment dwellers are prepared to pay a premium to to live near public open space (Dehring and Dunse, 2006). Research methods used in marketing (i.e. conjoint analysis) may be useful for this purpose. Knowledge obtained from this research could inform urban design decisions in new or established areas. However, from an equity perspective, this research should inform the value that 'society' places on public open space, to ensure that all groups in society—irrespective of their economic resources—have access to high quality public open space.

Conclusion

This chapter commenced with a Chinese proverb that 'One generation plants the trees, and another gets the shade'. This proverb speaks to the legacy of thoughtfully conceived planning policy that ensures equitable access to public open space. In this chapter, we reviewed evidence showing that access to high quality and proximate public open space designed to meet the needs of users across the life course is essential infrastructure that contributes to creating the conditions for the health and well-being of residents. With increasing urbanization and higher density housing, the provision of public open space has never been more important and there is a need to ensure that all residents—irrespective of age or their socioeconomic status—have access to public open space where they can recreate, walk, jog, play sport, or participate in active play. Irrespective of age, a physically active life is essential for health and well-being. Planners, urban designers, and landscape architects therefore have a critical role in ensuring that future generations enjoy the legacy of their professional work, through the thoughtful provision and design of public open space that fosters active living.

References

Astell-Burt, T., Feng, X., & Kolt, G. S. (2014). Green space is associated with walking and moderate-to-vigorous physical activity (MVPA) in middle-to-older-aged adults: findings from 203 883 Australians in the 45 and Up Study. *Br J Sports Med*, 48, 404–6.

Aspinall, P. A., Ward Thompson, C., Alves, S., Sugiyama, T., Brice, R., & Vickers, A. (2010). Preference and relative importance for environmental attributes of neighbourhood open space in older people. *Environ Plann B Plann Des*, 37, 1022–39.

Babey, S. H., Hastert, T. A., Yu, H., & Brown, E. R. (2008). Physical activity among adolescents. When do parks matter? *Am J Prev Med*, 34, 345–8.

Badland, H. M., Keam, R., Witten, K., & Kearns, R. A. (2010). Examining public open spaces by neighborhood-level walkability and deprivation. *J Phys Act Health*, 7, 818–24.

Barton, H. & Grant, M. (2006). A health map for the local human habitat. *J R Soc Promot Health*, 126, 252–3.

Bedimo-Rung, A. L., Mowen, A. J., & Cohen, D. A. (2005). The significance of parks to physical activity and public health: a conceptual model. *Am J Prev Med*, 28, 159–68.

Bell, J. F., Wilson, J. S., & Liu, G. C. (2008). Neighborhood greenness and 2-year changes in body mass index of children and youth. *Am J Prev Med*, 35, 547–53.

Beyer, K. M., Kaltenbach, A., Szabo, A., Bogar, S., Nieto, F. J., & Malecki, K. M. (2014). Exposure to neighborhood green space and mental health: evidence from the survey of the health of Wisconsin. *Int J Environ Res Public Health*, 11, 3453–72.

Bishop, B. (1999). *The National Strategy for an Ageing Australia: Background Paper*. Commonwealth of Australia.

Bohn-Goldbaum, E. E., Phongsavan, P., Merom, D., Rogers, K., Kamalesh, V., & Bauman, A. E. (2013). Does playground improvement increase physical activity among children? A quasi-experimental study of a natural experiment. *J Environ Public Health*, 2013, 109841.

Brockman, R., Fox, K. R., & Jago, R. (2011). What is the meaning and nature of active play for today's children in the UK. *Int J Behav Nutr Phys Act*, 8, 15.

CABE Space (2005). Start with the park: creating sustainable urban green spaces in Areas of H using Growth and Renewal. Commission for Architecture and the Built Environment (CABE), UK.

Cerin, E., Lee, K.-Y., Barnett, A., Sit, C. H. P., Cheung, M.-C., & Chan, W.-M. (2013). Objectively-measured neighborhood environments and leisure-time physical activity in Chinese urban elders. *Prev Med*, 56, 86–9.

Cleland, V., Crawford, D., Baur, L., Hume, C., Timperio, A., & Salmon, J. (2008). A prospective examination of children's time spent outdoors, objectively measured physical activity and overweight. *Int J Obes*, 32, 1685–93.

Cohen, D., Ashwood, J. S., Scott, M. M., et al. (2006a). Proximity to school and physical activity among middle school girls: The Trial of Activity for Adolescent Girls Study. *J Phys Act Health*, 3, S129–38.

Cohen, D. A., Ashwood, J. S., Scott, M. M., et al. (2006b). Public parks and physical activity among adolescent girls. *Pediatrics*, 118, e1381–9.

Cohen, D. A., Marsh, T., Williamson, S., et al. (2010). Parks and physical activity: Why are some parks used more than others? *Prev Med*, 50 (Suppl), S9–S12.

Coley, R. L., Sullivan, W. C., & Kuo, F. E. (1997). Where does community grow? *Environ Behav*, 29, 468–94.

Coombes, E., Jones, A. P., & Hillsdon, M. (2010). The relationship of physical activity and overweight to objectively measured green space accessibility and use. *Soc Sci Med*, 70, 816–22.

Crawford, D., Timperio, A., Giles-Corti, B., Ball, K., Hume, C., & Roberts, R. (2008). Do features of public open spaces vary according to neighbourhood socio-economic status? *Health Place*, 14, 889–93.

Dehring, C. & Dunse, N. (2006). Housing density and the effect of proximity to public open space in Aberdeen, Scotland. *Real Estate Economics*, 34, 553–66.

Dunton, G. F., Almanza, E., Jerrett, M., Wolch, J., & Pentz, M. A. (2014). Neighborhood park use by children: use of accelerometry and global positioning systems. *Am J Prev Med*, 46, 136–42.

Edwards, N., Hooper, P., Knuiman, M., Foster, S., & Giles-Corti, B. (2015). Associations between park features and adolescent park use for physical activity. *Int J Behav Nutr Phys Act*, 12, 21.

Edwards, N., Hooper, P., Trapp, G. S., Bull, F., Boruff, B., & Giles-Corti, B. (2013). Development of a Public Open Space Desktop Auditing Tool (POSDAT): A remote sensing approach. *Appl Geogr*, 38, 22–30.

Epstein, L. H., Raja, S., Gold, S. S., Paluch, R. A., Pak, Y., & Roemmich, J. N. (2006). Reducing sedentary behavior: the relationship between park area and the physical activity of youth. *Psychol Sci*, 17, 654–9.

Eronen, J., Von Bonsdorff, M., Rantakokko, M., & Rantanen, T. (2014). Environmental facilitators for outdoor walking and development of walking difficulty in community-dwelling older adults. *Eur J Ageing*, 11, 67–75.

Evenson, K. R., Wen, F., Hillier, A., & Cohen, D. A. (2013). Assessing the contribution of parks to physical activity using global positioning system and accelerometry. *Med Sci Sports Exerc*, 45, 1981–7.

Fjørtoft, I. (2004). Landscape as playscape: The effects of natural environments on children's play and motor development. *Children, Youth and Environments*, 14, 21–44.

Fjørtoft, I. (2001). The natural environment as a playground for children: The impact of outdoor play activities in pre-primary school children. *Early Child E J*, 29, 111–17.

Fjørtoft, I. & Sageie, J. (2000). The natural environment as a playground for children: Landscape description and analyses of a natural playscape. *Landsc Urban Plan*, 48, 83–97.

Floyd, M. F., Bocarro, J. N., Smith, W. R., et al. (2011). Park-based physical activity among children and adolescents. *Am J Prev Med*, 41, 258–65.

Foster, C., Hillsdon, M., Jones, A., et al. (2009). Objective measures of the environment and physical activity—results of the environment and physical activity study in english adults. *J Phys Act Health*, 6, S70–80.

Foster, S., Giles-Corti, B., & Knuiman, M. (2011). Creating safe walkable streetscapes: Does house design and upkeep discourage incivilities in suburban neighbourhoods? *J Environ Psychol*, 31, 79–88.

Foster, S., Giles-Corti, B., & Knuiman, M. (2012). Does fear of crime discourage walkers? A social-ecological exploration of fear as a deterrent to walking. *Environ Behav*, 46, 698–717.

Francis, J., Wood, L. J., Knuiman, M., & Giles-Corti, B. (2012). Quality or quantity? Exploring the relationship between Public Open Space attributes and mental health in Perth, Western Australia. *Soc Sci Med*, 74, 1570–7.

Gebel, K., Bauman, A., & Owen, N. (2009). Correlates of non-concordance between perceived and objective measures of walkability. *Ann Behav Med*, 37, 228–38.

Giles-Corti, B., Broomhall, M. H., Knuiman, M., et al. (2005a). Increasing walking: How important is distance to, attractiveness, and size of public open space? *Am J Prev Med*, 28, 169–76.

Giles-Corti, B., Bull, F., Knuiman, M., et al. (2013). The influence of urban design on neighbourhood walking following residential relocation: Longitudinal results from the RESIDE study. *Soc Sci Med*, 77, 20–30.

Giles-Corti, B., Kelty, S. F., Zubrick, S. R., & Villanueva, K. P. (2009). Encouraging walking for transport and physical activity in children and adolescents: how important is the built environment? *Sports Med*, 39, 995–1009.

Giles-Corti, B., Timperio, A., Bull, F., & Pikora, T. (2005b). Understanding physical activity environmental correlates: increased specificity for ecological models. *Exerc Sport Sci Rev*, 33, 175–81.

Gomez, L. F., Parra, D. C., Buchner, D., et al. (2010). Built environment attributes and walking patterns among the elderly population in Bogota. *Am J Prev Med*, 38, 592–9.

Gong, Y., Gallacher, J., Palmer, S., & Fone, D. (2014). Neighbourhood green space, physical function and participation in physical activities among elderly men: the Caerphilly Prospective study. *Int J Behav Nutr Phys Act*, 11, 40.

Grose, M. (2009). Changing relationships in public open space and private open space in suburbs in south-western Australia. *Landsc Urban Plan*, 92, 53–63.

Gunn, L., Lee, Y., Geelhoed, E., Shiell, A., Giles-Corti, B. (2014). The cost-effectiveness of installing sidewalks to increase levels of transport-walking and health. *Prev Med*, 67, 322–9.

Hall, T. (2010). *The Life and Death of the Australian Backyard*. Collingwood, VIC, Australia: CSIRO Publishing.

Hanibuchi, T., Kawachi, I., Nakaya, T., Hirai, H., & Kondo, K. (2011). Neighborhood built environment and physical activity of Japanese older adults: results from the Aichi Gerontological Evaluation Study (AGES). *BMC Public Health*, 11, 657.

Hino, A. A. F., Reis, R. S., Sarmiento, O. L., Parra, D. C., & Brownson, R. C. (2011). The built environment and recreational physical activity among adults in Curitiba, Brazil. *Prev Med*, 52, 419–22.

Kaczynski, A. T. & Henderson, K. A. (2007). Environmental correlates of physical activity: a review of evidence about parks and recreation. *Leisure Sciences*, 29, 315–54.

Kaczynski, A. T., Koohsari, M. J., Stanis, S. A. W., Bergstrom, R., & Sugiyama, T. (2014). Association of street connectivity and road traffic speed with park usage and park-based physical activity. *Am J Health Promot*, 28, 197–203.

Kaczynski, A. T., Potwarka, L. R., & Saelens, B. E. (2008). Association of park size, distance, and features with physical activity in neighborhood parks. *Am J Public Health*, 98, 1451–6.

Kaczynski, A. T., Potwarka, L. R., Smale, B. J. A., & Havitz, M. E. (2009). Association of parkland proximity with neighborhood and park-based physical activity: variations by gender and age. *Leis Sci*, 31, 174–91.

Kahlmeier, S., Kelly, P., Foster, C., *et al.* (2014). Health economic assessment tool (HEAT) for cycling and walking. Geneva, Switzerland: World Health Organization.

Kellett, J. & Rofe, M. W. (2009). Creating active communities: how can open and public spaces in urban and suburban environments support active living? A literature review. The Institute for Sustainable Systems and Technologies, University of South Australia to SA Active Living Coalition.

Klinker, C. D., Schipperijn, J., Christian, H., Kerr, J., Ersbøll, A. K., & Troelsen, J. (2014). Using accelerometers and global positioning system devices to assess gender and age differences in children's school, transport, leisure and home based physical activity. *Int J Behav Nutr Phys Act*, 11, 8.

Koohsari, M. J., Badland, H., & Giles-Corti, B. (2013a). (Re)Designing the built environment to support physical activity: Bringing public health back into urban design and planning. *Cities*, 35, 294–8.

Koohsari, M. J., Karakiewicz, J. A., & Kaczynski, A. T. (2013b). Public open space and walking: the role of proximity, perceptual qualities of the surrounding built environment, and street configuration. *Environ Behav*, 45, 706–36.

Lee, I.-M., Shiroma, E. J., Lobelo, F., Puska, P., Blair, S. N., & Katzmarzyk, P. T. (2012). Effect of physical inactivity on major non-communicable diseases worldwide: an analysis of burden of disease and life expectancy. *Lancet*, 380, 219–29.

Lee, S. & Christiansen, M. (1999). The cognition of playground safety and children's play-A comparison of traditional, contemporary, and naturalized playground types. State College, PA: Pennsylvania State University: Center for Hospitality, Tourism & Recreation Research.

Li, F. Z., Fisher, K. J., & Brownson, R. C. (2005a). A multilevel analysis of change in neighborhood walking activity in older adults. *J Aging Phys Act*, 13, 145–59.

Li, F. Z., Fisher, K. J., Brownson, R. C., & Bosworth, M. (2005b). Multilevel modelling of built environment characteristics related to neighbourhood walking activity in older adults. *J Epidemiol Community Health*, 59, 558–64.

Liu, G. C., Wilson, J. S., Qi, R., & Ying, J. (2007). Green neighborhoods, food retail and childhood overweight: differences by population density. *Am J Health Promot*, 21, 317–25.

Loukaitou-Sideris, A. & Stieglitz, O. (2002). Children in Los Angeles parks: a study of equity, quality and children's satisfaction with neighbourhood parks. *Town Plan Rev*, 73, 467–88.

Lozano, R., Naghavi, M., Foreman, K., *et al.* (2012). Global and regional mortality from 235 causes of death for 20 age groups in 1990 and 2010: a systematic analysis for the Global Burden of Disease Study 2010. *Lancet*, 380, 2095–128.

Maas, J., Verheij, R. A., De Vries, S., Spreeuwenberg, P., Schellevis, F. G., & Groenewegen, P. P. (2009). Morbidity is related to a green living environment. *J Epidemiol Community Health*, 63, 967–73.

Martin, K. & Wood, L. (2012). 'We live here too'.... What makes a child friendly neighbourhood? In: Burton, E., & Cooper, C. (eds) *Wellbeing: A Complete Reference Guide*. Oxford, UK: Wiley-Blackwell.

Mccormack, G. R., Rock, M., Toohey, A. M., & Hignell, D. (2010). Characteristics of urban parks associated with park use and physical activity: a review of qualitative research. *Health Place*, 16, 712–26.

Mccurdy, L., Winterbottom, K., Mehta, S., & Roberts, J. (2010). Using nature and outdoor activity to improve children's health. *Curr Probl Pediatr Adolesc Health Care*, 40, 102–17.

Michael, Y. L., Perdue, L. A., Orwoll, E. S., Stefanick, M. L., Marshall, L. M; Osteoporotic Fractures in Men Study Group. (2010). Physical activity resources and changes in walking in a cohort of older men. *Am J Public Health*, 100, 654–60.

Mitchell, R. & Popham, F. (2007). Greenspace, urbanity and health: relationships in England. *J Epidemiol Community Health*, 61, 681–3.

Moran, M., Van Cauwenberg, J., Hercky-Linnewiel, R., Cerin, E., Deforche, B., & Plaut, P. (2014). Understanding the relationships between the physical environment and physical activity in older adults: a systematic review of qualitative studies. *Int J Behav Nutr Phys Act*, 11, 79.

Morris, J. N., Heady, J., Raffle, P., Roberts, C., & Parks, J. (1953). Coronary heart-disease and physical activity of work. *Lancet*, 262, 1053–7.

Norman, G. J., Nutter, S. K., Ryan, S., Sallis, J. F., Calfas, K. J., & Patrick, K. (2006). Community design and access to recreational facilities as correlates of adolescent physical activity and body-mass index. *J Phys Act Health*, 3, S118.

OECD (2012). *Compact City Policies*. Paris, France: OECD Publishing.

Pereira, G., Christian, H., Foster, S., *et al.* (2013). The association between neighborhood greenness and weight status: an observational study in Perth Western Australia. *Environ Health*, 12, 49.

Pereira, G., Foster, S., Martin, K., *et al.* (2012). The association between neighborhood greenness and cardiovascular disease: an observational study. *BMC Public Health*, 12, 466.

Potwarka, L., Kaczynski, A., & Flack, A. (2008). Places to play: association of park space and facilities with healthy weight status among children. *J Community Health*, 33, 344–50.

Quigg, R., Reeder, A. I., Gray, A., Holt, A., & Waters, D. (2011). The effectiveness of a community playground intervention. *J Urban Health*, 89, 171–84.

Reed, J. A., Arant, C., Wells, P., Stevens, K., Hagen, S., & Harring, H. (2008). A descriptive examination of the most frequently used activity settings in 25 community parks using direct observation. *J Phys Act Health*, 5, S183.

Ribeiro, A. I., Mitchell, R., Carvalho, M. S., & De Pina, M. D. F. (2013). Physical activity-friendly neighbourhood among older adults from a medium size urban setting in Southern Europe. *Prev Med*, 57, 664–70.

Rodríguez, D. A., Cho, G. H., Evenson, K. R., *et al.* (2012). Out and about: Association of the built environment with physical activity behaviors of adolescent females. *Health Place*, 18, 55–62.

Roemmich, J. N., Epstein, L. H., Raja, S., Yin, L., Robinson, J., & Winiewicz, D. (2006). Association of access to parks and recreational facilities with the physical activity of young children. *Prev Med*, 43, 437–41.

Rundle, A., Quinn, J., Lovasi, G., *et al.* (2013). Associations between body mass index and park proximity, size, cleanliness, and recreational facilities. *Am J Health Promot*, 27, 262–9.

Saelens, B. E. & Handy, S. L. (2008). Built environment correlates of walking: a review. *Med Sci Sports Exerc*, 40, S550.

Sallis, J. F., Cerin, E., Conway, T. L., *et al.* (2016). Physical activity in relation to urban environments in 14 cities worldwide: a cross-sectional study. *Lancet*, 387, 2207–17.

Sallis, J. F., Cervero, R. B., Ascher, W., Henderson, K. A., Kraft, M. K., & Kerr, J. (2006). An ecological approach to creating active living communities. *Annu Rev Public Health*, 27, 297–322.

Sallis, J. F., Nader, P. R., Broyles, S. L., *et al.* (1993). Correlates of physical activity at home in Mexican-American and Anglo-American preschool children. *Health Psychol*, 12, 390.

Sallis, J., Prochaska, J., & Taylor, W. (2000). A review of correlates of physical activity of children and adolescents. *Med Sci Sports Exerc*, 32, 63–75.

Salmon, J. & Timperio, A. (2007). Prevalence, trends and environmental influences on child and youth physical activity. *Med Sport Sci*, 50, 183–99.

Schipperijn, J., Bentsen, P., Troelsen, J., Toftager, M., & Stigsdotter, U. K. (2013). Associations between physical activity and characteristics of urban green space. *Urban For Urban Greening*, 12, 109–16.

Shiels, G. (1989). More quality, less quantity in open space planning. *Australian Parks and Recreation*, 25, 12–14.

Sugiyama, T., Francis, J., Middleton, N. J., Owen, N., & Giles-Corti, B. (2010). Associations between recreational walking and attractiveness, size, and proximity of neighborhood open spaces. *Am J Public Health*, 100, 1752–7.

Sugiyama, T., Giles-Corti, B., Summers, J., Du Toit, L., Leslie, E., & Owen, N. (2013). Initiating and maintaining recreational walking: a longitudinal study on the influence of neighborhood green space. *Prev Med*, 57, 178–82.

Sugiyama, T., Paquet, C., Howard, N. J., *et al.* (2014). Public open spaces and walking for recreation: Moderation by attributes of pedestrian environments. *Prev Med*, 62, 25–9.

Sugiyama, T. & Ward Thompson, C. (2008). Associations between characteristics of neighbourhood open space and older people's walking. *Urban For Urban Greening*, 7, 41–51.

Sutton, S. B. (ed.) (1971). *Civilizing American Cities: A Selection of Frederick Law Olmsted's Writings on City Landscapes*. Cambridge, MA: MIT Press.

Takano, T., Nakamura, K., & Watanabe, M. (2002). Urban residential environments and senior citizens' longevity in megacity areas: The importance of walkable green spaces. *J Epidemiol Community Health*, 56, 913–18.

Taylor, A. F., Wiley, A., Kuo, F. E., & Sullivan, W. C. (1998). Growing up in the inner city—Green spaces as places to grow. *Environ Behav*, 30, 3–27.

Tester, J. & Baker, R. (2009). Making the playfields even: evaluating the impact of an environmental intervention on park use and physical activity. *Prev Med*, 48, 316–20.

Timperio, A., Ball, K., Salmon, J., Roberts, R., & Crawford, D. (2007). Is availability of public open space equitable across areas?. *Health Place*, 13, 335–40.

Timperio, A., Crawford, D., Telford, A., & Salmon, J. (2004). Perceptions about the local neighborhood and walking and cycling among children. *Prev Med*, 38, 39–47.

Todd, C. & Skelton, D. (2004). What are the main risk factors for falls among older people and what are the most effective interventions to prevent these falls?. Copenhagen, Denmark: WHO Regional Office for Europe.

Troped, P. J., Wilson, J. S., Matthews, C. E., Cromley, E. K., & Melly, S. J. (2010). The built environment and location-based physical activity. *Am J Prev Med*, 38, 429–38.

United Nations (UN) (2011). Sixty-sixth Sessions. Political Declaration of the High-level Meeting of the General Assembly on the Prevention and Control of Non-communicable Diseases. A/66/L. 1. New York, NY: United Nations.

United Nations (UN) (2013). World Population Ageing 2013.

US Department of Health and Human Services (2008). Physical activity guidelines advisory committee report, 2008. Washington, DC: US Department of Health and Human Services.

Veal, A. J. (2012). Open space planning standards in Australia: in search of origins. *Australian Planner*, 50, 224–32.

Veitch, J., Bagley, S., Ball, K., & Salmon, J. (2006a). Where do children play? A qualitative study of parents' perceptions of influences on children's active free play. *Health Place*, 12, 383–93.

Veitch, J., Bagley, S., Ball, K., & Salmon, J. (2006b). Where do children usually play? A qualitative study of parents' perceptions of influences on children's active free-play. *Health Place*, 12, 383–93.

Veitch, J., Salmon, J., & Ball, K. (2008). Children's active free play in local neighbourhoods: A behavioural mapping study. *Health Educ Res*, 23, 870–9.

Veitch, J., Salmon, J., Carver, A., *et al.* (2014). A natural experiment to examine the impact of park renewal on park-use and park-based physical activity in a disadvantaged neighbourhood: the REVAMP study methods. *BMC Public Health*, 14, 600.

Wheeler, B. W., Cooper, A. R., Page, A. S., & Jago, R. (2010). Greenspace and children's physical activity: A GPS/GIS analysis of the PEACH project. *Prev Med*, 51, 148–52.

Wilkinson, P. F. (1985). The golden fleece: the search for standards. *Leisure Studies*, 4, 189–203.

Wood, L., Martin, K., & Carter, M. (2010). Child's play: an investigation of child and parent outdoor play space preferences and Kings Park Naturescape. Perth, Australia: The University of Western Australia.

World Health Organization (WHO) (1998). Population ageing: a public helth challenge. Geneva, Switzerland: World Health Organization.

World Health Organization (WHO) (2002). Towards policy for health and ageing. Geneva, Switzerland: World Health Organization.

World Health Organization (WHO) (2009). Global health risks: mortality and burden of disease attributable to selected major risks. Geneva, Switzerland: World Health Organization.

World Health Organization (WHO) (2010). Global recommendations on physical activity for health. Geneva, Switzerland: World Health Organization.

World Health Organization (WHO) (2011). Global status report on noncommunicable diseases 2010. Geneva, Switzerland: World Health Organization.

World Health Organization (WHO) (2013). Global action plan for the prevention and control of noncommunicable diseases 2013–2020. Geneva, Switzerland: World Health Organization.

Zubrick, S., Wood, L., Villanueva, K., Wood, G., Giles-Corti, B., & Christian, H. (2010). Nothing but fear itself: Parental fear as a determinant impacting on child physical activity and independent mobility. Melbourne, Australia: Victorian Health Promotion Foundation.

Preventing stress and promoting mental health

Matilda van den Bosch, Catharine Ward Thompson, and Patrik Grahn

Stress as a mediator

The health-promoting or disease-preventing effects of natural environments are often attributed to the potential for recreation and stress relief. This chapter will discuss how, through the mediating effect of stress relief, nature may contribute to preventing mental disorders.

The associations between nature, stress, and mental health are not straightforward, but are expressed through several interacting steps (see Fig. 3.2.1). This means that visiting nature may not directly affect the biological processes behind, for example, depression, but by reducing the negative effects of stress on mental health, nature may protect people from developing mental disorders.

Even though the effects of nature's stress-relieving capacity on an individual may be small, the impact at a population level, and for public health in general, can be large, as mental disorders have a vast impact on the global burden of disease (GBD).

Mental disorders constitute a major public health issue

The World Health Organization's (WHO) classification of mental disorders includes depression, bipolar affective disorder, schizophrenia, anxiety disorders, dementia, substance use disorders, intellectual disabilities, and developmental and behavioural disorders. Similar types of disorders occur across cultures and disability occurs both in young and in older segments of the population. About half of mental disorders begin before the age of 14 years and mental disorders are a significant source of lost years of healthy life. Depression and poor mental health in old age are also a major public health issue. With a globally ageing population and increasing concern over social isolation among older people, who may often find themselves living alone for the first time in their lives (e.g. in 2011, 36% of people in the United Kingdom aged over 65 lived alone), mental health is an important issue and depression may be underdiagnosed in people who also experience cognitive decline and/or dementia (WHO, 2005; 2013) (Box 3.2.1).

Mental health is a central component of an individual's well-being, inseparable from physical health. The level of co-morbidity is high; mental disorders increase the risk for many other diseases and, conversely, many health conditions increase the risk for mental disorders. Thus, there is a large potential for public mental health actions to save many healthy years. Such actions must be of an intersectoral, interdisciplinary kind, including engagement with aspects of the environments where people live.

Inequity in mental health

A particular aspect of mental and psychosomatic disorders is their unequal distribution between societies and population groups. Populations in poor socioeconomic circumstances are at increased risk of poor mental health, depression, and lower subjective well-being (Patel and Jané-Llopis, 2005). In light of this, it is important to acknowledge the environmental and social context of mental disorders and the need for strategically planned support for mental well-being, including aspects of the neighbourhood environment. In considering the role of nature and the physical environment in mental well-being, issues of social inclusion are linked with issues of environmental justice and socio-spatial inequalities, so that healthier environments are often correlated with wealthier populations and comparatively lower prevalence of mental illness (Pearce et al., 2010). Issues of social health determinants and socioeconomic health inequities in relation to the environment are further discussed in Chapter 6.3 'Vulnerable populations, health inequalities, and nature'.

The association between stress and mental health disorders

In a globally urbanizing world, there is concern that the benefits of urban living (such as better access to services, food, and healthcare) may be counteracted by stressful, technology-intense urban living (sometimes called 'techno-stress'; see Arnetz, 1996; Iwanaga et al., 2005) and associated unhealthy environments with high traffic density, poor air quality, and a lack of green spaces for restoration (Godfrey and Julien, 2005). Health impacts of a change from rural to urban living are discussed in Chapter 8.1 'The shift from natural living environments to urban: population-based and neurobiological implications for public health'.

As outlined in Chapter 1.4 'The physiology of stress and stress recovery', physiological stress reactions affect internal organ systems in many interactive ways and chronic stress is a risk factor for many different diseases. Not surprisingly, mental and psychosomatic

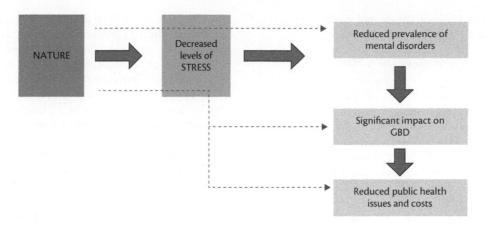

Fig. 3.2.1 Mental disorders are increasing all over the world, constituting one of the major threats to public health, and the costs for healthcare and society are substantial. This increase is partly due to increased stress. The potential capacity of nature to reduce stress is therefore important to explore further and acknowledge in public health actions aimed at promoting mental health.

(GBD = global burden of disease.)

Reproduced from Bengtsson A and Grahn P, 'Outdoor Environments in Healthcare settings: A quality evaluation tool for use in designing healthcare gardens,' *Urban Forestry and Urban Greening*, Volume 13, Issue 4, pp. 878–891, Copyright © 2014 The Authors. Published by Elsevier GmbH. Reproduced under a Creative Commons Attribution License (CC BY), https://creativecommons.org/licenses/by/3.0/.

disorders constitute the majority of disease categories thus affected; in several of these conditions, stress can be the critical factor for disease development. The high level of co-morbidity for mental disorders and the stress connected to physical diseases such as cancer also increases the risk of mental ill-health (Prince *et al.*, 2007). Thus, actions to prevent stress can reduce the level of co-morbidity. Such actions must include multilevel strategies, including creating restorative and tranquil urban environments.

Acute and post-traumatic stress disorders can be difficult to prevent, but nature can here be used as a treatment intervention. The intervention aspect is mainly dealt with in Chapter 4.1 'Using nature as a treatment option'. However, stress-related disorders are conditions where nature may also have a preventative effect.

Growing levels of stress in society in recent years, due to changing living environments, unhealthy workplaces, feelings of powerlessness, and lack of control and social support, are a global health concern. Even in developing countries, the prevalence of mental

health disorders is increasing, related, for example, to urban living (Risal *et al.*, 2016), psychosocial working conditions (Salas *et al.*, 2015), and other local physical, structural, and social stressors (Greif and Nii-Amoo Dodoo, 2015).

Promoting stress recovery and mental health through exposure to nature

Natural environments, and their implications for mental health and well-being, can be seen from a salutogenic perspective. That is to say, the value of being in natural environments is that it may stimulate, maintain, and reinforce our inner health (Antonovsky, 1996). This includes our capacity to cope with stress. Other protective factors against mental disorders are cognitive stimulation, exercise, pro-social behaviour, and self-esteem—all factors which have the potential to be improved by access to nature.

Indirect associations between nature and mental health

As discussed in Chapter 3.1 'Promoting physical activity—reducing obesity and non-communicable diseases', urban green spaces and natural environments may promote physical activity. Physical activity provides direct physical and cardiovascular benefits, but the positive effects on mood and stress levels are also well established (Penedo and Dahn, 2005). Thus, as nature supports physical activity, a spillover effect is likely to occur for mental health.

Chapter 3.3 'Promoting social cohesion and social capital—increasing well-being' discusses the opportunities for social interaction in green spaces. Social contact is also known to have positive effects on mood and stress level (Heinrichs *et al.*, 2003) and may be a mediating factor in mental health benefits from nature. A natural environment may also offer the opportunity to get away from socially demanding settings and allow people with mental health problems the chance to be alone, or at least in a peaceful context where social contact is not required (Ottosson and Grahn, 2008). Furthermore, natural environments are associated with people's sense of belonging to a place, which in turn predicts stress levels

---

Box 3.2.1 Facts about mental health (WHO)

- Persons with major depression or schizophrenia have a 40–60% higher risk of dying prematurely as compared to a general population.

- Mental illness represents three of the ten leading causes of disease burden in low- and middle-income countries, and four of the leading ten in high-income countries.

- More than 800,000 persons die from suicide each year.

- Globally, only 2.8% of the health budget is allocated to mental health.

- Depression affects one of five people over the age of 65.

Source: data from World Health Organization, *Mental health and older adults: Fact sheet*, Copyright © WHO 2016, available from http://www.who.int/mediacentre/factsheets/fs381/en/.

and may mediate links between nature and health (Lengen and Kistemann, 2012; Ward Thompson *et al.*, 2016).

Direct associations between nature, stress, and mental health

Intuitively, people often choose natural environments for recreation, suggesting that such places are well suited for stress reduction and mental relaxation (White *et al.*, 2013; Ulrich *et al.*, 1991). Visits to nature are commonly associated with decreases in self-reported stress (Annerstedt *et al.*, 2010). Viewing or being in a natural environment has also been shown to reduce physiological measures of stress, particularly if initial stress levels are high (Ulrich and Addoms, 1981; Ulrich *et al.*, 1989).

Recent research has enhanced our understanding of some of the mechanisms behind links between nature and stress. Much of this understanding has been gathered under experimental conditions, measuring varied biomarkers or using brain imaging techniques. Examples of psychophysiological measures and biomarkers of stress influenced by exposure to nature include blood pressure and heart rate (Hartig *et al.*, 2003; Ottosson and Grahn, 2005; Ulrich *et al.*, 1991), heart rate variability (Annerstedt *et al.*, 2013), respiratory sinus arrhythmia and pre-ejection period (van den Berg *et al.*, 2015), skin conductance and muscle tension (Ulrich *et al.*, 1991), and salivary and hair cortisol (Ward Thompson *et al.*, 2012; Gidlow *et al.*, 2016).

Beil and Hanes (2013) tested reactions to four different urban environments (ranging from very natural, mostly natural, mostly built, to very built). Greater benefits were reported from exposure to natural relative to built settings, as measured by pre-to-post changes in salivary amylase, cortisol, and self-reported stress.

In a Dutch study, allotment gardeners were assigned to experimental tasks before and after time spent gardening or indoor reading. This study used stress provocation tasks for inducing acute stress and the results demonstrated significantly steeper slopes of decreasing cortisol levels after engaging with nature (van den Berg and Custers 2011).

As with all studies using cortisol as biomarker, the reported results must be interpreted with the precaution in mind that the circadian patterns of cortisol may complicate analysis and interpretation, and that cortisol responses vary greatly in relation to different types of social stressors (Dickerson and Kemeny, 2004). A study in the United Kingdom (Ward Thompson *et al.*, 2012; see also Roe *et al.*, 2013) took into account circadian patterns of cortisol and avoided artificially induced stressors. Diurnal patterns of salivary cortisol were analysed, alongside self-reported stress, in relation to levels of green space in people's everyday living environments while participants undertook their normal daily activities. The sample consisted of adults not in work, aged 35–55, living in socially disadvantaged urban districts in Scotland. Negative relationships between higher green space levels and stress levels were found, as demonstrated by healthier cortisol rhythms. The studies were undertaken with deprived urban populations and the effects were found to be stronger among women. Recent methods have included brain imaging techniques, used in experimental studies on nature and stress. Recordings of people's brain activity measured by mobile EEG headsets as they walked from a busy street into a green park and out again showed brain patterns suggestive of lower frustration and higher meditation when in green space, versus when moving within retail and commercial urban areas

(Aspinall *et al.*, 2015). Such findings offer support for the Attention Restoration Theory described earlier (Kaplan, 1995) and suggest that one pathway to mental well-being from access to nature may lie in its capacity to encourage a positive emotional mindset and thus promote resilient cognitive and psychological resources.

These psychophysiological effects suggest that the natural environment may act biologically as a partial antidote to the negative effects of a stressful life, helping people cope better with demands as they arise (e.g. pressure at work) as well as helping them to reduce levels of stress post-hoc (Hartig, 2007). Read more about these mechanisms in Chapter 2.5, 'Biological mechanisms and neurophysiological responses to sensory impact from nature'.

Evidence for a relationship between access to nature and mental health

Population studies provide evidence on associations

A wide range of large population studies across the globe have delivered evidence on stress reduction and mental health benefits associated with access to green spaces, across the lifespan, and across strata of urbanization, socioeconomic status, and gender (Reklaitiene *et al.*, 2014; Triguero-Mas *et al.*, 2015; Sturm and Cohen, 2014). Given increasing global urbanization and the greater prevalence of mental disorders in urban than in rural areas (Peen *et al.*, 2010; Sundquist *et al.*, 2004), there is a specific need to provide access to green environments in cities, in order to offer opportunities for stress reduction and to contribute to prevention of mental illness, together with other multilevel strategies addressing, for example, psychosocial and cultural factors. Most relevant research is undertaken in urban areas, but there are also a few analyses of mental health benefits from access to suburban or rural green spaces (Annerstedt *et al.*, 2015; De Jong *et al.*, 2012).

The definition of access to urban green spaces is commonly based on distance estimations from residences to green areas, or estimations of the amount of green space within a geographical area. In practice, a five-minute walking distance, estimated to correspond to 300–400 m, is usually considered as good accessibility. There is as yet no definitive recommendation for adequate size of green space for mental health benefits, but some guidelines refer to a minimum of approximately 1–2 hectares (Handley *et al.*, 2003).

A Danish study, involving more than 10,000 participants, showed that those living more than 1 km away from green space (e.g. forests, parks, beaches, lakes) were more than 40% more likely to report high stress and had the worst scores on evaluations of general health, vitality, mental health, and bodily pain (Stigsdotter *et al.*, 2010). A large-scale (over 345,000) epidemiological study in the Netherlands, where fewer than 10% of inhabitants live in non-urban contexts, used household medical records and geographic information systems (GIS)-derived data for defining levels of green space in the living environment within a 3 km radius. It showed that residents with only 10% green space within 1 km had a 25% greater risk of depression and a 30% greater risk of anxiety disorders versus those with the highest amount of green space near the home (Maas *et al.*, 2009).

A study from the United Kingdom, including over 10,000 urban inhabitants, showed that both lower mental distress and higher well-being were associated with living in areas with more green space (White *et al.*, 2013), while a five-year longitudinal study of people from the same survey, who had moved home in the middle of the period under study, showed that moving to greener urban areas was correlated with sustained mental health improvements (Alcock *et al.*, 2014). Another European longitudinal study demonstrated a substantially decreased risk for women to develop mental illness (as measured by GHQ-12) if they lived in areas with high quality green spaces, especially in combination with good levels of physical activity (Annerstedt *et al.*, 2012). Cohen-Cline *et al.* (2015) used a twin-pair (monozygotic) design to show that greater access to green space was associated with less depression.

There are several studies indicating that the positive mental health effects of green spaces are more significant among women (Reklaitiene *et al.*, 2014). Green spaces have also been suggested to have a positive impact on the emotional and behavioural development of children (Amoly *et al.*, 2014; Balseviciene *et al.*, 2014; Dadvand *et al.*, 2015). However, a recently published study from Lithuania demonstrated somewhat contradictory results. Parenting stress and their children's mental health were studied. It showed that greater residential distance from city parks was associated with worse mental health in children whose mothers had a lower education level, while more residential greenness was associated with worse mental health in children whose mothers had a higher education level (Balseviciene *et al.*, 2014). Similar findings in terms of socioeconomic differences support the notion that the positive impact of nearby green space is particularly notable in poorer neighbourhoods (Flouri *et al.*, 2014).

Studies have considered the added benefit of physical exercise, known to have health benefits, if undertaken in a natural environment. Such activity in natural environments has been shown to be associated with a reduced risk of poor mental health to a greater extent than physical activity in other environments (Pretty *et al.*, 2005). It is suggested that each additional use of any natural environment per week is associated with about 6% lower risk of poor mental health (Mitchell, 2013). However, similar synergistic effects have not been found among children (Reed *et al.*, 2013).

Many factors affect mental health outcomes other than access to green spaces, such as previously mentioned social and cultural contexts. Some studies have considered the effect of green space accessibility in relation to other mediators. For example, the difference in depressive symptoms between an individual living in an environment with no tree canopy and an environment with 100% tree canopy is larger than the difference in symptoms associated with an individual who is uninsured compared to an individual with private insurance, according to a study from the United States including both urban and rural areas (Beyer *et al.*, 2014). Another study from the United States demonstrated that a nearby (<400 m) urban park was associated with the same mental health benefits as decreasing local unemployment rates by two percentage points (Sturm and Cohen, 2014).

Research challenges

One challenge for research on nature and health is that we don't yet know enough about moderating factors, such as the relative importance of length of stay in nature, or if certain features of the environment are specifically important for the stress-relieving effects. Nor do we fully understand the individual factors that may mediate the effects or differences between subgroups of a population. This makes it difficult to provide specific policy or planning recommendations; these must currently remain on a more general level, arguing for maintaining and developing green

spaces based on their multifunctionality, including their positive impact on mental health.

A theoretical framework for the association between nature, stress, and mental health

Supportive environments

The Supportive Environment Theory (SET) is based on the assumption that human beings, through evolution, are adapted to a life close to nature, in social and cultural interaction with a limited number of people (Pálsdóttir *et al.*, 2014). In such a context, people can comprehend, manage, and find meaning in their surrounding environment.

'Supportive environments' consist of physical environments (e.g. natural environments), social environments (e.g. work and leisure) and cultural environments (e.g. language, values, and lifestyle). A supportive environment is regarded as an important part of salutogenesis, supplying factors that contribute to an individual's health, regardless of whether the individual has been, or continues to be, exposed to potentially pathogenic physical, biological, and/or psychosocial stressors (Grahn *et al.*, 2010; Sahlin, 2014).

According to SET, people need supportive environments to maintain health physically (in their body, senses, muscles, locomotion) and mentally (in access to and experience of one's true feelings and thoughts). The hypothesis is that the physical environment can affect all human modalities in a direct way: sensations from the physical environment, particularly nature, are very varied, can affect all the senses, and can—often without any cognitive processing—instigate responses, for example in muscles and other parts of the body (Grahn *et al.*, 2010). This in turn affects functions, feelings, and behaviour.

The need for supportive environments varies depending on physical and mental capacity, situation, and state of mind (Grahn *et al.*, 2010); see Figure 3.2.2. The more an individual feels pressured, the greater the need for salutogenic environments. This means that an environment which is experienced as supportive by one individual is not necessarily experienced similarly by another (Ottosson, 2007; Ottosson and Grahn, 2008; Ottosson, 2001). The theory has been important when establishing nature-based rehabilitation in Scandinavia (Sahlin, 2014).

The framework of supportive environments has been used to study the relationship between environmental quality, older people's physical and mental capabilities (which often decline as they age), and the activities they want or need to undertake (Sugiyama and Ward Thompson, 2007; Bengtsson and Carlsson, 2006). The research explored how well the environment makes it easy and enjoyable to do things, or frustrates and hinders such activities. The relationship between perceived environmental support and quality of life was significant for older people (aged 65+) in outdoor activities that involved nature, but not for other activity types (Curl *et al.*, 2016).

One way of interpreting SET in relation to nature is through the theory of affordances (Gibson, 1977). An affordance is a property or characteristic of the environment in relation to an individual, concerning what options or opportunities it offers. Several studies have been conducted regarding what kind of outdoor environments people have the greatest need of and how these environments can be related to the support they provide (Kaplan *et al.*, 1998; Tyrväinen *et al.*, 2007; Ryan *et al.*, 2014). Since the 1980s, several studies have been carried out where the aim has been to examine how the most

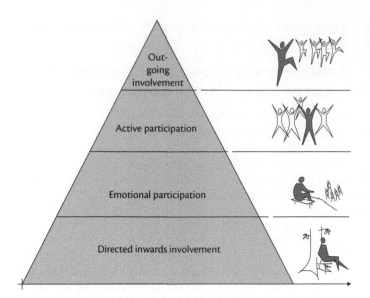

Fig. 3.2.2 The 'SET-pyramid' of physical/mental capacity. The y-axis 'level of executive function' indicates the capacity to cope with challenges and function in the surrounding world and the x-axis indicates the individual's "need for supportive environments". The pyramid shows that people's need for supportive environments is lower when they have a high capacity, ie high level of executive function. When people have a low capacity, the supportive environment should contain as little demanding information as possible, such as simple natural elements like sand, small pools of water, leaves, and sticks, while the most demanding is to meet people. At the lowest level of the pyramid, where the sensitivity to demand is very high, the environmental need mostly consists of simple natural elements. Following a gradual increase in demanding elements, the top level contains places where people can meet and socialize.

Reproduced from Bengtsson A and Grahn P, 'Outdoor Environments in Healthcare settings: A quality evaluation tool for use in designing healthcare gardens,' *Urban Forestry and Urban Greening*, Volume 13, Issue 4, pp. 878-891, Copyright © 2014 The Authors. Published by Elsevier GmbH. Reproduced under a Creative Commons Attribution License (CC BY), https://creativecommons.org/licenses/by/3.0/.

desired properties or needs can be combined under a smaller number of attributes that describe their basic characteristics. These studies have most often resulted in eight basic characteristics or affordances (Stigsdotter and Grahn, 2011; Grahn and Stigsdotter, 2010); see Box 3.2.2. Starting from people's needs and wishes relating to characteristics and affordances of green spaces, instead of their appearance, has proven to be a viable approach. People's aesthetic preferences differ depending on, for example, age, gender, cultural background, and so on. Their needs are, however, more common, making it possible to use the characteristics in different contexts and populations. The characteristics have been used in cities, as well as in rural contexts; and in epidemiological studies including large tracts of land, as well as in smaller rehabilitation gardens (Grahn *et al.*, 2010; de Jong *et al.*, 2012). They can, for example, be used to determine if green urban spaces in a city offer what is needed (Skärbäck *et al.*, 2014), or guide and support the design process of a therapeutic garden (Stigsdotter and Grahn, 2002; Grahn *et al.*, 2010). Certain properties, as the Kaplans (Kaplan *et al.*, 1998) and Ulrich (Ulrich *et al.*, 1991) argue are of crucial importance in a restorative setting, are among the eight characteristics (Grahn and Stigsdotter, 2010).

If large urban green areas continue to disappear, this will decrease the urban supply of important environmental characteristics for stress restoration. Resources regarding existing urban green spaces

Box 3.2.2 Eight perceived restorative characteristics of the environment

1. Refuge: for a severely stressed person, the most immediate need is to find a place of retreat where the individual can experience security; a transparent place, yet surrounded by greenery. This is an enclosed, safe, and secluded refuge for relaxation, with possibilities to oversee (or overhear) the surroundings.

2. Serenity: stressed individuals need an environment that is perceived as serene (places of peace with sounds of nature).

3. Nature: a place that is perceived as permissive and with an absence of people (Pálsdóttir *et al.*, 2014). This allows the individual to discover simple expressions of nature, and gradually become more and more fascinated by natural elements. The environment is perceived as untouched and developed without human intervention.

The above three affordances are found at the bottom of the SET-pyramid. These three characteristics are assumed to be needed for recovery and healing for those who are most stressed (Pálsdóttir *et al.*, 2014). These characteristics may also be used more generally in urban green spaces as a resource for those experiencing high levels of stress (Grahn and Stigsdotter, 2010).

4. Space: those who are moderately affected by stress are interested in discovering and being stimulated by the environment. For their well-being, they need to find a coherent space offering a restful feeling of entering another world, like for example the 'colonnade hall' of a beech forest or a wide open beach.

5. Rich in species: this group is also interested in finding and being fascinated by biodiverse places, with a variety of animal and plant species.

These two affordances belong to the second lowest level of the pyramid. Individuals at this level are not as sensitive to encountering other people, so long as they are not forced to socialize.

6. Culture: at the next level in the pyramid, there is a need to reflect on traces and vestiges of human labour, values, and culture.

7. Prospect: at this point, people also need the enjoyment of visiting open green places, offering vistas and social opportunities.

People at this level are only to a limited extent affected by stress and have a need to watch people in order to feel healthy. The presence of other people is thus positive, otherwise places may be perceived as desolate.

8. Social: the last affordance is about a need to find pleasurable, social environments where people meet, play, and interact. This becomes a prerequisite for well-being in a healthy, nonstressed individual, demonstrating the value of social contact for mental health (Fig. 3.2.3).

(continued)

Box 3.2.2 (Continued)

Studies have shown that urban green areas largely consist of Prospect, but offer less, for example, of Space, Nature, and Serenity (Qiu, 2014). This is despite the fact that the latter characteristics are in high demand for stressed people, while Prospect is much less so (Grahn and Stigsdotter, 2010). A supply of similarly designed urban green spaces leads to fewer people visiting nature for restoration and thus fewer opportunities for stress recovery (Björk et al., 2008; De Jong et al., 2012). In particular, Space and Nature are often only found in large green areas, yet these are in many cases threatened by urban densification aims (Skärbäck, 2014).

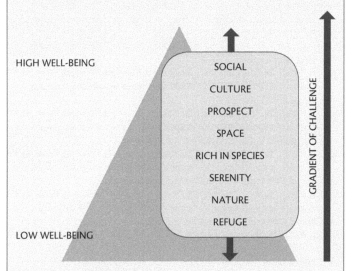

Fig. 3.2.3 The eight characteristics placed in the SET-pyramid of physical/mental capacity.

Reprinted from *Urban Forestry and Urban Greening*, Volume 13, Issue 4, Bengtsson A and Grahn P, 'Outdoor Environments in Healthcare settings: A quality evaluation tool for use in designing healthcare gardens,' pp. 878-891, Copyright © 2014 The Authors. Published by Elsevier GmbH. By permission of Elsevier, http://www.sciencedirect.com/science/journal/16188667

could be utilized better by analysing them, based on their correspondence to people's needs and abilities to offer stress recovery.

Conclusion

One of the key tasks for preventing mental disorders is to prevent stress and create opportunities for stress relief. The responsibility for this task must extend across disciplines and requires increased collaboration between different sectors in health, environment, and other institutions; and across different divisions of government and non-governmental agencies.

The evidence from a wide range of disciplines and sources has now reached a critical mass, where we can claim with some confidence that there is a significant relationship between mental health and exposure to natural environments, especially for women and for those living in socioeconomically deprived areas. Taking this evidence into account in public health strategies could offer various opportunities for primary mental illness prevention and early intervention, with a significant impact on the global burden of mental health disorders.

References

Alcock, I., White, M. P., Wheeler, B. W., Fleming, L. E., & Depledge, M. H. (2014). Longitudinal effects on mental health of moving to greener and less green urban areas. *Environ Sci Technol*, 48, 1247–55.

Amoly, E., Dadvand, P., Forns, J., et al. (2014). Green and Blue Spaces and Behavioral Development in Barcelona Schoolchildren: The BREATHE Project. *Environ Health Perspect*, 122, 1351–8.

Annerstedt, M., Jönsson, P., Wallergård, M., et al. (2013). Inducing physiological stress recovery with sounds of nature in a virtual reality forest—Results from a pilot study. *Physiol Behav*, 118, 240–50.

Annerstedt, M., Norman, J., Boman, M., Mattsson, L., Grahn, P., & Währborg, P. (2010). Finding stress relief in a forest. *Ecol Bull*, 53, 33–42.

Annerstedt, M., Östergren, P.-O., Björk, J., Grahn, P., Skärbäck, E., & Währborg, P. (2012). Green qualities in the neighbourhood and mental health—results from a longitudinal cohort study in Southern Sweden. *BMC Public Health*, 12, 337.

Annerstedt, M., Östergren, P.-O., Grahn, P., Skärbäck, E., & Währborg, P. (2015). Moving to Serene Nature May Prevent Poor Mental Health—Results from a Swedish Longitudinal Cohort Study. *Int J Environ Res Public Health*, 12, 7974–89.

Antonovsky, A. (1996). The salutogenic model as a theory to guide health promotion. *Health Promot Int*, 11, 11.

Arnetz, B. B. (1996). Techno-stress: A prospective psychophysiological study of the impact of a controlled stress-reduction program in advanced telecommunication systems design work. *J Occ Environ Med*, 38, 53–65.

Aspinall, P., Mavros, P., Coyne, R., & Roe, J. (2015). The urban brain: analysing outdoor physical activity with mobile EEG. *Br J Sports Med*, 49, 272–6.

Balseviciene, B., Sinkariova, L., Grazuleviciene, R., et al. (2014). Impact of residential greenness on preschool children's emotional and behavioral problems. *Int J Environ Res Public Health*, 11, 6757–70.

Beil, K. & Hanes, D. (2013). The influence of urban natural and built environments on physiological and psychological measures of stress— a pilot study. *Int J Environ Res Public Health*, 10, 1250–67.

Bengtsson, A. & Carlsson, G. (2006). Outdoor environments at three nursing homes: Focus group interviews with staff. *J Hous Elder*, 19, 49–69.

Beyer, K., Kaltenbach, A., Szabo, A., Bogar, S., Nieto, F., & Malecki, K. (2014). Exposure to neighborhood green space and mental health: evidence from the survey of the health of Wisconsin. *Int J Environ Res Public Health*, 11, 3453–72.

Björk, J., Albin, M., Grahn, P., et al. (2008). Recreational values of the natural environment in relation to neighbourhood satisfaction, physical activity, obesity and wellbeing. *J Epidemiol Community Health*, 62, e2.

Cohen-Cline, H., Turkheimer, E., & Duncan, G. E. (2015). Access to green space, physical activity and mental health: A twin study. *J Epidemiol Community Health*, 69, 523–9.

Curl, A., Ward Thompson, C., Alves, S., & Aspinall, P. (2016). Outdoor environmental supportiveness and older people's quality of life: a personal projects approach. *J Hous Elder*, 30, 1–17.

Dadvand, P., Nieuwenhuijsen, M. J., Esnaola, M., et al. (2015). Green spaces and cognitive development in primary schoolchildren. *Proc Natl Acad Sci*, 112, 7937–42.

de Jong, K., Albin, M., Skärbäck, E., Grahn, P., & Björk, J. (2012). Perceived green qualities were associated with neighborhood satisfaction, physical activity, and general health: Results from a cross-sectional study in suburban and rural Scania, southern Sweden. *Health Place*, 18, 1374–80.

Dickerson, S. & Kemeny, M. (2004). Acute stressors and cortisol responses: A theoretical integration and synthesis of laboratory research. *Psychol Bull*, 130, 355–91.

Flouri, E., Midouhas, E., & Joshi, H. (2014). The role of urban neighbourhood green space in children's emotional and behavioural resilience. *J Environ Psychol*, 40, 179–86.

Gibson, J. J. (1977). The theory of affordances. In: Shaw, R. B., J. (ed.) *Perceiving, Acting, and Knowing: Toward an Ecological Psychology*. Hillsdale, NJ: Lawrence Erlbaum Associates.

Gidlow, C. J., Randall, J., Gillman, J., Smith, G. R., & Jones, M. V. (2016). Natural environments and chronic stress measured by hair cortisol. *Landsc Urban Plan*, 148, 61–7.

Godfrey, R. & Julien, M. (2005). Urbanisation and health. *Clin Med*, 5, 137–41.

Grahn, P., & Stigsdotter, U. K. (2010). The relation between perceived sensory dimensions of urban green space and stress restoration. *Landsc Urban Plan*, 94, 264–75.

Grahn, P., Tenngart Ivarsson, C., Stigsdotter, U. K., & Bengtsson, I-L. (2010). Using affordances as a health-promoting tool in a therapeutic setting. In: Ward Thompson, C., Bell, S., & Aspinall, P (ed.) *Innovative Approaches to Researching Landscape and Health*. London, UK: Routledge.

Greif, M. J. & Nii-Amoo Dodoo, F. (2015). How community physical, structural, and social stressors relate to mental health in the urban slums of Accra, Ghana. *Health Place*, 33, 57–66.

Handley, J., Pauleit, S., Slinn, P., Barber, A., Baker, M., Jones, C., & Lindley, S. (2003). Accessible natural green space standards in towns and cities: a review and toolkit for their implementation. *English Nature Research Reports*. Peterborough, UK.

Hartig, T. (2007). Three steps to understanding restorative environments as health resources. In: Ward Thompson, C., Travlou, P (ed.) *Open Space: People Space*. Abingdon, UK: Taylor and Francis.

Hartig, T., Evans, G. W., Jamner, L. D., Davis, D. S., & Gärling, T. (2003). Tracking restoration in natural and urban field settings. *J Environ Psychol*, 23, 109–23.

Heinrichs, M., Baumgartner, T., Kirschbaum, C., & Ehlert, U. (2003). Social support and oxytocin interact to suppress cortisol and subjective responses to psychosocial stress. *Biol Psychiatry*, 54, 1389–98.

Iwanaga, K., Xin, X. L., Shimomura, Y., & Katsuura, T. (2005). Approach to human adaptability to stresses of city life. *J Physiol Anthropol Appl Human Sci*, 24, 357–61.

Kaplan, S. (1995). The restorative benefits of nature: Toward an integrative framework. *J Environ Psychol*, 15, 169–82.

Kaplan, R., Kaplan, S., & Ryan, R. L. (1998). *With People in Mind: Design and management of everyday nature*. Washington, DC: Island Press.

Lengen, C. & Kistemann, T. (2012). Sense of place and place identity: Review of neuroscientific evidence. *Health Place*, 18, 1162–71.

Maas, J., Verheij, R. A., De Vries, S., Spreeuwenberg, P., Schellevis, F. G., & Groenewegen, P. P. (2009). Morbidity is related to a green living environment. *J Epidemiol Community Health*, 63, 967–73.

Mitchell, R. (2013). Is physical activity in natural environments better for mental health than physical activity in other environments? *Soc Sci Med*, 91, 130–4.

Ottosson, J. (2001). The importance of nature in coping with a crisis: a photographic essay. *Landsc Res*, 26, 165–72.

Ottosson, J. (2007). *The importance of nature in coping. Acta Universitatis Agricultureae Sueciae* (Doctoral thesis). Uppsala, Sweden: Swedish University of Agricultural Sciences.

Ottosson, J. & Grahn, P. (2005). A comparison of leisure time spent in a garden with leisure time spent indoors: On measures of restoration in residents in geriatric care. *Landsc Res*, 30, 23–55.

Ottosson, J. & Grahn, P. (2008). The role of natural settings in crisis rehabilitation: how does the level of crisis influence the response to experiences of nature with regard to measures of rehabilitation? *Landsc Res*, 33, 51.

Pálsdóttir, A. M., Persson, D., Persson, B., & Grahn, P. (2014). The journey of recovery and empowerment embraced by nature—Clients' perspectives on nature-based rehabilitation in relation to the role of the natural environment. *Int J Environ Res Public Health*, 11, 7094–115.

Patel, V. & Jané-Llopis, E. (2005). Poverty, social exclusion and disadvantages groups. In: Hosman C, J.-L. E., Saxena, S. (eds) *Prevention of Mental Disorders: Effective Interventions and Policy Options*. Oxford, UK: Oxford University Press.

Pearce, J. R., Richardson, E. A., Mitchell, R. J., & Shortt, N. K. (2010). Environmental justice and health: the implications of the socio-spatial distribution of multiple environmental deprivation for health inequalities in the United Kingdom. *Trans Inst Br Geogr*, 35, 522–39.

Peen, J., Schoevers, R., Beekman, A., & Dekker, J. (2010). The current status of urban-rural differences in psychiatric disorders. *Acta Psychiat Scand*, 121, 84–93.

Penedo, F. J. & Dahn, J. R. (2005). Exercise and well-being: A review of mental and physical health benefits associated with physical activity. *Curr Opin Psychiatry*, 18, 189–93.

Pretty, J., Peacock, J., Sellens, M., & Griffin, M. (2005). The mental and physical health outcomes of green exercise. *Int J Environ Health Res*, 15, 319–37.

Prince, M., Patel, V., Saxena, S., *et al.* (2007). No health without mental health. *Lancet*, 370, 859–77.

Qiu, L. (2014). *Linking biodiversity and recreational merits of urban green spaces* (Doctoral thesis). Uppsala, Sweden: Swedish University of Agricultural Sciences.

Reed, K., Wood, C., Barton, J., Pretty, J. N., Cohen, D., & Sandercock, G. R. H. (2013). A repeated measures experiment of green exercise to improve self-esteem in UK school children. *PLoS One*, 8, e69176.

Reklaitiene, R., Grazuleviciene, R., Dedele, A., *et al.* (2014). The relationship of green space, depressive symptoms and perceived general health in urban population. *Scand J Public Health*, 42, 669–76.

Risal, A., Manandhar, K., Linde, M., Steiner, T. J., & Holen, A. (2016). Anxiety and depression in Nepal: Prevalence, comorbidity and associations. *BMC Psychiatry*, 16, 102.

Roe, J., Ward Thompson, C., Aspinall, P., *et al.* (2013). Green space and stress: evidence from cortisol measures in deprived urban communities. *Int J Environ Res Public Health*, 10, 4086–103.

Ryan, C. O., Browning, W. D., Clancy, J. O., Andrews, S. L., & Kallianpurkar, N. B. (2014). Biophilic design patterns: Emerging nature-based parameters for health and well-being in the built environment. *Archnet-IJAR*, 8, 62–76.

Sahlin, E. (2014). *To stress the importance of nature. Acta Universitatis Agriculturae Sueciae* (Doctoral thesis). Uppsala, Sweden: Swedish University of Agricultural Sciences.

Salas, M. L., Quezada, S., Basagoitia, A., *et al.* (2015). Working conditions, workplace violence, and psychological distress in andean miners: a cross-sectional study across three countries. *Ann Glob Health*, 81, 465–74.

Skärbäck, E., Björk, J., Stoltz, J., Rydell-Andersson, K., & Grahn, P. (2014). Green perception for wellbeing in dense urban areas—a tool for socioeconomic integration. *Nordic J Architectural Res*, 26, 179–205.

Stigsdotter, U., Ekholm, O., Schipperijn, J., Toftager, M., Kamper-Jørgensen, F., & Randrup, T. (2010). Health promoting outdoor environments-Associations between green space, and health, health-related quality of life and stress based on a Danish national representative survey. *Scand J Public Health*, 38, 411.

Stigsdotter, U., & Grahn, P. (2002). What makes a garden a healing garden. *J Ther Hort*, 13, 60–9.

Stigsdotter, U. K. & Grahn, P. (2011). Stressed individuals' preferences for activities and environmental characteristics in green spaces. *Urban For Urban Greening*, 10, 295–304.

Sturm, R. & Cohen, D. (2014). Proximity to urban parks and mental health. *J Ment Health Policy Econ*, 17, 19–24.

Sugiyama, T., & Ward Thompson C. (2005). Environmental support for outdoor activities and older people's quality of life. *J Hous Elder*, 19, 167–85.

Sundquist, K., Frank, G., & Sundquist, J. (2004). Urbanisation and incidence of psychosis and depression Follow-up study of 4.4 million women and men in Sweden. *Br J Psychiatry*, 184, 293–8.

Triguero-Mas, M., Dadvand, P., Cirach, M., *et al.* (2015). Natural outdoor environments and mental and physical health: Relationships and mechanisms. *Environ Int*, 77, 35–41.

Tyrväinen, L., Mäkinen, K., & Schipperijn, J. (2007). Tools for mapping social values of urban woodlands and other green areas. *Landsc Urban Plan*, 79, 5–19.

Ulrich, R. S. & Addoms, D. L. (1981). Psychological and recreational benefits of a residential park. *J Leisure Res*, 13, 43–65.

Ulrich, R., Simons, R., Losito, B., Fiorito, E., Miles, M., & Zelson, M. (1991). Stress recovery during exposure to natural and urban environments. *J Environ Psychol*, 11, 201–30.

Ulrich, R. S., Dimberg, U., & Driver, B. L. (1989). Psychophysiological indicators of leisure benefits. In: Driver, B. L., Brown, L. R., & Peterson, G. I. (eds) *Benefits of Leisure*. State College, PA: Venture Publishing.

van den Berg, A. E. & Custers, M. H. G. (2011). Gardening promotes neuroendocrine and affective restoration from stress. *J Health Psychol*, 16, 3–11.

van den Berg, M. M. H. E., Maas, J., Muller, R., *et al.* (2015). Autonomic nervous system responses to viewing green and built settings: Differentiating between sympathetic and parasympathetic activity. *Int J Environ Res Public Health*, 12, 15860–74.

Ward Thompson, C., Aspinall, P., Roe, J., Robertson, L., & Miller, D. (2016). Mitigating stress and supporting health in deprived urban communities: the importance of green space and the social environment. *Int J Environ Res Public Health*, 13, 440.

Ward Thompson, C., Roe, J., Aspinall, P., Mitchell, R., Clow, A., & Miller, D. (2012). More green space is linked to less stress in deprived communities: Evidence from salivary cortisol patterns. *Landsc Urban Plan*, 105, 221–9.

White, M. P., Pahl, S., Ashbullby, K., Herbert, S., & Depledge, M. H. (2013). Feelings of restoration from recent nature visits. *J Environ Psychol*, 35, 40–51.

World Health Organization (WHO) (2005). Mental health: facing the challenges, building solutions. Report from the WHO European Ministerial Conference. Copenhagen, Denmark: WHO Regional Office for Europe.

World Health Organization (WHO) (2013). Mental health and older adults. Available at: http://www.who.int/mediacentre/factsheets/fs381/en/ [Online].

Promoting social cohesion— increasing well-being

Birgit Elands, Karin Peters, and Sjerp de Vries

Defining social cohesion

Both green spaces and social cohesion contribute to (mental) health and well-being. The interrelation between social cohesion, green space, and health is complex and diverse. This chapter will discuss this relationship based on existing scientific evidence.

Social cohesion can be defined as the extent to which a geographical place achieves 'community' in the sense of shared values, cooperation, and interaction (Beckly, 1994), positive and friendly relationships (de Vries *et al.*, 2013), and feelings of being accepted and belonging (Forrest and Kearns, 2001; Elliot *et al.*, 2014). Social cohesion is thus about relationships between people, and as such it refers to the nature of a collective, rather than to that of a person. When discussing social cohesion, the terms 'sense of community', 'social ties', 'social networks', and 'social contacts' are often used as equivalents, and feelings of loneliness and shortage of social support as indicators for an absence of social cohesion. All terms refer to the extent residents living in the same neighbourhood have relations with each other. This can be understood as the width of social cohesion. It can also be interpreted through the meaning of these relations; that is, the extent to which people help each other or are concerned about or feel responsible for each other and/or the neighbourhood. We then speak of the depth of social cohesion (Veen *et al.*, 2015). We approach social cohesion as perceived by an individual person, as is the case in most scientific studies.

Social capital is often used in relation to social cohesion and is sometimes even considered to be similar to it. Social capital generally refers to resources, such as networks, norms, and trust that facilitate collaboration between people for mutual benefit (Putnam, 2000). Whereas social cohesion is generally perceived to be a community asset, social capital is generally perceived as an individual asset. Nevertheless, the definition of social cohesion sometimes includes (aspects of) social capital (Forrest and Kearns, 2001). In this chapter however, we will not elaborate on the notion of social capital any further.

Strengthening social cohesion

In order to understand the interrelation between social cohesion, green space, and health, we need to elucidate the mechanisms leading towards strengthening social cohesion. These mechanisms

indicate that green space invites people to go out, where they can have social interactions that potentially contribute to neighbourhood social cohesion (see Fig. 3.3.1).

The social cohesion of a neighbourhood is spatially anchored, as living together in an area implies meeting the same people in the same place in your daily life. In this chapter a neighbourhood is defined as a territory within a city or town, where people live, recreate, and interact socially (Kaźmierczak, 2013). Sometimes this territory coincides with the administrative unit used by municipalities. Neighbourhood open spaces, and green spaces in particular, provide opportunities for people to meet other people and interact. Green spaces can be defined as all areas that are predominantly natural, thus including elements such as lawns, trees, shrubs, flowerbeds, but also ponds, streams, fens, and lakes. As green spaces are often perceived as attractive places to visit, they offer good opportunities for residents to, by chance or not, meet other people.

Social interactions in public spaces are mostly informal and can provide relief from daily routines and alleviate tensions in a neighbourhood (Dines and Cattell, 2006). Public green spaces are often visited by various groups in society. Therefore, they are commonly acknowledged for their integrative potential as they offer the opportunity to become familiar with persons of different social and ethnic backgrounds (Lofland, 1998; Seeland *et al.*, 2009; Peters *et al.*, 2010). They can facilitate bonds between residents, and thus contribute to social cohesion.

This chapter aims at (i) discussing the importance and role of green spaces in promoting social cohesion and (ii) explaining how different forms of social interaction determine the relation between green spaces and social cohesion. In the following sections we will first explain the health and well-being aspects of social cohesion. We will then discuss different forms of social interaction in relation to green spaces. Finally, some important characteristics in the field of green space and health will be presented.

The mediating role of social cohesion

The association between having positive social relationships with others, and social cohesion on the one hand and one's well-being and health on the other, has been studied extensively. In general, this association is positive. Social cohesion is not only positively associated with mental health (De Silva *et al.*, 2005), but also with

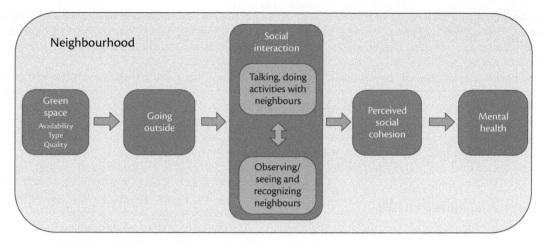

Fig. 3.3.1 Conceptual social cohesion framework.

physical health (Yang *et al.*, 2016). Moreover, it is associated with lower mortality rates (Holt-Lunstad *et al.*, 2010; Pantell *et al.*, 2013).

The neighbourhood is considered to be relevant as it has been shown that social cohesion within the neighbourhood is also positively associated with health and well-being (Rios *et al.*, 2012; Bjornstrom *et al.*, 2013; Pearson *et al.*, 2014). Especially in deprived neighbourhoods, a high level of social cohesion has been observed to have protective mental health effects (Fone *et al.*, 2014). Therefore, improving neighbourhood social cohesion, especially in deprived neighbourhoods, may help to reduce socioeconomic health disparities, a major issue within the public health domain.

Apart from neighbourhood characteristics, individual aspects of people living in the neighbourhood are also relevant. People with chronic illness are less likely to report deteriorating health when they experience high levels of social cohesion (Waverijn *et al.*, 2014). The relation between neighbourhood social cohesion and well-being varies also between age groups. Although there is a positive association for all age groups, it appears that the relation is stronger for older people. Qualitative interviews revealed that the importance of social cohesion for older people may be explained by the fact that they are more dependent on social ties within the neighbourhood, as they are less mobile and consider participation in local groups to be important (Elliot *et al.*, 2014).

The availability of green space contributes to neighbourhood social cohesion. As with health, in general this association is positive. In the 1990s, the first studies on the relationship between nearby green areas and social cohesion within the neighbourhood indicated that having green space very close at hand may contribute to social cohesion between neighbourhood members. Residents living in greener areas have been found to be more socially active, know more neighbours, and feel that their neighbours are more helpful and supportive (Kuo *et al.*, 1998; Kweon *et al.*, 1998). However, these studies have predominantly focused on the same and quite specific setting: a very poor segment of the population of a large city (Chicago), living in high-rise apartment buildings with scarce green.

This limitation was addressed by several studies that focus on representative samples within a country, thereby including a diversity of neighbourhoods and backgrounds of people. Objective measures of green, in terms of quantity and quality conditions,

proved to be related to social cohesion. In general, green spaces and public parks seem to strengthen social cohesion within a neighbourhood (Sugiyama *et al.*, 2008; Cohen *et al.*, 2008; Maas *et al.*, 2009; Kemperman and Timmermans, 2014; Kaźmierczak, 2013).

Given the evidence that social cohesion is positively associated with health and access to green space with social cohesion, is social cohesion an important link in the pathway from access to green space to health and well-being? A large-scale Dutch study indicates that it may be. In this study, people with more green space in their neighbourhood perceived less shortage of social support and loneliness, and reported better health (Maas *et al.*, 2009). More importantly, this study proved that shortage of social support, being an indicator for absent social cohesion, completely mediated the relation between green space and self-assessed risk of psychiatric morbidity. Also in other studies, social cohesion, among other factors, appeared to have a mediating role in the relation between quantity and quality of neighbourhood and streetscape greenery, and health indicators such as perceived general health, acute health-related complaints, and mental health (Sugiyama *et al.*, 2008; de Vries *et al.*, 2013).

Social interactions: from weak and one-off to strong and more structural

Social interactions between groups of people provide the basis for social cohesion. The use of public green space creates opportunities for informal social encounters or exchanges, which are often perceived as a key element in people's perception of their well-being (Cattell *et al.*, 2008). Social interaction can take different forms, from passing by other people while walking, to undertaking joint activities such as gardening or jogging. Interactions occur in any social situation in which persons are acting in awareness of others. These interactions also occur anonymously. Interactions can be formal (planned) or informal (casual, unplanned) (Kim and Kaplan, 2004). They can vary from weak and one-off, to strong and more structural interactions (Lofland, 1998).

Formal interactions are aimed at meeting familiar or known people and contributing to the maintenance of existing social ties (such as having a chat with a friend or picnicking with a group of friends in the park).

Informal interactions comprise a variety of interactions, starting from more *passive and one-off forms of interaction* (e.g. passing by other people while walking and watching children playing or elderly people sitting on a bench), to a *more focused attention form of interaction*, such as greeting an acquaintance or a short chat with vaguely known people or even strangers, extending to more *deliberate forms of interaction* (e.g. having a conversation with neighbours or undertaking a joint activity after meeting each other). From the perspective of social cohesion, in this chapter we focus merely on the informal relationships in green spaces with neighbourhood members, rather than with family members or friends living elsewhere.

Few interactions with unknown people

Green space invites socializing with other people. Observations of outdoor space use of residents living in apartment buildings in a large public housing development in Chicago revealed that green spaces attracted almost twice as many visitors and social activities as barren spaces (Coley *et al.*, 1997; Sullivan *et al.*, 2004). Social activities were defined as activities, such as talking and playing, taking place within a group of people. Greeting a neighbour without having a chat, however, was not considered to be a social activity. This study excluded the co-present and co-attention informal interactions, which (as discussed in the next section) are important for experiencing public familiarity.

Most visitors visit urban green space with their own friends, family, and relatives. They feel comfortable within their own social group and do not feel the need to interact with others. If people come to green space to socialize, it does not mean they want to meet new people. In a study of social interactions between native Dutch people and non-Western migrant groups in five urban parks, participant observations revealed that relatively few interactions occurred between social groups (Peters *et al.*, 2010). It became clear that interactions mainly occur due to external stimuli and impulses, such as ballgames, children, and dogs. Children played together for a while, parents chatted with each other, and balls were returned when needed. These interactions were defined by the visitors as 'small talk' and 'having a chat about a common interest'. However short, in general these interactions were valued positively. The valuation differed for people though. Whereas native Dutch people did not look for more interactions, some non-Western migrants did, although they did not take the initiative themselves. Similarly, for immigrants in Helsinki, the use of nearby urban nature was mainly motivated by spending time with their friends and relatives and not for creating new social ties. Nevertheless, spontaneous interactions did occur and were appreciated by the immigrants (Leikkilä *et al.*, 2013).

Through focused interaction, unknown people become familiar

Under certain circumstances, it is possible to familiarize with unknown visitors. Certain activities, such as playing and ballgames, are well-suited for the stimulation of multicultural encounters. In a comparative study on the potential of urban parks and forests in Zürich to make contacts and friends between different cultures, it was found that parks in particular have the potential to stimulate multicultural encounters as they are equally intensively used by both Swiss and immigrant young people. This is especially relevant for children of primary school age, while playing and doing sport. Older young people are more likely to visit urban forests for meeting friends and socializing, although in their own cultural group (Seeland *et al.*, 2009).

The fact that some activities are more favourable for getting to know strangers than others was confirmed in a study on the use of local parks in three inner-city neighbourhoods in Manchester (Kaźmierczak, 2013). Visitors of these parks explained that parks are not only places for meeting existing friends, but also for establishing new friendships. The recognition of the other and regular visits are important prerequisites for developing new friendships. They also indicated that short visits or visits focused on necessary activities (e.g. to pass through on the way elsewhere) may not support interactions with unknown people.

The Manchester study also examined to what extent park activities—among other factors—contributed to the number of friends and acquaintances in the neighbourhood. After distinguishing between necessary activities (e.g. to pass through on the way elsewhere), optional activities (e.g. relaxing or enjoying the nice scenery), and social activities (e.g. playing sports or games), analyses revealed that after length of residence, social activities were the most important. This is similar to the findings of Lund (2002) who identified that social cohesion was positively correlated with strolling trips in public spaces in the neighbourhood, and negatively correlated with destination trips.

Informal interactions create public familiarity

As discussed before, most people prefer to socialize in their own group. It is known that residents with a diverse background do not easily (wish to) establish social networks or make friends with each other. Nevertheless, this does *not* imply that casual encounters between people one may occasionally see are meaningless to residents.

On the basis of interviews with residents from two inner-city neighbourhoods in Berlin, it became evident that public familiarity (i.e. both recognizing other people, with whom one has no ties, and being recognized by other people) is highly important to people (Blokland and Nast, 2014). Living together in the same area implies meeting the same people in the same place in your daily life. This creates a joint understanding of neighbourhood life, stories, and boundaries. The familiarity with the neighbourhood creates a comfort zone, in which one knows the codes of conduct in public spaces and manoeuvres at ease. Moreover, this comfort zone embodies trust in other residents, who would help each other in need, and facilitates a feeling of belonging in their place of residence, even if they have no friends or family nearby in the neighbourhood, and even if they do not like the place where they live. In qualitative studies among residents in East London and Utrecht (NL) similar findings were obtained (Cattell *et al.*, 2008; Peters, 2011).

Multicultural neighbourhoods might benefit from public familiarity of its residents as it provides important grounds for experiencing ethnic and social variety on an everyday basis. It allows people to feel safe and comfortable in these places, thereby reducing intolerance and stimulating social integration (Dines and Cattell, 2006; Peters, 2011; Leikkilä *et al.*, 2013). Public familiarity is highly relevant for newly residing people with a different cultural background in a neighbourhood. For immigrants in Helsinki, the use of nearby urban nature helped them to understand the Finnish preference for less interaction and thus feel comfortable in their neighbourhood (Leikkilä *et al.*, 2013).

Importance of and motivation for social interaction varies

Although social interactions in public neighbourhood spaces are generally evaluated positively, they are not equally important to all residents. Those groups experiencing mobility or financial constraints, such as older people (Elliot *et al.*, 2014; Kemperman and Timmermans, 2014), children and youth (Seeland *et al.*, 2009), parents with young children, and unemployed people, attach greater value to social interactions in the neighbourhood than other groups do. Moreover, ethnic groups differ in this respect.

Evidence from a study on park use in Los Angeles revealed that Spanish-speaking Latinos and Asian/Pacific Islanders are more likely than whites to use parks for social interactions (Derose *et al.*, 2015). Similar results have been found in other US and European cities for other ethnic groups, among other African-Americans, Turkish, Moroccan, and Korean people.

Next, the importance people attach to social interaction is associated with the motives people have for using green space. From a study on community gardens two different types of gardeners could be distinguished, based on the dominant motives of their participants: interest-based motives and place-based motives. Whereas for the place-based gardener the harvest of vegetables and fruit is a by-product, for the interest-based gardener meeting other people is a by-product (Veen *et al.*, 2015). This shows that being in this kind of natural environment can enhance social interactions which are valued, even though developing relationships is not the main reason for visiting those places.

Moreover, social interactions may be stimulated by other factors such as place attachment. Feelings of belonging to a neighbourhood arise out of attachment to a particular place, as well as out of social interaction with neighbours (Kim and Kaplan, 2004). Green spaces seem to strengthen social cohesion also by way of increasing the place attachment of its residents (Kweon *et al.*, 1998; Maas *et al.*, 2009). Feeling attached to local green spaces is facilitated by organized events, active participation, and obtained memories (Peters, 2011).

Interactions can also be experienced negatively and this interrelates with the presence and motivations of users. This can occur when a specific group dominates the public space and acts hostile to other (groups of) people with different values, socioeconomic or cultural background, or practices. In the usage of everyday public spaces in a multiethnic area in East London, racism was one such negatively experienced interaction (Cattell *et al.*, 2008). Negative experiences in public spaces result in fewer subsequent contacts with local people (Dines and Cattell, 2006). The perception of safety within a neighbourhood has a large influence on social cohesion. Research links high crime or fear of crime with a lack of neighbourhood cohesion (Conklin, 1971; Rohe and Burby, 1988). Greenery positively influences this relation: the greener the neighbourhood, the stronger the social ties, and the lower the overall reported domestic violence levels. Also, crime levels were significantly lower in residences near natural spaces (Kuo *et al.*, 1998). This also relates to the fact that public familiarity, which is facilitated by casual encounters, leads to being able to 'read the environment' resulting in higher perceptions of safety.

Green matters: availability, type, and quality

When discussing the potential of green spaces for creating social cohesion, it is important to realize that certain characteristics of green space play a role in the extent to which public green spaces are of value.

Availability

We have argued that social cohesion is facilitated and stimulated by the availability of green spaces and the opportunities to have social interactions in these spaces. To fulfil its role in neighbourhood social cohesion, both the proximity and size of green are important.

Type

Although all green space types potentially facilitate social interaction, there are two types that are frequently discussed in scientific literature (i.e. urban parks and community and/or allotment gardens).

Urban parks are possibly favourable spaces for stimulating social cohesion as they contribute to the feeling of public familiarity of residents of the same neighbourhood and provide opportunities to perpetuate existing friendships and occasionally, develop new ones. The function of a park may vary. In smaller neighbourhood parks visitors more easily have small talks and develop new acquaintances. Larger urban parks, which attract a variety of people also beyond the own neighbourhood, are less suitable for direct interaction with other people. However, these parks also provide a vital locality where everyday experiences are shared and negotiated between a variety of cultural groups.

Some natural environments, such as community or allotment gardens, incorporate social interaction almost by definition. Gardens provide plenty of opportunities to socialize. Studies revealed that through involvement with other people, but also through contact with nature, social cohesion appeared to be particularly strong in such gardens. Besides, these often cross-cultural interactions diminish cultural boundaries and negative racial stereotypes (Bartolomei *et al.*, 2003; Holland, 2004; Wakefield *et al.*, 2007). Moreover, older gardeners reported having more contacts with friends and felt less lonely than did non-gardening neighbours in the same age category (Van den Berg *et al.*, 2010). Finally, in one study it was concluded that gardens contributed to physical and psychological health, at least partly mediated by social cohesion (Wakefield *et al.*, 2007).

Quality

The quality of green spaces determines largely whether people are going to use it and the extent to which it facilitates social cohesion (Francis *et al.*, 2012; de Vries *et al.*, 2013). Here it is argued that in order for green spaces to contribute to develop social ties, they must be easily accessible, aesthetically attractive, well maintained, perceived as safe, and provide good recreational facilities (Hartig *et al.*, 2014; Francis *et al.*, 2012; Kemperman and Timmermans, 2014; Kaźmierczak, 2013). Perceived safety is particularly crucial. This perception and other subjective perceptions of places might have an even stronger association with social cohesion than objective attributes of the environment (Francis *et al.*, 2012).

On a micro level, several studies showed that the presence of trees and grass in public spaces increased the use and number

Table 3.3.1 Green space characteristics facilitating social interaction

Factor	Examples
Availability	Proximity, size
Type	Urban parks (varying from neighbourhood parks to city parks)
	Community gardens
Quality	Design: good physical access, aesthetics, safety
	Vegetation: presence of trees and grass, variety of plant species (both native and exotic)
	Choreography of spaces: multifunctionality and multiuser groups
	Management: well-managed and room for self-organization

of individuals participating in social interaction in these spaces (Coley *et al.*, 1997; Kemperman and Timmermans, 2014; Sullivan *et al.*, 2004). Both grass and trees were most predictive for use; however, trees were the most important green elements as their presence predicted greater use and length of stay in public open spaces. Grass provides opportunities for social gathering, such as picnicking, hanging around, playing, ball games, and so on. Trees can also be considered as anchor points for social gatherings as they provide shade and intimacy/bordering group space.

Altogether, this shows that it is highly relevant to think about design issues, not only in terms of good physical access and welcoming spaces, but also by paying attention to the choreography of spaces. Green spaces should not be developed for singular activities or monocultural use, but designed to facilitate the needs of different neighbourhood groups and activities. It is known that people with varying socioeconomic and cultural backgrounds might vary in their preferences; for example, the type of plant species (native or exotic), the amount and type of ornamental infrastructure, and the level of management. Moreover, the design and maintenance should leave room for self-organization for local people. The fact that neighbourhood members had co-designed local parks increased the likelihood of social interactions between different (ethnic) groups (Risbeth, 2001; Peters *et al.*, 2010) (Table 3.3.1).

Conclusion

This chapter has discussed how green places contribute to well-being and health through social cohesion. Green spaces provide opportunities for people to meet other people and interact. These interactions are valued for becoming familiar with and understanding other people in the neighbourhood, thereby contributing to neighbourhood social cohesion. Although most green space visitors do not want to socialize with unknown others, they like to be there with other visitors. In this sense, green space contributes to the feeling of public familiarity among residents of the same neighbourhood.

Most social interactions are cursory; people have a short chat or just say hello. There are more weak and one-off interactions than strong and more structural interactions. Occasionally, green spaces provide opportunities to perpetuate existing friendships and develop new ones. This is particularly true for activities (e.g. playing soccer) or organized events, because these situations stimulate more intense interactions. However, it is important to realize that social cohesion is complex and multifactorial in its origin and green spaces can only play a facilitating role. In order to fulfil such a role, the type, quality, and design of green spaces are relevant. Aspects such as type of vegetation, safety, access, and availability of recreational facilities need to be considered carefully in the planning and management of green areas, not only by local authorities, but also, and maybe even more importantly, in collaboration with residents.

References

Bartolomei, L., Corkery, L., Judd, B., & Thompson S. M. (2003). *A Bountiful Harvest: Community Gardens and Neighbourhood Renewal in Waterloo.*, Sydney, Australia: NSW Department of Housing and University of New South Wales.

Beckly, T. (1994). Community stability and the relationship between economic and social well-being in forest dependent communities. *Soc Nat Resour*, 8, 261–6.

Bjornstrom, E. E., Ralston, M. L., & Kuhl, D. C. (2013). Social cohesion and self-rated health: the moderating effect of neighborhood physical disorder. *Am J Community Psychol*, 52, 302–12.

Blokland, T. & Nast J. (2014). From public familiarity to comfort zone: the relevance of absent ties for belonging in Berlin's mixed neigbourhoods. *Int J Urban Reg Res*, 38, 1142–59.

Cattell, V., Dines, N., Gesler, W., & Curtis, S. (2008). Mingling, observing, and lingering: everday public spaces and their implications for well-being and social relations. *Health Place*, 14, 544–61.

Cohen, D. A., Inagami, S., & Finch, B. (2008). The built environment and collective efficacy. *Health Place*, 14, 198–208.

Coley, R., Kuo, F., & Sullivan, W. (1997). Where does community grow? The social context created by nature in urban public housing. *Environ Behav*, 29, 468–92.

Conklin, J. (1971). Dimensions of community response to the crime problem, *Social Problems*, 18(3), 373–85.

Derose, K., Han, B., Williamson, S., & Cohen, D. B. (2015). Racial-ethnic variation in park use and physical activity in the city of Los Angelos. *J Urban Health*, 92, 1011–23.

De Silva, M. J., McKenzie, K., Harpham, T., & Huttly, S. R. A. (2005). Social capital and mental illness: a systematic review. *J Epidemiol Community Health*, 59, 619–27.

De Vries, S., Van Dillen, S. M. E., Groenwegen, P. P., & Spreeuwenberg, P. (2013). Streetscape greenery and health: Stress, social cohesion and physical activity as mediators. *Soc Sci Med*, 94, 26–33.

Dines, N. & Cattell, V. (2006). *Public spaces, social relations and well-being.* Bristol, UK: The Policy Press.

Elliot, J., Gale, S. R., Parsons, S., Kuh, D., & the HALCyon Study Team (2014). Neighbourhood cohesion and mental wellbeing among older adults: A mixed methods approach. *Soc Sci Med*, 107, 44–51.

Fone, D., White, J., Farewell, D., *et al.* (2014). Effect of neighbourhood deprivation and social cohesion on mental health inequality: a multilvel population-based longitudinal study. *Psychol Med*, 44, 2449–60.

Forrest, R. & Kearns, A. (2001). Social cohesion, social capital and the neighbourhood. *Urban Studies*, 38, 2125–43.

Francis, J., Giles-Corti, B., Wood, L., & Knuiman, M. (2012). Creating sense of community: the role of public space. *J Environ Psychol*, 32, 401–9.

Hartig, T., Mitchell, R., De Vries, S., & Frumkin, H. (2014). Nature and health. *Ann Rev Public Health*, 35, 207–28.

Holland, L. (2004). Diversity and connections in community gardens: a contribution to local sustainability. *Local Environ*, 9, 285–305.

Holt-Lunstad, J., Smith, T. B., & Layton, J. B. (2010). Social relationships and mortality risks: a meta-analytic review. *PloS Med*, 7, e1000316.

Kaźmierczak, A. (2013). The contribution of local parks to neighbourhood social ties. *Landsc Urban Plan*, 109, 31–44.

Kemperman, A. & Timmermans, H. (2014). Green spaces in the direct living environment and social contacts of the aging population. *Landsc Urban Plan*, 129, 44–54.

Kim, J. & Kaplan, R. (2004). Physical and psychological factors in sense of community: new urbanist Kentlands and nearby Orchard village. *Environ Behav*, 36, 313–40.

Kuo, F. E., Sullivan, W. C., & Wiley, A. (1998). Fertile ground for community: innercity neighborhood common spaces. *Am J Community Psychol*, 26, 823–51.

Kweon, B., Sullivan, W., & Wiley, A. (1998). Green common spaces and the social integration of inner-city older adults. *Environ Behav*, 30, 832–58.

Leikkilä, J., Faehnle, M., & Galanakis, M. (2013). Promoting interculturalism by planning of urban nature. *Urban For Urban Green*, 12, 183–90.

Lofland, L. H. (1998). *The Public Realm: Exploring the City's Quintessential Social Territory*. New York, NY, USA: Aldine de Gruyter.

Lund, H. (2002). Pedestrian environments and sense of community. *J Plan Educ Res*, 21, 301–12.

Maas, J., Van Dillen, S. M. E., Verheij, R. A., & Groenewegen, P. P. (2009). Social contacts as a possible mechanism behind the relation between green space and health. *Health Place*, 15, 586–95.

Pantell, M., Rehkopf, D., Jutte, D., et al. (2013). Social isolation: a predictor of mortality comparable to traditional clinical risk factors. *Am J Public Health*, 103, 2056–62.

Pearson, A. L., Ivory, V., Breetzke, G., & Lovasi, G. S. (2014). Are feelings of peace or depression the drivers of the relationship between neighbourhood social fragmentation and mental health in Aotearoa/New Zealand? *Health Place*, 26, 1–6.

Peters, K. (2011). *Living together in multi-ethnic neighbourhoods: The meaning of public space for issues of social integration* (Doctoral thesis). Wageningen, the Netherlands: Wageningen University.

Peters, K., Elands, B., & Buijs, A. (2010). Social interactions in urban parks: Stimulating social cohesion? *Urban For Urban Green*, 9, 93–100.

Putnam, R. D. (2000). *Bowling Alone: The Collapse and Revival of American Community*. New York, NY: Simon and Schuster.

Rios, R., Aiken, L. S., & Zautra, A. J. (2012). Neighborhood contexts and the mediating role of neighborhood social cohesion on health and psychological distress among Hispanic and non-Hispanic residents. *Ann Behav Med*, 43, 50–61.

Rishbeth, C. (2001). Ethnic minority groups and the design of public open space: an inclusive landscape? *Landscape Research*, 26(4), 351–66.

Rohe, W. & Burby, R. (1988). Fear of crime in public housing. *Environment and Behaviour*, 20 (6), 700–20.

Seeland, K., Dübendorfer, S., & Hansmann, R. (2009). Making friends in Zürich's urban forests and parks: the role of public green space for social inclusion. *For Policy Econ*, 11, 10–17.

Sugiyama, T., Leslie, E., Giles-Corti, B., & Owen, N. (2008). Associations of neighbourhood greenness with physical and mental health: do walking, social coherence and local social interaction explain the relationships? *J Epidemiol Community Health*, 62, e9.

Sullivan, W. C., Kuo, F. E., & DePooter, S. F. (2004). The fruit of urban nature. Vital neighbourhood spaces. *Environ Behav*, 36, 678–700.

Van den Berg, A. E., Van Winsum-Westra M., De Vries, S., & Van Dillen, S. M. E. (2010). Allotment gardening and health: a comparative survey among allotment gardeners and their neigbors without an allotment. *Environmental Health*, 9, 74.

Veen, E. J., Bock, B. B., Van den Berg, W., Visser, A. J., & Wiskerke, J. S. C. (2015). Community gardening and social cohesion: different designs, different motivations. *Local Environment*, 21, 1271–87.

Wakefield, S., Yeudall, F., Taron, C., Reynolds, J., & Skinner A. (2007). Growing urban health: community gardening in south-east Toronto. *Health Promot Int*, 22, 92–101.

Waverijn, G., Wolfe, M. K., Mohnen S., et al. (2014). A prospective analysis of the effect of neighbourhood and individual social capital on changes in self-rated health of people with chronic illness. *BioMed Central Public Health*, 14, 675.

Yang, Y. C., Boen, C., Gerken, K., et al. (2016). Social relationships and physiological determinants of longevity across the human life span. *Proc Natl Acad Sci*, 113, 578–83.

Public health impact of nature contact— intervention and rehabilitation

CHAPTER 4.1

Using nature as a treatment option

Anna María Pálsdóttir, Joe Sempik, William Bird, and Matilda van den Bosch

Defining treatment with nature

There is a wide range of interventions for health and well-being that use nature. These are sometimes distinguished according to how nature is used—either as a setting for the intervention, for nature-based interventions (NBIs), or as an integral part (a tool) of the therapeutic process, in nature-assisted interventions (NAIs). NBIs and NAIs have been developed in many different countries in different landscapes and natural settings of more or less managed character and there is a diversity of interventions for various conditions or disabilities. Apart from addressing a particular diagnosis, the aim is also to provide meaningful activities and structured routines during states of ill health.

NBI may take place in almost any type of natural outdoor environment, such as gardens, parks, mountains and highlands, forests, by lakes and seashores, and agricultural landscapes and farms. Various kinds of activities may be used, the fundament is that they take place in outdoor nature. NAI, on the other hand, may take place either outdoors or indoors and the activity is always directly related to the use of natural elements (e.g. planting a wood, designing a flowerbed, or cutting a hedge). However, the distinction between the two types is often blurred and in this chapter we will in, general, use the term NAI.

There is no single, standardized form of delivery of any of these interventions, but there seems to be a general understanding of intervention practices, based on both setting and activities. A type of treatment paradigm has been created through experience and literature, rather than through any formal arrangements. Some approaches may be more beneficial to one patient group than to another. Often this has been motivated by conceptual ideas and recognition that certain goals (e.g. development of work skills) can best be achieved by particular approaches (or by an emphasis on specific aspects of an individual approach). While no specific contraindications or negative side effects to NAIs have been identified, safety can be an issue for some client groups.

What types of nature-assisted interventions exist?

Depending on the type of natural setting and the type of activity or intervention, different categories of NAIs can be distinguished.

Some of those are interrelated and some programmes include several modalities, but broadly a few groups can be defined.

NAIs can include, for instance, care farming, horticultural therapy, and other interventions where nature is an integral part of the intervention process. These programmes can contain elements of healthcare, social rehabilitation, education, or employment opportunities (Sempik et al., 2010; Stigsdotter et al., 2011). Figure 4.1.1 provides an overview of the most common approaches and their relation to nature and therapy.

In the following paragraphs, various types of NAIs are outlined.

- *Horticultural therapy*. Horticultural therapy has been defined as 'the use of plants by a trained professional as a medium through which certain clinically defined goals may be met'(Growth Point, 1999). All interventions in this group include some sort of horticultural activity with plants and would commonly be described as a NAI. For example, garden therapy and sensory gardens in healthcare come under this category. Some particular aspects of horticultural therapy programmes in gardens include the design of the garden, which is supposed to stimulate and facilitate accessibility, activities, and sensory experiences, such as touch and smell, throughout the seasons. The edges of a garden are usually well defined, which helps the patients to feel safe and secure and to focus their attention and energy towards the natural elements. Furthermore, the garden is often deliberately and consciously planned, providing places and spaces for restoration, horticultural education, therapy, and social interactions, as well as refuge. Therapeutic horticulture and social and therapeutic horticulture are not necessarily directed at a defined clinical goal but intended towards improving the wellbeing of the individual in a more generalized way (Sempik et al., 2003).

- *Care farming*. This type of intervention can also be denoted as social farming or green care farming. It uses farms and agricultural landscapes and activities as means of intervention. While much variety occurs within the concept, care farms always include agricultural elements, working with, for example crops, livestock husbandry, use of machinery, or woodland management (Sempik et al., 2010). Many care farms are focused on production on a commercial level.

- *Green exercise*. While the health benefits of physical activity are widely recognized, it is only recently that the synergistic

Mapping the influence of nature–nature as care and therapy

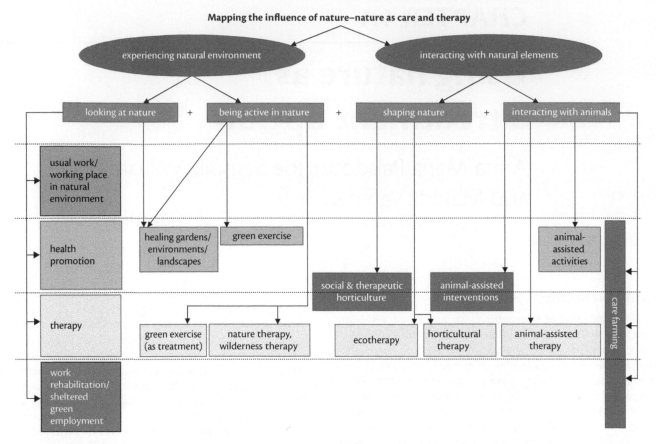

Fig. 4.1.1 Nature can be used in numerous intervention types with impact on different phases of well-being, therapy, or rehabilitation.

Reproduced from Sempik J, Hine R, and Wilcox D (Eds.), *Green Care: A Conceptual Framework*, A report of the Working Group on the Health Benefits of Green Care, COST Action 866, Green Care in Agriculture, Loughborough Centre for Child and Family Research, Loughborough University, UK, Copyright © 2010. Adapted from *The Journal of Science and Healing*, Volume 6, Issue 2, Dorit Karla Haubenhofer *et al.*, 'The Development of Green Care in Western European Countries,' pp. 106–111, Copyright © 2010 Elsevier Inc. with permission from Elsevier, http://www.sciencedirect.com/science/journal/15508307.

effects of physical activity in natural environments have been approached and studied. Research suggests that combining physical activity with exposure to nature results in significant improvements in self-esteem and mood measures, as well as reduced blood pressure (Pretty *et al.*, 2003; Pretty *et al.*, 2005; Hine *et al.*, 2008). Some studies show that this is even more efficient than prescribing physical activity alone (Peacock *et al.*, 2007). Read more about physical activity and nature in Chapter 3.1.

♦ *Ecotherapy.* This concept has been developed from the field of ecopsychology and now usually implies a type of intervention that embraces the complex field of ecohealth, stressing the interdependence between human health and the health of surrounding ecosystems. It is not always directed towards a particular clinical goal, but can also be implied as a means for community well-being. The practice of ecotherapy is based on a range of active interactions within multifunctional green spaces, all with the goal of re-establishing the equilibrium of human and ecosystem well-being (Sempik *et al.*, 2010; Pedretti-Burls, 2007).

♦ *Wilderness therapy.* Various types of wilderness or adventure therapies have been in use in the United States for many years and more recently reached Europe as an established concept. The most recent definition states that wilderness therapy 'is an experiential program that takes place in a wilderness or remote outdoor setting' (Conner, 2007). This means that the wilderness is considered as a 'co-therapist' for any kind of professional therapy for the actual diagnosis. Programmes typically provide healthy exercise and diet through hiking and physical activity, individual and group therapy sessions, educational curricula, primitive skills, group-living with peers, opportunities for solo time and reflection, leadership training, and challenges resulting from 'back-to basics' living (Sempik *et al.*, 2010).

When is nature a treatment option?

NAIs have been applied to a wide range of patients with various clinical diagnoses and in many different settings. In a systematic review, Annerstedt and Währborg (2011) concluded that these kind of treatment options can have significant effects on psychological, social, physical, and intellectual therapeutic goals, with reduced measurable symptoms of disease. Patient groups, which have received NAI in various forms include, for example, schizophrenia, dementia, depression, and anxiety, substance abuse, obesity, myocardial infarction, and other types of heart conditions. In many cases, the treatment does not aim to cure the disease, but to relieve symptoms and improve rehabilitation.

In the following sections, some examples of different types of interventions are provided and how they can be used for patients and clients with different diagnoses and conditions.

Mental disorders

Farming and gardening have long histories as activities for people with mental health problems (Berget *et al.*, 2012; Gallis, 2013). For example, in the United Kingdom, farms and gardens were features of many mental hospitals until the late 1950s. They did not only provide food for patients and staff, but were also sources of meaningful activities and diversion, something that was considered as therapeutic and promoting rehabilitation. Similar approaches existed also in many other countries. From this tradition, various NAIs have developed as treatment options for mental disorders (Murray and Elsay, 2015; Sempik *et al.*, 2005). These usually include care farming, therapeutic horticulture or horticultural therapy.

Current evidence suggests that care farming and therapeutic horticulture can be effective in reducing symptoms of depression and increasing self-efficacy (Berget *et al.*, 2008; Berget *et al.*, 2011; Pedersen *et al.*, 2012). While people with mental health problems may sometimes suffer from social exclusion and isolation, care farming seems to provide meaningful occupation, a daily routine, a sense of identity and purpose, physical activity, opportunities for employment, and social inclusion (Elsey *et al.*, 2016; Sempik *et al.*, 2005). These are all important aspects for promoting mental health.

Typical mental health problems that have been addressed with NAI include affective disorders (anxiety and depression), bipolar disorder, and a few cases of psychotic disorders (Kamioka *et al.*, 2014). It has, for example, been shown to improve social functioning in patients with schizophrenia (Um *et al.*, 2002; Prema *et al.*, 1986), affecting capacities such as interpersonal relationships and development of friendships.

Therapeutic horticulture has been reported to reduce levels of depression, sometimes with sustained effect after a completed intervention programme (Gonzalez *et al.*, 2011; Gonzalez *et al.*, 2010; Gonzalez *et al.*, 2009). Research suggests that not only are the social opportunities important, but that the natural surroundings of the garden in the therapy programme can act as a restorative environment (Gonzalez *et al.*, 2010). This has been considered in the context of Attention Restoration Therapy (ART) (Kaplan and Kaplan, 1989) and the dimensions of *being away* and *fascination* may be important mediators in the effect. See Chapter 2.1 for further elaborations around ART and other theories with bearing for NAIs.

In Sweden and Denmark, NAIs as rehabilitation programmes for individuals with stress-related mental disorders have been developed in different settings, including agricultural landscape and farms (Pálsdóttir *et al.*, 2012), forest sites (Nordh *et al.*, 2009; Sonntag-Öström *et al.*, 2014; Sonntag-Öström *et al.*, 2011), gardens and greenhouses (Adevi and Mårtensson, 2013; Pálsdóttir *et al.*, 2014; Tenngart Ivarsson, 2011), and the combination of garden and broadleaf forest (Sahlin *et al.*, 2012). These programmes usually rely on a multimodal rehabilitation team, including staff with various professions, such as physiotherapists, psychotherapists, and psychiatrists.

Among recognized effects are reduced healthcare consumption compared to control groups (Währborg *et al.*, 2014), improved function and perceived values of everyday occupations (Pálsdóttir *et al.*, 2014), and significant improvements regarding depression, exhaustion, and general health, including at follow-up (Sahlin, 2014). Empirical findings from these programmes and others have contributed to an expanding field of evidence-based health design for these patient groups (Grahn *et al.*, 2010; Jordan and Marshall, 2010; Millet, 2008; Sonntag-Öström *et al.*, 2011).

NAI has also been shown to be useful for patients suffering from post-traumatic stress disorders, PTSD (see Chapter 1.4. for a thorough review of this diagnosis) and other combat and stress-related conditions, improving both mental and physical well-being (Varning-Poulsen, 2015). Further, wilderness therapies, including canoeing, hiking, and other 'adventure-type' activities, have found resonance with this group (Westlund, 2014; Krasny *et al.*, 2014) possibly because they tend to be relatively young people who are generally physically fit, and who have trained and worked in challenging outdoor environments. However, less physically demanding farming (Westlund, 2014) and gardening (see, for example, High Ground http://highground-uk.org/) have also been used successfully with this group.

Learning disabilities

Although adults with learning or intellectual disabilities form one of the largest groups of users of therapeutic horticulture and horticultural therapy (Elings, 2012; Sempik *et al.*, 2005), their representation within research that measures outcomes is relatively low. They constitute a group of participants with a stable disability where the aim of therapeutic horticulture projects tends to be the provision of meaningful occupation as a form of day care, including long-term development of social and functional skills and preparation for possible employment if appropriate. Consequently, this group usually shows a long-term pattern of attendance (Sempik *et al.*, 2005).

Research suggests that horticultural therapy promotes social interaction (Kim *et al.*, 2012, Sempik *et al.*, 2014) and may also reduce stress among these users (Doxon *et al.*, 1987, Lee, 2010). People with learning difficulties are at an increased risk of developing physical health problems; for example, they are almost four times more likely to die from cardiovascular disease than the general population, and have significantly greater mortality due to respiratory disease (Harris and Barraclough, 1998). While some of the conditions associated with learning difficulties predispose the individuals to physical health problems, the increased physical activity associated with outdoor activities in a NAI programme may provide a beneficial and protective component.

Autism

While in many cases children and adults with autism have been included in NAI programmes alongside other disability groups (usually those with learning disabilities), the specific needs of autistic patients may benefit from specialist programmes with a high level of staffing and also specially designed environments. Etherington (2012) has described a programme of gardening activities for children with autism and has observed that this improves language and communication skills, in addition to reducing anxiety and aggression. Equally, Gaudion and McGinley (2012) described how a careful design of an outdoor garden space can promote exercise, occupation engagement, sensory experiences, social interaction, and a beneficial connection to nature for adults with autism. These are all components which help reduce symptoms associated with the condition.

Dementia and older people

Globally, the World Health Organization (WHO) estimates that around 47.5 million people suffer from chronic and progressive dementia. Among them, 58% live in low- and middle-income countries and the number of cases is expected to rise rapidly with an ageing population. This has, and will have a huge economic impact, and will also challenge healthcare systems. The condition affects central functions such as memory, thinking, behaviour, and ability to perform daily activities.

While pharmacological treatment may be of benefit to some patients, no single treatment has yet been defined which can efficiently prevent disease development or substantially improve the symptoms. In addition, existing treatment regimens often come with side effects, such as anxiety, falls, and stroke (Franchi, 2016). Therefore, supportive environments and explorations of alternative treatments are of high relevance.

Nature-assisted interventions have the potential to improve the lives of dementia sufferers by offering enjoyable, non-demanding activities that stimulate engagement and promote interactions with both the social and natural environments. It may also increase physical activity. While these activities may not prevent the progression of the condition, they support the quality of life and the well-being of the patients (Gigliotti et al., 2004).

Horticultural therapy and care farming have been used to promote well-being and reduce behavioural problems in patients suffering from dementia. Jarrott and Gigliotti (2010) demonstrated that participants with dementia in a horticultural therapy programme showed significantly greater active, passive, and 'other' engagement than the control group which carried out 'traditional activities'. Hewitt et al. (2013) also showed that social and therapeutic horticulture can contribute to improved well-being and provide enjoyment to people with dementia.

Horticultural programmes are suitable for older people and those with dementia because short sessions can be provided for those unable to manage longer ones, and these can be held indoors if necessary. Activities can be tailored to individual levels of cognitive ability and dexterity, and environments can be made safe and secure (for a guide to designing nature spaces for dementia patients, see Chalfont, 2007).

Specifically designed sensory gardens have been shown to modify behavioural issues and improve well-being related to participating (passive or active) in a garden programme. However, Gonzalez and Kirkevold (2015) specifically point out that we need more rigorous research with larger controlled studies that allow for causal conclusions on the effects and outcomes NAIs as treatment options for dementia before they can be broadly implemented.

While in the United Kingdom and United States horticultural therapy tends to be the most common programme for dementia, in the Netherlands, for example, care farming has been used for this group. Research suggests that it can improve nutritional status and provide a more varied programme than usual day care (de Bruin, 2009). In Sweden, gardens have been recognized as an important mediator for mental recovery in geriatric care (Ottosson and Grahn, 2005; Bengtsson, 2015).

The social enterprise Dementia Adventure (http://www.dementiaadventure.co.uk/) provides research-based access to nature for 'adventure'-type activities for dementia patients, such as sailing, coastal and woodland walks, and canal trips.

Behavioural problems and offending behaviour

Wilderness therapy, outdoor schools, and care farming have been used to support young people who are excluded from school and in danger of offending (or re-offending).

Wilderness programmes seek to address behavioural problems through experiential learning (Gass, 1993), that is, by direct experience of successfully completing physically demanding tasks and by engaging in the social dynamics of the group. They provide an environment that allows for self-reflection, and research suggests that they can be effective in reducing rates of recidivism of delinquency and behavioural problems (reviewed in Wilson and Lipsey, 2000), and may be more effective than some forms of conventional treatment (Williams, 2000). Evaluations of wilderness therapy programmes show improvements in behavioural and emotional problems (Russell, 2003; Russell, 2005) and positive changes in self-esteem and life quality (Roberts et al., 2016).

Care farming can also provide meaningful occupation for young people with symptoms of behavioural disturbance and can contribute to creating daily routines, developing work and social skills, and preparing for employment or further education. The care farm seems to provide a calm and structured environment and 'the feeling that the world is or can be meaningful, comprehensible and manageable' (Schreuder et al 2014). Research in the Netherlands (Elings, 2012) has indicated that residential care farm programmes can significantly increase well-being, reduce contact with the criminal justice system, and reduce drug use after completion of the treatment intervention. Care farming programmes for disaffected, disengaged, and disadvantaged youth have successfully been established in a number of different European countries (see, for example, Highfield Happy Hens, http://www.highfieldshappyhens. co.uk, described in Hine et al., 2008).

Research has also shown that nature-assisted interventions, for example, horticultural therapy, can be effective in helping to manage the behaviour of offenders within secure settings (Grimshaw and King, 2003). It has been reported to reduce feelings of hostility and reduce substance misuse (Rice and Remy, 1998) and to increase self-esteem and self-efficacy in violent sex offenders (Gibson and Hughes, 2000).

Many of those who come into contact with the criminal justice system have mental health issues and/or learning difficulties (Singleton et al., 1998; Bradley, 2009; Brooker et al., 2011). These individuals present a high risk of re-offending and show high rates of arrest and re-arrest. In recent years, liaison-diversion initiatives have been employed in many countries to identify individuals with mental health problems and learning difficulties at the point at which they come into contact with the criminal justice system and to provide support to divert them away from offending behaviour. A variety of approaches including NAI have been used to provide diversionary activities and meaningful occupation to this group of individuals. However, this aspect is in an early stage of development and more research is needed to explore the extent of its use and effectiveness.

While NAIs have been used to treat offenders, they have also been used to address the problems of those whose difficulties have been caused by offending behaviour. Renzetti et al. (2014) showed that a horticultural therapy programme reduced perceived anxiety, depression, and social isolation, in addition to improving the self-esteem and self-efficacy of women who had been the victims of domestic violence. There is a movement to introduce horticulture into prisons, to move from a pathogenic to a whole system approach, in addressing key health issues affecting prisoners and influencing wider social and environmental factors (Baybutt and Chemlal, 2016).

Physical rehabilitation

Garden activities form a part of many occupational therapy programmes, not only for those with mental health problems, but also those undergoing rehabilitation following injury, illness, or stroke. An early description of such use is in Colson's book *The Rehabilitation of the Injured* (1945). In this, he describes activities that he found of value in addressing specific conditions or providing particular levels of physical exertion. The practice of using horticulture and farming in physical rehabilitation has continued and is described in variety of publications—textbooks and practice guides, and also in specific programmes. For example, spinal rehabilitation programmes at the Royal National Orthopaedic Hospital in London, United Kingdom, make us of a therapy garden and a trained horticultural therapist (http://www.rnoh.nhs.uk/clinical-services/rehabilitation-and-therapy/occup/therapy-garden).

The inclusion of outdoor activities in rehabilitation programmes provides not only the opportunity to develop motor control and strength, but also addresses the psychological difficulties, social isolation, and fatigue that may follow, for example, injury or stroke. Ongoing randomized controlled trials seek to explore the effects of nature-assisted post-stroke rehabilitation as an add-on to standard management of post-stroke symptoms (Pálsdóttir *et al.*, 2015).

Physical disability

People with chronic physical disability also participate in nature-assisted therapies through, for example, the aid of adapted gardens and special tools. However, this tends to be a small client group (Sempik *et al.*, 2005). Limited research is available about this group and the ways in which individuals may benefit from these activities. This group may be small because individuals find support elsewhere and are able to engage with natural environments and activities in other ways (Von Benzon, 2011); or they do not suffer the same stigma and difficulties as other client groups, and hence do not have the same needs or experience the same levels of social isolation and exclusion as other groups. Organizations such as Thrive (http://www.thrive.org.uk/) in the United Kingdom provide support and advice for individuals to continue gardening despite physical disabilities and conditions (see also Carry on Gardening, http://www.carryongardening.org.uk/).

Non-communicable diseases

Pretty *et al.* (2003) first coined the term 'green exercise', which is defined as physical activity with direct exposure to nature. This has been used to help patients with NCDs to become more active. The use of parks and green spaces not only provide access to be more active, but also help reduce stress that in itself can be a barrier to becoming more active (Pretty *et al.*, 2005).

Conclusion

There is a variety of different NAIs that are suitable for people with various disabilities or disorders. Certain approaches appear to be more established (and perhaps more 'suitable') for particular conditions, and client groups and specific green care interventions have also been tailored to suit particular client groups, suggesting that it is a versatile and flexible approach.

While NAIs appear to be suitable as treatment options for many different conditions, there is a need to conduct rigorous research studies to explore mechanisms at play, to provide cost-effectiveness estimates and adequate comparisons with other treatment modalities. By establishing a firm evidence base for this type of treatments, wider implications and use in healthcare could be encouraged.

References

Adevi, A. A. & Mårtensson, F. (2013). Stress rehabilitation through garden therapy: The garden as a place in the recovery from stress. *Urban For Urban Greening*, 12, 230–7.

Annerstedt, M. & Währborg, P. (2011). Nature-assisted therapy: Systematic review of controlled and observational studies. *Scand J Public Health*, 39, 371–88.

Baybutt, M. & Chemlal, K. (2016). Health-promoting prisons: theory to practice. *Glob Health Promot*, 23, 66–74.

Bengtsson, A. (2015). From experiences of the outdoors to the design of healthcare environments. *Acta Universitatis Agriculturae Sueciae*, 66, 1652–6880. Swedish University of Agricultural Sciences.

Berget, B., Ekeberg, Ø., & Braastad, B. O. (2008). Animal-assisted therapy with farm animals for persons with psychiatric disorders: effects on self-efficacy, coping ability and quality of life, a randomized controlled trial. *Clin Pract Epidemiol Ment Health*, 4, 9.

Berget, B., Ekeberg, Ø., Pedersen, I., & Braastad, B. O. (2011). Animal-assisted therapy with farm animals for persons with psychiatric disorders: effects on anxiety and depression, a randomized controlled trial. *Occupational Therapy in Mental Health*, 27, 50–64.

Berget, B., Lidfors, L., Pálsdóttir, A. M., Soini, K., & Thodberg, K. (2012). Green care in the Nordic countries—a research filed in progress. Report from the Nordic research workshop in Green Care in Trondheim, June 2012. Ås, Norwegian University of Life Sciences.

Bradley, K. J. C. B. (2009). *The Bradley Report: Lord Bradley's review of people with mental health problems or learning disabilities in the criminal justice system*, London, UK: Department of Health London.

Brooker, C., Sirdifield, C., Blizard, R., *et al.* (2011). An investigation into the prevalence of mental health disorder and patterns of health service access in a probation population. Lincoln, UK: University of Lincoln.

Chalfont, G. (2007). *Design for Nature in Dementia Care*. London, UK: Jessica Kingsley Publishers.

Colson, J. H. C. (1945). *The Rehabilitation of the Injured*. London, UK: Cassell.

Conner, M. (2007). What is wilderness therapy and a wilderness program. Mentor Research Institute.

de Bruin, S. (2009). *Sowing in the Autumn season: Exploring benefits of green care farms for dementia patients*. Wageningen Universiteit (Wageningen University).

Doxon, L., Mattson, R., & Jurich, A. (1987). Human stress reduction through horticultural vocational training. *HortScience*, 22, 655–6.

Elings, M. (2012). Effects of care farms: Scientific research on the benefits of care farms for clients. Wageningen UR: Plant Research International.

Elsey, H., Murray, J., & Braggy, R. (2016). Green fingers and clear minds: prescribing 'care farming' for mental illness. *Br J Gen Pract*, 66, 99–100.

Etherington, N. (2012). *Gardening for Children with Autism Spectrum Disorders and Special Educational Needs: Engaging with Nature to Combat Anxiety, Promote Sensory Integration and Build Social Skills*. London, UK: Jessica Kingsley Publishers.

Franchi, B. (2016). Pharmacological management of behavioural and psychological symptoms of dementia. *J Pharm Pract Res*, 46, 277–85.

Gallis, C. (2013). *Green Care: For Human Therapy, Social Innovation, Rural Economy, and Education*. New York, NY: Nova Science Publishers.

Gass, M. A. (1993). *Adventure Therapy: Therapeutic Applications of Adventure Programming*. Bubuque, IA: Kendal Hunt Publishing Co.

Gaudion, K. & McGinley, C. (2012). Green spaces outdoor environments for adults with autism. London, UK: The Helen Hamlyn Centre for Design, The Royal College of Art.

Gibson, R. B. & Hughes, M. P. (2000). Treatment of the sexually violent predator: a horticultural approach. *J Ther Hort*, 11, 20–5.

Gigliotti, C. M., Jarrott, S. E., & Yorgason, J. (2004). Harvesting health: Effects of three types of horticultural therapy activities for persons with dementia. *Dementia*, 3, 161–80.

Gonzalez, M. T., Hartig, T., Patil, G. G., Martinsen, E. W., & Kirkevold, M. (2009). Therapeutic horticulture in clinical depression: A prospective study. *Res Theory Nurs Pract*, 23, 312–28.

Gonzalez, M. T., Hartig, T., Patil, G. G., Martinsen, E. W., & Kirkevold, M. (2010). Therapeutic horticulture in clinical depression: a prospective study of active components. *J Adv Nurs*, 66, 2002–13.

Gonzalez, M. T., Hartig, T., Patil, G. G., Martinsen, E. W., & Kirkevold, M. (2011). A prospective study of group cohesiveness in therapeutic horticulture for clinical depression. *Int J Ment Health Nurs*, 20, 119–29.

Gonzalez, M. T. & Kirkevold, M. (2015). Clinical use of sensory gardens and outdoor environments in norwegian nursing homes: a cross-sectional e-mail survey. *Issues Ment Health Nurs*, 36, 35–43.

Grahn, P., Tenngart Ivarsson, C., Stigsdotter, U. K., & Bengtsson, I.-L. (2010). Using affordances as a health-promoting tool in a therapeutic garden. London, UK: Taylor & Francis.

Grimshaw, R. & King, J. (2003). *Horticulture in Secure Settings: A Study of Horticultural Activities in Prisons and Secure Psychiatric Facilities.* Reading, UK: Thrive.

Growth_Point (1999). Your future starts here: practitioners determine the way ahead. *Growth Point*, 79, 4–5.

Harris, E. C. & Barraclough, B. (1998). Excess mortality of mental disorder. *Br J Psychiatry*, 173, 11–53.

Hewitt, P., Watts, C., Hussey, J., Power, K., & Williams, T. (2013). Does a structured gardening programme improve well-being in young-onset dementia? A preliminary study. *BJOT*, 76, 355–61.

Hine, R., Peacock, J., & Pretty, J. (2008). Care farming in the UK: contexts, benefits and links with therapeutic communities. *Therapeutic Communities*, 29, 245–60.

Jarrott, S. E. & Gigliotti, C. M. (2010). Comparing responses to horticultural-based and traditional activities in dementia care programs. *Am J Alzheimer Dis Other Demen*, 25, 657–65.

Jordan, M. & Marshall, H. (2010). Taking counselling and psychotherapy outside: Destruction or enrichment of the therapeutic frame? *Eur J Psychother Couns*, 12, 345–59.

Kamioka, H., Tsutani, K., Yamada, M., *et al.* (2014). Effectiveness of horticultural therapy: a systematic review of randomized controlled trials. *Compl Ther Med*, 22, 930–43.

Kaplan, R. & Kaplan, S. (1989). *The Experience of Nature: A Psychological Perspective.* New York, NY: Cambridge University Press.

Kim, B.-Y., Park, S.-A., Song, J.-E., & Son, K.-C. (2012). Horticultural therapy program for the improvement of attention and sociality in children with intellectual disabilities. *HortTechnology*, 22, 320–4.

Krasny, M. E., Pace, K. H., Tidball, K. G., & Helphand, K. (2014). Nature engagement to foster resilience in military communities. *Greening in the Red Zone.* Springer.

Lee, M.-J. (2010). Effects of various horticultural activities on the autonomic nervous system and cortisol response of mentally challenged adults. *HortTechnology*, 20, 971–6.

Millet, P. (2008). Integrating horticulture into the vocational rehabilitation process of individuals with exhaustion syndrome (burnout): A pilot study. *Int J Disability Manage*, 3, 39–53.

Murray, J. & Elsay, H. (2015). Green fingers clear minds. Striving to develop a strong evidence base on nature based interventions for people with ill-health. Findings and suggestions Report. Leeds Institute of Health Science, University of Leeds

Nordh, H., Grahn, P., & Währborg, P. (2009). Meaningful activities in the forest, a way back from exhaustion and long-term sick leave. *Urban For Urban Greening*, 8, 207–19.

Ottosson, J. & Grahn, P. (2005). A comparison of leisure time spent in a garden with leisure time spent indoors: on measures of restoration in residents in geriatric care. *Landscape Research*, 30, 23–55.

Pálsdóttir, A. M., Andersson, G., Grahn, P., *et al.* (2015). A randomized controlled trial of nature-based post-stroke fatigue rehabilitation ("the nature stroke study"(nastru)): study design and progress report. *Int J Stroke*, 10, 430.

Pálsdóttir, A. M., Persson, D., Persson, B., & Grahn, P. (2014). The journey of recovery and empowerment embraced by nature—Clients' perspectives on nature-based rehabilitation in relation to the role of the natural environment. *Int J Environ Res Public Health*, 11, 7094–115.

Pálsdóttir, A. M., Wissler, S., Nilsson, K., Petersson, I., & Grahn, P. (2012). Nature-based rehabilitation in peri-urban areas for people with stress-related illnesses-a controlled prospective study. XI International People Plant Symposium on Diversity: Towards a New Vision of Nature 1093, 31–5.

Peacock, J., Hine, R., & Pretty, J. (2007). The mental health benefits of green exercise activities and green care. Report for MIND.

Pedersen, I., Martinsen, E. W., Berget, B., & Braastad, B. O. (2012). Farm animal-assisted intervention for people with clinical depression: a randomized controlled trial. *Anthrozoös*, 25, 149–60.

Pedretti-Burls, A. (2007). Ecotherapy: a therapeutic and educative model. *Journal of Mediterranean Ecology*, 8, 19–25.

Prema, T., Devarajaiah, C., & Gopinath, P. (1986). Horticulture therapy: an attempt at Indianisation of psychiatric nursing. *Nurs J India*, 77, 154–56.

Pretty, J., Griffin, M., Sellens, M., & Pretty, C. (2003). Green exercise: Complementary roles of nature, exercise and diet in physical and emotional well-being and implications for public health policy. *CES Occasional Paper*, 1, 1–39.

Pretty, J., Peacock, J., Sellens, M., & Griffin, M. (2005). The mental and physical health outcomes of green exercise. *Int J Environ Health Res*, 15, 319–37.

Renzetti, C. M., Follingstad, D. R., & Fleet, D. (2014). From Blue to Green: The Development and Implementation of a Horticultural Therapy Program for Residents of a Battered Women's Shelter. CRVAW Faculty Presentations. Paper 1.

Rice, J. S. & Remy, L. (1998). Impact of horticultural therapy on psychosocial functioning among urban jail inmates. *J Offender Rehabil*, 26, 169–91.

Roberts, J., Barton, J., & Wood, C. (2016). Wilderness and youth at risk. In: Barton, J., Braggs, R., Wood, C., & Pretty, J. (eds) *Green Exercise: Linking Nature, Health and Well-being.* New York, NY & London, UK: Routledge, Taylor & Francis.

Russell, K. (2003). An assessment of outcomes in outdoor behavioral healthcare treatment. *Child & Youth Care Forum*, 32, 355–81.

Russell, K. C. (2005). Two years later: A qualitative assessment of youth well-being and the role of aftercare in outdoor behavioral healthcare treatment. *Child & Youth Care Forum*, 34, 209–39.

Sahlin, E. (2014). *To stress the importance of nature. Acta Universitatis Agriculturae Sueciae* (Doctoral thesis). Uppsala, Sweden: Swedish University of Agricultural Sciences.

Sahlin, E., Matuszczyk, J. V., Ahlborg, J. R., & Grahn, P. (2012). How do participants in nature-based therapy experience and evaluate their rehabilitation. *J Ther Hortic*, 22, 8–21.

Schreuder, E., Rijnders, M., Vaandrager, L., Hassink, J., Enders-Slegers, M.-J., & Kennedy, L. (2014). Exploring salutogenic mechanisms of an outdoor experiential learning programme on youth care farms in the Netherlands: untapped potential? *Int J Adolesc Youth*, 19, 139–52.

Sempik, J., Aldridge, J., & Becker, S. (2003). Social and therapeutic horticulture: evidence and messages from research. CCFR Family and Environment research programme.

Sempik, J., Aldridge, J., & Becker, S. (2005). *Health, Well-being and Social Inclusion, Therapeutic Horticulture in the UK.* Bristol, UK: The Policy Press.

Sempik, J., Hine, R., & Wilcox, D. (2010). Green Care: A Conceptual Framework; A report of the Working Group on the Health Benefits of Green Care. COST Action 866, Loughborough University.

Sempik, J., Rickhuss, C., & Beeston, A. (2014). The effects of social and therapeutic horticulture on aspects of social behaviour. *BJOT*, 77, 313–19.

Singleton, N., Gatward, R., & Meltzer, H. (1998). *Psychiatric Morbidity Among Prisoners in England and Wales*. London, UK: Stationery Office.

Sonntag-Öström, E., Nordin, M., Lundell, Y., *et al.* (2014). Restorative effects of visits to urban and forest environments in patients with exhaustion disorder. *Urban For Urban Greening*, 13, 344–54.

Sonntag-Öström, E., Nordin, M., Slunga Järvholm, L., Lundell, Y., Brännström, R., & Dolling, A. (2011). Can the boreal forest be used for rehabilitation and recovery from stress-related exhaustion? A pilot study. *Scand J For Res*, 26, 245–56.

Stigsdotter, U. K., Pálsdóttir, A-M., Burls, A., Chermaz, A., Ferrini, F., & Grahn, P. (2011). Nature-based therepautic interventions, In: Nilsson, K., Sanger, M., Gallis, C., Hartig, T., de Vries, S., Seeland, K., & Schipperijn, J. (eds) *Forest, Trees and Human Health*, pp. 309–42. New York, Dordrecht, Heidelberg and London: Springer.

Tenngart Ivarsson, C. (2011). *On the Use and Experience of a Health Garden* (Dctoral thesis). Uppsala, Sweden: Swedish University of Agricultural Sciences.

Um, S., Kim, S., Song, J., Kwack, H., & Son, K. (2002). Effect of horticultural therapy on the changes of self-esteem and sociality of individuals with chronic schizophrenia. XXVI International Horticultural Congress: Expanding Roles for Horticulture in Improving Human Well-Being and Life Quality 639, 185–91.

Varning-Poulsen, D. (2015). *How war veterans with post-traumatic stress disorder experience nature-based therapy in a forest therapy garden*. Københavns UniversitetKøbenhavns Universitet, Det Natur-og Biovidenskabelige FakultetFaculty of Science, Institut for Geovidenskab og NaturforvaltningDepartment of Geosciences and Natural Resource Management, Landskabsarkitektur og planlægningLandscape Architecture and Planning.

Von Benzon, N. (2011). Who's afraid of the big bad woods? Fear and learning disabled children's access to local nature. *Local Environment*, 16, 1021–40.

Währborg, P., Petersson, I. F., & Grahn, P. (2014). Nature-asisted rehabilitation for reactions to severe stress and/or depression in a rehabilitation garden: Long-term folow-up including comparisons with a matched population-based reference cohort. *J Rehabil Med*, 46, 271–6.

Westlund, S. (2014). *Field Exercises: How Veterans are Healing Themselves Through Farming and Outdoor Activities*. Gabriola Island, BC, Canada: New Society Publishers.

Williams, B. (2000). The treatment of adolescent populations: An institutional vs. a wilderness setting. *J Child Adolesc Group Ther*, 10, 47–56.

Wilson, S. J. & Lipsey, M. W. (2000). Wilderness challenge programs for delinquent youth: A meta-analysis of outcome evaluations. *Eval Program Plan*, 23, 1–12.

The human–animal bond and animal-assisted intervention

Aubrey H. Fine and Shawna J. Weaver

The human–animal bond

Humans have long co-existed, with animal domestication dating back thousands of years. The positive nature of many human–animal relationships can be felt intuitively and is apparent in the high percentage of households with pets. In the United States, for example, more than 60% of the population has a household pet. There are many justifications for these relationships, including both health and psychological benefits derived from positive interactions between humans and animals. These benefits may result from what is known as the human–animal bond.

The first official use of the term human–animal bond appeared in the Proceedings of the Meeting of the Group for the Study of Human–Companion Animal Bond in Dundee, Scotland in March of 1979 (Fine, 2014; Group for the Study of the Human/Companion Animal Bond, 1979). The American Veterinary Medical Association's Committee on the Human–Animal Bond now defines it as 'a mutually beneficial and dynamic relationship between people and other animals that is influenced by behaviours that are essential to the health and well-being of both. This includes, but is not limited to, emotional, psychological, and physical interactions of people, other animals, and the environment' (JAVMA, 1998).

Animal-assisted intervention: a brief introduction

The broad field of animal-assisted interventions is rooted in the context of the human–animal bond. Animal-assisted interventions (AAIs) are activities that involve working and interacting with animals in a therapeutic setting. The premise of AAI is that bonding with animals is beneficial to humans. The established description provided by the International Association for Human–Animal Interaction Organizations (IAHAIO) states that animal-assisted intervention is a goal-oriented intervention that intentionally includes animals in health, education, and human services (e.g. social work) for the purposes of therapeutic gains in humans. This definition was incorporated in their recent white paper (Jegatheesan et al., 2014) on defining AAI, which also included guidelines for the wellness of the animals involved. While AAI is a relatively new therapeutic approach, there is already a wide spectrum of settings in which AAI is utilized, and a wide array of disorders and issues for which AAI seem to be effective.

Animal-assisted intervention includes both animal-assisted therapy (AAT) and animal-assisted education (AAE). Another related approach is that of animal-assisted activities (AAA), which are informal and non-goal oriented. For further definitions, see Table 4.2.1.

The logistics of animal-assisted intervention

AAI incorporates human/animal teams in formal human service. Placed under this rubric of AAI is a spectrum of alternatives incorporating animals, ranging from informal visitation programmes to very specific intervention designed by professionals. Different types of interventions can be applied, depending on the setting, professional training, patient diagnosis, and treatment goals. Professionals in various fields such as psychology, nursing, physical and occupational therapy, and speech and language therapy may find working with animals to be beneficial. There is a range of standards and guidelines depending on the field and the intended activities.

It is critical not only to consider the value for human well-being, but also include animal welfare concerns when practising AAI. There are a few organizations throughout the world focused on training professionals and volunteers in AAI. These organizations generally educate people on animal well-being, on various interventions, and offer certification. Local laws and regulations legitimate AAI in practice or in programmes.

The history of animal-assisted intervention

AAI finds its influence in healthcare practices dating back hundreds of years. There are early accounts of physicians and nurses recognizing the value of animals for accelerated healing and alleviation of boredom or loneliness.

In the 1960s, the child psychotherapist Boris Levinson discovered that bringing along his pet dog to therapy seemed to soften the children's reactions to their interaction with him. He first published a paper on his findings (Levinson, 1962) and eventually described his experiences of how withdrawn and uncommunicative children interacted more positively around a dog in the two volumes—*Pet-Oriented Child Psychotherapy* (1969) and *Pets and Human Development* (1979). What was initially a serendipitous discovery ended up becoming the modern initiation of this field.

Table 4.2.1 Description of animal-assisted intervention (including animal-assisted therapy and animal-assisted education) and animal-assisted activities

AAI: The umbrella term for goal-oriented interventions that intentionally include or incorporate animals in health, education, and human service for the purpose of human therapeutic gains.

AAT: therapy is goal oriented, planned, and structured; delivered by health, education, and human service professionals. Progress is measured and included in professional documentation. AAT is delivered by a formally trained (including licensure, degree, or equivalent) professional.	AAE: education is goal oriented, planned, and structured; delivered by educational and related service professional. It is conducted by teachers, focusing on academic goals, pro-social skills, and cognitive functioning. Students' progress is measured and documented.

AAA: activities are informal interactions and visits, often conducted by volunteers. It is not goal-driven, and the volunteer teams (of person and animal) have received at least introductory training. These teams may also work formally with a professional in an AAI format.

(AAI = animal-assisted intervention, AAT = animal-assisted therapy, AAE = animal-assisted education, AAA = animal-assisted activities.)

Adapted with permission from Brinda Jegatheesan (Chair), International Association of Human-Animal Interaction Organizations (IAHAIO) White Paper, *The IAHAIO Definitions for Animal Assisted Interventions and Animal Assisted Activity and Guidelines for Wellness of Animals Involved, Final Report*, Copyright © IAHAIO 2014, http://www.iahaio.org/new/fileuploads/9313IAHAIO%20WHITE%20PAPER%20TASK%20FORCE%20-%20FINAL%20REPORT.pdf

Many practitioners and researchers followed the lead of Levinson and added their unique contribution to the growing interest in animals as support for people. For example, Samuel Corson, a professor of psychiatry and biophysics at Ohio State University, suggested that animals could act as a social lubricant in the therapeutic process. He observed that patients seemed to open up, became calmer, communicated more, and were less resistant to the therapeutic intervention. Since those early years, many have engaged in incorporating AAI as an alternative therapy for various patient groups (Fine, 2010). Today, AAI is growing in popularity and research within the field has increased.

Understanding animal-assisted intervention through the benefits of the human–animal bond

While the research field of structured AAI is still developing, there has been a wealth of research supporting the value of human–animal interactions in general. In the late 1970s, Erika Friedmann and her colleagues studied the positive effects of having a pet on a person's cardiovascular health (Friedmann *et al.*, 1980). In a paper published in 1990, Friedmann and colleagues postulated that having a pet leads to the following benefits: (a) improved fitness by stimulating physical activity; (b) decreased anxiety by providing a source of physical contact; and (c) decreased loneliness by providing companionship (Friedmann *et al.*, 1990). Since the innovative research of Friedmann and her colleagues, several international studies have confirmed that having a pet has a positive effect on people's well-being (e.g. Headey and Grabka, 2007). Moreover,

different studies have demonstrated that petting an animal can cause a decrease in blood pressure and heart rate (Eddie, 1996; Shiloh *et al.*, 2003). Karen Allen and her colleagues showed that the mere presence of a pet dog or cat can lower levels of heart rate and blood pressure in cognitively demanding situations, such as completing arithmetic tasks (Allen *et al.*, 2002).

Further research has demonstrated that attachment to a pet can reduce cortisol levels, and increase oxytocin levels. Oxytocin is a peptide hormone associated with making people feel happy, calm, patient, trusting, and sensitive to non-verbal forms of communication and social bonding. The earliest research on the impact of human–animal interactions and its impact on oxytocin was done by South African psychologist Johannes Odendaal. In his research, he observed that during interactions with their dogs, patients' endorphin (oxytocin and dopamine) levels increased significantly, and the inverse was found for cortisol levels, which significantly decreased. In 2003, Odendaal conducted a study that measured the levels of oxytocin in dogs and humans when they interacted with each other (Odendaal and Meintjes, 2003). They discovered that blood pressure levels decreased and oxytocin levels almost doubled after the interaction occurred.

Since this influential work, several other studies have found an increase of oxytocin in the blood and urine levels of both dogs and humans after interaction. Miho Nagasawa (2008) research found that focused eye contact between humans and dogs increased oxytocin levels in the human (measured in the urine). In an additional study, Nagasawa and his colleagues (Romereo *et al.*, 2014) found that when sprayed with oxytocin, dogs showed a higher desire for affiliation towards their owners than when sprayed with a placebo. Findings from the research showed that the dogs' oxytocin blood and urine levels increased most when the dogs' affiliative efforts were reciprocated. Suzanne Miller and colleagues (Miller *et al.*, 2009) studied changes of a person's plasma oxytocin as a consequence of the interaction with the pet dog after coming home from work and not having seen their dog during the day. Interestingly, interacting with the dog led to an increase in plasma oxytocin in women, but not men. Linda Handlin and associates also found that an increase in oxytocin occurs for both people and dogs by petting, while kissing the dog was found to be associated with an even higher increase (Handlin *et al.*, 2011; 2012). Overall, this suggests that parts of the positive effects of AAI might be mediated through oxytocin release, an area that requires more research.

Theories explaining the benefits of the human–animal bond and animal-assisted intervention

The literature seems to be conclusive in suggesting that interactions with animals offer psychological and physiological benefits to humans. The question that remains is why this is the case. There are three major theories that explain this phenomenon, namely theories dealing with: (i) animals acting as a social support; (ii) attachment; (iii) and the biophilia hypothesis. Fine and Beck (2010) suggest that the theories of attachment and animals acting as social support provide a logical explanation for why so many people engage in the care of a dependent animal.

Social support

Social support is a generic term covering the emotional, practical, and informal support offered through a person's network of supportive relationships. These relationships need not be with other humans to offer the necessary feedback, presence, physical touch, or emotional enhancement people naturally desire (McNicholas and Collis, 2001). However, research has identified numerous roles that animals can take in providing social support. For example, a study by Strand (2004) found that children who have pets in their home often turn to their pets for comfort during high stress situations. In essence, the pet acts as a buffer and helps young children use self-calming techniques to reduce those stressors. Animals may at times even replace the social support generally offered by other people, enabling humans who lack a strong social network to still enjoy the companionship of another being (Van Houte and Jarvis, 1995).

The social support offered by animals may go beyond the simple joys of companionship. Other benefits animals offer through social support include recreational activities that help people stay physically active and thus healthier. For example, walking a dog enables both the person and the dog to be outside getting exercise (Zeltman and Johnson, 2011). Such activities may also increase social interactions with other people who are encountered during that time. Additionally, having a pet may improve the social support among family members, as individuals come together to care for their pet. Strengthening human relationships is an effect of the human–animal bond that is also seen in AAI.

Attachment theory

This second supporting theory was developed by John Bowlby (1969), a British psychologist, psychiatrist, and psychoanalyst who was among the more influential psychologists of the twentieth century. The attachment theory explains the need for humans to protect and be protected (Sable, 1995). Attachment patterns tend to start early, as babies already become attached and come to see the importance of secure attachment. Relationships and experiences throughout life shape a person's attachment to others, and fuel the emotional and psychological benefits experienced through attachment. According to Sigal Zilcha-Mano and her colleagues, the attachments among people and animals relate to Bowlby's attachment theory: proximity seeking, seeing the connection as a safe haven, feeling secure, and separation distress (Zilcha-Mano et al., 2011). These features suggest that relationships with animals mirror parent–child relationships (Barba, 1995). Human–animal relationships are enhanced because of the pet's dependence on the caretaker for its physical well-being, just as parent–child relationships are enhanced because of the child's dependence (Bowlby, 1980).

While attachment to other people can in certain situations and for some individuals be anxiety provoking, attachment with an animal may be an easier and simpler task (Smokovic et al., 2012). This might explain why some studies show that human–pet relationships can be more stable than human relationships with other people (Beck and Madresh, 2008). This effect can be important in a therapeutic relationship, where the neutralizing influence of an animal may stabilize the therapeutic relation.

Biophilia hypothesis

A third theory, the biophilia hypothesis, offers additional insights into human relationships with other species of beings. The hypothesis refers to humans' innate desire to connect with other living organisms. Coined by one of the world's pre-eminent biologists and naturalists Edward O. Wilson, biophilia is defined as the inherent need of humans to understand and relate with nature (Wilson, 1984). Even in these modern times, humans are intimately reliant on the environment for survival (Kellert, 1993). Chapter 8.3 discusses the biophilia hypothesis and biophilic design in detail. Increased time spent in cities and inside buildings, decreased exposure to natural settings, and changing relationships to other animals have all influenced the human–nature connection. It is plausible that AAI may work at a deeper level, or within other dimensions of reconnecting people with nature to re-establish a balanced attachment and increased well-being for both people and nature. The concept of biophilia proposes several biophilic responses. Such responses can be considered within AAI.

The humanistic response

The humanistic response helps foster individual relationships and companionship. Humans crave kinship and affection, and developing a relationship with an animal can contribute to a person's physical health and emotional well-being. Of all the responses, the work of AAI perhaps best appeals to the humanistic response to nature. Through AAI, practitioners can promote a natural and inherent relationship with an animal in a safe and predictable space. This can aid patients in relationship building and fulfil emotional needs. This can be transferred to other relationships in life.

The moralistic response

The moralistic response encourages people to be kind and helpful, and to act according to ethical or moral beliefs. This response encourages sharing of resources and collaboration. However, it can also be a source of guilt, regret, anxiety, and worry. A sense of responsibility for nature and worry about the current state of the environment is today a source of anxiety for many people (Bernstein, 2005).

The moralistic response can be applied therapeutically to help clients consider how their actions affect others, and how engaging in service can alleviate emotional pain. This may promote stronger empathy, compassion, and responsibility for their actions.

The naturalistic response

This response enables enrichment of the mind and body when experiencing nature. The naturalistic response is evident in people's desire to be a part of nature for the sake of adventure and immersion. Children display the naturalistic response by playing in the woods and letting their imaginations run wild with their surroundings. This is a valuable component of AAI—to reconnect with nature through play. Practitioners can foster this connection through unstructured play and conversation in the presence of the therapy animal, and even better, with sessions outside. The naturalistic response fosters a sense of belonging and can enrich a person's experience through all five senses.

The symbolic response

The symbolic response to nature offers humans a way of creating connection and communicating emotion, as the symbolic response is a reflection of intellectual growth and adaptation. Communication is critical to survival, but its importance goes beyond survival, including enrichment through mental stimulation. Humans communicate through symbolism in writing, music, art, and speech, not just to survive but to communicate emotion and intellectual thought.

The presence of an animal assistant may help people feel more comfortable in communicating and sharing their creative expression. An animal will not judge, critique, or ask questions. Combining AAI with another form of holistic therapy like art, music, or play therapy can potentially work synergistically to improve the therapeutic session.

The aesthetic response

The aesthetic response occurs, for instance, when people react to flowers in bloom, to autumn colours, or to a beautiful sunset. This visual appreciation for the environment engages positive and calming emotions. A peaceful environment suggests an absence of storms or predators. Patients can experience the same aesthetic response of peace, reassurance, and relaxation next to a calm therapy animal. The animal can communicate that there is nothing around to pose a threat and the patient can thus feel safe.

The scientific response

Another source of security for people is knowledge. The scientific response is the desire to increase knowledge of how and why the environment works in the ways it does. Knowledge about the world increases knowledge about one's self, as well as one's confidence and self-efficacy. When conducting AAI sessions, practitioners can utilize the therapy animal as a model or example, such as what the animal's emotional needs are, to help explain the patient's needs. For instance, a practitioner can discuss how dogs find ways to relax, that they need to sleep and recover, or how their health is compromised without good nutrition. An ageing animal can help a practitioner breach difficult topics like bereavement, serious illness, and dying. Knowledge often brings a sense of control to a person, and learning in the presence of, or through the example of an animal can make the information feel less threatening and more normalized.

Evidence for animal-assisted intervention

Over the past 50 years, AAI has become a more accepted therapeutic alternative for supporting individuals with various needs and diagnoses. While there continues to be a demand for more evidence, researchers in the field have made important progress in support of the work within AAI, and especially since 2008 significant progress has been made in filling the research agenda with more rigorous studies (McCune et al., 2014).

The field continues to grow and is increasingly applied in numerous alternative settings. This rapid growth requires the continuation of research, education, and training. Furthermore, growth in AAI should include further analysis of the logistics, expectations, and guidelines of the various interventions applied. More studies in specific settings, for specific populations, and looking into specific quantitative factors will offer important insights. In a study analysing whether therapy dogs are a negative distraction or positive influence during cognitive behaviour therapy, for example, Hunt and Chizkov (2014) found that dogs offer positive emotional support and do not seem to negatively affect the session as a distraction. It is anticipated that more high-quality research studies in future years will eventually provide even more evidence and prove what many people already believe and experience; that a therapeutic connection with an animal can improve health.

The spectrum of disorders and animal-assisted intervention treatment

As the body of quantitative research on AAI evolves, qualitative studies, including case studies, appear to be a good source for understanding the underlying mechanisms of AAI in treating various disorders. Some examples of disorders and where studies have shown AAI to have a positive effect will be discussed next.

In 2012, Marguerite E. O'Haire conducted a meta-analysis of research studies on AAI and autism spectrum disorders. While these studies had some limitations (such as small sample sizes or the many varying approaches to AAI), the researcher found AAI to be a promising and positive contributor of treatment for autism spectrum disorders. The studies found a decrease in autistic severity and stress levels and noted an increase in social interaction and communication (O'Haire, 2012).

Several case studies have also highlighted the efficacy of AAI for treating victims of assault, resulting in, for example, improved emotional health and faster return to normal life. For example, a case described by mental health nurses concludes that an assault victim with bipolar disorder experienced increased well-being and functioning through taking care of a therapy dog for several hours a day. The patient experienced faster rehabilitation and mood stabilization. Meanwhile, the nurses found no negative effect of including a therapy dog in the rehabilitation program (Sockalingam et al., 2008).

A number of studies have been carried out on the physical, emotional, and mental benefits of AAI for older people. Research suggests that AAI improves social interaction, communication, and coping ability among older people (including those affected by dementia). In a review by Bernabei et al. (2013) it was concluded that the presence of a therapy animal (and even a robot animal) was beneficial to mood, social interaction, cognition, agitation reduction, and other symptoms. While some cases include highly structured interventions, the mere presence of and unstructured interactions with animals offer significant benefits. In other research done with elderly participants, ample evidence shows that animals act as important social supports during spousal bereavement and difficult treatments such as cancer therapy (McNicholas and Collis, 2006).

Implementation of animal-assisted intervention

Fibromyalgia, anxiety, depression, obesity, eating disorders, and recovery from cardiovascular disorders are other illnesses and disorders where AAI has been applied successfully (Le Roux and Kemp, 2009; Prothmann et al., 2006). However, there are many factors that must be considered in determining if AAI is a valuable intervention to apply. Clinicians must consider health risks including allergies, but also need to be aware of fears or aggression towards animals, and restrictions in some treatment settings. Beyond identifying these basic limitations, clinicians also need to consider the goals and objectives behind applying AAI. This process includes an analysis of the patient's physical, cognitive, behavioural, and emotional needs and assessing how AAI fits into the overall treatment plan. Treatment objectives will also be influenced by the clinician's professional orientation of practice, as well as perhaps how s/he views the animals being engaged in the therapy.

The following is a brief case study that demonstrates how a professional may incorporate therapy animals considering different perspectives: *'Sasha' is a fourteen-year-old female who has been directly affected by her parents' complicated and emotional separation. As the custody battle continues, Sasha is rarely able to see her father, with whom she'd had a positive relationship. She has moved into a small apartment where she shares a room with her sibling who is eight years old. Over the last six months, Sasha has become depressed and anxious. Her performance at school is declining and the teacher reports she is not engaged in her classroom. Lately, some disturbing suspicions have arisen about her interactions with some older acquaintances at school. Sasha has been referred to the school counsellor and a therapist to determine what is going on for Sasha socially and emotionally and how she can be helped.*

Considering the issues Sasha is facing, AAI may be relevant, based on the theories of social support, attachment, and biophilia. From a holistic perspective one may recognize the value of all three theoretical approaches in working with a girl like Sasha. The following will provide some insights of how the theories may apply in Sasha's case.

Animals as social supports in the treatment room

For practitioners who work with clients struggling with social support, there are many ways animals can be incorporated into the therapeutic milieu. In Sasha's case, the presence of an animal might facilitate the discussion of her difficult situation. The therapeutic environment may be perceived as less threatening in the presence of a therapy animal. Having an animal close may make it easier to open up. This is perhaps one of the initial discoveries made in the field of AAI—the animal acts as a social catalyst, allowing the client or patient to feel more at ease and supported. Once Sasha has developed a relationship with the therapy animal, her mother might be encouraged to bring a pet into the family (if it wouldn't add too much stress or hardship), to help support Sasha and her sibling in this transition. A pet—even a fish or other small pet—in the bedroom with Sasha and her sibling might ease the tension caused by sharing a space.

The attachment theory at work in animal-assisted intervention

Care taking is one aspect of the attachment theory evident in AAI. People who have responsibilities for an animal may experience the benefits of attachment by feeling a sense of belonging and importance to another being. Attachment to an animal also encourages patients to keep appointments and to continue treatment. Aubrey Fine (2014) reports that therapists using therapy animals seem to have more patients who come in time for the sessions, potentially because they don't want to miss interacting with the therapy animals.

Clinicians may also request that clients feed or groom the therapy animal and take it on a walk. The client can also be given responsibility to teach the animal a new behaviour. Providing these options allows clients to feel more engaged. Therapy animals who have also had struggles in their life, such as dogs who have been rescued or have physical disabilities, may have similar challenges that the client has experienced. For example, a child struggling with abuse

may feel an affiliation to an animal that was rescued from abuse. Such affiliations lead to stronger attachment.

In Sasha's case, a school counsellor may find it is easier to motivate her to check in if school routines are interrupted by a dog visit. If Sasha were able to develop an attachment to an animal (either in therapy or in her home), she may have an easier time coping with the loss of attachment to her father by focusing her energies on a new attachment with a pet. She can learn indirectly that she is a giver and that other beings still care for her. These opportunities may help her disclose her feelings and consider ways to work things through. If her social attachments at school are unhealthy, she may be encouraged to replace that undesirable source of support with a therapy animal while she re-establishes better peer relationships. Furthermore, therapeutic transfer between the therapy animal and the therapist may enable Sasha to feel more comfortable with a therapist, simply by becoming comfortable with the animal first. This position has been identified in the literature to be a strong benefit of therapy (Fine, 2010).

Biophilia hypothesis through a clinical lens

The biophilia hypothesis offers a rich perspective to psychology and AAI that appears to have not yet been fully explored. When working with animals in AAI, biophilic responses may become useful, relevant, and therapeutic within the relationship. Recognition of biophilic values can enrich the therapy by using innate responses to enhance or reframe a person's experience of nature and overall health. Because biophilia is a part of so many facets of human life, the theory of biophilia is valuable in many therapeutic situations. For instance, if people have a fear or phobia related to nature, biophilia principles can help therapists empower their client. Even in the simplest of approaches, the benefits of biophilia are experienced just in the presence of nature.

In Sasha's case, she may be seeking a new bond—a friend or confidant. As in the case of the theories of social support and attachment, biophilia also recognizes the human need to commune with others. The humanistic value, which is the value describing the human desire for relationship with animals, may spark Sasha's desire for friendship at a time when she may not have any reliable friends, and is also missing her father. In continued work with Sasha, a therapist may find other ways for Sasha to connect with nature to be helpful in the therapeutic process.

Altogether, AAI can offer various beneficial dimensions where the animal can act as a social lubricant to enhance the therapeutic relationship, as well as provide a dynamic impetus that may encourage therapeutic communication and change.

The importance of education

For AAI to be successfully integrated in a clinical setting, the professional must consider not only the client's or patient's health, but also animal welfare and the human–animal relationship. There is a need for accessible training for AAI around the world, although some colleges, universities, and organizations offer programmes related to AAI. This includes programmes that offer courses or entire degree programmes, workshops and training, and continuing education. Some examples of resources include the University of Denver in Colorado, Prescott College in Arizona, the International Society for Animal Assisted Therapy (ISAAT), Animal Assisted Interventions International, Pet Partners, and

Therapy Dogs International. Universities and various organizations usually offer many critical training components in AAI. This training may include skill development in working with animals, animal welfare, legal considerations, and public policies, logistics and protocol development of AAI in different settings, animal selection, and basic skills for interacting with people in need. By establishing an evidence-based education and licensing, the practice of AAI may increase in the medical community. This in turn may lead to improved access to more hospitals, schools, nursing homes, and other facilities where AAI could be beneficial and needed. With an increased use of AAI, there will be a need for stronger training, quality assessment, and for national or even international standards.

Conclusion

Animal-assisted interventions may become a useful alternative and complementary form of therapy for certain patient groups. Research progress made in the past 30 years has started to unravel some of the mysteries of how animals can therapeutically enhance our quality of life. The field is now at a crossroads and is in need of more empirical evidence. This evidence could help demonstrate the efficacy of human–animal interactions and the value of animal-assisted interventions. It has for long been a common notion that animals are good for our well-being. With improved studies and identification of best practice, this may develop into an established and valid therapeutic alternative with importance for a range of patient groups.

References

Allen, K., Blascovich, J., & Mendes, W. B. (2002). Cardiovascular reactivity and the presence of pets, friends, and spouses: the truth about cats and dogs. *Psychosom Med*, 64, 727–39.

Barba, B. E. (1995). A critical review of research on the human/companion animal relationship. *Anthrozoös*, 8, 9–15.

Beck, L. & Madresh, E. A. (2008). Romantic partners and four-legged friends: An extension of attachment theory to relationships with pets. *Anthrozoös*, 21, 43–56.

Bernabei, V., Ronchi, D. D., Ferla, T. L., *et al.* (2013). Animal-assisted interventions for elderly patients affected by dementia or psychiatric disorders: A review. *J Psychiatr Res*, 47, 762–73.

Bernstein, J. (2005). *Living in the borderland: the evolution of consciousness and the challenge of healing trauma*. New York, NY: Routledge.

Bowlby, J. (1969). Disruption of affectional bonds and its effects on behavior. *Canada's Mental Health Supplement*, 69, 1–17.

Bowlby, J. (1980). *Attachment and Loss*. New York, NY: Basic Books.

Eddie, T. J. (1996). RM and Beaux: Reduction in cardiac response in response to a pet snake. *J Nerv Ment Dis*, 184, 573–5.

Fine, A. H. (2014). *Our Faithful Companions: Exploring the Essence of Our Kinship with Animals*. Loveland, CO: Alpine Publications Incorporated.

Fine, A. H. (ed.) (2010). *Handbook on Animal-Assisted Therapy: Theoretical Foundations and Guidelines for Practice*, 3rd edition. San Diego, CA: Academic Press.

Fine, A. H. & Beck, A. (2010). Understanding our kinship with animals: input for health care professionals interested in the human/animal bond. In: Fine, A. H. (ed.) *Handbook on Animal-Assisted Therapy: Theoretical Foundations and Guidelines for Practice*, 3rd edition. San Diego, CA: Academic Press.

Friedmann, E., Locker, B. Z., & Lockwood, R. (1990). Perception of animals and cardiovascular responses during verbalization with an animal present. *Anthrozoös*, 6, 115–34.

Friedmann, E., Katcher, A. H., Lynch, J. J., & Thomas, S. A. (1980). Animal companions and one year survival of patients after discharge from a coronary care unit. *Public Health Rep*, 95, 307–12.

Group for the Study of the Human/Companion Animal Bond (1979). Proceedings of a meeting held at the University of Dundee, 23–25th March 1979. Scotland: the group.

Handlin L., Hydbring-Sandberg, E., Nilsson, A., Ejdeback, M., Jansson, A., & Uvnas-Moberg, K. (2011). Short-term interaction between dogs and their owners: effects of oxytocin, cortisol, insulin and heart rate. *Anthrozoös*, 24, 301–15.

Handlin, L., Nilsson, A., Ejdeback, M., Hydbring-Sandberg, E., & Uvnas-Moberg, K. (2012). Associations between the Psychological characteristics of the human-dog relationship and oxytocin and cortisol levels. *Anthrozoös*, 25, 215–28.

Headey, B. & Grabka, M. M. (2007). Pets and human health in Germany and Australia: National longitudinal results. *Soc Indic Res*, 80, 297–311.

Hunt, M. G., & Chizkov, R. R. (2014). Are therapy dogs like Xanax? Does animal-assisted therapy impact processes relevant to cognitive behavioral psychotherapy? *Anthrozoös*, 27, 457–69.

Jegatheesan, B., Beetz, A., Choi, G., *et al.* (2014). The IAHAIO Definitions for Animal Assisted Interventions and Animal Assisted Activity and Guidelines for Wellness of Animals Involved, Final Report. Presented at the 2014 IAHAIO meeting in Amsterdam, Netherlands. 24–26th July, 2014.

Journal of the American Veterinary Medical Association (JAVMA) (1998). Statement from the committee on the human-animal bond. *JAVMA*, 212, 1675.

Kellert, S. R. (1993). The biological basis for human values of nature. In: Kellert, S. R. & Wilson, E. O. (eds) *The Biophilia Hypothesis*. Washington, DC: Clearwater Press.

Le Roux M. & Kemp, R. (2009). Effect of a companion dog on depression and anxiety levels of elderly residents in a long-term care facility. *Psychogeriatrics*, 9, 23–6.

Levinson, B. (1962). The dog as a 'co-therapist'. *Ment Hyg*, 46, 59–65.

Levinson, B. (1969). *Pet-Oriented Child Psychotherapy*. Springfield, IL: Charles Thomas.

Levinson, B. (1979). *Pets and Human Development*. Springfield, IL: Charles Thomas.

McCune, S., Kruger, K. A., Griffin, J. A., *et al.* (2014). Evolution of research on the mutual benefits of human-animal interaction. *Animal Frontiers*, 4, 49–58.

McNicholas, J. & Collis, G. M. (2001). Children's representations of pets in their social networks. *Child Care Health Dev*, 27, 279–94.

McNicholas, J., & Collis, G. M. (2006). Animals as social supports: Insights for understanding animal assisted therapy. In: Fine, A. (ed.) *Handbook on Animal Assisted Therapy*, 2nd edition. San Diego, CA: Academic Press.

Miller S. C., Kennedy C., Devoe D., Hickey M., Nelson T., & Kogan L. (2009). An examination of changes in oxytocin levels in men and women before and after interaction with a bonded dog. *Anthrozoös*, 22, 31–42.

Nagasawa, M., Kikusui, T., Onaka, T., & Ohta, M. (2008). Dog's gaze at its owner increases owner's urinary oxytocin during social interaction. *Horm Behav*, 55, 434–51.

Odendaal, J. S. J., & Meintjes, R. A. (2003). Neurophysiological correlates of affiliative behaviour between humans and dogs. *Vet J*, 165, 296–301.

O'Haire, M. E. (2012). Animal-assisted intervention for autism spectrum disorder: A systematic literature review. *J Autism Dev Disord*, 43, 1606–22.

Prothmann, A., Bienert, M., & Ettrich, C. (2006). Dogs in child psychotherapy: Effects on state of mind. *Anthrozoös*, 19, 265–77.

Romereo, T., Nagaswa, M., Mogi, K., Hasegawa, T., & Kikusui, T. (2014). Oxytocin promotes social bonding in dogs. *Proc Natl Acad Sci U S A*, 111, 9085–90.

Sable, P. (1995) Pets, attachment, and well-being across the life cycle. Social Work, 40, 334–341.

Shiloh, S., Sorek, G., & Terkel, J. (2003). Reduction of state-anxiety by petting animals in a controlled laboratory experiment. *Anxiety, Stress and Coping*, 16(4), 387–395.

Smokovic, I., Fajfar, M., & Mlinaric, V. (2012). Attachment to pets and interpersonal relationships: Can a four-legged friend replace a two-legged one? *J Eur Psychol Stud*, 3, 15–23.

Sockalingam, S., Li, M., Krishnadev, U., *et al.* (2008). Use of animal-assisted thearpy in the rehabilitation of an assault victim with a concurrent mood disorder. *Issues Ment Health Nurs*, 29, 73–84.

Strand, E. (2004). Interparental conflict and youth maladjustment: The buffering effects of pets. *Stress Trauma and Crisis Trauma*, 3, 151–68.

Van Houte, B. A. & Jarvis, P. A. (1995). The role of pets in preadolescent psychosocial development. *J Appl Dev Psychol*, 16, 463–479.

Wilson, E. O. (1984). *Biophilia: The Human Bond with Other Species*. Cambridge, MA: Harvard University Press.

Zeltman, P., & Johnson, R. A. (2011). *Walk a Hound, Lose a Pound: How You and Your Dog Can Lose Weight, Stay Fit, and Have Fun* (New Directions in the Human-Animal Bond). West Lafayette, IN: Purdue University Press.

Zilcha-Mano, S., Mikulincer, M., & Shaver, P. R. (2011). Pet in the therapy room: An attachment perspective on animal-assisted therapy. *Attachment and Human Development*, 13S, 541–61.

CHAPTER 4.3

Similarities, disparities, and synergies with other complex interventions—stress as a common pathway

Cecilia Stenfors, Eva Bojner Horwitz, Töres Theorell, and Walter Osika

Cultural, contemplative, and nature-related activities—promising measures for major public health challenges

Mental and psychosomatic health problems currently constitute one of the greatest public health issues. Apart from individual suffering, this causes long-term absenteeism and high societal costs. Common mental disorders involve problems with mood and emotion regulation, as well as with cognitive capacity, such as executive functioning and episodic memory. There is also a significant co-morbidity with major somatic diseases, like cardiovascular diseases and dementia. Furthermore, all of these conditions seem to be related to maladaptive stress signalling (including prolonged, excessive, or deficient response of the stress system), at both central and peripheral levels. For a thorough review of stress physiology, see Chapter 1.4.

Contemplative practices, like mindfulness and compassion training, and cultural activities have all been used to improve or prevent some of these health problems. Such practices seem to have in common with nature-assisted or based interventions (NA/BI) that they facilitate exploration and cultivation of the inner, personal experiences, and outer 'landscapes', respectively.

In this chapter, factors that may underlie some of the common mental health problems are discussed and put into a context to reveal reasons for why various complex interventions, including nature-assisted or based interventions, may share a mechanistic background. This is followed by a review of contemplative practices and cultural activities as health-promoting activities. Then similarities, differences, and possible synergies between NA/BI, contemplative, and cultural activities will be elaborated on.

Potential risk factors of common psychological health problems

Chronic activation of both conscious and unconscious negative thoughts may be a major cause of psychological and somatic disorders. This process is mediated via prolonged, excessive, or deficient responses of various physiological stress systems (Brosschot, 2010).

As outlined in Chapter 1.4, stress responses are activated when an internal or external stimulus is appraised as threatening to the individual's well-being. This appraisal may be conscious, but often it happens automatically based on previous learned or conditioned responses (LeDoux, 2000).

Depending on the interpretation of the stimulus as associated with threat or not, the initial reaction can be upregulated or down-regulated, that is, reappraised, by 'higher' order cognitive control processes in the prefrontal cortex of the brain, particularly if there is an awareness of the incoming stimulus and one's reaction to it. The interpretations, both the initial and subconscious, as well as conscious reappraisals, are also impacted by earlier experiences (Jamieson et al., 2012). This constitutes the neurophysiological background for behavioural modification by both contemplative and cultural activities, as well as NA/BI.

As chronic stress and lack of restoration are among the major risk factors of many common mental disorders (Stenfors et al., 2013), facilitating prevention, restoration from, or resiliency against these processes may have significant benefits to public health.

Complex interventions as measures to handle stress

During human evolution several practices have been developed, which have been used to enable resilient ways to handle different stressors. We will present some examples in the following sections.

Contemplative practices

In nearly all major religions and also in several philosophical traditions, different forms of contemplative exercises have been core parts of the practice (Ricard et al., 2014). For example, the medieval Christian European worldview recognized two orientations to life;

one was termed *vita activa*, and the other *vita contemplative*. Most of medieval society was focused on production, whether handcrafts or agriculture, which would adhere to *vita active*. In the monasteries, by contrast, the few were aiming for a life of prayer and contemplation (*vita contemplative*) (Zajonc, 2009). Also in other religious traditions, such as Judaism, Sufism, and Buddhism, there is a history of cultivation of stillness in order to facilitate reverence and prayers, and in the case of Buddhism also an insight in how the mind (in its interactions with the outside world) creates suffering (Wallace, 2009).

Nowadays, if one wishes to recover, or even flourish, as a result of contemplative practices, most of us simultaneously have to live an active life, as we cannot hide behind monastery walls or be on retreats in infinitum. The complexity of the world and the high volumes of information we have to cope with have grown exponentially. In order to handle this increase of stressors in an integrative way, by also using parts of the old contemplative practices, different measures have been developed. Globally, different contemplative practices are now increasingly being used in healthcare, and several universities conduct investigations of contemplative neuroscience. There is also a noticeable increase of scientific publications regarding functional and structural neural mechanisms associated with meditation and mindfulness (Marchand, 2014; Fröding and Osika, 2015).

Meditation practice

The brain is less skilled in distinguishing real stimuli or threats from the ones we only imagine (Gilbert *et al.*, 2006). Hence, our inner thought processes might feed fruitless ruminating processes in obsessive loops, fuelling stress activating processes, unless we find tentative solutions and let those distressing thoughts go. The ability to notice such thoughts, to inhibit subsequent emotions and dysfunctional behaviour, to stay on target and resist distraction depends on the current level of attentional control. This capacity is also connected to better cognitive performance, and operates in the frontal and prefrontal cortex (Davidson *et al.*, 2012).

In general, a meditation 'novice' is often instructed to initially utilize focused attention practice by paying attention to, for example, the breath as an object of attention. By choosing to focus on only one object or phenomenon, it is intended to enhance awareness also of one's emotional and cognitive states while developing attentional skills (Lutz *et al.*, 2008). Training of attention skills enhances the capability to sustain awareness of one's thinking patterns, emotions, and sensory perceptions. This awareness facilitates distance from thoughts and emotions, such that they become less powerful and compelling.

Mindfulness

The current mainstream understanding of what mindfulness is, refers to a quality that involves bringing one's complete attention to the present experience on a moment-to-moment basis, nonjudgementally. Meditation exercises, but also yoga (e.g. hatha yoga) and body awareness training are part of mindfulness practice (Kabat-Zinn, 1990; Kabat-Zinn and Davidson, 2012). These exercises involve paying attention to the body and bodily sensations in a gradual sweeping of attention through the body from feet to head. When thoughts arise and attention wanders, the practice is to return the attention to the intended focus.

To attend to visceral, momentary sensations may be helpful or harmful to a person depending on how such awareness is understood. Under the right conditions, contemplative practices may have a therapeutic impact. On the other hand, interoceptive signals may also be catastrophized in panic and related disorders.

If a person spends a great deal of time pursuing idealized, interoceptive states, rather than learning to more subtly achieve and maintain such states, she will require greater effort to achieve feelings of presence. Body-focused contemplative practices may alter interoceptive processing by increasing bottom-up integration of what is happening in the body rather than attempting to alter body sensations to fit the top-down expectations of what should happen in the body (Mehling *et al.*, 2012).

As interoceptive signals inform emotional experience, contemplative practice may promote a cycle of awareness of the contingencies between environmental triggers, bodily responses, cognitive appraisals, and emotional experiences. This can subsequently improve performance and emotional well-being.

Cognitive flexibility and meta-skills

Mindfulness practice can increase meta-skills, that is, the ability to notice emotions, thoughts, and intentions from a more 'distanced' perspective, and integrate this into purposeful activities, leading to optimized executive functioning.

Working memory capacity has been described as the 'bottle neck' for several higher cognitive functions. It is responsible for the transient holding and processing of new and already stored information, an important process for learning, decision-making, and memory updating. It could be hypothesized that the number of possible meta-skill levels is related to the working memory capacity and effectiveness of the central executive function (Jankowski and Holas, 2014). Accordingly, mindfulness training has been associated both with better working memory capacity, increased cognitive flexibility, and better metacognitive skills (Moore and Malinowski, 2009).

In 'normal' cognitive development, metacognitive abilities develop as the prefrontal cortex (PFC) matures and executive functions develop. Therefore it is particularly interesting that some meditation effects are mediated partly through the growth and activity in the left PFC (Brefczynski-Lewis *et al.*, 2007).

Emotional regulation and compassion training

Emotional regulation, which is disrupted in most mental disorders, has been shown to improve after mindfulness training (Goyal *et al.*, 2014). However, becoming better at detecting difficult experiences might lead to a subsequent increase in anxiety and suffering (Kerr *et al.*, 2011). Some clinicians therefore argue that it is wise to actually start one's meditation practice with exercises that improve the functioning of the (self)-soothing system (Gilbert, 2014). Soothing is a complex and multicomponent process involving complex interactions between soothing systems and threat systems. Hence, feeling safe, reassured, and soothed can arise not just via the absence of threat cues, but from specific cues that activate the soothing system. The focus is thus on cues that help us feel safe (e.g. connectedness to supportive people or a safe external environment). Intimate soothing cues relate to affection cues such as physical touch, cuddling, and hand holding, with evidence that these can affect the opiate systems. More general soothing cues of safeness relate to non-verbal communication (facial expressions, voice tones, and postures), reflective attentiveness, and empathy.

Empathetically resonating with others' suffering can initiate processes of emotional exhaustion or burnout, in fact, a kind of empathy 'fatigue', or an emotional shut down, which has been shown in numerous studies (e.g. of medical students). On the other hand, meditational practice focused on love and compassion is associated with an improved ability to handle experiences of watching others suffer, preventing 'empathy fatigue' (Klimecki et al., 2014), and the field of compassion research is currently expanding substantially.

Similarities and disparities between NA/BI and contemplative practices

The experience of being in nature often manifests as a psychological state in which an individual's sense of self and time are eclipsed by absorption in the moment. Many people's most contemplative and meaningful experiences are reported to have occurred amid nature, for example the temporary absence of one's own mind-chatter, experienced along a shoreline of a silent lake, while walking in a mindful pace and mood, or the state of narrowed perceptual focus when weeding or planting in the garden (which resembles the experience of focused attention training described earlier).

Henry David Thoreau investigated the reciprocal effects between nature and the human mind in his book *Walden* (Thoreau, 1854/1997). He acknowledged the difficulties to capture in words what he had experienced so powerfully. Ralph Waldo Emerson, another early theorist and researcher at the interface of nature and mind, concluded that: 'There are no fixtures in nature. The universe is fluid and volatile. Permanence is but a word of degrees ... behind the course effect, is a fine cause, which, being narrowly seen, is itself the effect of a finer cause. Everything looks permanent until its secret is known' (Emerson, 1841/1981). This description is quite similar to some first person accounts of meditation practice: 'Consciousness does not appear to itself chopped up in bits. Such words as 'chain' or 'train' do not describe it fitly as it presents itself in the first instance. It is nothing jointed; it flows. A 'river' or a 'stream' are the metaphors by which it is most naturally described. In talking of it hereafter let us call it the stream of thought, of consciousness, or of subjective life' (James, 1890).

Both mindfulness and NA/BI have the potential to reduce psychological and physiological stress, improve mood (Kaplan, 2001; Annerstedt et al., 2013; Goyal et al., 2014), and improve or replenish cognitive functioning, especially executive functioning (Kaplan and Berman, 2010; Lutz et al., 2008; Jha et al., 2007).

For example, Berman et al. (2008) found that walking in nature or viewing pictures of nature, compared to urban environment exposures, improved both mood and directed attention abilities in healthy individuals. Similar studies on individuals suffering from major depression found that both cognition and mood improved more after a nature walk, relative to an urban walk, among depressed individuals (Berman et al., 2012).

There are a number of pathways and mechanisms through which both NA/BI and mindfulness activities may generate effects on stress, mood, and cognitive functioning. Among these are greater exposure to stimuli that trigger positive concepts, representations, and feelings, enabling greater presence in the here-and-now, reduced load on directed attention resources, increased feelings of connectedness (to nature, the world, or to other people in general) and increased perspective-taking.

At the brain level, mindfulness meditation has been associated with certain structural and functional patterns. That is, PFC regions important for executive cognitive functioning are thicker and appear to operate more effectively in meditators compared to non-meditators (Brefczynski-Lewis et al., 2007).

Furthermore, the amygdala has been found to be less reactive in meditators (Hölzel et al., 2013). This parallels findings on the brain patterns of people living in more natural environments, compared to those living in urban environments, as these were associated with decreased neural reactivity in the amygdala in response to emotional stress (see Chapter 8.1) (Lederbogen et al., 2011). Similarly, nature exposure seem to decrease rumination, a maladaptive pattern of self-referential, negative thoughts that increase the risk for depression. Walking in nature decreases both self-reported rumination and neural activity in an area of the brain linked to risk for mental illness (subgenual PFC) (Bratman et al., 2015). This seems to correlate to the enhanced capacity to take distance from yourself and being functionally compassionate after mediation practice (Klimecki et al., 2014).

A difference between meditation and NA/BI regarding positive effects on cognitive functions is that meditation involves active practice in controlling one's attention and switching between different types of attentional states, such as directed or focused top-down attention versus bottom-up 'open monitoring' (Malinowski, 2013; Hasenkamp et al., 2014).

NA/BIs, on the other hand, seem to facilitate restoration of executive cognitive resources, especially effortful directed attention, as an effect of the ways in which this type of external stimuli softly tap effortless bottom-up attention, versus do not tap effortful top-down attentional processes (Kaplan and Kaplan, 1989) (see Chapter 2.1 for more insights in these theories).

However, attentional replenishment may also increase the capacity to train cognitive functions and improve learning, including cognitive strategies and mindfulness skills. Research on the environmental effect on children's cognitive ability suggest this may be the case, as an association has been found between school 'greenness' and children's cognitive development and school performance (Mårtensson et al., 2009; Dadvand et al., 2015). Additionally, similar to the replenishment of directed attention resources by nature exposure (Kaplan and Berman, 2010), actively putting your mind and body into a state of open awareness can also facilitate restoration of these resources (Kaplan, 2001). Moreover, increasing the capacity to filter out internal and external distractions, or 'resisting interference' (practised in focused attention exercises), may prevent fatigue of directed attentional resources.

Nature contains less cues of social processes, like judgement or comparison, compared to many other (e.g. urban) environments. Such social signals can be distracting and interfere with cognitive tasks that demand focused attention. This may cause attentional fatigue. Negative social signals are also powerful stressors, which can evoke enhanced amygdala activity and other stress responses. This can also inhibit PFC-dependent functions, such as executive functions and emotion regulation.

In conclusion, NA/BI may provide relief from social stressors and instead offer feelings of connectedness to the environment. NA/BI can also enable prosocial behaviour (Howell et al., 2011;

Zhang *et al.*, 2014) as well as stimulating the soothing system (Gilbert, 2014). This is especially interesting when comparing NA/BI with self-compassion, which is less associated with social comparison, rumination, and anger, compared with self-esteem (Neff and Vonk, 2009). Self-esteem refers to the degree to which we evaluate ourselves positively and it is often based on comparisons with others. In contrast, self-compassion is not based on positive judgements or evaluation—it is a way of relating to ourselves. People feel self-compassion because they are human beings, not because they are special and above average. It emphasizes interconnection rather than separateness (Goetz *et al.*, 2010; Neff, 2011). Feelings of connectedness to something other and greater than oneself have in other areas been found to be positively related to well-being. Nature connectedness can also support greater perspective taking, which may also reduce self-referential negative ruminations, or at least buffer against the negative impact of such thoughts (Bratman *et al.*, 2015).

In mindfulness, relief from negative social signals or thought can also be gained from the training of attention skills and non-judgemental awareness of one's thinking patterns, emotions, and sensory perceptions. Attentional skills enhance the capability to sustain non-judgemental awareness. This awareness facilitates perspective taking and distance from thoughts and emotions, such that these become less powerful and compelling. In particular, mindfulness supports the recognition of automatic thinking patterns, awareness of outer and inner stimuli, as well as learning to direct ones attention to those stimuli that one values and considers constructive.

Cultural activities and health

Lately, there has been a growth of interest and research in the role of culture in both healthcare and in community-based public health initiatives (Clift, 2012). In the Scandinavian countries, as well as in the United States, large cohort studies of cultural participation have been undertaken to explore potential links between culture and health (Hyyppä and Mäki, 2001; Wilkinson *et al.*, 2007; Cuypers *et al.*, 2012).

Well-performed and controlled studies have demonstrated that a high level of cultural participation (as, for example, measured by indexes based on visiting the theatre, concerts, arts exhibitions, museums, and sports events) is associated with a decreased mortality risk (Bygren *et al.*, 1996; Konlaan *et al.*, 2000). Annamaria Laaksonen, research manager at the International Federation of Arts Councils and Culture Agencies Australia, describes how the arts sector can also contribute to other sectors, for example health and management (Laaksonen, 2011).

Dance

Embodiment

In dance, but also in other forms of fine arts and cultural activities, the whole body reacts to the activity (Koch and Bräuninger, 2005). This is valuable as embodied knowledge (and memory) plays an important role in our perception (Cross *et al.*, 2011). The acknowledgement of such phenomena has contributed to a broadening of the research focus in cognitive neuroscience, from a solely abstract and analytical view of the mind, to an integration of the view of the mind as 'embodied' (Varela *et al.*, 1992; Bojner Horwitz *et al.*, 2013). The quintessence of the term is that all human beings exist intrinsically as embodied beings, and that mental functions cannot be fully understood without reference to our physical body, as well as to the environment we are experiencing, and vice versa.

When using dance to promote health, the term 'embodiment' is for example used for investigating the impact of different movement qualities on perception. In other forms of fine arts and cultural activities such as visual art, music, poetry, and theatre, there is also a connection to the whole body response, where embodied knowledge (and memory) plays an important role in our perception (Kirsch *et al.*, 2013). When analysing bodily health effects after a cultural activity or NA/BI, there seems to be a link to the embodied mind and its response to the effects. We can train the awareness of our embodied mind using contemplation and reflection, regardless if it is a cultural or nature-related activity.

Alexithymia

'Alexithymia' is the inability to discriminate emotion in others and self. Engagement in dance seems to enhance this capacity, being associated with emotional competence in interplay with others (Bojner Horwitz *et al.*, 2015). Participation in dance might enable emotional nuances of movement patterns and increase the perception and discrimination of emotions. These improvements may be due to the multimodal stimulation from dance and music, possibly by also activating the brain's mirror systems (Freedberg and Gallese 2007). This may facilitate contact with emotions and experiences that are otherwise difficult to reach by only cognitive means.

Different movements seem to carry different emotional implications. Similarly, different shapes and patterns in our external environment, and in nature, affect us in various ways (see for example Chapter 2.5).

On parallels between nature and culture in health promotion

Studying experiences of nature poses some similar difficulties as studying experiences of culture, both having an ephemeral existence. How are we to define and describe the temporal and spatial, but non-verbal experience of such phenomena? Language is ill-equipped to convey experience in the first person for the description of cultural and nature-related activities (Levinson *et al.*, 1991).

That said, the experience of culture—including music, theatre, dance, visual arts, and literature, as well as, for example, beautiful nature—seem to have the potential to be revitalizing and to promote admiration and reflection (Wikström *et al.*, 1993; Theorell *et al.*, 2013; Zhang *et al.*, 2014; Viding *et al.*, 2015).

Art

Nature has long been an inspiration for art, and already in the more than 17,000-year-old paintings in the Lascaux caves in France, the horses, deer, bulls, and other animals that once roamed the land were depicted. Paintings from the Ming Dynasty show the important role of nature in Chinese art, where in particular mountains were revered as the manifestation of 'qi'—nature's power.

There seems to be variability in what reactions art invokes in humans. For example, abstract paintings tend to evoke stress reactions among patients in hospitals, while paintings of natural landscape induce calmness and harmony (Lankston *et al.*, 2010). This seem to relate to the calming effect of viewing fractals of a certain dimension, abundant in nature and some art styles (Taylor *et al.*, 2014). Read Chapter 2.5 for more insights in this interesting topic.

Music

Musical group activities are important for generating cohesiveness in a group—which is *per se* of value for collective survival. Similarly to the potential of calm nature or the sound of birdsong (Annerstedt *et al.*, 2013) in curbing stress reactions (see Chapter 2.5 on natural soundscapes), slow, soft music with harmonic chords induces heart rate reduction (for a review see Theorell, 2014). Music during surgical procedures decreases sedative requirements during anaesthesia (Lepage *et al.*, 2001). However, the possible health promoting effects of nature and arts are not limited to 'calming' effects. More often music, for instance, is needed when we need a boost of energy. Energizing music or pieces of art may help a student facing an exam to keep awake during tedious studying. Music has also been reported to improve work efficiency of medical personnel (George *et al.*, 2011). This reasoning could be applied to emotions in general—when strong emotions are needed as triggers. For instance, during funerals music is constructed to facilitate emotional reactions, which are part of mourning processes, and marches are used in order to energize military troops.

Synergies between NA/BI, cultural activities, and contemplative practices

Being in a tranquil natural environment may ease and support a mindful state or mindfulness meditation, as some natural environments appear to support calmness of the mind, also shown by corresponding brain network activity (Hunter *et al.*, 2010). Contemplative and cultural activities are often located to tranquil and beautiful nature environments, and combining these experiences may facilitate and strengthen the effects of each activity.

For example, integrating programmes of art therapy into the environment of healing gardens seems to have synergistic effects on reducing symptoms of depression in older people (McCaffrey, 2007). Houses of worship have been described as restorative environments (Herzog *et al.*, 2013), and there might be synergies in performing prayers or reflection if they are situated in a tranquil environment.

Conclusion

The cultivation of attentional control through mindfulness could enhance the ability to create *imagined* restorative and supporting environments, as well as increase the restorative effects that this imagery produces. In fact, contemplative practices, including mindfulness, often involve exercises with focused imagery. These can concern imagery that help to foster focus and clarity of mind (e.g. visualizing thoughts as clouds floating by, to not get caught up by them), provide the meditator with support (e.g. imagine when you were successful at something or felt support), be soothing, or provide rest (e.g. imagine a calm tranquil place).

On the other hand, greater degrees of mindfulness may also amplify the experience of real natural environments, as well as enhance the positive effects that these environments have on cognition, emotions, and stress levels via the increased ability to be immersed in and attentive to the experience of being in nature.

Different types of nature (e.g. serene and calm vs. more dramatic nature) may similarly have different effects on psychological and somatic states, which could be utilized to tailor the NA/BI to current individual needs.

References

Annerstedt, M., Jönsson, P., Wallergård, M., *et al.* (2013). Inducing physiological stress recovery with sounds of nature in a virtual reality forest—Results from a pilot study. *Physiol Behav*, 118, 240–250.

Berman, M. G., Jonides, J., & Kaplan, S. (2008). The cognitive benefits of interacting with nature. *Psychol Sci*, 19, 1207–12.

Berman, M. G., Kross, E., Krpan, K. M., *et al.* (2012). Interacting with nature improves cognition and affect for individuals with depression. *J Affect Disord*, 140, 300–5.

Bojner Horwitz, E., Lennartsson A-K., Theorell TP., & Ullén, F. (2015). Engagement in dance is associated with emotional competence in interplay with others. *Front Psychol*, 31, 1096.

Bojner Horwitz, E., Stenfors, C., & Osika, W. (2013). Contemplative inquiry in movement: managing writers´s block in academic writing. *Int J Transpers Stud*, 32, 16–26.

Bratman, G. N., Hamilton, J. P., Hahn, K. S., Daily, G. C., & Gross, J. J. (2015). Nature experience reduces rumination and subgenual prefrontal cortex activation. *Proc Natl Acad Sci*, 112, 8567–72.

Brefczynski-Lewis, J. A., Lutz, A., Schaefer, H. S., Levinson, D. B., & Davidson, R. J. (2007). Neural correlates of attentional expertise in long-term meditation practitioners. *Proc Natl Acad Sci U S A*, 104, 11483–8.

Brosschot, J. F. (2010). Markers of chronic stress: Prolonged physiological activation and (un) conscious perseverative cognition. *Neurosci Biobehav Rev*, 35, 46–50.

Bygren, L. O., Konlaan, B. B., & Johansson, S. E. (1996). Attendance at cultural events, reading books or periodicals, and making music or singing in a choir as determinants for survival: Swedish interview survey of living conditions. *BMJ*, 313, 1577.

Clift, S. (2012). Creative arts as a public health resource: moving from practice-based research to evidence-based practice. *Perspect Public Health*, 132, 120–7.

Cross, E. S., Kirsch, L., Ticini, L. F., & Schütz-Bosbach, S. (2011). The impact of aesthetic evaluation and physical ability on dance perception. *Front Hum Neurosci*, 5, 102.

Cuypers, K., Krokstad, S., Holmen, T. L., Knudtsen, M. S., Bygren, L. O., & Holmen, J. (2012). Patterns of receptive and creative cultural activities and their association with perceived health, anxiety, depression and satisfaction with life among adults: the HUNT study, Norway. *J Epidemiol Community Health*, 66, 698–703.

Dadvand, P., Nieuwenhuijsen, M. J., Esnaola, M., *et al.* (2015). Green spaces and cognitive development in primary schoolchildren. *Proc Natl Acad Sci*, 112, 7937–42.

Davidson, R. J., Begley, S., & Amari, F. (2012). *The Emotional Life of Your Brain*. Brilliance Audio.

Emerson, R. W. (1981). *The Portable Emerson: New Edition*. London, UK: Penguin.

Freedberg, D. & Gallese, V. (2007). Motion, emotion and empathy in esthetic experience. *Trends Cogn Sci*, 11, 197–203.

Fröding, B. & Osika, W. (2015). Neuroenhancement: how mental training and meditation can promote epistemic virtue. New York, NY: Springer.

George, S., Ahmed, S., Mammen, K. J., & John, G. M. (2011). Influence of music on operation theatre staff. *J Anaesthesiol Clin Pharmacol*, 27, 354.

Gilbert, P. (2014). The origins and nature of compassion focused therapy. *Br J Clin Psychol*, 53, 6–41.

Gilbert, P., Baldwin, M. W., Irons, C., Baccus, J. R., & Palmer, M. (2006). Self-criticism and self-warmth: An imagery study exploring their relation to depression. *J Cogn Psychother*, 20, 183–200.

Goetz, J. L., Keltner, D., & Simon-Thomas, E. (2010). Compassion: an evolutionary analysis and empirical review. *Psychol Bull*, 136, 351.

Goyal, M., Singh, S., Sibinga, E. M., *et al.* (2014). Meditation programs for psychological stress and well-being: a systematic review and meta-analysis. *JAMA Intern Med*, 174, 357–68.

Hasenkamp, W. (2014). Using first-person reports during meditation to investigate basic cognitive experience. In: *Meditation–Neuroscientific*

Approaches and Philosophical Implications. pp. 75-93. Springer International Publishing.

Herzog, T. R., Gray, L. E., Dunville, A. M., Hicks, A. M., & Gilson, E. A. (2013). Preference and tranquility for houses of worship. *Environ Behav*, 45, 504–25.

Howell, A. J., Dopko, R. L., Passmore, H. A., & Buro, K. (2011). Nature connectedness: Associations with well-being and mindfulness. *Pers Individ Dif*, 51, 166–71.

Hölzel, B. K., Hoge, E. A., Greve, D. N., *et al.* (2013). Neural mechanisms of symptom improvements in generalized anxiety disorder following mindfulness training. *Neuroimage Clin*, 2, 448–58.

Hunter, M. D., Eickhoff, S. B., Pheasant, R. J., *et al.* (2010). The state of tranquility: Subjective perception is shaped by contextual modulation of auditory connectivity. *Neuroimage*, 53, 611–18.

Hyyppä, M. T. & Mäki, J. (2001). Why do Swedish-speaking Finns have longer active life? An area for social capital research. *Health Promot Int*, 16, 55–64.

James, W. (1890/2004). *The Principles of Psychology (Volume 1 of 2).* Digireads.com Publishing, p. 239.

Jamieson, J. P., Nock, M. K., & Mendes, W. B. (2012). Mind over matter: reappraising arousal improves cardiovascular and cognitive responses to stress. *J Exp Psychol Gen*, 141, 417.

Jankowski, T., & Holas, P. (2014). Metacognitive model of mindfulness. *Conscious Cogn*, 28, 64–80.

Jha, A. P., Krompinger, J., & Baime, M. J. (2007). Mindfulness training modifies subsystems of attention. *Cogn Affect Behav Neurosci*, 7, 109–19.

Kabat-Zinn, J. (1990). *Full Catastrophe Living: Using the Wisdom of Your Mind and Body to Face Stress, Pain, and Illness.* London, UK: Piatkus.

Kabat-Zinn, J. & Davidson, R. (eds). (2012). *The Mind's Own Physician: A Scientific Dialogue with the Dalai Lama on the Healing Power of Meditation.* Oakland, CA: New Harbinger Publications.

Kaplan, R. & Kaplan, S. (1989). *The Experience of Nature: A Psychological Perspective.* Cambridge, UK: Cambridge University Press Archive.

Kaplan, S. (2001). Meditation, restoration, and the management of mental fatigue. *Environ Behav*, 33, 480–506.

Kaplan, S. & Berman, M. G. (2010). Directed attention as a common resource for executive functioning and self-regulation. *Perspect Psychol Sci*, 5, 43–57.

Kerr, C. E., Josyula, K., & Littenberg, R. (2011). Developing an observing attitude: an analysis of meditation diaries in an MBSR clinical trial. *Clin Psychol Psychother*, 18, 80–93.

Kirsch, L., Drommelschmidt, K. A., & Cross, E. S. (2013). The impact of sensorimotor experience on affective evaluation of dance. *Frontiers in human neuroscience*, 7, 521.

Klimecki, O. M., Leiberg, S., Ricard, M., & Singer, T. (2014). Differential pattern of functional brain plasticity after compassion and empathy training. *Soc Cogn Affect Neurosci*, 9, 873–9.

Koch, S. C., & Bräuninger, I. (2005). International dance/movement therapy research: Theory, methods, and empirical findings. *Am J Dance Ther*, 27, 37–46.

Konlaan, B. B., Bygren, L. O., & Johansson, S. E. (2000). Visiting the cinema, concerts, museums or art exhibitions as determinant of survival: a Swedish fourteen-year cohort follow-up. *Scand J Public Health*, 28, 174–8.

Laaksonen, A. (2011). Creative partnerships: intersections between the arts, culture and other sectors. a discussion paper prepared for the 5th World Summit on Arts & Culture Melbourne, 3–6 October, 2011. *IFACCA D'art Report*, (41).

Lankston, L., Cusack, P., Fremantle, C., & Isles, C. (2010). Visual art in hospitals: case studies and review of the evidence. *J R Soc Med*, 103, 490–9.

Lederbogen, F., Kirsch, P., Haddad, L., *et al.* (2011). City living and urban upbringing affect neural social stress processing in humans. *Nature*, 474, 498–501.

LeDoux, J. (2000). Emotion circuits in the brain. *Annu Rev Neurosci*, 23, 155–84.

Lepage, C., Drolet, P., Girard, M., Grenier, Y., & DeGagné, R. (2001). Music decreases sedative requirements during spinal anesthesia. *Anesth Analg*, 93, 912–16.

Levinson, A., Acocella, J. R., & Garafola, L. (1991). *André Levinson on Dance: Writings From Paris in the Twenties.* Middletown, CT: Wesleyan University Press.

Lutz, A., Slagter, H. A., Dunne, J. D., & Davidson, R. J. (2008). Attention regulation and monitoring in meditation. *Trends Cogn Sci*, 12, 163–9.

Malinowski, P. (2013). Neural mechanisms of attentional control in mindfulness meditation. *Front Neurosci*, 7, 8.

Marchand, W. R. (2014). Neural mechanisms of mindfulness and meditation: evidence from neuroimaging studies. *World J Radiol*, 6, 471.

McCaffrey, R. (2007). The effect of healing gardens and art therapy on older adults with mild to moderate depression. *Holistic Nurs Pract*, 21, 79–84.

Mehling, W. E., Price, C., Daubenmier, J. J., Acree, M., Bartmess, E., & Stewart, A. (2012). The multidimensional assessment of interoceptive awareness (MAIA). *PLoS One*, 7, e48230.

Moore, A. & Malinowski, P. (2009). Meditation, mindfulness and cognitive flexibility. *Conscious Cogn*, 18, 176–86.

Mårtensson, F., Boldemann, C., Söderström, M., Blennow, M., Englund, J. E., & Grahn, P. (2009). Outdoor environmental assessment of attention promoting settings for preschool children. *Health Place*, 15, 1149–157.

Neff, K. D. (2011). Self-compassion, self-esteem, and well-being. *Soc Pers Psychol Compass*, 5, 1–12.

Neff, K. D. & Vonk, R. (2009). Self-compassion versus global self-esteem: Two different ways of relating to oneself. *J Pers*, 77, 23–50.

Ricard, M., Lutz, A., & Davidson, R. J. (2014). Mind of the meditator. *Scientific American*, 311(5), 38–45.

Stenfors, C., Magnusson Hanson, L., Oxenstierna, G., Theorell, T., & Nilsson, L. G. (2013). Psychosocial working conditions and cognitive complaints among Swedish employees. *PloS One*, 8, e60637.

Taylor, R. P., Spehar, B., Van Donkelaar, P., & Hagerhall, C. M. (2014). Perceptual and physiological responses to Jackson Pollock's fractals. *Brain and Art*, 43.

Theorell, T. (2014). *Psychological Health Effects of Musical Experiences: Theories, Studies and Reflections in Music Health Science.* Berlin, Germany: Springer Science and Business.

Theorell, T., Osika, W., Leineweber, C., Hanson, L. L. M., Horwitz, E. B., and Westerlund, H. (2013). Is cultural activity at work related to mental health in employees? *Int Arch Occup Environ Health*, 86, 281–8.

Thoreau, H. D. (1854/1997). *Walden*. Fender, S. (ed.) Oxford, UK: Oxford University Press.

Varela, F. J., Thompson, E., & Rosch, E. (1992). *The Embodied Mind.* CogNet. Available at: http://cognet.mit.edu/ [Online].

Viding, C. G., Osika, W., Theorell, T., Kowalski, J., Hallqvist, J., & Horwitz, E. B. (2015). "The Culture palette"-a randomized intervention study for women with burnout symptoms in Sweden. *Br J Med Practitioners*, 8, a813.

Wallace, B. A. (2009). *Contemplative Science: Where Buddhism and Neuroscience Converge.* New York, NY: Columbia University Press.

Wikström, B. M., Theorell, T., & Sandström, S. (1993). Medical health and emotional effects of art stimulation in old age. *Psychother Psychosom*, 60, 195–206.

Wilkinson, A. V., Waters, A. J., Bygren, L. O., & Tarlov, A. R. (2007). Are variations in rates of attending cultural activities associated with population health in the United States? *BMC Public Health*, 7, 226.

Zajonc, A. (2009). *Meditation as Contemplative Inquiry: When Knowing Becomes Love.* Herndon VA: Lindisfarne Books.

Zhang, J. W., Piff, P. K., Iyer, R., Koleva, S., & Keltner, D. (2014). An occasion for unselfing: beautiful nature leads to prosociality. *J Environ Psychol*, 37, 61–72.

SECTION 5

Public health impact of varied landscapes and environments

The great outdoors: forests, wilderness, and public health

Qing Li and Simon Bell

Definitions of forest and wilderness

In many ways, forests and wilderness areas represent the places which are most different from and offer the greatest contrast to the urban environment where the majority of the population live. But what exactly is a forest? To most people it is probably an area of land covered in trees and other woody vegetation. The Food and Agriculture Organization (FAO) of the United Nations defines it as 'land area of more than 0.5 ha, with a tree canopy cover of more than 10%, which is not primarily under agricultural or other specific non-forest land use' (FAO).

The use of the word 'forest' in English may convey a different meaning and etymology to that from other languages. In English, however, it comes from the Latin term 'forestis silva' meaning the woodland (silva) outside (forestis), in this case meaning outside civilisation—the wild, untamed places used for hunting and by outlaws (such as the legendary Robin Hood). These forests are also the settings for fairy tales and are often scary places to be avoided in myth and legend (Harrison, 1992; Schama, 1995). Such cultural associations are still strong and affect our relationship with forests to this day.

A further aspect of the relationship of forests to civilisation is provided by Giambattista Vico's writing in the eighteenth century, in his *Scienza Nuova* (*New Science*). He claimed: 'This is the order of human institutions: first, the forests, after that the huts, then the villages, next the cities, and finally the academies' (Vico, 1725).

This provides a metaphor for the human relationship with forests which were, and continue to be, cleared to make way for agriculture which has enabled civilisations to arise and so to develop into the urban-dominated environment of today. However, it also suggests that we have a historic relationship with forests which, apart from supplying timber fuel and forage, also provide us with other values—spiritual, aesthetic, or recreational, for example (Bell and Ward Thompson, 2013).

This link with the natural world has been recognized as important for urban dwellers for as long as cities have existed, it would seem; as reflected in Martial's concept of *rus in urbe* in ancient Roman times and in mediaeval discussions of the virtues of access to green and wooded landscapes for good health (Ward Thompson, 2011) (Fig. 5.1.1).

Forests are not homogeneous places and there are different categories which have different potentials and possibilities for human engagement and for playing a role in human health and well-being (Bell and Ward Thompson, 2013).

1. Firstly, there are protected 'natural' forests, variously categorized as reserves, wilderness areas, or parks. These present possibilities to escape from cities and for unmediated, direct contact with nature—perhaps 'red in tooth and claw'.

2. Secondly, there are vast areas of managed natural forests, which may be old primary growth or mainly second growth, and which may be managed under industrial conditions primarily for timber or under multiple-objective regimes. If accessible through road systems, these provide many opportunities for walking, cycling, and skiing, even if the aesthetic quality may not be very high.

3. Thirdly, there are countries and regions where historical clearances of forests for agriculture and urban expansion have led to more recent reforestation programmes, initially for timber production but increasingly to provide multipurpose forests for a wide range of social and ecological purposes. These may seem more artificial to many people, and not as natural as the previously described forms, but may represent a major resource for outdoor access in some countries.

4. Fourthly, there are forests close to or within urban areas. These may be tracts of forest which were protected in some way, such as former hunting parks or forests that have become incorporated into the urban fabric, or they may be areas specially planted to benefit the urban population. These can be under significant pressure from numbers of people and may seem less 'natural' owing to the external influences, such as urban sights and noise, or level of provision of facilities.

What is wilderness? In conceptual terms the description provided by the WILD Foundation (2014) sums it up:

- 'A place that is mostly biologically intact; and,

- A place that is legally protected so that it remains wild, and free of industrial infrastructure, and open to traditional indigenous use, or low impact recreation.'

The foundation goes on to say: 'The essence of a wilderness area is that it is a place where humans can maintain a relationship with wild nature. Whether that relationship is characterized by recreational use or traditional, indigenous use does not matter, so long

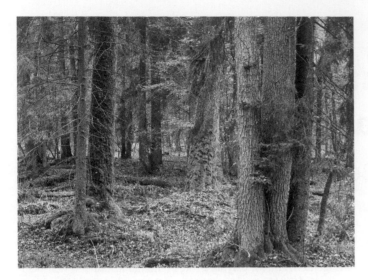

Fig. 5.1.1 Białowieża National Park in Eastern Poland is a large tract of what may be as close to the original primaeval forest in Europe as it is possible to get, complete with large herbivores such as the European bison.
Image courtesy of Simon Bell.

as the relationship is predicated on a fundamental respect for—and appreciation of—wild nature' (The WILD Foundation, 2014).

There are also various definitions as to how an area can be identified or designated as a wilderness—for example being 7 km from a road of any sort. In some countries, such as Scotland, in the United Kingdom, the term 'wildland' is used, since according to the strict definition there is no wilderness (Scottish Natural Heritage, 2014) or in the US Forest Service where wilderness areas are a special land use category (US Forest Service, 2014).

Wilderness as an idea was very much promoted by the early conservationist John Muir in his Wilderness Discovery books. In 1901 he wrote: 'Thousands of tired, nerve shaken, overcivilised people are beginning to find that going to the mountains is going home; that wilderness is a necessity; and that mountain parks and reserves are useful not only as fountains of timber and invigorating rivers but as fountains of life' (Muir, 1901) which we can easily see is an early recognition of the value of nature for restoring ourselves and overcoming stress.

Visiting wilderness and forest areas, including mountains, started in the Romantic era, at the turn of the eighteenth and nineteenth centuries, with the inspiration of the poets, writers, and painters such as Turner and Wordsworth attracted to the sublime qualities of the English Lake District (Bell, 2012). The American national parks were also selected for their sublime qualities following the inspiration of John Muir and the Sierra Club.

More recently, the view of wilderness as remote, untouched places has been challenged with the emergence of ideas of wilderness as being associated with processes of natural vegetation colonization and development. Ingo Kovarik and Stefan Körner (2005) describe the 'four natures approach', where the first nature is the primaeval type before human settlement; the second nature is the cleared agricultural landscape; the third nature is the designed park; and the fourth nature is the re-colonization of urban areas in the post-industrial era. Kovarik recently argued for the wilderness quality of abandoned areas in Berlin, for example (Kovarik,

2013). The sublime qualities of urban wilderness have also been explored recently (Unt *et al.*, 2013). This is significant for this chapter's theme, as there may be aspects of health associated with urban wilderness, as well as 'true' wilderness.

However, while quite simple terms, these may mean different things to different people or in different cultures (read more in Chapter 6.4 about cultural influences on nature experience). Nowadays, since the majority of the terrestrial surface of the globe has been affected in one way or another by human activity, truly wild areas, in the sense that they are untouched by human activity or are free from human elements, are very rare indeed. Nevertheless, there are many environments which are *relatively* free from human intervention or elements and which *appear* to be wild.

This chapter will present and discuss the current state of evidence for the health benefits of forests and wilderness. Given the fast moving state of research, we will refer to a number of recent or ongoing projects whose results may not be fully documented, although they will be referenced. Some specific projects will also be highlighted which relate to some particular aspect, target group, or research method.

Public health aspects of forests and wilderness: theories and concepts

Human engagement with—or disengagement from—forests and wilderness clearly goes back a long way. In the context of urbanized societies in Western societies we might be less concerned with the contribution that forests may make to the basic requirements of survival and more with what Abraham Maslow and others have termed 'higher level' needs in a kind of 'hierarchy of needs' (Maslow, 1954). These needs are associated with well-being, fulfilment, and pleasure. However, in developing parts of the world, forests are still important assets for provisioning (e.g. timber supply) and regulating (e.g. climate regulation) ecosystem services and needs.

Engagement with forests and wilderness for health and well-being can be direct or indirect, active or passive, external (viewing the forest as part of the landscape) or internal (being within it), or a combination of these (Bell and Ward Thompson, 2013). This section refers to a selection of theories which have been used to frame, explain, or support the research evidence to be presented later. This provides a complement to Chapter 2.1, which gives a full overview of theories of environmental psychology.

We have to start from how we engage with an environment—a forest or wilderness—and this is through our senses. Perception of the environment and its subsequent or concurrent association with other experiences, our mood, cultural background, and so on depends on our sensory apparatus—sight, smell, taste, sound, and the haptic senses (touch, temperature, humidity, and so on). In part, this provides us with aesthetic experiences—the pleasure of beauty or the powerful feeling of the sublime—which is one aspect at the heart of obtaining a positive psychological benefit.

A sublime experience occurs when our senses are swamped by the magnitude of a landscape that is difficult to comprehend and which suggests limitlessness (Bell, 2012). The imagination and capacity for judgement are also overwhelmed by this impression, in a similar way to trying to comprehend the notion of the infinity of the universe. This is usually the initial feeling experienced by many people on first visiting the Rocky Mountains or standing on a cliff while a storm surges in the sea beneath us. We tend to feel very small, humble and helpless in the face of the scale of these scenes or the awesome power of processes such as storms. The feeling of potential, but not actual, danger gives the experience an extra sharpness, such as might be felt when looking over the parapet into the depths of the Grand Canyon. This psychological response may be one way in which we are able to gain a sense of perspective when we are stressed or feeling overwhelmed by problems.

The ecological theory of perception (Gibson, 1979) roots environmental preferences in the context of 'affordances'. The concept of affordances is very powerful (Heft, 2010) and offers a way into understanding how the different aspects of landscapes—in this case forests and wilderness—provide different individuals or user groups with possibilities for use, which may be much wider than the obvious purposes for which the areas are managed (such as timber production or biodiversity protection) (Bell, 2010). If we take two different groups, children/young people and older people, the affordances for physical activity of a specific forest for one group may be different than for the other—children may clamber on rocks, which are more suited for sitting on by an older person, for example.

Theories on the 'restorative' effects of natural environments apply to our understanding of the impacts of forests and wilderness on our well-being. These theories are presented in Chapter 2.1.

Physiological aspects of health in forests and wilderness: the research evidence

The forest environment has long been enjoyed for its quiet atmosphere, beautiful scenery, calm climate, pleasant aromas, and clean fresh air. Forest settings may reduce stress and have a relaxing effect.

Although theories and the data on physiological effects support the notion of forests as health promoting, most studies only compare the effect between forest environments and urban environments. There is still a lack of comparison of the effects of forest environments with other natural environments, and the evidence of forests as unique environments for specific health effects is scarce.

In this section, we review studies on the physiological effects of forests and wilderness. Much research on nature and health refers to stress relief as a pathway. Several studies have been conducted in forest environments, investigating effects on the neuroendocrine immune system.

Researchers in for example Japan have tried to identify the preventive effect of forests and wilderness on lifestyle-related diseases and have proposed a new concept called *Shinrin-yoku* or 'forest bathing' (Li *et al.*, 2007). A forest bathing trip is a short leisurely visit to a forest, for the purpose of relaxation (*shinrin* means forest and *yoku* means bathing in Japanese) (Li *et al.*, 2007; Li, 2012). Forest bathing as a relaxation and/or stress management activity and a method of preventing disease and promoting health is now gaining increased public attention in Japan (Li, 2012). Forest environments have been shown to produce various effects on the neuroendocrine immune system in comparison with urban environments (Li, 2012), although we cannot, with certainty, rule out that

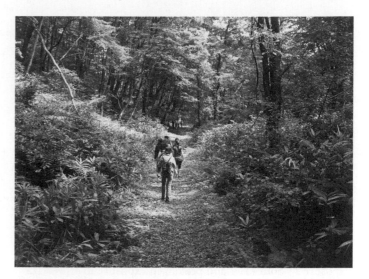

Fig. 5.2.2 Japanese subjects partaking in Shinrin-yoku in a forest, within a study to test its effects on the physiological health of people.
Image courtesy of Qing Li.

the same would apply for another natural environment or another type of relaxing exposure (Fig. 5.2.2).

Effects of forests and wilderness on the autonomous nervous system

Cortisol and other common biomarkers of stress

As described in Chapter 1.4, the autonomous nervous system affects the endocrine and immune systems by releasing neurotransmitters through the hypothalamus. Further on, through transmission and feedback loops, the endocrine system affects the nervous and immune systems by secreting hormones. Moreover, the immune system feeds back to the nervous and endocrine systems through cytokines.

Forest environments act on the endocrine system to reduce stress hormone levels showing stress recovery effects. Its potential for stress management deserves further clarification and attention. It has been reported that in comparison with urban environments, visiting forest environments can reduce sympathetic and increase parasympathetic nervous activity, as demonstrated by reduced blood pressure, heart rate, salivary, and blood cortisol (Park *et al.*, 2010; Tsunetsugu *et al.*, 2010; Lee *et al.*, 2011; Li *et al.*, 2011; Song *et al.*, 2015). These effects may influence health via the neuroendocrine immune system, inducing a reduction in urinary dopamine, adrenaline, and/or noradrenaline and an enhancement in natural killer (NK) cell activity in peripheral blood (Li *et al.*, 2007; 2008ab; 2009; 2010; Li and Kawada, 2011; Li, 2012).

Gen-Xiang Mao and colleagues (2012) reported that forest bathing has therapeutic effects on hypertension in older people and induces inhibition of the renin-angiotensin system and inflammation, thus aiding its preventive efficacy against cardiovascular disorders. Moreover, Chorong Song and colleagues (2013) found that there are individual differences in blood pressure after forest bathing between type A and type B behaviour patterns and that type B showed more of an effect than type A. Recently, Hiroko Ochiai and colleagues (2015) pointed out that spending time in a forest is a promising treatment strategy for reducing and maintaining blood pressure at an optimal range and possibly preventing a progression to clinical hypertension in middle-aged males with normal to high blood pressure.

Forests protect health through increased adiponectin and dehydroepiandrosterone sulphate (DHEA-S)

Adiponectin is a serum protein hormone produced by adipose tissue with for example cardio-protective, anti-obesity, and anti-diabetic properties (Bjørnerem et al., 2004). Low levels of serum adiponectin are associated with several metabolic disorders (Simpson and Singh, 2008). Dehydroepiandrosterone sulphate (DHEA-S) is an immunoprotective steroid hormone (Bauer, 2005; Buford and Willoughby, 2008) which has been related to higher levels of resilience (Morgan Iii et al., 2009; Petros et al., 2013), and protects against the damaging effects of excessive cortisol excretion (do Vale et al., 2011). DHEA-S levels decline after exposure to both brief and prolonged exposure to stress (Izawa et al., 2012).

Forest environments have been found to significantly increase both serum adiponectin and DHEA-S levels in comparison with urban environments (Li et al., 2011). However, forest environments do not appear to affect serum estradiol and progesterone levels in females, or serum insulin, free triiodothyronine, and thyroid-stimulating hormone levels in males (Li, 2012).

Effects of forests and wilderness on the immune system and cancer

The immune system, including NK cells, plays an important role in bodily defence against bacteria, viruses, and tumours. People with higher NK activity have shown a lower incidence of cancers, and vice versa (Imai et al., 2000). In comparison to urban environments, forests have been shown to act directly on the immune system by increasing the number of NK cells and intracellular levels of anticancer proteins, such as perforin, granulysin, and granzymes in both male and female subjects. The increased NK activity has been shown to last for more than 30 days after a trip to a forest (Li et al., 2007; 2008a; 2008b; 2010; Li and Kawada, 2011). This suggests that a forest bathing trip once a month may promote a higher level of NK activity and consequently have a preventive effect on cancer. Conversely, taking an urban trip has not been shown to increase human NK activity or the expression of selected intracellular antcancer proteins. perforin, granulysin, and granzymes A/B, indicating that the increased NK activity effect of a forest bathing trip is not mediated by physical activity and the trip itself, but may be particularly due to the forest environment (Li et al., 2008a).

Furthermore, stress hormones inhibit immune function (Li et al., 2005) and since forest environments seem to reduce stress hormone levels, it may be that forest environments also indirectly act on the immune system to increase NK activity as mediated by reduced levels of stress hormones (Li, 2010; 2012).

Research has shown an association between living in areas with lower forest coverage and higher standardized mortality ratios (SMRs) of cancer. Additionally, there are significant inverse correlations between the percentage of forest coverage and the SMRs of lung, breast, and uterine cancers in females, and the SMRs of prostate, kidney, and colon cancers in males in all prefectures in Japan,

even after controlling for the effects of smoking and socioeconomic status (Li et al., 2008c).

Effects of forests and wilderness on lifestyle-related diseases

Stress is one factor contributing to increased prevalence of many lifestyle-related diseases, such as hypertension, ischaemic heart disease, gastrointestinal ulcer, and depression (see Chapter 1.4). As exposure to forest environments has been associated with reduced stress levels, they may have a preventive effect on such disorders. In addition, Yoshinori Ohtsuka and colleagues (1998) reported that forest walking can reduce blood glucose levels in diabetic patients. Moreover, forest bathing has been associated with decreased scores for anxiety, depression, anger, fatigue, and confusion, and also increased feelings of vigour (Li and Kawada, 2014).

Taken together, when compared with the urban environment, forests may produce various beneficial physiological effects on human health through the neuro-endocrine-immune system and therefore contribute to disease prevention. At the moment it is considered to be a combined effect of non-specific and specific responses to forest environments and forest bathing.

Physical activity benefits associated with forests and wilderness: the research evidence

As presented earlier and elsewhere in this book (Chapter 3.1), the sedentary lifestyle of modern Western societies contributes to the epidemics of obesity and poor cardiovascular health. Motivating people to be more physically active is a central but challenging public health task. Part of the obstacle in doing so may be due to unhealthy environments or barriers such as costs or accessibility of places in which to exercise. Urban and peri-urban forests may play a certain role in this context, due to their accessibility to large parts of the population.

A forest may provide a pleasant ambience for physical activity and, if it is large enough, it can accommodate a range of different forms of recreation which promote physical health, mental restoration, and aesthetic pleasure all at once. Research on local woodland use by communities in Scotland showed that the predominant use is for walking and cycling (Ward Thompson et al., 2004; 2005). Compared with streets or small open spaces, forests provide an environment with less pollution, cleaner air to breathe while exercising, and potentially also the beneficial effects of aromatic hydrocarbons. However, the specific benefits of forests are yet not elucidated and more studies are needed.

Cultural differences in using forests and wilderness

In countries with a strong cultural association with forests, such as Finland, forests may be the location of choice for outdoor recreation and exercise and children are brought up able to ski cross-country and be comfortable with the forest environment. This familiarity means that they frequently develop the habit of visiting forests and gain multiple benefits from this (Bell and Ward Thompson, 2013). In other countries where there is less forest and a reduced cultural connection forests may be less attractive, thus people use them less frequently as noted in a division of Europe into 'forest culture' zones (Bell et al., 2005).

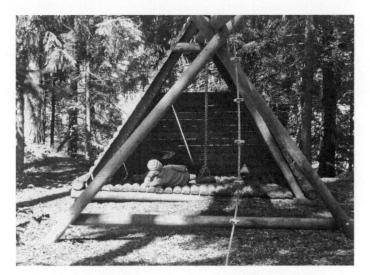

Fig. 5.3.3 A forest kindergarten in Austria. The children here spend each day outside and benefit from close contact with nature. Advocates of such kindergartens claim that the children benefit physiologically—by building up their immune system, physically, through constant activity and psychologically, by being in close contact with nature.

Image courtesy of Simon Bell.

Another aspect of this is that when the familiarity with forest environments is low, the perceived risks may prevent people from visiting them. Fear of crime, of being attacked, or getting lost may be a major barrier, especially to women in some urban woodlands, while children may be discouraged or prevented from playing in woods owing to safety concerns (Ward Thompson *et al.*, 2004). However, introducing children to forests and wilder areas at an early age seems to help them to become accustomed to such landscapes and may provide a range of benefits of the types described here which are retained throughout their lives. Forest kindergartens and forest schools are proving increasingly popular and help to overcome barriers (Fig. 5.3.3). Read more about risks and risk perception in interactions with nature in Chapter 7.4.

Barriers preventing physical activity in forests and wilderness

Assuming that recreation in forests and wilderness areas is associated with elevated levels of physical activity and thus better health, physical barriers need to be considered in research. Forests and wild places are by their nature the least tamed environments and are found in sometimes inhospitable but usually rough and challenging terrain. Research with physically disabled people and deaf or hearing impaired people in Scotland (Bell *et al.*, 2006; Bell, 2007) concerning access to forests and wild areas shows that members of these groups want to visit them and appreciate the special qualities of being out in nature away from their normally restricted home environments. Facilitating aspects such as information, trail quality, parking, and toilet facilities are more important to them. If the facilities are there they will, to a greater extent, visit and obtain the associated benefits (OPENspace, 2007).

Even if the benefits of increased physical activity in forests and wilderness are demonstrated to be positive to a statistically significant degree, there is as yet no information as to how much of this environmental 'dose' is adequate to achieve the benefits.

Psychological benefits associated with forests and wilderness: the research evidence

Mental health benefits from activity in forests and wilderness

An epidemiological study of a large, general population sample from across Scotland has shown that physical activity in natural environments is associated with a reduction in the risk of poor mental health to a greater extent than physical activity in other environments, and that regular users of woodlands or forests for physical activity were at about half the risk of poor mental health of non-users (although a large part of the effect was attributed to the physical activity itself) (Mitchell, 2012).

Forest settings have also been shown to benefit children and adolescents, especially those with behavioural problems and mental disorders who can be highly disruptive in conventional school settings. A comparative study with children aged from 10 to 13 years showed that the forest setting was advantageous to mood in all behaviour groups, but particularly in those children suffering from a 'mental disorder' (Roe and Aspinall, 2011a). Detailed analysis of a small group of children with severe behavioural problems illustrated how the forest setting offered opportunities for curiosity, creativity, exploration, and challenge, opportunities largely missing in these young people's lives to date, and how the setting allowed therapeutic processes to occur naturally, without professional intervention (Roe and Aspinall, 2011b). Read more about forest-based and other nature-based interventions in Chapter 4.1.

Forest medicine has emerged as a new interdisciplinary science area and become a focus of public attention. Forest medicine belongs to the categories of alternative, environmental, and preventive medicine and is the study of the effects of forest environments on human health (Li, 2012). It may contribute to establish a new preventive strategy on lifestyle-related diseases and cancers.

Conclusion

Taken together, from the evidence discussed in this chapter we can make the following conclusions:

1. In comparison with urban environments, forest and wilderness can decrease indicators of sympathetic nervous activity, such as blood pressure, heart rate, and levels of stress hormones, for example urinary adrenaline and noradrenaline. In addition, forests seem to increase parasympathetic nervous activity.

2. In comparison with urban environments, forest and wilderness can increase the activity and number of human NK cells and the intracellular levels of anticancer proteins, suggesting it has a preventive effect on cancers.

3. In comparison with urban environments, forests and wilderness can decrease scores for anxiety, depression, anger, fatigue, and confusion and increase vigour, showing psychological benefits, suggesting a potential for preventing mental disorders.

4. Forests and wilderness also show some physical activity benefits contributing to health promotion.

5. The preventive effects of forest and wilderness should be confirmed by further interdisciplinary and clinical studies in order to clarify the health benefits.

6. Further studies comparing the effects of forest and wilderness with other natural environments or restorative settings are also necessary.

Acknowledgements

This work was supported in part by the Council for Science, Technology and Innovation (CSTI), Cross-ministerial Strategic Innovation Promotion Program (SIP), 'Technologies for creating next-generation agriculture, forestry and fisheries' (funding agency: Bio-oriented Technology Research Advancement Institution, NARO).

References

Bauer, M. E. (2005). Stress, glucocorticoids and ageing of the immune system. *Stress*, 8, 69–83.

Bell, S. (2007). Accessibility and Disability: Making Woods More Accessible Edinburgh, OPENspace report for the Forestry Commission: 13.

Bell, S. (2010) Challenges for research in landscape and health. In: Ward Thompson, C., Aspinall, P., and Bell, S. (Eds) *Innovative approaches to researching landscape and health*. Abingdon, UK: Routledge.

Bell, S. (2012). *Landscape: Pattern, Perception and Process*, 2nd edition. Abingdon, UK: Routledge.

Bell, S. & Ward Thompson, C. (2013). Human engagement with forest environments: implications for physical and mental health and wellbeing. In: Fenning, T. (ed.) *Challenges and Opportunities for the World's Forests in the 21st Century*. Berlin, Germany: Springer Verlag.

Bell, S., Blom, D., Rautamaki, M., Castel-Branco, C, Simson, S., & Olsen, E. A. (2005). Design of urban forests. In: Konijnendijk, C., Nilsson, K, Randrup, T. B., & Schipperijn, J. (eds). *Urban Forests and Trees*. Berlin, Germany: Springer Verlag.

Bell, S., Findlay, C., & Montarzino, A.; OPENspace Research Centre (2006). Access to the countryside by deaf visitors. Scottish Natural Heritage Commissioned Report No. 171(ROAME No. F03AB05).

Bjørnerem, A., Straume, B., Midtby, M., et al. (2004). Endogenous sex hormones in relation to age, sex, lifestyle factors, and chronic diseases in a general population: The Tromso Study. *J Clin Endocrinol Metab*, 89, 6039–47.

Buford, T. W. & Willoughby, D. S. (2008). Impact of DHEA(S) and cortisol on immune function in aging: a brief review. *Appl Physiol Nutr Metab*, 33, 429–33.

Gibson, J.J. (1979). *The ecological approach to visual perception*. New York, NY: Houghton Mifflin.

Harrison, R. P. (1992). *Forests: The Shadow of Civilization*. Chicago, IL: University of Chicago Press.

Heft, H. (2010) Affordances and the perception of landscape: an inquiry into environmental perception and aesthetics. In: Ward Thompson, C., Aspinall, P., and Bell, S. (Eds) *Innovative approaches to researching landscape and health*. Abingdon, UK: Routledge.

Imai, K., Matsuyama, S., Miyake, S., Suga, K., & Nakachi, K. (2000). Natural cytotoxic activity of peripheral-blood lymphocytes and cancer incidence: an 11-year follow-up study of a general population. *Lancet*, 356, 1795–9.

Izawa, S., Saito, K., Shirotsuki, K., Sugaya, N., & Nomura, S. (2012). Effects of prolonged stress on salivary cortisol and dehydroepiandrosterone: a study of a two-week teaching practice. *Psychoneuroendocrinology*, 37, 852–8.

Kovarik, I. (2013). Cities and wilderness: a new perspective. *Int J Wilderness*, 19, 32–6.

Kovarik, I. & Körner, S. (2005). *Wild Urban Woodlands: New Perspective for Urban Forestry*. Berlin, Germany: Springer.

Lee, J., Park, B. J., Tsunetsugu, Y., Ohira, T., Kagawa, T., & Miyazaki, Y. (2011). Effect of forest bathing on physiological and psychological responses in young Japanese male subjects. *Public Health*, 125, 93–100.

Li, Q. (2010). Effect of forest bathing trips on human immune function. *Environ Health Prev Med*, 15, 9–17.

Li, Q. (2012). Forest medicine. In: Li Q (ed.) *Forest Medicine*, pp. 1–316. New York, NY: Nova Science Publishers, Inc.

Li, Q. & Kawada, T. (2011). Effect of forest environments on human natural killer (NK) activity. *Int J Immunopathol Pharmacol*, 24 (S1), 39–44.

Li, Q. & Kawada, T. (2014). The possibility of clinical applications of forest medicine. *Nihon Eiseigaku Zasshi*, 69, 117–21.

Li, Q., Liang, Z., Nakadai, A., & Kawada, T. (2005). Effect of electric foot shock and psychological stress on activities of murine splenic natural killer and lymphokine-activated killer cells, cytotoxic T lymphocytes, natural killer receptors and mRNA transcripts for granzymes and perforin. *Stress*, 8, 107–16.

Li, Q., Morimoto, K., Nakadai, A., et al. (2007). Forest bathing enhances human natural killer activity and expression of anti-cancer proteins. *Int J Immunopathol Pharmacol*, 20, 3–8.

Li, Q., Morimoto, K., Kobayashi, M., et al. (2008a). Visiting a forest, but not a city, increases human natural killer activity and expression of anti-cancer proteins. *Int J Immunopathol Pharmacol*, 21, 117–28.

Li, Q., Morimoto, K., Kobayashi, M., et al. (2008b). A forest bathing trip increases human natural killer activity and expression of anti-cancer proteins in female subjects. *J Biol Regul Homeost Agents*, 22, 45–55.

Li, Q., Kobayashi, M., & Kawada, T. (2008c). Relationships between percentage of forest coverage and standardized mortality ratios (SMR) of cancers in all prefectures in Japan. *The Open Public Health Journal*, 1, 1–7.

Li, Q., Kobayashi, M., Wakayama, Y., et al. (2009). Effect of phytoncide from trees on human natural killer cell function. *Int J Immunopathol Pharmacol*, 22(4), 951–9.

Li, Q., Kobayashi, M., Inagaki, H., et al. (2010). A day trip to a forest park increases human natural killer activity and the expression of anti-cancer proteins in male subjects. *J Biol Regul Homeost Agents*, 24, 157–65.

Li, Q., Otsuka, T., Kobayashi, M., et al. (2011). Acute effects of walking in forest environments on cardiovascular and metabolic parameters. *Eur J Appl Physiol*, 111, 2845–53.

Mao, G. X., Cao, Y. B., Lan, X. G., et al. (2012). Therapeutic effect of forest bathing on human hypertension in the elderly. *J Cardiol*, 60, 495–502.

Maslow, A. (1954). *Motivation and Personality*. New York, NY: Harper and Row.

Mitchell, R. (2012). Short report: Is physical activity in natural environments better for mental health than physical activity in other environments? *Soc Sci Med*, 91, 130–4.

Morgan, C. A. 3rd, Rasmusson, A., Pietrzak, R. H., Coric, V., & Southwick, S. M. (2009). Relationships among plasma dehydroepiandrosterone and dehydroepiandrosterone sulfate, cortisol, symptoms of dissociation, and objective performance in humans exposed to underwater navigation stress. *Biol Psychiatry*, 66, 334–40.

Muir, J. (1901). *The Eight Wilderness Discovery Books*. London, UK: Diadem Books.

Ochiai, H., Ikei, H., Song, C., et al. (2015). Physiological and psychological effects of forest therapy on middle-aged males with high-normal blood pressure. *Int J Environ Res Public Health*, 12, 2532–42.

Ohtsuka, Y., Yabunaka, N., & Takayama, S. (1998). Shinrin-yoku (forest-air bathing and walking) effectively decreases blood glucose levels in diabetic patients. *Int J Biometeorol*, 41, 125–7.

OPENspace (2007). Enhancing the Forest Sector's contribution to equal access for disabled people to recreation goods, facilities and services in Scottish Forests: Good practice examples of access to forests or countryside Edinburgh, UK. Report for Forestry Commission Scotland: 33.

Park, B. J., Tsunetsugu, Y., Kasetani, T., Kagawa, T., Miyazaki, Y. (2010). The physiological effects of Shinrin-yoku (taking in the forest atmosphere or forest bathing): evidence from field experiments in 24 forests across Japan. *Environ Health Prev Med*, 15, 18–26.

Petros, N., Opacka-Juffry, J., & Huber, J. H. (2013). Psychometric and neurobiological assessment of resilience in a non-clinical sample of adults. *Psychoneuroendocrinology*, 38, 2099–108.

Roe, J. & Aspinall, P. (2011a). The restorative outcomes of forest versus indoor settings in young people with varying behaviour states. *Urban For Urban Greening*, 10, 205–12.

Roe, J. & Aspinall, P. (2011b). The emotional affordances of forest settings: an investigation in boys with extreme behavioural problems. *Landsc Res*, 36, 535–52.

Schama, S. (1995). *Landscape and Memory*. New York, NY: Knopf.

Scottish Natural Heritage (2014). Available at: http://www.snh.gov.uk/protecting-scotlands-nature/looking-after-landscapes/landscape-policy-and-guidance/wild-land/ (accessed 16 July 2014) [Online].

Simpson, K. A. & Singh, M. A. (2008). Effects of exercise on adiponectin: a systematic review. *Obesity*, 16, 241–56.

Song, C., Ikei, H., Lee, J., Park, B. J., Kagawa, T., & Miyazaki, Y. (2013). Individual differences in the physiological effects of forest therapy based on Type A and Type B behavior patterns. *J Physiol Anthropol*, 32, 14.

Song, C., Ikei, H., Kobayashi, M., *et al.* (2015). Effect of forest walking on autonomic nervous system activity in middle-aged hypertensive individuals: a pilot study. *Int J Environ Res Public Health*, 12, 2687–99.

The WILD Foundation (2014). Available at: http://www.wild.org/main/how-wild-works/policy-research/what-is-a-wilderness-area/ (accessed 16 July 2014) [Online].

Tsunetsugu, Y., Park, B. J., & Miyazaki, Y. (2010). Trends in research related to "Shinrin-yoku" (taking in the forest atmosphere or forest bathing) in Japan. *Environ Health Prev Med*, 15, 27–37.

Unt, A.-L., Travlou, P., & Bell, S. (2013). Blank space: Exploring the sublime qualities of urban wilderness at the former fishing harbour in Tallinn, Estonia. *Landsc Res*, 39, 267–86.

U. S. Department of Health and Human Services (2008). 2008 Physical Activity Guidelines for Americans. Available at: https://www.health.gov/paguidelines (accessed 17 June 2014) [Online].

United States Forest Service (2014). Wilderness areas. Available at: http://www.fs.fed.us/recreation/programs/cda/wilderness.shtml (accessed 16 July 2014) [Online].

do Vale, S., Martin Martins, J., Fagundes, M. J., & do Carmo, I. (2011). Plasma dehydroepiandrosterone-sulphate is related to personality and stress response. *Neuro Endocrinol Lett*, 32, 442–8.

Vico, G. (1725) *Scienza Nuova* (the new Science). Napoli, Italy: Stamperia Museana.

Ward Thompson, C. (2011). Linking landscape and health: the recurring theme. *Landsc Urban Plan*, 99, 187–95.

Ward Thompson, C., Aspinall, P., Bell, S., Findlay, C., Wherrett, J. & Travlou, P. (2004) *Open Space and Social Inclusion: Local Woodland Use in Central Scotland*. Edinburgh, UK: Forestry Commission.

Ward Thompson, C., Aspinall, P., Bell, S., & Findlay, C. (2005) "It gets you away from everyday life": local woodlands and community use—what makes a difference? *Landsc Res*, 30, 109–46.

CHAPTER 5.2

Blue landscapes and public health

Mathew P. White, Rebecca Lovell, Benedict W. Wheeler, Sabine Pahl, Sebastian Völker, and Michael H. Depledge

A brief historical reflection

Water drives many of the environmental processes which support life on earth. For humans it is a truly fundamental determinant of health; we cannot survive for more than three to four days without access to water.

Beyond the necessity of water for biological function, humankind has valued water and blue elements of landscapes such as rivers, lakes, and the sea for their health-giving properties throughout history. The ancient Sumerian, Egyptian, and Greek civilizations prized water within landscapes, with places such as Epidaurus and its mineral springs becoming sites for healing, drawing in people from across the classical world.

Water was and is also crucial to many of the world's major religions. In the Islamic and Judeo-Christian traditions water plays an essential symbolic role. Consider for example customs such as the immersion of the body during baptisms for Christians and before marriage within Judaism, and ritual washing within Islam. These practices appear to have been incorporated in many modern day secular rituals too, for example annual lake and sea bathing events (Foley, 2011).

In Europe the notion of blue features within the landscapes as being healthful is evident in the practices of mediaeval Augustinian monks who viewed river walks as restorative activities, the siting of preventoria in the early twentieth century near rivers and lakes, and the taking of the sea air in the Victorian and Edwardian periods. Today, some of our most prized and beloved cultural artefacts, such as Constable's *The Haywain* and Monet's *Waterlillies*, depict watery landscapes and we spend much time and resources seeking our own salutogenic first-hand experiences of blue spaces.

However, despite the centrality of water to human culture, it is surprising that relatively little environment-health research has specifically considered 'blue' landscapes and how they may contribute positively to health and well-being (Völker and Kistemann, 2011).

This chapter aims to explore whether there is evidence that blue landscapes provide a specific positive contribution to human health and well-being. We outline four types of research that use quite different methodological approaches: (a) preference-based approaches; (b) experiential approaches; (c) experimental approaches; and d) quantitative spatial approaches (see Table 5.2.1).

The following sections briefly summarize selected work within each of these paradigms.

Preference-based approaches

Preference-based approaches fall into two broad categories; revealed preferences and stated preferences.

Revealed preferences are inferred from an individual's behaviour, in particular their willingness to pay to experience something (e.g. a blue landscape view). It is assumed the more they are willing to pay, the more utility (i.e. well-being) they must derive from it. This approach has been used to analyse house prices and hotel room rates, and confirms that, all else being equal, people are willing to pay between 10% and 15% more for similar homes/rooms with water views (Luttik, 2000; Lange and Schaeffer, 2001).

Stated preferences refer to what people say they like. For instance, when asked openly about the features of landscapes they like, or when asked to rate specific images or photographs, people often prefer blue landscapes including rivers, lakes, and the sea (see e.g. Herzog, 1985). Put simply, people reveal their preferences, without needing to state them, through their choices.

Building on this earlier work, some of the authors of this chapter used a stated preference approach in a series of studies exploring preferences for blue landscapes in more detail, including both rural and urban landscapes. This research demonstrated a higher preference for urban landscapes containing water (e.g. images of Amsterdam) than when they saw urban landscapes without water. Moreover, these preferences for urban water scenes were not significantly different from rural landscapes without water, suggesting that urban landscapes could be significantly enhanced by the addition of aquatic elements (White et al., 2010). These findings were replicated using black and white images of the same landscapes (White et al., 2014a). This was important because there is evidence that the colour blue is preferred, even in isolation (Palmer and Schloss, 2010), and thus eliminating the colour blue from the images allowed for the exploration of preferences independent of colour.

Despite these generally positive findings for water landscapes using preference approaches, we also note several boundary conditions such as the effect of visible environmental degradation. Margo Wilson and colleagues (1995), for instance, manipulated images of

Table 5.2.1 Approaches to exploring the relationships between blue landscapes and public health

	Preference-based approach	Experiential approach	Experimental approach	Quantitative spatial approach
Main research questions	Which (blue) landscapes do people like/dislike?	How do people feel when they spend time in (real) blue landscapes?	What are the relative benefits of different types of blue landscape compared to other settings?	Are there cumulative health and well-being benefits from living near blue landscapes?
Methods (examples)	Revealed preferences (e.g. house prices). Stated preferences (e.g. photo ratings).	Post visit surveys and interviews. Experience sampling (*in situ*).	Controlled comparison of reactions to different environmental settings. Often have a stress induction to explore 'restorative' properties of blue space.	Analysis of large datasets where health data has been merged with and geographical information based on residence. Exploration of mechanisms such as physical activity.

blue landscapes to include various indicators of poor quality such as surface foam and algal blooms. As predicted, people were less willing to visit the contaminated versions of the scenes. Blue landscapes might be particularly vulnerable to contamination or littering impacts because any signs of contamination to water might be indicative of broader threats to health and well-being. Researching boundary conditions such as these is important because current levels of marine litter and other forms of pollution are often very high.

A further boundary condition is weather. In one study, we presented participants with images of landscapes with and without water under either sunny conditions or cloudy/rainy conditions (White *et al.*, 2014b). Blue landscapes were highest in preference ratings compared to landscapes without water, even under inclement weather conditions. However, the difference between cloudy and sunny conditions was significantly greater for blue landscapes than for either rural or urban environments without water. This means that preferences for blue landscapes seem to be relatively more sensitive to weather conditions. Along with the contaminated water studies, the findings remind us that we should be careful in extrapolating from research which exposes people to idealized versions of blue landscapes in laboratory conditions. Further, they also highlight the need for protecting the quality and integrity of blue landscapes for public health beyond simply the quality of drinking water, focusing also on the importance of blue landscape aesthetics.

In sum, the results of many decades of preference-based work suggest that people like being near (clean) blue landscapes. If such preferences are justified, then we should see tangible benefits to health and well-being following specific instances of exposure to these settings and among those with ready access to such environments.

The experiential and experimental approaches both hypothesize that there should be demonstrable benefits to health and well-being from specific exposures to blue landscapes, and the quantitative spatial approach assumes that such benefits will be cumulative and thus those who live near blue landscapes should be healthier and happier than those who live further away.

Experiential approaches

Experiential studies take several forms but have, at their heart, the aim of collating people's lived experiences in different landscapes, thus providing insight into the health and health behaviour-related choices people make. Some studies have asked people to recollect recent visits to blue, and other, landscapes and say how they felt or what they did (e.g. Barton and Pretty, 2010; Korpela *et al.*, 2010; White *et al.*, 2013a). In others, more in-depth and open-ended surveys and/or interviews are used to explore experiences of freshwater or coastal landscapes (Völker and Kistemann, 2013; Ashbullby *et al.*, 2013). Finally, developing communication technology is allowing researchers to ask people how they are feeling *in situ* across a range of settings including blue landscapes (MacKerron and Mourato, 2013).

In one study, Kalevi Korpela and his colleagues (2010) surveyed over a thousand Finnish people about their 'favourite' places within 15 km of their homes to examine the extent to which visiting these places helped respondents feel 'restored', contrary to stress associated with the hustle and bustle of modern life. The three types of favourite place that were associated with the highest restoration scores were exercise/activity areas (e.g. playing fields), extensively managed nature areas, and waterside environments. We extended these findings in the United Kingdom by showing that coastal environments in particular may be especially good at promoting restorative experiences, at least when people are asked to reflect upon a specific visit made in the last week (White *et al.*, 2013b). Thus when asked to recall how they feel in general about visiting certain places, or about a specific visit, blue landscapes are among those associated with the most positive memories.

A similar conclusion emerged from a different approach adopted by Jo Barton and Jules Pretty (2010). These researchers monitored people's experiences of activities in different natural environments. The overall picture suggested that just a single experience of contact with nature did significantly improve both mood and self-esteem. Of particular importance here was the finding that '*for both measures, waterside habitats showed the greatest changes*'.

While Barton and Pretty monitored psychological states *before and after* the visit, George MacKerron and Susana Mourato (2013) measured emotional states *during* the visit. They applied a mobile phone app (www.mappiness.co.uk) that used an *experience sampling approach* to 'beep' people over the course of the day to ask them what they were doing, who they were with, and how they felt. Using over one million responses from over 20,000 participants the researchers used geolocation to pin-point exactly where participants were based on the phone signals. Controlling for a host of variables such as weather, companions, activities, and individual level fixed effects, the findings suggested that people were 'happiest' in 'marine and coastal margins'. The next 'happiest' environment was uplands (mountains/moorlands/heaths).

Other studies have used interpretivist approaches to explore the health-related 'affordances' of blue landscapes in more depth. Katherine J. Ashbullby and colleagues (Ashbullby *et al.*, 2013), for instance, interviewed parents and children about their trips to a beach. One particularly strong recurring theme was the way in which spending time at the beach was seen as 'good quality family time' where parents and children played together. As one 11-year-old boy put it: 'Instead of the adults just sitting somewhere on a bench while the kids do activities they get up and they play Frisbee or cricket and football and sometimes go swimming with them.'

Simon Bell and colleagues (2015) also considered the value of blue spaces using in-depth interview techniques, and found that participants expressed strong and enduring connections to the local coastlines, with different locations perceived to cater for different therapeutic needs and interests. That is, there was individual heterogeneity in the kinds of therapeutic value different local blue spaces were perceived to deliver and a sense of familiarity and place emerged as key considerations.

Focusing on urban promenades alongside the river Rhine in the cities of Cologne and Düsseldorf in Germany, Sebastian Völker and Thomas Kistemann (2013) found that alongside feelings of restoration, also cultural determinants of health were important among visitors—from the aesthetic 'bright light and the glistening of the sun on the water', to the symbolic cultural and historical significance of German rivers (e.g. 'Father Rhine'). A subsequent qualitative study compared people's health-related discourse in relation to time spent in these blue space promenades with discourse related to urban green spaces in the same cities. This suggested that health- and well-being-related reactions varied across the different settings. In particular, a number of specifically 'blue' space health effects emerged, such as enhanced contemplation and greater emotional bonding, which were less evident in the cities' green spaces (Völker and Kistemann, 2015).

Finally, as with the preference-based work, it is also apparent that any potentially beneficial effects of blue space for public health are likely to be moderated by quality of the environment. In the United States, for instance, Aaron Hipp and Oladele Ogunseitan (2011) found that visitors to coastal parks reported their visit to be significantly more restorative when they perceived higher levels of air and water quality. Further, Martin Dallimer and colleagues (2012) found that visitors to riparian parks in Sheffield, United Kingdom, reported greater well-being in riverside locations with greater species diversity representative of ecological 'quality'. Actual or perceived biodiversity may be an important part of the health value of riparian natural environments and aquatic zones might be conceived of as a health-related intervention in attracting wildlife.

In sum, people report a range of positive health-related outcomes in blue landscapes whether we ask them to reflect on favourite places or specific visits and whether we monitor changes in the emotional states before and after, or even during a specific visit. Open-ended approaches can be useful in revealing features which might be overlooked using survey techniques (e.g. cultural and social aspects). Finally, it is important to note the detrimental effects of pollution or poor levels of actual or perceived biodiversity. To the extent that lower quality may undermine the benefits, this may help justify improvements based also on salutogenic health promotion grounds, over and above the perhaps more obvious ones associated with disease prevention.

Experimental approach

A potential criticism of the experiential work relates to selection effects. People tend to go to places they already know they like, so perhaps the samples reporting positive experiences in blue landscapes are unrepresentative, making it hard to generalize the findings. One way to address this issue is to use an experimental approach that randomly assigns people to experience different environments or exposes them to several environments and compares their reactions to each.

Much of the experimental work around emotional and physiological outcomes by blue exposure has been inconclusive. Although environments including water seem to attract more interest and attention, this has not been possible to objectify with physiological measurements and particularly any difference between blue and green environments has been hard to capture.

However, we conducted one experimental study (White *et al.*, 2015) that did report at least some distinct effects of blue versus green landscapes. We asked older women to exercise under laboratory conditions for 15 minutes while watching projections of urban, green, or blue landscapes on to a wall (or while facing the blank wall as a control condition). There was no significant difference between the green and blue landscapes in terms of psychological outcomes. However, a difference was found for time perception and willingness to repeat the exposure. Specifically, the only condition where time seemed to pass significantly quicker (suggesting less boredom and more 'flow') than staring at a blank wall was the blue landscape condition. Moreover, twice as many participants were willing to repeat exercising in the blue than green landscape.

In sum, work conducted using the experimental approach to exploring blue landscapes and well-being related outcomes to date has offered less support for the notion that blue landscapes offer particular psychophysiological benefits over and above green landscapes. Nonetheless, despite the lack of psychophysiological effects, participants appear to be more willing to repeat the blue landscape experience echoing the stated preference work. In this sense, they may be experiencing certain benefits from blue landscapes that enable people to enter a state of flow.

Quantitative spatial approach

The quantitative spatial approach is fundamentally different and tends to rely on large secondary datasets, assessing relationships between residential neighbourhood environments and health outcomes. A good example is the landmark study in the Netherlands by Sjerp de Vries and colleagues (2003) where the researchers merged two data sets; one containing public health data (n >10,000) and the other a national spatial database of land cover, classifying 25 m grid squares into types including urban green, agricultural green space, and fresh and salt water areas (referred to as 'blue space'). Findings indicated that people living in areas with a greater percentage of blue space reported significantly fewer symptoms of ill health, supporting the assumption that preferences for blue landscapes were associated with tangible health benefits. The researchers did not, however, report better overall or mental health scores as a function of blue space in the local area.

A series of similarly designed studies were subsequently conducted in several countries. In Ireland, for instance, Finbarr Brereton and colleagues (2008) found that people who lived within

2 km of the coast had significantly greater life satisfaction than those living more than 5 km from the coast. In the United Kingdom, Ben Wheeler and his colleagues (2012) revealed a similar coastal proximity gradient in self-reported health, and also demonstrated that this was more pronounced in socioeconomically deprived neighbourhoods. In other words, living near the sea benefited those in poorer neighbourhoods most, which might contribute to reducing sociodemographic health inequalities (see also Wheeler *et al.*, 2015; and Mitchell and Popham, 2008 for similar effects for urban green space) (see Fig. 5.2.1). In a study in Barcelona, Spain, it was found that children who spent more time at local beaches had better social and behavioural skills than those who spent relatively little time there, even after controlling for a range of sociodemographic factors (Amoly *et al.*, 2014). This has particular significance, as both social and behavioural skills are known to correlate with health outcomes in later life. Finally, using longitudinal data from England, we showed that people reported significantly higher self-reported health and significantly lower mental health problems (as measured by General Health Questionnaire, GHQ) in years when they lived within 5 km of the coast (compared to further inland) (White *et al.*, 2013a). They did not however replicate the findings for inland water from de Vries *et al.* (2003), or the life satisfaction findings of Brereton *et al.* (2008).

Why should living near blue landscapes be beneficial for health? This may be related to some of the generally recognized pathways between nature and health (see chapters in for example Section 3 of this book); (a) ecosystem services and environmental quality; (b) increased physical activity; (c) stress recovery; or (d) improved social capital. We discuss the first of these two issues in a little more detail below. As we have already outlined the relationship between blue landscapes and mental health-related outcomes, often associated with stress, we don't expand further on the third pathway. Finally, given the paucity of research on the relationships between blue space and social relations, we exclude this potential pathway from the chapter.

Although relatively little work in this field has yet looked at regulating ecosystem services and improved environmental quality, a number of environmental features of blue spaces may be important. For instance, in a meta-analysis of several studies, mainly from China and other Asian countries, looking at the potential of blue spaces to reduce the urban heat island effect, Völker and his colleagues (Völker *et al.*, 2013) compared air temperatures at a variety of urban blue spaces such as ponds, lakes, and rivers with non-blue reference sites at defined distances in the same city. The analysis suggested an average cooling effect of $2.5°$ Kelvin attributed to urban blue space sites during the warmest months, with larger water bodies providing the largest differential in temperature. Given predicted changes in climate, improved integration of open water systems within urban environments may be a key mitigation and adaptation mechanism for reducing heat-related morbidity. Similar effects of urban green spaces have been demonstrated (Bowler *et al.*, 2010). Read more about the cooling effect of urban green spaces in Chapter 8.5.

A rather different mechanism that might be beneficial for the health of particularly Northern coastal communities was suggested in a recent UK study (Cherrie *et al.*, 2015). Specifically, it was found that coastal locations tend to have higher environmental levels of ultraviolet (UV) radiation (from sunshine), and that this may be related to higher levels of blood serum vitamin D among coastal dwellers (since sunlight is one of the main sources of vitamin D in humans). This is potentially important for health, since vitamin D is associated with a range of positive health outcomes, not only skeletal, but also extraskeletal, such as preventing autoimmune and cardiovascular diseases and some cancers. However, as acknowledged by the authors, the health risks from sunlight and UV radiation (e.g. skin cancer) must also be taken into account when attempting to assess the overall health effect of greater UV exposure by blue space accessibility.

Finally, there has also been some discussion in the literature about the potential of aquatic environments, especially coastal waters, to be particularly high in 'negative ions' which some researchers have suggested might help with a range of psychological symptoms such as depression and also affect blood pressure (e.g. Ryushi *et al.*, 1998). For instance, the concentration of negative ions

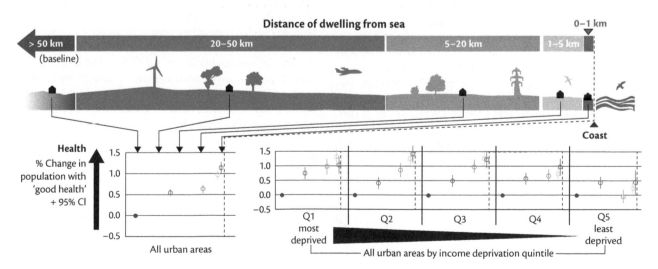

Fig. 5.2.1 The coast and good health in urban areas. Age-standardized percentage of population stating 'good health' relative to those in areas furthest from the coast (450 km)—adjusted regression coefficients with 95% confidence intervals; total and by income de privation quintile.

was found to be up to four times higher in coastal than inland urban areas (Pawar *et al.*, 2012), a finding attributed mainly to greater levels of UV radiation (see previous discussion in this chapter of Cherrie *et al.*, 2015), but one which might also be due to breaking waves. Negative air ions have also been found, in non-aquatic settings, to be associated with lower aerosols and pollen concentrations (e.g. Yan *et al.*, 2015). However, the direct effects of negative ions on human health are disputed and empirical evidence is weak. For instance, in their review of the literature, Perez and colleagues (2013) found no evidence of positive psychological effects attributable to negative air ions, except for lower depression scores under high-density exposure conditions. Given this paucity of good quality evidence linking negative ions and human health, we remain extremely cautious about this being a potential mechanism linking blue space and health.

Evidence for the link between living near blue landscapes and increased physical activity is, however, stronger. First, surveys in Denmark (Schipperjin *et al.*, 2010) and England (White *et al.*, 2014b) have shown that people who live near aquatic environments are indeed more likely to visit them than those who live far from them. Second, evidence from Australia (Bauman *et al.*, 1999), New Zealand (Witten *et al.*, 2008), and England (White *et al.*, 2014b) suggests that people who live near the coast are more likely to engage in regular physical activity. Finally, because people tend to spend longer on visits to blue space than other kinds of natural environments, the amount of energy expended tends to be greater (Elliott *et al.*, 2015). Together, these strands of evidence suggest that people living near blue spaces visit them more often for health-promoting physical activity, possibly because these preferred environments are more accessible for them.

In short, there is a growing body of evidence suggesting that people living near blue landscapes do tend to be healthier and happier than those who do not live near water and this might be through relatively simple mechanisms such as getting out more and engaging in more exercise, precisely because people like spending time in these environments. Despite consistently positive findings, it is important to note that effect sizes in these studies are often relatively small. In our (Wheeler *et al.*, 2012) census analysis, for instance, living within 1 km versus 50 km of the sea, increased the prevalence of 'good health' by only about 1%. Nevertheless, although these results appear small, it is also important to put them in the context of the relative influence of other factors on self-reported health that people might suppose are highly important. For instance, in our own analysis of panel data, living ≤5 km as compared to >50 km, was associated with about a quarter of the impact of being employed versus unemployed on self-reported health (White *et al.*, 2013a). Moreover, given that over eight million people live within 5 km of the English coast, small differences at the individual level may still mean substantive gains at the population level.

Intriguingly, in one study where quality was explored (Wheeler *et al.*, 2015), results suggested that freshwater ecological quality was actually inversely associated with self-reported health. That is, populations living in areas with poorer surface water quality reported better health than those living in areas of good water quality. The authors suggest that 'the inverse association between water quality and health ... may be ... indicative of the 'environmentalist's paradox'. If degraded surface water quality is indicative of human activity (such as intensive agriculture) in the surrounding catchment, but that human activity is a source of social and economic benefit, then there may be population health and wellbeing gain at the cost of environmental degradation' (Wheeler *et al.*, 2015). Again, these findings suggest that caution is needed in interpreting research findings examining the relationships between blue landscapes, as well as other natural landscapes and public health because the picture is often more complex than is first apparent.

Conclusion

The present chapter summarized some insights and evidence into the positive, salutogenic effects of blue landscapes, such as rivers and coastlines, on human health and well-being. Although positive effects seem to have been recognized throughout history, there has been relatively little systematic empirical work, compared to study of woodlands or urban green space. What little that has been done tends, we argue, to fall under one of four broad paradigms: the preference, experiential, experimental, and quantitative spatial approaches. Generally speaking, there seems to be more evidence in support of an association between exposure to blue landscapes and positive health outcomes in the preference, experiential, and quantitative spatial approaches than the experimental approach; however, boundary conditions were noted across all approaches. While selective, our review does not suggest that blue landscapes are always and everywhere good for public health, and issues such as the weather, pollution, and biodiversity may play a role in any benefits experienced.

Further work is now needed to link up some of these disparate strands and to integrate findings from the different approaches into a systematic body of work recognizing that blue landscapes are not simply a part of 'green' landscapes, but may have important, specific properties in terms of the benefits they might convey for public health. This work could usefully address several questions, such as: (a) Why do people continue to express preferences for blue landscapes even when there is relatively little experimental evidence that they confer any psychophysiological benefits over and above green landscapes?; (b) Given the relatively small effect sizes for health benefits associated with living near blue landscape areas, are there potential therapeutic benefits of exposure to blue landscapes for certain health conditions?; and (c) What impact might further degradation in the quality of blue landscapes (e.g. marine litter and loss of biodiversity) have on public health, for example through impacting on motivation to visit such environments for stress reduction, physical activity, and quality family time (over and above direct impacts of poor quality aquatic environments on illness and disease)? These less tangible benefits of blue landscapes are only just beginning to be realized, and we look forward to further work exploring their potential importance for public health in the future.

Acknowledgements

The writing of the current chapter was supported by the BlueHealth project, which has received funding from the European Union's Horizon 2020 research and innovation programme under grant agreement No. 666773.

References

Amoly, E., Dadvand, P., Forns, J., *et al.* (2014). Green and blue spaces and behavioral development in Barcelona schoolchildren: the BREATHE Project. *Environ Health Perspect*, 122, 1351.

Ashbullby, K. J., Pahl, S., Webley, P., & White, M. P. (2013). The beach as a setting for families' health promotion: A qualitative study with parents and children living in coastal regions in Southwest England. *Health Place*, 23, 138–47.

Barton, J. & Pretty, J. (2010). What is the best dose of nature and green exercise for improving mental health? A multi-study analysis. *Environ Sci Technol*, 44, 3947–55.

Bauman, A., Smith, B., Stoker, L., Bellew, B., & Booth, M. (1999). Geographical influences upon physical activity participation: evidence of a 'coastal effect'. *Aust N Z J Public Health*, 23, 322–4.

Bell, S. L., Phoenix, C., Lovell, R. & Wheeler, B. W. (2015). Seeking everyday wellbeing: The coast as a therapeutic landscape. *Soc Sci Med*, 142, 56–67.

Bowler, D. E., Buyung-Ali, L., Knight, T. M., & Pullin, A. S. (2010). Urban greening to cool towns and cities: A systematic review of the empirical evidence. *Landsc Urban Plan*, 97, 147–55.

Brereton, F., Clinch, J. P., & Ferreira, S. (2008). Happiness, geography and the environment. *Ecol Econ*, 65, 386–96.

Cherrie, M. P. C., Wheeler, B., White, M. P., Sarran, C. E., & Osborne, N. J. (2015). Coastal climate is associated with elevated solar irradiance and higher 25(OH)D level in coastal residents. *Environ Int*, 77, 76–84.

Dallimer, M., Irvine, K.N., Skinner, A.M.J. *et al.* (2012). Biodiversity and the feel-good factor: Understanding associations between self-reported human wellbeing and species richness. *Bioscience*, 64, 47–55.

de Vries, S., Verheij, R. A., Groenewegen, P. P., & Spreeuwenberg, P. (2003). Natural environments-healthy environments? An exploratory analysis of the relationship between greenspace and health. *Environ Plann*, 351717–32.

Elliott, L.R., White M.P., Taylor, A.H. & Herbert, S. (2015). Energy expenditure on recreational visits to different natural environments: Implications for public health. *Soc Sci Med*, 139, 56–60.

Foley, R. (2011). Performing health in place: The holy well as a therapeutic assemblage. *Health Place*, 17, 470–9.

Herzog, T. R. (1985). A cognitive analysis of preference for waterscapes. *J Environ Psychol*, 5, 225–41.

Hipp, J. A. & Ogunseitan, O. A. (2011). Effect of environmental conditions on perceived psychological restorativeness of coastal parks. *J Environ Psychol*, 31, 421–9.

Korpela, K. M., Ylén, M., Tyrväinen, L., & Silvennoinen, H. (2010). Favorite green, waterside and urban environments, restorative experiences and perceived health in Finland. *Health Promot Int*, 25, 200–9.

Lange, E. & Schaeffer, P. V. (2001). A comment on the market value of a room with a view. *Landsc Urban Plan*, 55, 113–120.

Luttik, J. (2000). The value of trees, water and open space as reflected by house prices in the Netherlands. *Landsc Urban Plan*, 48, 161–7.

MacKerron, G. & Mourato, S. (2013). Happiness is greater in natural environments. *Glob Environ Chang*, 23, 992–1000.

Mitchell, R. & Popham, F. 2008. Effect of exposure to natural environment on health inequalities: an observational population study. *Lancet*, 372, 1655–60.

Palmer, S. E. & Schloss, K. B. (2010)An ecological valence theory of human color preference. *Proc Natl Acad Sci*, 107, 8877–82.

Pawar, S. D., Meena, G. S., & Jadhav, D. B. (2012). Air ion variation at Poultry-farm, coastal, mountain, rural and urban sites in India. *Aerosol Air Qual Res*, 12, 440–51.

Perez, V., Alexander, D. D., & Bailey, W. H. (2013). Air ions and mood outcomes: a review and meta-analysis. *BMC Psychiatry*, 13, 29.

Ryushi, T., Kita, I., Sakurai, T., Yasumatsu, M., Isokawa, M., Aihara, Y., & Hama, K., (1998). The effect of exposure to negative air ions on the recovery of physiological responses after moderate endurance exercise. *Int J Biometeorol*, 41, 132–6.

Schipperijn, J., Ekholm, O., Stigsdotter, U.K., Toftager, M., Bentsen, P., Kamper- Jørgensen, F., Randrup, T.B., (2010). Factors influencing the use of green space: results from a Danish national representative survey. *Landsc. Urban Plan*, 95, 130–137.

Völker, S., Baumeister, H., Claßen, T., Hornberg, C., & Kistemann, T. (2013). Evidence for the temperature-mitigating capacity of urban blue space—a health geographic perspective. *Erdkunde*, 67, s355–71.

Völker, S., & Kistemann, T. (2011). The impact of blue space on human health and well-being—Salutogenetic health effects of inland surface waters: A review. *Int J Hygiene Environ Health*, 214, 449–60.

Völker, S. & Kistemann, T. (2013). "I'm always entirely happy when I'm here!" Urban blue enhancing human health and well-being in Cologne and Düsseldorf, Germany. *Soc Sci Med*, 78, 113–24.

Völker, S. & Kistemann, T. (2015). Developing the urban blue: Comparative health responses to blue and green urban open spaces in Germany. *Health Place*, 35, 196–205.

Wheeler, B. W., Lovell, R., Higgins, S. L., *et al.* (2015). Beyond Greenspace: An ecological study of population general health and indicato of natural environment type and quality. *Int J Health Geogr*, 14, 17.

Wheeler, B., White, M. P., Stahl-Timmins, W., & Depledge, M. H. (2012). Does living by the coast improve health and wellbeing? *Health Place*, 18, 1198–201.

White, M., Smith, A., Humphryes, K., Pahl, S., Snelling, D., and Depledge, M. (2010). Blue space: The importance of water for preference, affect, and restorativeness ratings of natural and built scenes. *J Environ Psychol*, 30, 482–493.

White, M. P., Alcock, I., Wheeler, B. W., & Depledge, M. H. (2013a). Coastal proximity and health: A fixed effects analysis of longitudinal panel data. *Health Place*, 23, 97–103.

White, M. P., Pahl, S. Ashbullby, K. J., Herbert, S., & Depledge, M. H. (2013b). Feelings of restoration from recent nature visits. *J Environ Psychol*, 35, 40–51.

White, M. P., Wheeler, B. W., Herbert, S., Alcock, I., & Depledge, M. H. (2014a). Coastal proximity and physical activity. Is the coast an underappreciated public health resource? *Prev Med*, 69, 135–140.

White, M. P., Cracknell, D., Corcoran, A., Jenkinson. G., & Depledge, M. H. (2014b). Do preferences for waterscapes persist in inclement weather conditions and extend to sub-aquatic scenes? *Landsc Res*, 39, 339–58.

White, M. P., Pahl, S. Ashbullby, K. J., Burton, F., & Depledge, M. H. (2015). The effects of exercising in different natural environments on psycho-physiological outcomes in post-menopausal women: A simulation study. *Int J Environ Res Public Health*, 12, 11929–53.

Wilson, M. I., Robertson, L. D., Daly, M., & Walton, S. A. (1995). Effects of visual cues on assessment of water quality. *J Environ Psychol*, 15, 53–63.

Witten, K., Hiscock, R., Pearce, J., & Blakely, T. (2008). Neighbourhood access to open spaces and the physical activity of residents: a national study. *Prev Med*, 47, 299–303.

Yan, X., Wang, H., Hou, Z., Wang, S., Zhang, D., Xu, Q., & Tokola, T. (2015). Spatial analysis of the ecological effects of negative air ions in urban vegetated areas: A case study in Maiji, China. *Urban For Urban Greening*, 14, 636–45.

CHAPTER 5.3

Technological nature and human well-being

Peter H. Kahn, Jr.

Two movements that are restructuring human existence

Two world movements are radically restructuring human existence. One is the degradation and destruction of large parts of the natural world. As evidence shows—some of it presented in this volume—we depend on and need interaction with nature for our physical and psychological well-being. We have for hundreds of thousands of years, for as long as we've been a species. The second movement is that as a world culture we are now engaged in unprecedented technological growth, both in terms of its computational sophistication and pervasiveness. The important point to understand here is that this growth is not a linear function, but exponential. If we took a dollar and doubled it every day, that is an example of an exponential function. After a week we would have $64. After a month of such doubling, our lay intuition says to expect a lot more money, of course: maybe many hundreds of thousands of dollars. But in fact the amount would be over a billion dollars. At some point in that money growth curve, the growth begins to 'explode' upward. That's what's happening with our technology on our planet right now, but we don't really see it.

At the intersection of these two movements lies what I have termed *technological nature*: technologies that in various ways mediate, augment, and simulate our experience of the natural world. For example, many of us have grown up watching nature videos of pristine landscapes, and of animals that we find charismatic—such as lions, elephants, pandas, and wolves. Digital hearths loop on digital displays with the crackling of a wood fire. Cancer wards have begun to bring into their sterile environments photos of nature, and even faux skylights. Many of us, perhaps not worrying about cancer, use tanning beds to access a form of technological sunshine. We snap photos in nature and then upload them to Facebook, often in real time. Millions of people *geocache*: they use GPS and mobile devices to find hidden caches, often in natural settings. Inexpensive robotic pets mimic our companion animals. Some years ago, you could telehunt in Texas. You would go online from your computer in New York City or Miami or anywhere on this planet and control a mounted rifle through a web interface and hunt and kill a live animal. The animal would then be gutted and skinned, by the owner of the establishment, and the meat shipped to your doorstep. Texas outlawed telehunting, but teleshooting still exists, using targets instead of animals.

Does it matter that we are replacing direct forms of human interaction with nature with technologically mediated, simulated, and augmented forms of these interactions? In other words, does it matter that we are replacing nature with technological nature?

In this chapter, I will want to suggest that the answer is *yes*. I'll present emerging research to make this case, and argue that as we move to an increasingly technological world with at best technological nature as a substitute for the real thing, we will be shifting the baseline downward—as we have already—for what can be considered as physically and psychologically healthy humans.

Three forms of technological nature

A technological nature window

Windows with a nature view have been shown to promote physical and psychological health (Kaplan and Kaplan, 1989). In one often-cited study, for example, Ulrich (1984) examined the potential differences in the recovery of patients after gall bladder surgery depending on whether the patients were assigned to a room with a view of a natural setting (a small stand of deciduous trees) or a view of a brown brick wall. Results showed that patients with the natural window view required less potent painkillers, tended to have fewer postsurgical complications, and most importantly had shorter postoperative hospital stays (cf. Moore, 1981; Kuo and Sullivan, 2001; Taylor *et al.*, 2002). Moreover, even pictures of nature have been shown to have beneficial effects (Coss, 1990, summarized in Ulrich, 1993; Heerwagen, 1990). Read more about these kind of positive health effects from nature views in other sections of this book, for example Section 3.

Based on this body of research, my colleagues and I began to wonder: What if the view of nature was neither a 'real' view out a window, nor a static picture of nature in an inside setting? Instead, what if we could leverage current technologies and reinvent the nature window by means of a real time digital display of nature (a *technological nature window*) in the place of an actual window? Could we garner similar psychological effects?

Toward investigating this question, we conducted two studies that displayed real time high-definition television (HDTV) views of the immediate outside natural environment on a 50-inch plasma display. In both studies that follow—*The Field Study* and *The Experimental Study*—the view was a normal window view from the building overlooking a nature scene that included water in the foreground, as part of a public fountain area, and then extended to include stands of deciduous trees on one side, and a grassy expanse that allowed a visual 'exit' on the other. The HDTV camera sat on top of the university building. The view was chosen to include features that people usually find aesthetically pleasing and restorative in nature (Kaplan and Kaplan, 1989).

The field study

In this study, we installed in seven offices of faculty and staff at the University of Washington the plasma window described above and shown in Figure 5.3.1.

Utilizing a naturalistic field study methodology, data was collected over a 16-week period: six weeks with the inside office 'as is'; six weeks with the large display window and live video feed installation; and four weeks following the removal of the display window with the office returned to its original state. Across the 16-week period, each participant completed seven 30–45 minute semi-structured interviews which focused on the participant's (a) impressions and use of the large display window; (b) perceived effects of the real time views of the outdoor scene; (c) awareness of people walking through the plaza area (the indirect stakeholders); (d) assessment of the importance of the large display window; (e) intuitions about work performance and health; (f) social interaction related to the large display window; and (g) experiences, reflections, and comments on any other related topics. In total, 30+ hours of interviews were conducted and yielded 652 pages of interview transcripts. In addition, each participant completed 10 work satisfaction surveys, 10 mood surveys, 10 office perception surveys, journal entries, and responses to email queries.

The results from this field study are reported elsewhere (Friedman et al., 2008). Here I highlight three of the central findings: (i) participants made a shift in thinking of the technological nature window from something static to something dynamic, like a real window. Participants often took brief mental breaks and stared out the technological nature window, and said that they returned to their work a bit more refreshed and refocused. Through looking out the technological nature window, participants also spoke of feeling connected to the outdoors, and to the wider social community. (ii) Participants in the field study felt less isolated and alienated in their inside offices,

and more connected to the people they helped to serve. The technological nature window also connected participants to the wider social functioning of their institution, providing meaning to their work. (iii) After six weeks of using the technological nature window, the participants in this field study unanimously recommended it to other co-workers with inside offices, and—four weeks after the installation was removed—were clear that they themselves would choose to have one again in their inside offices.

Many buildings have inside spaces, such as inside offices and basement facilities, where it is difficult—if not impossible—to provide people with visual access to the outside environment. In such situations, this study supports the proposition that some psychological benefits can be had through utilizing a technological nature window. However, an important question needs to be addressed: How does such a technological nature window compare to an actual window with a nature view?

The experimental study

Toward addressing this question—of how looking at a technological nature window compares to an actual nature window view—we set up a between-subject experiment that involved three conditions (Kahn, et al., 2008). Each condition employed the same office on a university campus. In one condition, the view was the normal window view from the office overlooking a nature scene (the same view described in the above field study). In a second condition, a 50-inch plasma screen was inserted into the office window, entirely covering it. We then used the above-mentioned HDTV camera and displayed on the plasma display essentially the same glass window view one would see from inside the office itself. In the third condition, we sealed off the original glass window with light-blocking material, and covered it with drapes, in effect turning the space into an inside office. Ninety undergraduate participants were randomly assigned to one of the three office conditions. We measured their physiological recovery from low level stress. We also conducted a second-by-second coding of what people did with their eyes.

Briefly, our key results were as follows: there was more rapid heart rate recovery in the glass window condition compared to the blank wall condition. In turn, there was no difference in the heart rate recovery between the technological nature window condition and the blank wall condition. In terms of eye gaze behaviour, both windows just as frequently garnered participants' attention, and on this measure our results showed equivalent functionality between the two windows. But the glass window view held participants' attention longer than the technological nature window view. Finally, when participants spent more time looking at the glass window, their heart rate tended to decrease more rapidly; that was not the case with the technological nature window.

Taking both studies together, the results suggest that a technological nature window is better than no window (the inside office in the field study), but not as good as an actual window with a nature view.

Robot pets as technological nature

Let's now switch to a different form of technological nature. Instead of technological nature views, let's consider robot pets. They mimic biological pets. And interaction with biological pets, as is well documented, provide children and adults with many physical and psychological health gains (Barker and Wolen, 2008; Beck and Katcher, 1996; Melson, 2001). As a species, we have very roughly

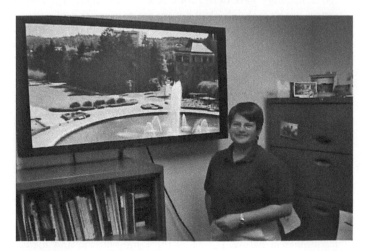

Fig. 5.3.1 Lecturer with her real time technological nature window (in an inside office) of local nature outside the building.

Image reproduced courtesy of Peter H. Kahn Jr.

around 10 thousand years of having social relationships with domestic animals. Can we have social relationships with technological nature robot animals?

In one study, my colleagues and I investigated people's relationships with Sony's robot dog AIBO through analysing 6,438 spontaneous postings of 182 members of three online AIBO discussion forums (Friedman *et al.*, 2003). Results showed that AIBO psychologically engaged this group of people. In particular, these members of the discussion forums often conceptualized AIBO not only as a technology but as having a lifelike biology, as having mental states, and as being capable of engendering social rapport. As one member wrote: 'I do view him as a companion, among other things he always makes me feel better when things aren't so great.' Moreover, the relationship members described with AIBO often appeared similar to the relationship people have with live dogs. As another member wrote:

'Aibo is so much more than just a robot doggy, he is a 'real' animal, and species, and brings people together, and brings much happiness to those that come in contact with him'

Reprinted from "*Hardware companions?* ..." Friedman, Kahn, Hagman, Proceedings of CHI '03, © ACM, Inc.

In a second study, we found some evidence for social interaction with AIBO by three- to five-year-old children (Kahn *et al.*, 2006). Thus in a third study, we investigated whether children with autism could benefit by interacting with AIBO (Stanton *et al.*, 2008). Our results showed that they did. Eleven children diagnosed with autism (ages 5–8) interacted with the robotic dog AIBO and, during a different period within the same experimental session, a simple mechanical toy dog (Kasha), which had no ability to detect or respond to its physical or social environment. Results showed that, in comparison to Kasha, the children spoke more words to AIBO, and more often engaged in three types of behaviour with AIBO typical of children without autism: verbal engagement, reciprocal interaction, and authentic interaction. In addition, we found suggestive evidence that the children interacted more with AIBO, and, while in the AIBO session, engaged in fewer autistic behaviours.

A large question for our purposes here is how AIBO stacks up to its biological counterpart. To investigate this question, we investigated 72 children's interactions with and reasoning about AIBO compared to one of two Australian Shepherd dogs (Melson *et al.*, 2009). We found these participants more often affirmed that a live dog, in comparison to AIBO, had mental states (83% live dog, 56% AIBO), could be a companion (91% live dog, 70% AIBO), and had moral standing (86% live dog, 76% AIBO). But what is particularly interesting is not just that AIBO was not as compelling as a live dog, but that AIBO was as compelling as it was. Those are the second set of numbers in the parentheses—ranging from 56% to 76%. That said, during the unstructured play period, the majority of children explored AIBO as an artefact, poking and touching AIBO as they would an unfamiliar toy. Only about a quarter of the children ever touched the biologically live dog in this way, and they did so infrequently. Also, compared with the biologically live dog, children much less frequently engaged toward AIBO in gentle, affectionate social touch, particularly with petting and scratching.

Thus in certain contexts, such as with children with autism, their appears to be possible beneficial uses of this form of technological nature. However, even here we need to be careful in generalizing in so far as the children with autism study did not directly compare interactions with AIBO to a biologically live dog.

A telegardan as technological nature

Let's consider the psychological effects of interacting with one additional form of technological nature with what is called a telegarden. You know about a telephone. You know about telesurgery, where a surgeon in one location can control a robotic surgical instrument in a physically different location and perform surgery. In turn, a telegarden is an installation that allows people to plant and tend seeds in a distant garden by controlling a robot system through a web-based interface. One such telegarden was developed under the codirection of Ken Goldberg and Joseph Santarromana, and eventually housed in the Ars Electronica Center in Linz, Austria. Many thousands of people throughout the world activated the robot arm in the telegarden remotely, viewed the garden through a camera, and planted seeds in the garden, watered their plants, and if successful as a telegardener, tended to their plants. The installation also had an accompanying online chat room. In turn, colleagues and I conducted a line-by-line analysis of three months of chat data (Kahn *et al.*, 2005). The central question we investigated was: How well did this telegarden work as a means to connect people to nature?

Our answer, put simply, was: not so well. Quantitatively, only 6% of 16,504 posts referred to people's discussion of the nature within the telegarden; and only an additional 7% referred to people's discussion of nature beyond the telegarden. And even here, the qualitative data showed a 'thin' connection. People did not, for example, talk about the plants in the telegarden in biocentric terms of deserving care or respect (Kahn, 1999). People did not talk about talking to their plants; rather, the nature discourse sounded more like 'My watering is done', 'Hold on a sec, let me plant one real quick', 'What is the plant at sector p8?' That's not rich nature discourse. The interactions did not seem satisfy the mind, heart, and spirit of what most gardeners presumably experience.

Several questions about technological nature now and into the future

At this junction, I would like to address a few questions that the reader might have.

1. **As technology gets better and better, and engages multiple senses, won't technological nature get as good as real nature?** Granted, technological advances will increasingly allow technological nature to have greater veracity, and it will also engage more of our senses. Likely enough, more psychological and health benefits will emerge. For example, a study by Annerstedt *et al.* (2013) found enhanced stress recovery in virtual nature that had virtual nature sounds versus no virtual nature sounds. Will future technologies close the gap between the artificial and the real? In my view, the answer in part remains an empirical one, awaiting future technologies and future psychological studies. But the point I would want to emphasize is that in these future studies, we need to hold out the right benchmarks (Kahn *et al.*, 2007). It's not enough to say that a particular technology meets this technological specification or that technological specification. Rather, does interacting with the newest form of technological nature accord us the same physical and mental health benefits as interacting with its actual nature counterpart? Does the technological nature refresh us as well? Are we equally creative through such interactions? Does it give space for our

imaginations? Does it satisfy our deepest longings for connection and authenticity? Does it allow us access to the quiet spaces just behind our busy world and busy minds? Nature does all of this, and more. We need to hold technological nature to the same standards.

2. **Why are we building—and tempted by—technological nature?** As I have argued elsewhere (Kahn, 2011), we are a technological species and we have always been one. Technologies have helped us to survive. Flint. Scrapers. Bows and arrows. But for hundreds of thousands of years, our technologies were rudimentary. And then during the start of the Neolithic period, and the rise of agriculture, our technologies began to increase in their complexity and capacities. As Kurzweil (2005) argues compellingly, this rate of change has been going on at exponential rate, and we are now at the 'knee' of an exponential function where the rate of change is almost impossible for us to comprehend with our minds. We are drawn to technology not only because of incessant manipulative advertising by global corporations, but because we love it, likely because technological innovation was highly adaptive during the Neolithic period. We need to 'own' our love of technology, even as we recognize that we're out of control with it, and hardly know it. Unless we design and employ technological systems that allow us to flourish, and unless we check our desires for unending and increasingly sophisticated and pervasive technology in our lives, then what started with a great upside in our evolutionary history will lead us not just astray, but potentially to our collapse on a worldwide level (Diamond, 2005).

3. **If we were actually getting seriously harmed by the loss of nature in an increasingly technological world, wouldn't we know it?** I don't think so, not easily. A large part of the reason involves what I have termed *environmental generational amnesia*. The basic idea here is that each generation constructs a conception of what is environmentally normal based on the natural world encountered in childhood. With each generation the amount of environmental degradation increases, but each generation tends to take that degraded condition as the nondegraded condition, and as the normal experience. I remember an early study a colleague and I conducted in Houston, Texas interviewing black children in an economically impoverished neighbourhood (Kahn and Friedman, 1995). The majority of children understood about air pollution in general, but significantly fewer children believed that Houston had air pollution, even though Houston was at the time one of the most polluted cities in the United States. How could this be? My explanation is that to understand the idea of pollution one needs to compare existing polluted states to those that are less polluted. But if one's only experience is with a certain amount of pollution, then that becomes not pollution, but the norm against which more polluted states are measured. What happened with these black children in Houston is what's happening this very moment on a worldwide level. Because of our own inaccurately constructed baseline, it's very difficult for us experientially to believe that we've lost as much as we have, both in terms of interaction with nature, and human health and well-being.

Conclusion

Based on the research reviewed in this article, and other research discussed elsewhere (Kahn, 2011) it appears that in terms of physical and psychological human health that interaction with technological nature is better than no nature, but not as good as the real thing. If that's the case, then we should be moved to preserve and rewild the nature we have, and to bring more of it into our daily lives (Kahn and Hasbach, 2012; 2013). Walking alongside an urban lake. Breathing fresh air through an open window. Singing with the songbirds. Swimming in a mountain stream. Running with one's dog along the beach. Gardening. Hands in earth. Sun on skin. Smelling the flowers. A campfire. Looking up into the night sky, awed by the million stars overhead.

People sometimes say that we don't need to worry about the loss of nature. They say that adaptation is how we evolved as a species, and that we'll adapt—especially through our technological innovations—and so we'll be fine.

My response is that it's true that we're an adaptive species. But not all adaptations are good for us. Elephants in a zoo adapt to concrete confines the size of a small parking lot. But that doesn't mean they do well. They stamp their feet for hours on end in neurotic patterns of disease. They shut themselves down emotionally. They become distant shells of their former and flourishing ancestral selves. A similar result would happen to all of us if we were put in prison for the rest of our lives. We would adapt, as most prisoners do. But we would suffer physically and psychologically. If our children were born in the prison, then they, too, would suffer. They might not know it as vividly as we do because they wouldn't have had the experience of being free. But that wouldn't change an objective account of their affliction.

I would like to suggest that most of us are already in such a prison: a massive urban prison. The world talks about sustainability. And perhaps it's true, though I doubt it, that seven or ten billion of us can live sustainably over thousands of upcoming years on this planet. But even if we could, it would be an underwhelming and dispiriting form of living. We would be like biological meat, like cattle in a feedlot. That's just the plain truth. Through scientific evidence, rationality, and the sheer intuitive knowing of our deeper selves, I hope we can wake from our amnesia to know so, and to change course.

References

Annerstedt, M., Jönsson P., Wallergård M., *et al.* (2013). Inducing physiological stress recovery with sounds of nature in a virtual reality forest—results from a pilot study. *Physiol Behav*, 118, 240–50.

Barker, S. B., & Wolen, A. R. (2008). The benefits of human-companion animal interaction: A review. *J Vet Med Educ*, 35, 487–95.

Beck, A. M., & Katcher, A. H. (1996). *Between pets and people: The importance of animal companionship*. West Lafayette: Purdue University Press.

Coss, R. G. (1990). Picture perception and patient stress: A study of anxiety reduction and postoperative stability. Unpublished manuscript, Department of Psychology, University of California, Davis.

Diamond, J. M. (2005). *Collapse: How Societies Choose to Fail or Succeed.* New York, NY: Penguin.

Friedman, B., Freier, N. G., Kahn, P. H., Jr., Lin, P., & Sodeman, R. (2008). Office window of the future?—Field-based analyses of a new use of a large display. *Int J Hum Comput Stud*, 66, 452–65.

Friedman, B., Kahn, P. H. Jr., & Hagman, J. (2003). Hardware companions?: What online AIBO discussion forums reveal about the human-robotic relationship. *Proceedings Conference on Human Factors in Computing Systems* (pp. 273–280). New York, NY: Association for Computing Machinery Press.

Heerwagen, J. (1990). The psychological aspects of windows and window design. In: Anthony, K. H., Choi, J., and Orland, B. (eds.). *Proceedings of the 21st Annual Conference of the Environmental Design Research Association*. Oklahoma City, OK: EDRA.

Kahn, P. H. Jr. (1999). *The Human Relationship with Nature: Development and Culture*. Cambridge, MA: MIT Press.

Kahn, P. H. Jr. (2011). *Technological Nature: Adaptation and the Future of Human Life*. Cambridge, MA: MIT Press.

Kahn, P. H., Jr., & Friedman, B. (1995). Environmental views and values of children in an inner-city Black community. *Child Development*, 66, 1403–17.

Kahn, P. H., Jr., Friedman, B., Alexander, I. S., Freier, N. G., and Collett, S. L. (2005). The distant gardener: What conversations in the Telegarden reveal about human-telerobotic interaction. *Proceedings of the 14th International Workshop on Robot and Human Interactive Communication (RO-MAN '05)* (pp. 13–18). Piscataway, NJ: Institute of Electrical and Electronics Engineers (IEEE).

Kahn, P. H., Jr., Friedman, B., Gill, B., *et al.* (2008). A plasma display window?—The shifting baseline problem in a technologically-mediated natural world. *J Environ Psychol*, 28, 192–9.

Kahn, P. H., Jr., Friedman, B., Perez-Granados, D. R., & Freier, N. G. (2006). Robotic pets in the lives of preschool children. *Interaction Studies*, 7, 405–36.

Kahn, P. H. Jr., & Hasbach, P. H. (eds) (2013). *The Rediscovery of the Wild*. Cambridge, MA: MIT Press.

Kahn, P. H. Jr., & Hasbach, P. H. (2012). (eds). *Ecopsychology: Science, Totems, and the Technological Species*. Cambridge, MA: MIT Press.

Kahn, P. H. Jr., Ishiguro, H., Friedman, B., *et al.* (2007). What is a human?—Toward psychological benchmarks in the field of human-robot interaction. *Interaction Studies*, 8, 363–90.

Kaplan, R. & Kaplan, S. (1989). *The Experience of Nature: A Psychological Perspective*. New York, NY: Cambridge University Press.

Kuo, F. E. & Sullivan, W. C. (2001). Aggression and violence in the inner city: Effects of environment via mental fatigue. *Environ Behav*, 33, 543–71.

Kurzweil, R. (2005). *The Singularity is Near*. New York, NY: Viking.

Melson, G. F. (2001). *Why the Wild Things Are: Animals in the Lives of Children*. Cambridge, MA: Harvard University Press.

Melson, G. F., Kahn, P. H. Jr., Beck, A. M., *et al.* (2009). Children's behavior toward and understanding of robotic and living dogs. *J Appl Dev Psychol*, 30, 92–102.

Moore, E. O. (1981). A prison environments' effect on health care service demands. *J Environ Syst*, 11, 17–34.

Stanton, C. M., Kahn, P. H., Jr., Severson, R. L., Ruckert, J. H., & Gill, B. T. (2008). Robotic animals might aid in the social development of children with autism. *Proceedings of the 3rd ACM/IEEE International Conference on Human-Robot Interaction 2008* (pp. 97–104). New York, NY: Association for Computing Machinery.

Taylor, A. F., Kuo, F. E., & Sullivan, W. C. (2002). Views of nature and self-discipline: Evidence from inner city children. *J Environ Psychol*, 22, 49–63.

Ulrich, R. S. (1984). View through a window may influence recovery from surgery. *Science*, 224, 420–1.

Ulrich, R. S. (1993). Biophilia, biophobia, and natural landscapes. In: Kellert, S. R. & Wilson, E. O. (eds) *The Biophilia Hypothesis*, pp. 73–137. Washington, DC: Island Press.

SECTION 6

Varied populations and interactions with nature

CHAPTER 6.1

Children and nature

Nancy M. Wells, Francesqca E. Jimenez, and Fredrika Mårtensson

Children's disconnection from nature

Children are disconnected from the natural world. Increasingly, children spend more time on indoor pursuits—watching television, using computers, and playing video games (Rideout et al., 2010), and less time outdoors (Hofferth, 2009; Louv, 2005). Disconnection from nature may contribute to poor knowledge of the natural world or 'ecological illiteracy' (Balmford et al., 2002; Bebbington, 2005), and ultimately, diminished later-life environmental attitudes and behaviours (Wells and Lekies, 2006) which could have long-term implications for the health of the planet.

For public health professionals, children's disconnection from nature has urgent ramifications as nature is associated with a wide variety of positive human health outcomes and, conversely, disconnection from nature is linked to a range of negative health outcomes. This chapter aims to outline linkages between the natural environment and children's health.

A variety of interwoven factors are implicated in children's disconnection from nature. These include urbanization and the loss of natural areas, parental fear of crime and 'stranger danger', children's hyper-programmed lives, and the prevalence of computers and other media sources (Ginsburg, 2007; Strife and Downey, 2009; Louv, 2005). While an extensive examination of these contributing factors is beyond the scope of this chapter, to begin with we briefly examine recent changes in play, recess, and screen time. We then briefly introduce issues of socioeconomic status (SES) and ethnic disparity in nature access for children.

Play

Along with children's divorce from nature has come concern about children engaging in less outdoor free play. Despite evidence of the developmental importance of play (Ginsburg, 2007), children today spend markedly less time playing outdoors than previous generations. A 2004 study found that while 70% of mothers reported spending time outdoors 'every day' in their own childhood, only 31% of their children reported spending time outdoors 'every day' (Clements, 2004). While these finding may be somewhat susceptible to the inaccuracies of retrospective memory, they are consistent with evidence based on daily diary data. Hofferth (2009) reports that in 1997, 16% of US children (ages 6–12) participated in outdoor activities weekly, but by 2003 the percentage dropped to 10%. In 1997, children spent 36 minutes on average per week outdoors; by 2003 that number had dropped to 25 minutes per week (Hofferth, 2009). The decline of play is purportedly due to a variety of factors including a focus on academic performance, prioritization of extracurricular enrichment programmes, busy lifestyles, and changing family structure (Ginsburg, 2007) (Box 6.1.1).

Recess

In the United States, the trend towards reduced school recess may contribute to children's disconnection from nature and to less time spent in play. A 1989 US survey conducted by the National Association of Elementary School Principals found that 96% of participating school systems had at least one recess period; a decade later, only 70% of kindergarten classes had a recess period (Ginsburg, 2007; Pellegrini and Bohn, 2005). Similar declines have been documented in England (Pellegrini and Bohn, 2005). In 2006, a national survey conducted by the US Centers for Disease Control and Prevention found that only 12% of states required elementary schools to provide daily recess. Fifty-seven per cent (57%) of school districts required, and 33% recommended, daily recess (Robert Wood Johnson Foundation, 2012).

Screen time: computers and home media

The growth of home media may contribute to disconnection from nature. While only 9% of US families had televisions in 1950 (Andreason, 1994) by 2009, 99% of families had one or more (Rideout et al., 2010). On average, US households have 3.8 TVs (Rideout et al., 2010). By 2009, TV consumption constituted 4.5 hours per day among children age 8 to 18 (Rideout et al., 2010). In 1999, less than half (47%) of children age 8–18 had used a computer the previous day and spent, on average, 27 minutes per day using the computer for recreation. By 2009, US children spent 1.29 hours daily using the computer (Rideout et al., 2010).

Displacement theory suggests that media activities displace other activities that are of developmental importance (Anderson et al., 2001; Hofferth, 2010). Although this theory has received relatively little attention, a 2003 study found that while most young children who spent time on computer-based activities spent no less time engaged in sports and outside play than children who did not have computers. Meanwhile, for children who used computers more than eight hours per week, there was an inverse association with time spent engaged in sports and outdoor activities (Attewell et al., 2003).

Box 6.1.1 OPEC—a landscape configuration with potential for play by Fredrika Mårtensson

Planning departments need to know what types of ground is suitable for children's play and how play environments can be designed and furnished to be made more useful. Objective standards for assessing outdoor environments are important for research. The Outdoor Play Environment Categories (OPEC) tool describes a configuration of a set of environmental characteristics that were developed with this twofold intention (Mårtensson, 2013). Swedish studies show that preschool children with access to outdoor settings high in OPEC are reported being more physically active (Boldemann et al., 2011), better able to concentrate (Mårtensson et al., 2009, and having better well-being and sleep; Söderström et al., 2009). Below, the development of the tool is outlined.

Spacious, green, and varied

The challenge was to develop an environmental assessment tool taking into account how the complexity of a landscape is reflected in children's play behaviour. The overall landscape configuration of a green and varied spacious outdoor environment deemed high in quality was specified into three different aspects: (i) the total size of the outdoor area; (ii) the proportion of area with shrubs, trees or hilly terrain, including areas with more nature-like ground but not plain lawns; and (iii) the integration between vegetation, open areas, and more permanent play settings implying a mix of different types of ground well distributed over the area.

Research offers some ideas of why and how such outdoor environments can be beneficial to children´s health. The proximity to greenery has documented cognitive effects, but one also needs to take into account what type of activity takes place at a site. Children use their entire body when playing outdoors, making them more physically active and more likely to seek out settings that make them comfortable (e.g. leafy shade under trees when it is hot weather). Rachel Sebba (1991) has described a mental state characteristic for children outdoors when concurrently attentive to signals from their bodies and the events going on around them. The literature on nature-based therapy describes how practices of mindfulness connecting mind and body can improve the capacity to regulate psychological, physical, and social needs (von Essen and Mårtensson, 2014). When many children are outdoors together in a high-quality environment, this attentiveness toward the surroundings adds certain characteristics to their play.

The flow of outdoor play

In high-quality environments, children now and then get the urge to run as fast as they possibly can. They tend to switch between energetic running games and pretend play or contemplative recuperation. Their activity is dominated by place-related movement in intimate and joyful interaction with their surroundings. They are singing, chatting, and making up new stories. How do we recognize this 'play of flux and transformation' and how does it build up?

When children go outdoors they are attentive towards the possibility of exploring the yet undiscovered, and are likely experiencing 'extent', as Rachel Kaplan and Stephen Kaplan once described

it (read about Kaplan and Kaplan in Chapter 2.1 'Environmental psychology'). Children take an interest in the affordances allowing them to do exciting things, like spinning, balancing, swaying, and rolling objects or their own bodies. An abundance of loose material adds flexibility to play, allowing more options, and facilitating negotiation and conflict resolution.

Children can make an outdoor place their own for a day or more by repeated use or slight modification by a tree, a stone, or a fence. Children need secure play-bases to set forth in more rapid play sequences. The open spaces in-between are vital for their ability to navigate and coordinate the next step; for example, when making a quick dash through an open stretch or zigzagging through a bosket of trees. They also use the configuration of play spaces to elaborate on vital themes in human development, as dependence/independence when making a journey by going around a corner, or 'taming horses' in the fringe.

The Outdoor Play Environment Categories, OPEC, illustrate a combination of basic factors important for children's opportunity to health-promoting outdoor play. Playgrounds with a lot of equipment can house many affordances for physical activity, but can still have an overall design that does not support children's dynamic play-flow. Fencing delimiting mobility and protective mats replacing sand or woodchip further thwart the flexibility of the space. Children benefit from having space in-between play areas and an abundance of loose material to help them navigate and negotiate. Natural environments are useful and barren environments gain in play potential with some rain or snow. How the play potential of outdoor environments varies across regions—with their specific landscape and climate—is still little explored, but important to recognize in any development of health-promoting environmental assessment for children.

The criteria of the OPEC tool

With the OPEC tool, three environmental categories are evaluated from 1 to 3 points for each setting, with 1 point indicating the lowest quality and 3 points the highest quality. The two alternatives for size are adjusted to the regions studied, the first one in Stockholm area, Sweden, and the second Malmoe, Sweden and Raleigh in North Carolina, United States.

A. Total size of the outdoor area:

  1 point: <1,200 m^2

  2 points: 1,200–3,000 m^2

  3 points: >3,000 m^2

Alternative (depending on context)

  1 point: <2,000 m^2

  2 points: 2,000–6,000 m^2

  3 points: >6,000 m^2

B. Proportion of surfaces with trees, shrubbery, or hilly terrain:

  1 point: Little/non-existent

  2 points: <half of the area

  3 points: ≥ half of the area

(continued)

> **Box 6.1.1** (Continued)
>
> C. Integration between vegetation, open areas, and play areas:
>
>   1 point: No integration. Open spaces, vegetation, and play areas in separate parts of the environment.
>
>   2 points: Either of the following characteristics
>
>   a) trees or shrubbery are adjacent to play areas
>
>   b) the open spaces are located in-between the play areas
>
>   3 points: Both 2a and 2b above are fulfilled
>
> Criteria for OPEC tool reproduced courtesy of Fredrika Mårtensson.

Social equity: socioeconomic status and ethnic disparities in nature access

Compounding the concern that children are disconnected from the natural environment is a realization that nature access is often particularly limited among low-income and ethnic minority youth; this inequity may be among the factors contributing to health disparities (see reviews: Strife and Downey, 2009; Evans and Kantrowitz, 2002). The notion of nature access as an environmental justice issue was highlighted during the 2013 New York City mayoral election with candidate Bill De Blasio's characterization of New York City as a 'tale of two cities'—of 'haves' and 'have-nots'. Among the issues to be addressed, according to De Blasio, was the lack of equity in the park system: the lowest income communities receive the least funding for parks (Dolesh, 2014).

Studies from around the globe suggest ethnic and economic disparities in access to nature and outdoor opportunities are not uncommon. Data from 1989 for New York City, for example, indicate that poor children live in neighbourhoods with, on average, 17 square yards of park space per child, compared to 40 square yards per non-poor child (Sherman, 1994). In an analysis of Baltimore, Maryland parks, Boone and colleagues (2009) find that unlike many other US cities, a higher proportion of blacks have walking access to parks than whites, however whites have access to greater acreage of parks; and the parks to which blacks have access are often hazardous or polluted. In Tampa, Florida, street trees are less prevalent in black, low-income, and rental neighbourhoods (Landry and Chakraborty, 2009). A 1999 study examining 45 randomly selected New York City playgrounds found that those in low-income areas had more hazards than those in high-income communities (Suecoff et al., 1999). Strife and Downey (2009) point out that physical proximity to green space may not tell a full story if fear of crime or hazards impair use of parks and natural areas. Councilmember Mark Levine responded to the NYC green space equity controversy, 'We have to push back on the idea that parks are a luxury and an amenity. .... parks [are] essential infrastructure ... ' (Dolesh, 2014).

Read more about nature, health, and inequalities in Chapter 6.3 'Vulnerable populations, health inequalities, and nature'.

Research evidence: linking nature to children's health and well-being

In light of the evidence indicating children's disconnection from the natural world, along with the socioeconomic and ethnic disparities exacerbating that disconnection, the purpose of this chapter is to document evidence that nature matters; that nature access has critical implications for children's health, functioning, and well-being. We do not present an exhaustive review of the literature, but rather, attempt to provide both breadth and depth, relying, in part, on prior review articles in the interest of space. The specific aims of this chapter are: (i) to review evidence linking nature access to children's health and well-being, with particular attention to socioeconomic and racial disparities; (ii) to consider gaps in the evidence and directions for future research; (iii) to describe promising programmes and interventions aimed at promoting children's connection to the natural environment.

In this section, we review evidence that links nature to children's health, function, and well-being. We include aspects of both mental and physical health, and address the following outcomes: social interaction and social cohesion; cognitive restoration and academic performance; symptoms of attention deficit hyperactivity disorder; myopia; physical activity and obesity; and vitamin D deficiency.

Social interaction and social cohesion

The natural environment draws people together and fosters social cohesion (see also Chapter 3.3 'Promoting social cohesion and social capital– increasing well-being'). In studies comparing barren and vegetated outdoor spaces within inner-city Chicago, Illinois public housing complexes, Faber Taylor and her colleagues (1998) found that outdoor spaces with high levels of vegetation were more supportive of children's play and facilitated children's interaction with adults more than comparable spaces lacking vegetation. In green spaces, children were more likely to interact with both family and unrelated adults. These findings relate to earlier studies indicating that green outdoor public spaces, with trees and vegetation, are used more by both youth and adult residents, in contrast to barren spaces devoid of trees and grass (Coley et al., 1997). Sullivan and his colleagues (2004) report that nearly double the number of people used green spaces than barren spaces, and 83% more social activities occurred in green, compared to barren, spaces.

Among the Chicago public housing studies are those that take advantage of a natural experiment. Over time, trees and vegetation around some buildings diminished, while around others, they thrived. Because the buildings are architecturally identical and residents are assigned to buildings in a near-random manner, the studies allow researchers a quasi-experimental look at the influence of nature. Kuo and her colleagues (1998) found that residents of green buildings had stronger neighbourhood social ties than residents of buildings devoid of vegetation. These researchers also documented that the vegetation–social ties relation was mediated by social interaction. In other words, nature draws people together and facilitates social interaction, which, over time, weaves a community fabric, and contributes to the development of social networks. While these studies focus on adults, community cohesion is likely to benefit children as well.

Studies of children's play in nature reinforce the value of nature for social well-being. Communication skills and relationships among children improve through play in nature (Pyle, 2002; Bixler et al., 2002; Moore, 1986). Children who play together in naturescapes build positive relationships with one another (Moore, 1996; Moore and Wong, 1997), and such play may reduce bullying or violent behaviour (Malone and Tranter, 2003). Evaluations of schoolyard greening projects indicate that diverse vegetative landscapes promote cooperation, civility, and harmony (Dyment and Bell, 2008; Moore and Cosco, 2000) whereas other schoolyard designs may lead to competition for access to equipment (Malone and Tranter, 2003). Further, play in natural spaces fosters children's creative play (Cobb, 1977; Faber Taylor et al., 1998) which in turn, fosters language development and cooperation (Fjortoft and Sageie, 2000; Moore and Wong, 1997).

Cognitive functioning and academic performance

Views of, and access to nature bolster cognitive functioning. This evidence is grounded the in Attention Restoration Theory (ART) developed by Stephen Kaplan (1995) (see also Chapter 2.1 'Environmental psychology' for more discussion around theories of nature health association). ART is based, in part, on the work of the early American psychologist William James (1892), who purported that humans have two types of attention: involuntary attention, which is effortless, and involuntary or 'directed' attention, which requires effort and concentration. With prolonged use, attentional capacity becomes depleted and a person experiences 'directed attention fatigue' (DAF) characterized by difficulty concentrating, distractibility, and often, irritability. Nature engages involuntary attention, allows neural inhibitory mechanism that underlie directed attention to rest, and thereby facilitates recovery from DAF.

A growing number of studies have examined the impact of the natural environment on children's cognitive functioning. Wells (2000) followed children whose families relocated to new homes in greener neighbourhoods. From pre-move to post-move, improvements in children's cognitive functioning were statistically explained by increases in the amount of nearby nature, and not by improvements in housing quality. A subsequent study examined the effect of nature window views on three aspects of self-discipline: concentration, inhibition, and delayed gratification among children living in Chicago public housing. Among girls, the amount of nature viewed from the apartment unit was systematically related to all three measures of self-discipline, suggesting that exposure to nature bolsters cognitive functioning, or specifically, executive functioning of the brain. Among boys however, no such pattern was found. The absence of a relation with respect to boys is likely due to boys spending less time in and near the home environment and having a larger territorial range (Faber Taylor et al., 2002). Similarly, among preschool children, playing in green space with trees and varied terrain was linked to less frequent inattentive behaviour (Mårtensson et al., 2009).

Recent research examines linkages between near-school nature and school performance. Matsuoka (2010) evaluated high schools with landscapes and views ranging from 'all natural' to 'all built'. Controlling for a variety of variables, schools' views of trees and shrubs from the cafeteria was positively associated with standardized test scores, graduation rates, percentages of children planning on attending four-year colleges, as well as fewer incidences of criminal behaviour. Similarly, a study from Barcelona demonstrated a positive relation between school greenness and cognitive development over a year, only partly mediated by air pollution levels (Dadvand et al., 2015).

Attention deficit disorder/attention deficit hyperactivity disorder

Globally, 5.3% of children age 18 years and younger are affected by attention deficit hyperactivity disorder (ADHD) (Polanczyk et al., 2007). According to the US Centers for Disease Control and Prevention (CDC), US rates of ADHD have increased from 7.8% in 2003 to 11% in 2011 (Visser et al., 2014). ADHD affects children's attentional capacity and is associated with poor academic performance as well as poor peer and familial relations (Daley, 2006).

Building on the research linking nature exposure with cognitive functioning, researchers have examined the potential role of the natural environment in the reduction of symptoms among children with ADHD. This line of inquiry is based on behavioural and perhaps physiological parallels between DAF and ADHD (Faber Taylor et al., 2001; Kuo and Faber Taylor, 2004; Faber Taylor and Kuo, 2009). DAF and ADHD share symptoms including difficulty concentrating and completing tasks, impairment of impulse control, and inability to delay gratification. Parents of children with ADHD reported that their children function better and exhibit fewer symptoms of ADHD after activities in green outdoor settings, in contrast to indoor and built outdoor settings (Faber Taylor et al., 2001; Kuo and Faber Taylor, 2004).

In a recent true experiment, 17 school-age children diagnosed with attention deficits (ADD or ADHD) were randomly assigned to the order in which they took three 20-minute walks (on different days): in a park, in a neighbourhood, and downtown. Children concentrated better following the park walk than after neighbourhood or downtown walks of similar duration (Faber Taylor and Kuo, 2009). Van Den Berg and Van Den Berg (2010) found similar results in a study of children attending a farm for children with ADHD. Given the complex aetiology of ADHD (Daley, 2006) including a significant genetic component, the natural environment is not presented as a 'cure' but rather, as a potential tool to reduce symptoms.

Myopia

Around the globe, rates of myopia or nearsightedness have surged. In the United States, among youth age 12–17 years, myopia has increased from 24% to 34% from 1971/1972 to 1999/2004 (Vitale et al., 2009). In Asia, increases are more dramatic. In Taiwan, for example, in 1983, 6% of 7-year-olds and 37% of 12-year-olds were myopic, while in 2000, rates were 21% and 61%, respectively (Lin, 2004). The onset of myopia at a young age is associated with increased risk of later-life glaucoma, cataracts, and blindness. The World Health Organization indicates that myopia is among the top priorities aimed at preventing avoidable blindness by 2020 (Mccurdy et al., 2010).

Although many myopia cases can be attributed to inheritance, environmental factors are believed to be the primary explanation of recent increases (Sherwin et al., 2012). Studies suggest an inverse relation between time outdoors and the incidence or progression of myopia. Among both 12-year-olds in Sydney, Australia and 11- to 20-year olds in Singapore, China, levels of outdoor activity show a strong inverse correlation with myopia prevalence (Rose et al., 2008; Dirani et al., 2009). In a meta-analysis of seven cross-sectional studies linking time outdoors inversely with myopia, Sherwin and colleagues (2012) concluded that each additional hour that a child spent outdoors per week translated into a 2% drop in the odds of developing or worsening myopia. Additional analysis of five prospective studies revealed that after adjusting for the number of myopic parents and reading, the odds ratio for developing myopia was 0.91 for every one hour of sport/outdoor activity per week. The difference between non-myopes' and future myopes' time spent outdoors per week was 11.65 versus 7.98 hours per week (Sherwin et al., 2012). Together, the evidence suggests that increasing time outdoors is an appropriate strategy to mitigate this trend.

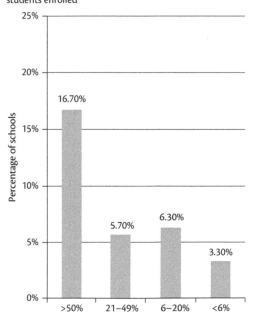

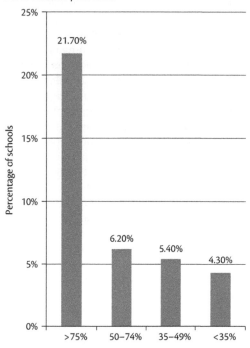

Physical activity and childhood obesity

Childhood obesity is a global epidemic with profound societal implications. From the 1970s to the 1990s, the prevalence of childhood overweight and obesity has doubled or tripled in Australia, Brazil, Canada, Chile, Finland, France, Germany, Greece, Japan, the United Kingdom, and the United States (Wang and Lobstein, 2006). Globally, in 2010, an estimated 42 million children under the age of five were overweight or obese (World Health Organization). Obesity is linked to a variety of health problems including hypertension, type 2 diabetes, sleep apnoea, and depression (Mccurdy et al., 2010); and childhood obesity is linked to later-life obesity (Guo et al., 2002). Children in low-income communities and ethnic minority youth are disproportionately at risk for obesity (CDC, 2010; Ogden et al., 2014).

Most children in the United States are not achieving recommended levels of physical activity (Pate et al., 2002). Among US children ages 6–11, only 42% achieve the recommended one hour of moderate-to-vigorous physical activity (MVPA) per day (Troiano et al., 2008). Like childhood obesity, increased sedentary behaviour is a global phenomenon evident not only in Western countries, but also in China (Chen et al., 2014) and developing countries like Vietnam (Trang et al., 2013) and South Africa (Mcveigh and Meiring, 2014).

Time spent outdoors is a consistent and positive predictor of children's physical activity (Sallis et al., 2000; Hinkley et al., 2008). During the school day, outdoor recess time contributes significantly to total daily MVPA (Council on School Health, 2013; Robert Wood Johnson Foundation, 2007; Robert Wood Johnson Foundation, 2012; Chen et al., 2014). From 1997 to 2003, the amount of time children (age 6–12) spent outdoors, on average, declined from 36 to 25 minutes per week (Hofferth, 2009).

Proximity to parks, natural areas, and recreational facilities has been linked to both physical activity and, inversely, to obesity; (see also Chapter 3.1 'Promoting physical activity—reducing obesity and other non-communicable diseases'). Higher neighbourhood greenness has been associated cross-sectionally with lower child and youth body mass index (BMI) but only in high population density areas (Lui et al., 2007). Bell et al. (2008) examined the relation between neighbourhood greenness and children's BMI both cross-sectionally and longitudinally. With a sample of predominantly African American, low-income youth, the researchers found an inverse, cross-sectional association between neighbourhood greenness and BMI z-scores. Moreover, children in greener neighbourhoods were less likely to increase their BMI over the two-year study period, compared to children in less green neighbourhoods. These analyses controlled for various covariates such as race and gender.

More recently, in an eight-year longitudinal study, Wolch et al. (2011) found that among more than 3,000 children aged 9–10 years, those with access to parks within 500 m of their homes and to recreation programmes within 10 km had reduced risk of obesity at age 18.

Despite efforts to combat childhood inactivity and obesity across the population and to target low-income and ethnic minority communities specifically, these communities are often least likely to have the physical and policy infrastructure to get children outdoors engaged in physical activity. Daily recess policies in the United States provide one example. Low-income schools are most likely to have no recess (Robert Wood Johnson Foundation, 2012; Slater et al., 2012). As illustrated in Figure 6.1.1, more than a fifth (22%) of schools with 75% or more of children qualifying for free or reduced price meals (FRPM, a school-level metric of community poverty)

Fig. 6.1.1 Percentage of schools reporting no recess by per cent ethnic minority and by per cent eligible for free or reduced price meals.

report having no recess compared with 6% of schools with 50–74% FRPM (Robert Wood Johnson Foundation, 2012). Similarly, schools educating predominantly ethnic minority youth are less likely than predominantly white schools to have daily recess (Slater et al., 2012). Daily diary data indicate that among African American students, 39% had no recess on the diary day, while among white and other minority students, rates were 15% and 25%, respectively (Roth et al., 2003).

Vitamin D deficiency

Public health researchers report that vitamin D deficiency has reached pandemic levels worldwide and greatly harms children's physical health and development (Holick and Chen, 2008). According to NHANES 2001–2004 data, in the United States, 7.6 million children and adolescents are deficient in vitamin D, while an additional 50.8 million are insufficient (Kumar et al., 2009). An increase in paediatric vitamin D deficiency and insufficiency is seen even in countries with high sun exposure like India, the Middle East, and Australia (Holick, 2008). Dubbed the 'sunshine vitamin', vitamin D synthesis begins in the human body when ultraviolet rays (UVR) penetrate the skin. Because melanin in the skin can inhibit absorption of sunlight, individuals with more pigmentation in their skin such as African Americans and other people of colour (Holick, 2008), are more likely to be vitamin D deficient. While campaigns to prevent incident of skin cancer by encouraging the proper use of sun protection have likely inadvertently affected vitamin D levels, increased time indoors undoubtedly contributes to the crisis. Kumar et al. (2009) note that youths who spend more than four hours a day watching television, playing video games, or using computers are more likely to be vitamin D deficient. Since only about 10% of RDA of vitamin D comes from food sources, skin exposure to sunlight 15 minutes twice a day is crucial to achieving optimal levels without supplementation (Holick and Chen, 2008).

Research is starting to show the many ways vitamin D affects health in childhood through adulthood. Historically, vitamin D deficiency among children has most commonly been linked to rickets, a childhood disease that causes softening of the bones that can lead to increase fracture and deformity. Rickets is caused when vitamin D deficiency results in imbalances of calcium and phosphate whereby these minerals then leach from the bones. Rickets, although remaining common in developing countries, was nearly eradicated in industrialized counties after the nineteenth century. However, it has recently re-emerged as a global paediatric health concern (Huh and Gordon, 2008). Yet, vitamin D also plays a role in non-skeletal diseases such as cancer and autoimmune disease (Holick, 2008). Particularly, because of clustering in northerly latitudes, researchers hypothesize that vitamin D deficiency may increase risk for colorectal cancers, and multiple sclerosis (Holick, 2008), however causation has not been confirmed. In children, vitamin D deficiency also may be connected to metabolic and related disorders such as insulin insensitivity, diabetes, obesity, cardiovascular disease, and asthma (Huh and Gordon, 2008). If untreated, suffering these diseases in childhood increases some disease likelihood throughout the lifecourse. A 31-year cohort study conducted in Finland showed that children who were given 2000 IU of vitamin D per day during their first year of life were 78% less likely to develop type 1 diabetes than children who were not given this supplement (Hypponen et al., 2001).

Future research and implications for public health

Despite the growing evidence that nature matters to children's health, there are various outstanding research questions that are of both practical and theoretical interest. Here we briefly highlight two: nature as a buffer and the dose-response relation of nature and health.

Nature as a buffer

Aside from the considerable evidence that nature has direct beneficial effects on children's health, there is growing evidence that access to nature may moderate the impact of stressors or other negative factors. Wells and Evans (2003) found that access to nearby nature moderated the detrimental effects of stressful live events (e.g. being picked on at school, being subject to peer pressure, having a grandparent die, and so on) on children's psychological distress. The more nature children had near their homes, the less profound was the effect of stressful life events on psychological distress. Importantly, this moderating or buffering effect was most pronounced for the most vulnerable children—those exposed to the greatest number of stressful life events (see Fig. 6.1.2). Similarly, Mitchell and Popham (2008) found that among adults, proximity to nearby nature moderated the association between socioeconomic status and mortality risk. If nature can indeed mitigate the negative effects of both stressful life events and SES on mental and/or physical health outcomes, further research is needed to examine this notion more broadly—with respect to a variety of stressors or negative environmental factors.

This notion of nature as a buffer, that natural views and nature access might dampen or mitigate various negative effects of stress and adversity, may have profound implications for public health. Recently parallels have been drawn between the childhood resilience literature (e.g. Masten, 2001; Luthar, 2006) and the empirical

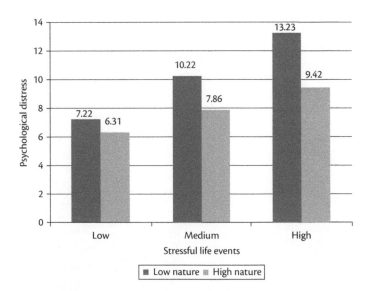

Fig. 6.1.2 Nature moderates the effects of stressful life events on children's psychological distress.

Reproduced with permission from Wells NM and Evans GW, 'Nearby nature: A buffer of life stress among rural children,' *Environment and Behavior*, Volume 35, Number 3, pp. 311-330, Copyright © 2003 Sage Publications.

evidence connecting nature access to children's well-being (Wells, 2012). Relatively speaking, nature is a low-cost intervention strategy that might help to level the playing field for youth who face adversity—be it poverty or other forms of disadvantage.

Dose-response relation

Research has not yet clearly illuminated the issue of how much nature access or nature exposure is needed to yield a benefit. What 'daily dose' of nature is necessary to yield cognitive benefits? How proximate should green infrastructure, such as parks and greenways, be to a neighbourhood to promote residents' physical activity? Research in this arena will further theory and also provide practical guidance to landscape architects and urban planners in their decision-making regarding design and policy.

Programmes: promotion, prevention, and intervention

The evidence clearly indicates myriad health benefits of nature access for children; and detrimental effects of disconnection from nature. While there can be negative consequences of time outdoors (such as sunburn, bug bites, and poison ivy), on the whole, there is an urgent need for children to connect with the natural environment. A variety of programmes have appeared internationally to address this need. Below we highlight five: 'playworkers', adventure playgrounds, outdoor classrooms, 'Parks Rx', and school gardens.

Playworkers

'Playwork' is an established and expanding profession in the United Kingdom dedicated to facilitating play among children and young people, and its tenets are gaining practice internationally. Children learn and progress in their development through play. Playwork defines play as 'a set of behaviours that are freely chosen, personally directed, and intrinsically motivated' (Wilson, 2010). Many recognized, and popular forms of childhood play do not fulfil a child's innate desire for creative, spontaneous, free play. Playworkers train professionally to facilitate play and to create play areas that are safe yet challenging and encourage a sense of adventure. Their work is meant to be unobtrusive and invisible to children, therefore they intervene only when necessary to prevent injury or harm. The oxymoron of *playwork* (Wilson, 2010) is deliberate, as the profession consciously recognizes that in an ideal world it should not exist.

Adventure playgrounds

Adventure playgrounds, originally developed a half century ago, are enjoying a global resurgence and may be one compelling strategy to reconnect children with the outdoors. Adventure playgrounds are play areas in which children engage in unstructured play and are able to learn to take calculated risks. Children engage with the natural landscape and 'loose parts', such as wood, empty boxes, and old tyres, that they can manipulate, move, and imagine to be anything (see Fig. 6.1.3).

Danish landscape architect Carl Theodora Sorenson originally conceived a 'junk playground' when he noticed that children preferred to play in spaces other than those he had designed. The first junk playground opened in Copenhagen in 1943. Following the Second World War, British landscape architect, Lady Allen of

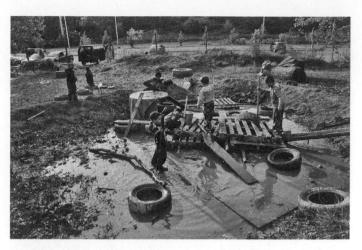

Fig. 6.1.3 Children in the 'Anarchy Zone' adventure playground in Ithaca Children's Garden, Ithaca NY, United States.
Reproduced with permission. Copyright © Rusty Keeler.

Hurtwood, expanded the concept of junk playgrounds to exclude all asphalt and to include more natural characteristics, such as knolls, water, and vegetation. The adventure playground movement began in the United Kingdom in 1946 and spread throughout Europe, where today there are more than 1,000 adventure playgrounds, facilitated by playworkers.

One of the defining, yet controversial, characteristics of adventure playgrounds is that they bring to light the potential dangers children face in self-directed play, and spur the discussion about overprotective parenting styles and its consequences for children's development. It should be noted that adventure playgrounds are no more dangerous than conventional playgrounds (Rosin, 2014).

Outdoor classrooms

Forest schools provide children access to, and education through, nature. The forest school model supplements regular classroom learning with trips to woodlands, meadows, or beaches. At most forest schools, students spend at least one day a week outside of the classroom in natural settings. The purpose of these field trips is to not only expose children to nature, but to allow for exploration and education through direct contact with the natural world. Udeskole or 'outdoor school', which is popular in Denmark, follows this paradigm. Designed primarily for children ages 7 to 16, udeskole uses nature as a classroom, as well as an interdisciplinary education tool. Children are encouraged to reflect on and write about nature, or to learn mathematics and science skills in hands-on interaction with plants and vegetation.

The ideological basis of forest schools is also shared by forest kindergartens, popular in Germany. Kindergarten translates to 'children's garden'. And indeed, when Friedrich Wilhelm August Froebel first envisioned kindergartens he intended that children spend as much time outdoors as possible, as he had a child. Over time, Froebel's conception changed to a classroom education model. However, in Germany there are over 1,000 forest kindergartens or waldkindergartens that eschew the classroom model completely. These schools are held almost entirely outdoors, year round, in all kinds of weather. Daily, children gather at a shelter and then spend the day walking and exploring in the woods. Teachers are present to provide guidance and ensure safety, but an emphasis is placed on self-directed learning and social interaction.

School gardens

School gardens have a long, international history, dating back to the 1800s in Austria and elsewhere. In the United States, school gardens were common during the First and Second World Wars as part of the victory garden movement (Hayden-Smith, 2014). In recent years, there has been a resurgence of school gardens across the United States. In Berkeley, California, Chef Alice Water's Edible Schoolyard project (http://edibleschoolyard.org/) has contributed to the growing momentum. Thousands of gardens worldwide are now registered on the edible schoolyard website. In 2007, as part of the PlaNYC, New York City Mayor Michael Bloomberg set the goal of establishing a garden in every school (Learn to Grow). Along with outdoor classrooms, school gardens may be a mechanism to bring learning outdoors and to diminish the notion that learning only happens indoors.

School gardens have been employed to educate students in a range of topics including science, environmental studies, nutrition, language arts, and math (Graham *et al.*, 2005). In addition, school gardens, along with a garden-based curriculum, have the potential to improve children's health and health behaviours (Ozer, 2007; Twiss *et al.*, 2003). In fact, gardens are unique in their potential to impact both sides of the energy balance equation: diet and physical activity. Recent evidence from a New York State study suggests that school gardens can significantly increase the time children spend engaged in MVPA during the school day (Wells *et al.*, 2014).

Parks Rx

The term 'green prescription' has been used to refer to medical doctors prescribing physical activity (Swinburn *et al.*, 1998). More recently, 'Parks Rx' and 'Nature Rx' programmes have emerged, with a more explicit focus on prescribing time outdoors, particularly for children as described in chapter 10.1 (NRPA, 2014). Further, these programmes encourage a dialogue between doctors and patients about the importance of active living and engaging with nature. In the United States, Parks Rx programmes have sprouted across the country from Washington DC to San Diego, California (National Recreation and Park Association, 2014). The partnership between the healthcare community and parks' services underlying Parks Rx demonstrates an evolving understanding of the link between public health and public spaces.

Initial feedback from these programmes has cast light on some of the barriers preventing patients from fulfilling their Parks Rx, which has led to further intervention strategies linking healthcare, outdoor recreation, and community organizations. For example, in order to address patient concerns about park safety and 'lack of familiarity with parks' (National Recreation and Park Association, 2014), the city of Baltimore implemented their Docs In the Park (DITP) programmes in 2011. Between 2011 and 2013 more than 400 youths participated in DITP events. In 2013, that number increased to 600 young people when DITP expanded in an effort to continue outreach to underserved families. Through Portland, Oregon's PlayRx programme, more than 200 prescriptions are dispensed yearly to youths, granting them a scholarship to parks and recreation activities. The city has noted that fulfilment of PlayPx has increased not only among the targeted youth, but that whole families are now utilizing the parks' services.

Conclusion

Children need nature. Nature is not optional; not a mere amenity, but rather, has important implications for children's health and well-being. Moreover, the natural environment is 'essential infrastructure' to which all citizenry ought to have access.

Acknowledgements

Our thanks go to Aaron Ong and Krista Galie for research assistance on this chapter.

References

Anderson, D., Huston, A., Schmitt, K., Linebarger, D., & Wright, J. (2001). Early childhood televison viewing and adolescent behavior. *Monogr Soc Res Child Dev*, 66, I–VIII, 1–147.

Andreason, M. S. (1994). Patterns of family life and television consumption from 1945 to the 1990's. In: Zillmann, D., Bryant, J., & Huston, A. C. (eds.) *Media, Children, and the Family*. Hillsdale, NJ: Lawrence Erlbaum Associates.

Attewell, P., Suazo-Garcia, B., & Battle, J. (2003). Computers and young children: Social benefit or social problem? *Social Forces*, 82, 277–96.

Balmford, A., Clegg, L., Coulson, T., & Taylor, J. (2002). Why conservationist should heed pokeman. *Science*, 295, 2367.

Bebbington, A. (2005). The ability of A-level students to name plants. *J Biol Educ*, 39, 62–7.

Bell, J. F., Wilson, J. F., & Liu, G. C. (2008). Neighborhood greenness and 2-year changes in body mass index of children and youth. *Am J Prev Med*, 35, 547–53.

Bixler, R. D., Floyd, M. F., & Hammitt, W. E. (2002). Environmental socialization: Quantitative tests of the childhood play hypothesis. *Environ Behav*, 34, 795–818.

Boldemann C, Dal H, Mårtensson F, Cosco N, Moore R, Bieber B. (2011) Preschool outdoor play environment may combine promotion of children's physical activity and sun protection. Further evidence from Southern Sweden and North Carolina. *Science & Sports*, 26,72–82.

Boone, C. G., Buckley, G. L., Grove, J. M., & Sister, C. (2009). Parks and people: An environmental justice inquiry in Baltimore, Maryland. *Ann Assoc Am Geogr*, 99, 767–87.

CDC. (2010). *Childhood Obesity* [Online]. CDC. Available at: http://www.cdc.gov/HealthyYouth/obesity/ (accessed 19 May 2010).

Chen, Y., Zheng, Z., Yi, J., & Yao, S. (2014). Associations between physical inactivity and sedentary behaviors among adolescents in 10 cities in China. *BMC Public Health*, 14, 744.

Clements, R. (2004). An investigation of the state of outdoor play. *Contemporary Issues in Early Childhood*, 5, 68–80.

Cobb, E. (1977). *The Ecology of Imagination in Childhood*. New York, NY: Columbia University Press.

Coley, R. L., Sullivan, W. C., & Kuo, F. E. (1997). Where does community grow? The social context created by nature in urban public housing. *Environ Behav*, 29, 468–94.

Council on School Health (2013). Policy statement: The crucial role of recess in school. *Pediatrics*, 131, 183–8.

Dadvand, P., Nieuwenhuijsen, M. J., Esnaola, M., *et al.* (2015). Green spaces and cognitive development in primary schoolchildren. *Proc Natl Acad Sci*, 112, 7937–42.

Daley, D. (2006). Attention deficit hyperactivity disorder: A review of the essential facts. *Child Care Health Dev*, 32, 193–204.

Dirani, M., Tong, L., & Gazzard, G. (2009). Outdoor activity and myopia in Singapore teenage children. *Br J Ophthalmol*, 2009, 997–1000.

Dolesh, R. J. (2014). *Equity in the Big Apple*. Ashburn, VA: National Recreation and Park Association (NRPA).

Dyment, J. E. & Bell, A. C. (2008). Grounds for movement: Green school grounds as sites for promoting physical activity. *Health Educ Res*, 23, 952–62.

Evans, G. W. & Kantrowitz, E. (2002). Socioeconomic status and health: The potential role of environmental risk exposure. *Ann Rev Public Health*, 23, 303–31.

Faber Taylor, A. & Kuo, F. E. (2009). Children with attention deficits concentrate better after walk in the park. *J Attention Disord*, 12, 402–9.

Faber Taylor, A., Kuo, F. E., & Sullivan, W. C. (2001). Coping with ADD the surprising connection to green play settings. *Environ Behav*, 33, 54–77.

Faber Taylor, A., Kuo, F. E., & Sullivan, W. C. (2002). View of nature and self-discipline: Evidence from inner city children. *J Environ Psychol*, 22, 49–63.

Faber Taylor, A., Wiley, A., Kuo, F. E., & Sullivan, W. C. (1998). Growing up in the inner city: Green spaces as places to grow. *Environ Behav*, 30, 3–27.

Fjortoft, I. & Sageie, J. (2000). The natural environment as a playground for children: Landscape description and analysis of a natural landscape. *Landsc Urban Plan*, 48, 83–97.

Ginsburg, K. R. (2007). The importance of play in promoting healthy child development and maintaining strong parent-child bonds. *Pediatrics*, 119, 182–91.

Graham H, Beall DL, Lussier M, McLaughlin P, Zidenberg-Cherr S. (2005) Use of school gardens in academic instruction. *J Nutr Educ Behav.*, 37(3), 147–151.

Guo, S. S., Wu, W., Chumlea, W. C., & Roche, A. F. (2002). Predicting overweight and obesity in adulthood from body mass index values in childhood and adolescence. *Am J Clin Nutr*, 76, 653–8.

Hayden-Smith, R. (2014). *A brief history of school gardens* [Online]. Kitchen Gardeners International. Available at: http://kgi.org/blogs/rose-hayden-smith/brief-history-school-gardens (accessed 23 September 2014) [Online].

Hinkley, T., Crawford, D., Salmon, J., Okely, A. D., & Hesketh, K. (2008). Preschool children and physical activity—A review of correlates *Am J Prev Med*, 34, 435–41.

Hofferth, S. L. (2009). Changes in American children's time—1997 to 2003. *Electron Int J Time Use Res*, 6, 26–47.

Hofferth, S. L. (2010). Home media and childrens' achievement and behavior. *Child Dev*, 81, 1598–619.

Holick, M. F. (2008). The vitamin D deficiency pandemic and consequences for nonskeletal health: Mechanisms of action. *Mol Aspects Med*, 29, 361–8.

Holick, M. F. & Chen, T. C. (2008). Vitamin D deficiency: A worldwide problem with health consequences. *Am J Clin Nutr*, 87, 1080S–6S.

Huh, S. Y. & Gordon, C. M. (2008). Vitamin D deficiency in children and adolescents: Epidemiology, impact and treatment. *Rev Endocr Metab Disord*, 9, 161–70.

Hypponen, E., Laara, E., Jarvelin, M. R., & Virtanen, S. M. (2001). Intake of vitamin D and risk of type 1 diabetes: A birth-cohort study. *Lancet*, 358, 1500–3.

James, W. (1892). *Psychology: A Briefer Course*. New York, NY: Holt.

Kaplan, S. (1995). The restorative benefits of nature: Toward an integrative framework. *J Environ Psychol*, 15, 169–82.

Kumar, J., Muntner, P., Kaskel, F. J., Hailpern, S. M., & Melamed, M. L. (2009). Prevalence and associations of 25-Hydroxyvitamin D deficiency in US children: NHANES 2001–2004. *Pediatrics*, 124, e362–70.

Kuo, F. E. & Faber Taylor, A. (2004). A potential natural treatment for attention-deficit/ hyperactivity disorder: Evidence from a national study. *Am J Public Health*, 94, 1580–6.

Kuo, F. E., Sullivan, W. C., & Wiley, A. (1998). Fertile ground for community: Inner-city neighborhood common spaces. *Am J Community Psychol*, 26, 823–51.

Landry, S. M. & Chakraborty, J. (2009). Street trees and equity: evaluating the spatial distribution of an urban amenity. *Environment and Planning*, 41, 2651–70.

Learn to Grow. Available at: http://growtolearn.org/ (accessed 23 September 2014) [Online].

Lin, L. L. K. (2004). Prevalence of myopia in Taiwanese schoolchildren: 1983 to 2000. *Ann Acad Med Singapore*, 33, 27–33.

Louv, R. (2005). *Last Child in the Woods: Saving Our Children from Nature-Deficit Disorder*. Chapel Hill, NC: Algonquin Books.

Lui, G. C., Wilson, J. S., Qi, R., & Ying, J. (2007). Green neighborhoods, food retail and childhood overweight: differences by population density. *Am J Health Promot*, 21, 317–25.

Luthar, S. S. (2006). Resilience in development: A synthesis of research across five decades. In: Cicchetti, D. & Cohen, D. J. (eds.) *Developmental Psychopathology: Risk, Disorder, and Adaptation*. Hoboken, NJ: Wiley.

Malone, K. & Tranter, P. (2003). Children's environmental learning and the use, design and management of schoolgrounds. *Children, Youth and Environments*, 13, 87–137.

Masten, A. (2001). Ordinary magic: Resilience processes in development. *Am Psychol*, 53, 205–20.

Matsouka, R. H. (2010). Student performance and high school landscapes: Examining the links. *Landsc Urban Plan*, 97, 273–82.

Mccurdy, L. E., Winterbottom, K. E., Mehta, S. S., & Roberts, J. R. (2010). Using nature and outdoor activity to improve children's health. *Curr Probl Pediatr Adolesc Health Care*, 5, 102–17.

Mcveigh, J. & Meiring, R. (2014). Physical activity and sedentary behavior in an ethnically diverse group of South African school children. *J Soc Sci Med*, 13, 371–8.

Mitchell, R. & Popham, F. (2008). Effect of exposure to natural environment on health inequalities: an observational population study. *Lancet*, 372, 1655–60.

Moore, R. C. (1986). The power of nature orientations of girls and boys toward biotic and abiotic play settings on a reconstructed schoolyard. *Children's Environments Quarterly*, 3, 52–68.

Moore, R. C. (1996). Compact nature: The role of playing and learning gardens on children's lives. *Therapeutic Horticulture*, 8, 72–82.

Moore, R. C. & Cosco, N. G. (2000). Developing an earth-bound culture through design of childhood habitats, natural learning initiative. A Global View of Community Gardening. *People, Land, and Sustainability*. University of Nottingham.

Moore, R. C. & Wong, H. 1997. *Natural learning: Rediscovering nature's way of teaching*, Berkeley, CA, MIG Communications.

Mårtensson, F., Boldemann, C., Söderström, M., Blennow, M., Englund, J. E., & Grahn, P. (2009). Outdoor environmental assessment of attention promoting settings for preschool children. *Health Place*, 15, 1149–57.

Mårtensson, F, (2013) Guiding environmental dimensions for outdoor play, Journal of Social medicine, 90 (4) 658-665, http://socialmedicinsktidskrift.se/index.php/smt/article/view/1047/849

National Recreation and Park Association (NRPA) (2014). *Prescribing Parks for Better Health: Success Stories*. Ashburn, VA: National Recreation and Park Association.

Ogden, C. L., Carroll, M. D., Kit, B. K., & Flegal, K. M. (2014). Prevalence of childhood and adult obesity in the United States, 2011–2012. *J Am Med Assoc*, 311, 806–14.

Ozer, E. J. (2007). The effects of school gardens on students and schools: conceptualization and considerations for maximizing healthy development. *Health Educ Behav*, 34, 846–63.

Pate, R. R., Freedson, P. S., Sallis, J. F., *et al*. (2002). Compliance with physical activity guidelines: prevalence in a population of children and youth. *Annals of Epidemiology*, 12, 303–8.

Pellegrini, A. D. & Bohn, C. M. (2005). The role of recess in children's cognitive performance and school adjustment. *Educ Res*, 34, 13–19.

Polanczyk, G., Silva De Lima, M., Horta, B. L., Biederman, J., & Rohde, L. A. (2007). The worldwide prevalence of ADHD: A systematic review and metaregression analysis. *Am J Psychiatry*, 164, 942–8.

Pyle, R. (2002). Eden in a vacant lot: Special places, species and kids in community of life. *Children and Nature: Psychological, Sociocultural and Evolutionary Investigations*. Cambridge, MA: MIT Press.

Rideout, V., Foehr, U., & Roberts, D. (2010). *Generation M2: Media in the lives of 8- to 18-year olds*. Menlo Park, CA: Henry J. Kaiser Family Foundation.

Robert Wood Johnson Foundation (2007). Recess Rules: Why the undervalued playtime may be America's best investment for healthy kids and healthy schools. Robert Wood Johnson Foundation. Available at: http://www.rwjf.org/en/library/research/2007/09/recess-rules.html [Online].

Robert Wood Johnson Foundation 2012. *Increasing Physical Activity through Recess*. Robert Wood Johnson Foundation. Active Living Research. Available at: http://activelivingresearch.org/increasing-physical-activity-through-recess [Online].

Rose, K. A., Morgan, I. G., Ip, J., *et al.* (2008). Outdoor activity reduces the prevalence of myopia in children. *Ophthalmology*, 115, 1279–85.

Rosin, H. (2014). The Overprotected Kid. *The Atlantic.* 19 March 2014.

Roth, J. L., Brooks-Gunn, J., Linvar, M. R., & Hofferth, S. L. (2003). Time diaries from a national sample of elementary school teachers. *Teachers College Record*, 105, 317–43.

Sallis, J., Prochaska, J., & Taylor, W. (2000). A review of correlates of physical activity of children and adolescents. *Med Sci Sports Exercise*, 32, 963–75.

Sherman, A. (1994). *Wasting America's Future.* Boston MA: Beacon Press.

Sherwin, J. C., Reacher, M. H., Keogh, R. H., Khawaja, A. P., Mackey, D. A., & Foster, P. J. (2012). The association between time spent outdoors and myopia in children and adolescents. *Ophthalmology*, 119, 2141–51.

Slater, S. J., Nicholson, L., Chriqui, J., Turner, L., & Chaloupka, F. (2012). The impact of state laws and district policies on physical education and recess practices in a nationally representative sample of US public elementary schools. *Arch Pediatr Adolesc Med*, 166, 311–16.

Söderström M, Boldemann C, Sahlin U, Mårtensson F, Raustorp A, Blennow M. 2012. The quality of the outdoor environment influences children's health. -A cross-sectional study of preschools. (2012) Acta Paediatr 5. doi: 10.1111/apa.12047)

Strife, S. & Downey, L. (2009). Child development and access to nature: A new direction for environmental inequality research. *Organ Environ*, 22, 99–122.

Suecoff, S. A., Avner, J. R., Chou, K. J., & Crain, E. F. (1999). A comparison of New York City playground hazards in high and low income areas. *Arch Pediatr Adolesc Med*, 153, 363–6.

Sullivan, W. C., Kuo, F. E., & Depooter, S. F. (2004). The fruit of urban nature: vital neighborhood spaces. *Environ Behav*, 36, 678–700.

Swinburn, B. A., Walter, L. G., Arroll, B., Tilyard, M. W., & Russell, D. G. (1998). The green prescription study: A randomized controlled trial of written exercise advice provided by general practitoners. *Am J Public Health*, 88, 288–91.

Trang, N. H., Hong, T. K., van der Ploeg, H. P., Hardy, L. L., Kelly, P. J., & Dibley, M. J. (2013). Longitudinal sedentary behavior changes in adolescents in Ho Chi Minh City. *Am J Prev Med*, 44, 223–30.

Troiano, R. P., Berrigan, D., Dodd, K. W., Masse, L. C., Tilert, T., & Mcdowell, M. (2008). Physical activity in the United States measured by accelerometer. *Med Sci Sports Exerc*, 40, 181–8.

Twiss, J., Dickinson, J., Duma, S., Kleinman, T., Paulsen, H., & Rilveria, L. (2003). Community gardens: lessons learned from california healthy cities and communities. *Am J Public Health*, 93, 1435–8.

van den Berg, A. E. & van den Berg, C. G. (2010). A comparison of children with ADHD in a natural and built setting. *Child Care Health Dev*, 37, 430–9.

Visser, S. N., Danielson, M. L., Bitsko, R. H., *et al.* (2014). Trends in the parent-report of health care provider-diagnosed and medicated attention-deficit/hyperactivity disorder: United States, 2003–2011. *J Am Acad Child Adolesc Psychiatry*, 53, 34–46.

Vitale, S., Sperduto, R. D., & Ferris, F. L. (2009). Increased prevalence of myopia in the United States between 1971–1972 and 1999–2004. *Arch Ophthalmol*, 127, 1632–9.

von Essen, E., & Mårtensson, F. (2014). Young adults' use of food as a self-therapeutic intervention *Int J Qual Stud Health Well-being.*, 9:23000, 1-9. doi: 10.3402/qhw.v9.23000

Wang, Y. & Lobstein, T. (2006). Worldwide trends in childhood overweight and obesity. *Int J Pediatr Obes*, 1, 11–25.

Wells, N. M. (2000). At home with nature: Effects of "greenness" on children's cognitive functioning. *Environ Behav*, 32, 775–95.

Wells, N. M. (2012). The role of nature in children's resilience: cognitive and social processes. In: Krasny, K. T. M. (ed.) *Greening in the Red Zone.* Berlin, Germany: Springer.

Wells, N. M. & Evans, G. W. (2003). Nearby nature: A buffer of life stress among rural children. *Environ Behav*, 35, 311–30.

Wells, N. M. & Lekies, K. S. (2006). Nature and the life course: Pathways from childhood nature experiences to adult environmentalism. *Children, Youth and Environments*, 16, 1–24.

Wells, N. M., Myers, B. M., & Henderson, C. R. (2014). School gardens and physical activity: A randomized controlled trial of low-income elementary schools. *Prev Med*, 69, S27–S33.

Wilson, P. (2010). The playworker primer. College Park, MD: Alliance for Childhood (NJ3a).

Wolch, J., Jerrett, M., Reynolds, K., *et al.* (2011). Childhood obesity and proximity to urban parks and recreational resources: A longitudinal cohort study. *Health Place*, 17, 207–14.

World Health Organization. *Global strategy on diet physical activity and health* [Online]. Available at: http://www.who.int/dietphysicalactivity/childhood/en/ (accessed 15 September 2014) [Online].

CHAPTER 6.2

Nature-based treatments as an adjunctive therapy for anxiety among elders

Mark B. Detweiler, Jack Carman, and Jonna G. Meinersmann-Detweiler

Nature and quality of life among elders

The science and role of nature-based treatment in geriatric medicine is rarely part of the medical school curricula or geriatric residency programmes. The role of nature in improving the quality of life (QoL) in the frail elderly by providing pleasant surroundings and activities has in large part been delegated to non-medical specialties such as horticulture and landscape architecture. Quantitative studies demonstrating positive outcomes of nature-based treatment modalities are rarely discussed in medical journals.

Assessing and approaching the burden associated with anxiety on cognitive and functional capacities in ageing and disease may contribute to improving QoL by optimizing environmental designs and including nature-based treatments to improve outcomes. This chapter will focus on some of the evidence supporting the role of nature, gardens, and horticulture in modulating anxiety in frail elders with the aim of heightening the profile of nature as a stabilizing and healing component of geriatric care.

Prevalence of anxiety among elders

In the United States and Europe by 2050, it is predicted that one in three persons will be 65 years or older, a huge demographic change as compared with one in five in 2011 (Lenze and Wetherell, 2011). Late-life anxiety disorders have been referred to as the 'geriatric giant', due not only to it's long-term repercussions on cognition and function (Andrews-Hanna et al., 2007; Cassidy and Rector, 2008; Vytal et al., 2012), but also to its impact on QoL, morbidity, and mortality, especially in persons with co-morbid medical problems. Common anxiety disorders among elders include generalized anxiety disorder (GAD), post-traumatic stress disorder, social phobia, panic disorder, specific phobias, obsessive-compulsive disorder, agoraphobia, and fear of falling (FoF) (Scheffer et al., 2007). GAD is the most frequent late-life anxiety disorder (Chou, 2009). The burden resulting from the high prevalence and chronicity of GAD alone, without any co-morbidities, presents a public health imperative to develop management strategies for this often undiagnosed and untreated disorder among elderly (Porensky et al., 2009).

Anxiety occurs more frequently in the elderly population than does depression and dementia. Some studies place the prevalence of anxiety among older adults at 10–20%, twice as common as dementia (8%) and four to eight times more prevalent than major depressive disorders (1–3%) (Cassidy and Rector, 2008). The prevalence of anxiety is estimated to be 15 to 56% in clinical settings and 15 to 52% in community settings (Bryant et al., 2008). Nonetheless, anxiety is often overlooked by family members and health professionals (Lenze and Wetherell, 2011). Late-life anxiety may be difficult to diagnose as older people tend to express psychiatric problems as physical complaints (D'Arrigo, 2013). Also, standardized anxiety assessment tools have been developed for younger age groups, not older people (Bryant et al., 2008).

The hidden anxiety diagnosis

Diagnosing underlying anxiety in frail elders is complicated by today's fast paced office visits and in hospital settings when medical symptoms may sometimes be triaged higher than anxiety symptoms (Tesar et al., 2010). For example, the symptoms of attention deficits, tachycardia, hypertension, headache, and pain may have both physical or psychiatric origins. Moreover, signs of diminished attention often indicate underlying anxiety (Rankin et al., 1995). Arrhythmias may convert into primary psychiatric disorders such as a panic attacks (Frommeyer et al., 2013). A two-decade study demonstrated that persons who experience symptoms of anxiety are at increased risk of developing hypertension (Mercante et al., 2011). In addition, a common clinical presentation is anxiety with co-morbid headaches. In anxiety disorder patients, particularly those with GAD, the diagnosis of primary headache can improve patient management and clinical outcomes. Regarding the relationship between anxiety and pain, Ploghaus et al. demonstrated that the hippocampal entorhinal cortex of the brain may respond differentially to identical painful stimuli, dependent on whether the perceived pain intensity is augmented by pain-relevant anxiety (Ploghaus et al., 2001).

Neurobiology of anxiety disorders

Normal ageing and other biological, physical, or chemical stressors may accelerate neurodegenerative changes, possibly leading to reduced functional neural connectivity and clinical anxiety. Late-onset anxiety probably follows the same neurobiological model (Vink et al., 2008). The level of anxiety may be related to the degrees of disruption among the amygdala, anterior cingulate cortex, dorsolateral and ventromedial prefrontal cortices parts of the brain (Lenze and Wetherell, 2011; Andrews-Hanna et al., 2007; Aupperle and Paulus, 2010). Significant to older people, chronic stress, such as anxiety, disrupts cognition due to selective volume loss of the CA3/dentate gyrus subfields of the hippocampus (Wang et al., 2010).

A broad spectrum of biopsychosocial variables among older people may increase the risk of acquiring anxiety disorders (Coolidge et al., 2000). When compared with a non-anxious elder cohort, persons with GAD have worse health-related QoL and greater healthcare utilization, even without concurrent psychiatric co-morbidity (Porensky et al., 2009). The diagnosis of co-morbid disorders with anxiety is important, as concurrence increases the risk of cognitive and functional impairment, disability, and suicidality (Simon, 2009). GAD is one of the most common co-morbid conditions with medical disorders (Noyes, 2001). Frequent co-morbidities of GAD include other anxieties (e.g. panic disorder, phobias, and compulsions), major depressive disorder, bipolar disorder, and substance abuse. Anxiety is the most common psychiatric co-morbidity of major depressive disorder (47.5%) (Beekman et al., 2000).

The role of nature in reducing anxiety among elders

There are a variety of therapies for the treatment of anxiety. Pharmacological or psychotherapeutic treatments have been shown to improve the QoL for patients with panic disorder, social phobia, and post-traumatic stress disorder. Benzodiazepines are frequently utilized for the treatment of anxiety in older people. However, they may increase the risk of cognitive impairment, Alzheimer's disease, and falls (de Gage et al., 2014), as well as eventually polluting the environment.

Inclusive anxiety protocols should address the possible lifestyle contributors, such as excessive caffeine, chocolate, alcohol, cannabis; over-the-counter medications; herbal medications; insufficient exercise; poor diet; and poor sleep hygiene. In some cases, treatment of anxiety may consist of a combination of medications, psychotherapy, behavioural therapy, and alternative medical methods such as horticulture, meditation, or acupuncture.

Nature seems to be among the most effective alternative treatments of anxiety. For example, as discussed in Chapter 2.1, 'Environmental psychology', it has been hypothesized that human beings have an automatic and subconscious positive response when perceiving nature (Relf, 1998; Ulrich, 1983). Dzhambov and Dimitrova assessed whether 'awareness of nature experiences' was a significant modifier of the beneficial effects of the interaction of older people with urban green spaces. They confirmed their hypothesis that elders' personal history of purposeful and conscious interaction with nature formulated an internal cognitive model of 'self' in natural settings that diminishes health anxiety when they visited urban parks (Dzhambov and Dimitrova, 2014). Several studies have

suggested that being able to view, experience or interact with nature has a positive impact on health, anxiety, and aggression in older people (Namazi and Johnson, 1992; Mather et al., 1997; McMinn and Hinton, 2000). Incorporating safe gardens into the designs of assisted living centres, rehabilitation centres, and dementia residences encourages autonomy, sensory stimulation, and ambulation (Detweiler et al., 2008; Mooney and Nicell, 1992).

A dementia unit with minimal opportunities for decision-making and without access to a garden may contribute to residents' feelings of helplessness, consequently increasing the risk of anxiety and inappropriate behaviours (McMinn and Hinton, 2000). It is not uncommon to find the residents of dementia units wandering throughout the unit searching for an unlocked door in the attempt 'to go home'. Providing elderly residents liberal access to outdoor gardens often diminishes the anxiety of being locked inside without perceived escape (Dzhambov and Dimitrova, 2014; Detweiler et al., 2008). The incorporation of a garden in a dementia residence can improve the daily QoL of both the residents and the staff by contributing to the reduction of disruptive behaviours (Namazi and Johnson, 1992; Detweiler et al., 2008). In general, dementia residents seem to experience less anxiety and agitated behaviours with garden access (Namazi and Johnson, 1992; McMinn and Hinton, 2000; Mooney and Nicell, 1992).

The characteristics of plants, trees, water, and wildlife provide an infinite spectrum of shapes, colours, textures, and sounds to stimulate the visual, auditory, tactile, and olfactory senses (Koura et al., 2010). In doing so, there is a focusing of attention and varying increase in cognitive load depending on the novelty and affective connection of the natural environment to the individual (Simpson et al., 2001). The work of Dvorak-Bertsch et al. provides some theoretical support to the contribution of nature in anxiety reduction (Dvorak-Bertsch et al., 2007). They report that individual differences in anxiety levels and emotional processing may be influenced by the level of attentional focus and cognitive load. Anxiety may be reduced by heightening the experiential cognitive load and redirecting attentional focus away from anxiety-provoking internal or external triggers.

A prospective observational study investigated the effect of a dementia garden specifically designed for residents in a locked facility (Detweiler et al., 2008; Edwards et al., 2013; Detweiler et al., 2009). Based on Cohen-Mansfield Agitation Inventory (CMAI) scores, anxiety, as indexed by agitation, decreased during the 12 months when the garden was accessible. Frequent users of the garden were found to have the most improved CMAI scores, but both frequent and infrequent garden visitors had better mean CMAI scores by the end of the observation year. Gardens and outdoor spaces may contribute to reduced FoF anxiety by promoting ambulation, exercise, and reducing falls (Detweiler et al., 2008; Detweiler et al., 2009; Gagnon et al., 2005). Moreover, preliminary study results suggest that increased utilization of a dementia garden may decrease the number of falls and fall severity by approximately 30% (Detweiler et al., 2009), thus lowering FoF anxiety.

Nature, gardens, and horticulture in elders' environment and residences

One of the fears of the ageing population is to lose their independence with the result of transition to institutional homes for older poeple. Yeunsook et al. (2012) explored housing alternatives that would enable older people to live in places with the most natural social integration available, including proper spatial planning to promote holistic health of the fragile aged. They explored the ideal design of a community home for elders with dementia, with appropriate scales for easy management, connections with the local community, and natural green environments for healing that will ease local residents' aversion towards elder housing.

Residents in elder housing may derive a sense of well-being and life satisfaction from both passive (window view of garden or green space) and active (active gardening) components of interaction with the green environment (Brascamp and Kidd, 2004; Joseph *et al.*, 2005). Large windows allowing those domiciled in residences to view a garden can reduce stress and anxiety by reminding them of the possibility of visiting the garden, in addition to promoting positive reminiscences (Simpson *et al.*, 2001; Epstein *et al.*, 2007). Purposeful involvement led by dementia unit staff members in horticultural and garden activities can increase garden utilization (Chapman *et al.*, 2007). Increased garden and green space utilization may in turn contribute to improvements in depression (Rappe and Kivelä, 2005), quality of life (Dvorak-Bertsch *et al.*, 2007), and physical and cognitive rehabilitation (McMinn and Hinton, 2000; Jonveaux *et al.*, 2013) with the benefit of emotional, physical, and spiritual renewal (Milligan *et al.*, 2004).

Appropriately designed gardens have an important therapeutic role for older people experiencing the stresses of ageing, including anxiety accompanied by co-morbid medical and psychiatric problems (Gulwadi, 2006). Specialists in the field maintain that an environment that includes greater than 70% lush greenery and gardens with pleasant smells, colours, and shapes, in addition to less complex visual stimuli such as manmade hardscape, may reduce anxiety (Marcus, 2008). When exposed to a herb garden and a simple landscaped area planted with one tree, older people respond more favourably, in terms of mood and cardiac physiology, as compared to a structured garden (Goto *et al.*, 2013). In urban areas, communal gardening on allotment sites may promote elders' healthy ageing by improving socialization (Jorgensen and Anthopoulou, 2007; van den Berg *et al.*, 2010).

There are a variety of therapeutic garden settings that have evolved over the past two decades. Healing gardens are designed for specific patient populations, such as burns victims (Legacy Emanuel Medical Center, Portland, OR) and patients with AIDS (Terence Cardinal Cook Health Center, NY, NY). Regarding the development of therapeutic gardens in senior care communities, there are several garden types, including physical therapy gardens, Alzheimer's gardens, and other specialized gardens.

One example of a successfully designed residence and garden for older people is the Saint John Neumann Nursing Home in Philadelphia, Pennsylvania, United States, a Catholic non-profit, 226-bed, skilled nursing facility located on 12 acres of campus. The Sensory Garden is a secure interior courtyard area that does not have access to the exterior areas of the building. It is not dementia specific and is open to everyone in the facility 24 hours a day as the doors are unlocked. This garden has been designed to meet the physical, psychological, social, and spiritual needs of the older adults living within the nursing home (see Fig. 6.2.1).

The garden has been named the 'Sensory Garden' because it has been designed to positively affect a person's senses. The garden was designed to enable maximized use in all seasons, as well as at all times of the day and night. The plants have been selected for their

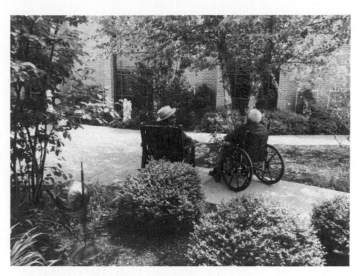

Fig. 6.2.1 Older people enjoying the Sensory Garden, engaging in a quiet conversation.
Image reproduced courtesy of Jack Carman, FASLA, RLA, CAPS, Design for Generations, LLC, United States.

seasonal interest. The exfoliating bark of the River Birch tree and the colours of the Coral Bark Maple tree make these plants visually appealing during the winter months, while the tender perennials that attract humming birds in the summer months provide a delightful scene. The 'Memory Bells' that have soft pleasant sounds when the wind blows also alert a person to outdoor breezes. Lavender and other fragrant herbs provide pleasant smells and can be used in the horticultural therapy programmes. The feel of Lambs Ear, a non-toxic herb, can bring a smile to anyone's face as it feels like the edge of a blanket the residents may have had as a child.

The Sensory Garden is accessible by all residents regardless of their ambulation status. People using wheelchairs, walkers, or canes are able to enjoy the garden. A positive design aspect of the Sensory Garden is that it is surrounded on three sides by full length windows. This enables residents who may not be able to go outside, or who choose not to, to sit by the windows enjoying nature and watching the garden events. There are no steps. All the paths are level with tinted concrete to reduce glare and have a minimum width of five feet, making them broad enough for people in wheelchairs to pass other persons walking along the paths. The garden area is easily navigable as the paths all loop around with no dead ends. Low voltage lighting along the paths and under the trees, allows the staff to take people outside at any time of the night. This style of lighting creates a softer, more residential feel, as opposed to spot lights and taller lamp post light fixtures.

Access to nature for all of the elders and their caregivers was one of the core principals in designing the Sensory Garden. Many of the activities and programmes that occur within the senior living community are able to take place in the garden. Staff meetings, barbecues, special events, religious ceremonies, nature programmes, and other activities occur on an almost daily basis. Administrator Michelle Bieszczad notes, 'There is hardly a time when the garden is not being used'. Regarding the effect of the garden on anxiety, Bieszczad stated, the 'staff will take a person outside if they are anxious or agitated, weather permitting. Many of the residents will calm down after being outside'. Recreation specialists, physical therapists, and other nursing home department personnel work with residents in the garden. Physical therapists take their patients for walks outside instead of walking indoors in the halls. There is an exercise class that meets on a regular basis and is moved outside whenever the weather is pleasant. Family members who come to visit may spend time together with the resident in a quiet corner of the garden. In addition, the garden allows caregivers to relax during lunch or during their breaks in a natural environment. Stress reduction from a garden accessible to staff of elder housing may reduce staff turnover, thus increasing the quality of care. The garden supports these individual and collective nursing home needs.

Conclusion

In conclusion, outside of the purview of the geriatric allopathic community, there is a growing body of evidence to support the incorporation of nature-based adjunctive treatment protocols and environmental designs in geriatric care plans. This evidence demonstrates the role of nature, gardens, and horticulture as healing components in modulating anxiety in frail elders. The diagnostic, treatment, and research curricula in university geriatric education programmes and geriatric medical residencies would benefit from an expanded effort to integrate evidence-based studies that delineate the role of nature in improving QoL by reduction of elders' daily anxiety. Adjunctive medical treatment modalities, housing design, green space design, and healthy activities are essential to consider for the present and future care of our burgeoning worldwide geriatric population.

References

Andrews-Hanna, J. R., Snyder, A. Z., Vincent, J. L., et al. (2007). Disruption of large-scale brain systems in advanced aging. Neuron, 56, 924–35.

Aupperle, R. L. & Paulus, M. P. (2010). Neural systems underlying approach and avoidance in anxiety disorders. Dialogues Clin Neurosci, 12, 517–31.

Beekman, A. T., de Beurs, E., van Balkom, A. J., et al. (2000). Anxiety and depression in later life: Co-occurrence and communality of risk factors. Am J Psychiatry, 157, 89–95.

Brascamp, W. & Kidd, J. L. (2004). Contribution of plants to the well-being of retirement home residents. Acta Horticulturae, 639, 145–50.

Bryant, C., Jackson, H., & Ames, D. (2008). The prevalence of anxiety in older adults: methodological issues and a review of the literature. J Affect Disord, 109, 233–50.

Cassidy, K. L. & Rector, N. A. (2008). The silent geriatric giant: anxiety disorders in late life. Geriatrics & Aging, 11, 150–6.

Chapman, N. J., Hazen, T., & Noell-Waggoner, E. (2007). Gardens for people with dementia: Increasing access to the natural environment for residents with Alzheimer's. Journal of Housing for the Elderly, 21, 249–63.

Chou, K. L. (2009). Age at onset of generalized anxiety disorder in older adults. Am J Geriatr Psychiatry, 17, 455–64.

Coolidge, F. L., Segal, D. L., Hook, J. N., et al. (2000). Personality disorders and coping among anxious older adults. J Anxiety Disord, 14, 157–72.

D'Arrigo, T. (2013). Finesse required to treat anxiety in the elderly. American College of Physicians Internist. Available at: http://www.acpinternist.org (accessed 2 August 2014) [Online].

de Gage, S. B., Moride, Y., Ducruet, T., et al. (2014). Benzodiazepine use and risk of Alzheimer's disease: case-control study. BMJ, 349, g5205.

Detweiler, M. B., Murphy, P., Myers, L. C., et al. (2008). Does a wander garden influence inappropriate behaviors in dementia residents? Am J Alzheimers Dis Other Demen, 23, 47–56.

Detweiler, M. B., Murphy, P. F., Kim, K. Y., et al. (2009). Scheduled medications and falls in dementia patients utilizing a wander garden. Am J Alzheimers Dis Other Demen, 24, 322–32.

Dvorak-Bertsch, J. D., Curtin, J. J., Rubinstein, T. J., et al. (2007). Anxiety modulates the interplay between cognitive and affective processing. Psychol Sci, 18, 699–705.

Dzhambov, A. M. & Dimitrova, D. D. (2014). Elderly visitors of an urban park, health anxiety and individual awareness of nature experiences. Urban For Urban Greening, 13, 806–13.

Edwards, C. A., McDonnell, C., & Merl, H. (2013). An evaluation of a therapeutic garden's influence on the quality of life of aged care residents with dementia. Dementia, 12, 494–510.

Epstein, M., Hansen, V., & Hazen, T. (2007). Therapeutic gardens: Plant centered activities meet sensory, physical and psychosocial needs. Oreg J Aging, 9, 8–14.

Frommeyer, G., Eckardt, L., & Breithardt G. (2013). Panic attacks and supraventricular tachycardias: the chicken or the egg? Neth Heart J, 21, 74–7.

Gagnon, N., Flint, A. J., Naglie, G., et al. (2005). Affective correlates of fear of falling in elderly persons. Am J Geriatr Psychiatry, 13, 7–14.

Goto, S., Park, B. J., Tsunetsugu, Y., et al. (2013). The effect of garden designs on mood and heart output in older adults residing in an assisted living facility. HERD, 6, 27–42.

Gulwadi, G. B. (2006). Seeking restorative experiences. Environ Behav, 38, 503–20.

Jonveaux, T. R., Batt, M., Fescharek, R., et al. (2013). Healing gardens and cognitive behavioral units in the management of Alzheimer's disease patients: The Nancy experience. J Alzheimers Dis, 34, 325–38.

Jorgensen, A. & Anthopoulou, A. (2007). Enjoyment and fear in urban woodlands—Does age make a difference? Urban For Urban Greening, 6, 267–78.

Joseph, A., Zimring Harris-Kojetin, L., & Kieferc, K., et al. (2005). Presence and visibility of outdoor and indoor physical activity features and participation in physical activity among older adults in retirement communities. J Hous Elderly, 19, 141–65.

Koura, S., Oshikawa, T., Ogawa, N., et al. (2010). Utilization of horticultural therapy for elderly persons in the urban environment. Acta Horticulturae, 881, 865–8.

Lenze, E. J. & Wetherell, J. L. (2011). A lifespan view of anxiety disorders. Dialogues Clin Neurosci, 13, 381–99.

Marcus, C. C. (2008). Ratio of lush greenery to hardscape of 7:3. Healthcare Garden Design Certificate Program, Chicago Botanic Garden.

Mather, J. A., Nemecek, D., & Oliver, K. (1997). The effect of a walled garden on behavior of individuals with Alzheimer's. Am J Alzheimers Dis, 12, 252–7.

McMinn, B. G. & Hinton, L. (2000). Confined to barracks: The effects of indoor confinement on aggressive behavior among inpatients of an acute psychogeriatric unit. Am J Alzheimers Dis Other Demen, 15, 36–41.

Mercante, J. P. P., Peres, M. F. P., & Bernik, M. A. (2011). Primary headaches in patients with generalized anxiety disorder. J Headache Pain, 12, 331–8.

Milligan, C., Gatrell, A., & Bingley, A. (2004). 'Cultivating health': Therapeutic landscapes and older people in northern England. Soc Sci Med, 58, 1781–93.

Mooney, P. & Nicell, P. L. (1992). The importance of exterior environment for Alzheimer's residents: effective care and risk management. Healthcare Forum, 5, 23–9.

Namazi, K. H. & Johnson, B. D. (1992). Pertinent autonomy for residents with dementias: Modification of the physical environment to enhance independence. Am J Alzheimers Care Relat Disord Res, 7, 16–21.

Noyes, R. Jr. (2001). Comorbidity in generalized anxiety disorder. Psychiatr Clin North Am, 24, 41–55.

Ploghaus, A., Narain, C., Beckmann, C. F., et al. (2001). Exacerbation of pain by anxiety is associated with activity in a hippocampal network. J Neurosci, 15, 9896–903.

Porensky, E. K., Dew, M. A., Karp, J. F., *et al.* (2009). The burden of late-life generalized anxiety disorder: effects on disability, health-related quality of life, and healthcare utilization. *Am J Geriatr Psychiatry*, 17, 473–82.

Rankin, E. J., Gilner, F. H., Gfeller, J. D., *et al.* (1995). Anxiety states and sustained attention in a cognitively intact elderly sample: preliminary results. *Psychol Rep*, 75, 1176–778.

Rappe, E. & Kivelä, S. L. (2005). Effects of garden visits on long-term care residents as related to depression. *HortTechnology*, 15, 298–303.

Relf, P. D. (1998). People-plant relationship. In: Simson, S. P. & Straus, M. C. (eds) *Horticulture as Therapy Principals and Practice*, pp. 23–42. New York, NY: Food Products Press, an Imprint of Hawthorn Press.

Scheffer, A. C., Schuurmans, M. J., van Dijk, N., *et al.* (2007). Fear of falling: measurement strategy, prevalence, risk factors and consequences among older persons. *Age Ageing*, 37, 19–24.

Simon, N. M. (2009). Generalized anxiety disorder and psychiatric comorbidities such as depression, bipolar disorder, and substance abuse. *J Clin Psychiatry*, 70(Suppl 2), 10–14.

Simpson, J. R., Snyder, A. Z., Gusnard, D. A., *et al.* (2001). Emotion-induced changes in human medial prefrontal cortex: I. During cognitive task performance. *Proc Natl Acad Sci*, 98, 683–7.

Tesar, G. E., Austerman, J., Pozuelo, L., *et al.* (2010). Behavioral Assessment of the General Medical Patient. Cleveland Clinic Center for Continuing Education. Available at: http://www.clevelandclinicmeded.com/medicalpubs/diseasemanagement/psychiatry-psychology/behavioral-assessment-of-medical-patient/ (accessed 14 August 2014) [Online].

Ulrich, R. S. (1983). Aesthetic and affective response to natural environment. *Human Behavior & Environment*, 6, 85–125.

van den Berg, A. E., van Winsum-Westra, M., de Vries, S., *et al.* (2010). Allotment gardening and health: A comparative survey among allotment gardeners and their neighbors without an allotment. *Environmental Health*, 9, 74.

Vink, D., Aartsen, M. J., & Schoevers, R. A. (2008). Risk factors for anxiety and depression in the elderly: a review. *J Affect Disord*, 106, 29–44.

Vytal, K., Cornwell, B., Arkin, N., *et al.* (2012). Describing the interplay between anxiety and cognition: From impaired performance under low cognitive load to reduced anxiety under high load. *Psychophysiology*, 49, 842–52.

Wang, Z., Neylan, T. C., Mueller, S. G., *et al.* (2010). Magnetic resonance imaging of hippocampal subfields in posttraumatic stress disorder. *Arch Gen Psychiatry*, 67, 296–303.

Yeunsook, L., Yoon, H., Lim, S., *et al.* (2012). Housing alternatives to promote holistic health of the fragile aged. *Indoor and Built Environment*, 21, 191–204.

CHAPTER 6.3

Vulnerable populations, health inequalities, and nature

Richard Mitchell, Julia Africa, and Alan Logan

How and why should we think about vulnerable populations in relation to nature?

Health scientists have long studied our environment, principally to discern and mitigate wide ranging threats to public health, including those from contaminants to socially mediated instability and injustice. The likelihood of being exposed to, and affected by, more health damaging environments is not spread equally across society (Brulle and Pellow, 2006). Less advantaged, more vulnerable groups are often more exposed to adverse environments and this is an important pathway which can help explain why members of these groups have a disproportionately high risk of premature, poorly addressed, and unresolved health outcomes (WHO, 2008).

Increasingly, this is discussed as environmental inequity or injustice. The exclusive focus on harm from the environment is, however, now under challenge. The idea that aspects of the physical environment can make a positive contribution to health and well-being is something of a turnaround for health sciences, changing the perspective from risks to opportunities. One of the central tenets of this book is that natural environments, specifically, may be good for our health and well-being. How does this paradigm shift change how we support the health of vulnerable populations, and is it reasonable to re-use existing perspectives on environment, health, and vulnerability when thinking about nature?

In this chapter we will examine three key ideas. First, we will explore ways in which vulnerability might affect the likelihood of beneficial contact with nature. Second, we will explore the idea that the health benefits of contact with nature may be greater for more vulnerable populations than for others. This highlights the potential nature has for generating an additional avenue for reducing health inequalities. Third, we will consider changes in our relationships with nature over time, and their potential implications both for vulnerability and health.

Defining vulnerability

For most of this chapter we will define vulnerability in conventional public health terms. Vulnerable people are those whose characteristics and settings tend to render them less able to stay healthy and well, either because of their limited resources or abilities, and/or

because of systematic discrimination by wider society and economy. We might, for example, define vulnerability by possession of one or more of: low socioeconomic position; membership of particular minority ethnic groups; residence in poor quality housing; low level of education; physical or mental impairment; diminished political agency; or very young or very old age, but we note that this is not an exhaustive list. We will also make frequent reference to the 'use of nature'. Examples of the use of nature are provided elsewhere in this book (e.g. in Section 3 and 5) but include individual or team recreational activities, social gatherings, community gardening, ecological education, and idle relaxation in nature.

We acknowledge that these definitions focus most attention on urban dwelling citizens of economically developed countries. Many other people around the world have a different relationship with nature, one that is primarily for basic economic needs, for example providing food, fuel, and fresh water, and one which may include cultural practices and beliefs that are not utilitarian in spirit. Their vulnerabilities, and the role of nature in creating or ameliorating them, are arguably not well covered either by the research we have drawn upon here.

Inequalities in access to and use of nature

The most straightforward aspects of the relationship between vulnerable populations, nature, and health align with a simple equation. Contact with nature protects and enhances our health -> beneficial contact with nature is not evenly distributed and more vulnerable people may get less -> those with relatively less contact may be at a health disadvantage. This equation prompts questions; do vulnerable populations tend to have less beneficial contact with nature? If so, how and why does that occur? There are at least two routes: nature is less available to more vulnerable people, and/or where nature is available they use it less. Let's explore these in turn.

There's a vast body of literature on inequitable access to natural environments, where access is defined by residential proximity or quantity, particularly within an urban setting (see, for example Abercrombie et al., 2008; Astell-Burt et al., 2014; Dai, 2011; Pedlowski et al., 2002; Wolch et al., 2014; Zhou and Kim, 2013). This work often sits within the traditions of environmental justice which has, more conventionally, explored the relationship between vulnerability and greater exposure to pathogens like air pollution or contaminated land (Brulle and Pellow, 2006; Jennings et al., 2012).

The environmental justice research is dominated, numerically at least, by American studies which define vulnerability in terms of race (Wolch *et al.*, 2014). European and Australasian studies have tended to use socioeconomic definitions of vulnerability. Summarizing this large body of research is difficult since study designs, methodologies, and findings are mixed (Jennings *et al.*, 2012). The literature as a whole indicates that, in general, vulnerable populations have less salutogenic natural environments available and more often reside in areas with abundant environmental stressors, like air and soil pollution. Wolch *et al.*'s (2014) brief review of the literature for example, concludes 'there is abundant evidence of environmental injustice in the distribution of urban green space. A variety of other studies show that racial/ethnic minorities and low-income people have less access to green space, parks, or recreational programs than those who are White or more affluent' (Wolch *et al.*, 2014).

As always, there are exceptions to the rule and a few studies find little or no evidence for systematic inequality in the distribution of, or access to, urban nature. Barbosa *et al.* (2007), for example, found that those enjoying the best access to green spaces in the city of Sheffield in the United Kingdom, included more deprived groups and older people, while Zhou and Kim's (2013) study in Illinois found no significant racial/ethnic difference in terms of access to parks. Given the heterogeneity of cities, the histories of their social, economic, and spatial development and the ways in which nature and green environments might be measured, some inconsistency in evidence about equality of access to nature is not surprising. Overall though, the evidence suggests inequality is the norm (Jennings and Gaither, 2015; Dobbs *et al.*, 2014).

The environmental justice literature is also concerned with *how* these spatial, structural inequalities occur. Joassart-Marcelli's (2010) elegant exploration of funding for urban green spaces in the Los Angeles region, for example, demonstrates how wider fiscal inequalities determine and maintain inequalities in park access and quality. Access to nature may, in some locations, be just another example of how social and economic systems create, maintain, and compound vulnerability and inequality. This may also have a historical background, as discussed later in this chapter.

There is also some evidence that, even where natural environments are available, vulnerable populations use them less (Jones *et al.*, 2009), though the findings are inconsistent (Ghandehari *et al.*, 2012). Distance and time have been identified as 'practical' barriers, which may be more keenly perceived by those from low socioeconomic positions (Jones *et al.*, 2009; Macintyre *et al.*, 2008). Others have focused on whether the characteristics of the space, its quality, or the services it offers, are influential (Cohen *et al.*, 2013; Mitchell and Popham, 2007; Bruton and Floyd, 2014). Bruton and Floyd (2014) found evidence that park facilities and their cleanliness varied between both minority and non-minority neighbourhoods, and more and less wealthy neighbourhoods. For example, areas for sitting and resting were less clean in minority areas, and parks located in more affluent areas (with less minority residents) had more wooded areas and overall tree canopy.

Yet, it also seems that broader cultural and attitudinal factors are important. Some vulnerable groups perceive natural spaces as controlled by, or existing for, dominant economic or ethnic groups and identify those spaces with use by a 'white' or affluent 'elite' (Jennings

and Gaither, 2015; Byrne, 2012). Others see them as threatening spaces or as simply not being suitable for the uses that they desire, including active and passive recreation and interaction with nature (Byrne, 2012). Cultural background may also be associated with particular views on the suitability of natural spaces for fishing or hunting for example, and these views may also be in contrast to those of park managers and other users.

Byrne's study of the 'cultural politics' of park use among Latino populations in Los Angeles sheds a particularly sharp light on some of these issues (Byrne, 2012). His respondents 'reported feeling 'out of place', 'unwelcome' or excluded from these parks. They identified the predominantly White clientele of parks; the ethno-racial profile of park-adjacent neighbourhoods; a lack of Spanish-language signs; fears of persecution; and direct experiences of discrimination as exclusionary factors' (Byrne, 2012). Strife and Downey (2009) echo these sentiments, noting that facets of the park and its staff may make minority and low-income youth and families feel unwelcome.

Fear of green spaces is also a significant barrier, particularly for women. While this may not be specific to vulnerable populations, it remains an important contributor to their under-representation (Byrene, 2009; Ward Thompson *et al.*, 2008; Jansson *et al.*, 2013). The perception of fear and risks in nature are topics further discussed in Chapter 7.4 'Risk and perception of risk in interactions with nature'.

As with the environmental justice literature, we note that there are mixed findings in terms of whether vulnerable populations are more or less likely to use natural environments. The association between use of green spaces and vulnerability may also be culturally and geographically specific. A 2012 report by Ghandehari *et al.*, for example, noted that people with low income were *more* likely to be park users in their study in northern Iran.

Read more about cultural identity and relation to nature in Chapter 6.4 'Responses to nature from populations of varied cultural background'.

The importance of childhood experiences in 'normalizing' the use of green spaces may underpin and perpetuate some of these cultural inequalities. Catharine Ward Thompson and colleagues' (2008) finding that the most important predictor of woodland use in adulthood was regular use in childhood reveals how inequalities in use might persist intergenerationally and therefore become part of a vulnerable group's culture. At the start of an outdoor education experience in the United Kingdom, children from the poorest circumstances were six times more likely to have never visited a wild open space than more affluent children (Mitchell and Shaw, 2008). This is a clear example of how social factors and environmental injustice may determine an individual's health behaviours throughout the life course from a very early age and relates to the paradigm of the Developmental Origins of Health and Disease (DOHaD) (see Chapter 1.2 'A life course approach to public health: why early life matters' for an overview of this topic).

There is a surprisingly small literature on access to, use of, and perceptions of nature by disabled people (Burns *et al.*, 2009). Both mentally and physically disabled people are under-represented in natural environments, but to focus solely on the physical accessibility of natural spaces as both explanation and solution is unhelpful (Tregaskis, 2004). Burns *et al.* (2009), for example, argue that this grossly simplifies and underestimates both the range of impairments faced by people, and their needs for accessing natural spaces. Others have shown that preferences for natural environments among disabled people are very similar to those without disability and, as in any population, there is a considerable variety in opinion within 'the disabled population' about whether and how they would like natural spaces to be rendered more accessible to them (Brown *et al.*, 1999; Seeland and Nicolè, 2006). Given the suggestions from studies of both patient and free-living populations that contact with nature may be of particular and profound benefit to mental health (Mantler and Logan, 2015; Mitchell *et al.*, 2015), there is a particular need to pay attention to the needs and perspectives of those rendered vulnerable by mental health problems.

There is, therefore, good evidence that vulnerable populations may have relatively worse access to high quality natural environments, particularly in urban settings, and that even where nature is available they may be less likely to use it. However, this is not *always* the case; relationships between vulnerability and use of natural spaces are likely to depend on the specific combination of personal history, location, and vulnerability. Overall, the evidence argues for establishing, maintaining, and promoting urban green spaces of high quality in deprived areas.

In the next section, we explore the idea that natural environments may be particularly beneficial for vulnerable populations. If an apparently greater benefit of contact with nature for more vulnerable populations can be established, it raises the prospect that contact with nature can have a role as an intervention to reduce health inequalities.

Mitigation of health inequalities by nature exposure

Although many of the deeply entrenched social and economic inequalities faced by disadvantaged populations may not be directly addressed by equitable access to quality green and blue space environments, they may provide a critical buffer against the higher burden of negative health outcomes. As described elsewhere in this text, the ability of natural environments to potentially offset higher non-communicable disease (NCD) risks may be mediated by a reduction in the physiological wear and tear encountered by collective exposure to physical, social, and psychological stressors (Logan *et al.*, 2015). Put simply, there is already good reason to suspect that natural environments offer particularly salient health benefits for vulnerable populations.

As explored in this book, an increasingly robust body of research indicates that contact with nature has a beneficial influence on health and well-being, although not typically addressing vulnerable populations *per se*. Many of the NCDs, for which contact with nature seem to have a positive impact, are far more common among vulnerable populations. If equitable access to safe natural environments could help to encourage physical activity, improve mental outlook, and reduce psychological stress, the argument in favour of natural environments being a more critical variable for vulnerable populations is at least structurally sound (Lachowycz & Jones, 2014).

Some epidemiological studies have begun to specifically explore this idea and have found that populations with higher access to natural environments experience better health outcomes across all groups, but also particularly among the most vulnerable groups. For example, when objective green space measurements were

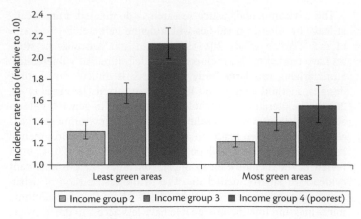

Fig. 6.3.1 Contrasting income-related mortality inequality in more and less green neighbourhoods of England.
Adapted from *The Lancet*, Volume 372, Issue 9650, Mitchell R and Popham F, 'Effect of exposure to natural environment on health inequalities: an observational population study,' pp. 1655-1660, Copyright © 2008 Elsevier Ltd, with permission from Elsevier, http://www.sciencedirect.com/science/journal/01406736.

compared with the national mortality records from the United Kingdom Office for National Statistics, an independent association was observed between residence in the greenest areas with lower rates of circulatory disease and all-cause mortality. Vulnerable populations living in areas with the lowest indicators of natural environment density experienced cardiovascular mortality rates twice that of those living in more affluent areas. In contrast, when a primary indicator of vulnerability (low income) was paired with high levels of residential-area urban green space, mortality rates versus the less vulnerable populations were significantly narrowed (Mitchell and Popham, 2008). Figure 6.3.1 illustrates these findings and shows the risk of mortality for successively poorer income groups, relative to the wealthiest income group, under two scenarios: lowest and highest levels of green space. The inequality in mortality is much smaller in areas with the highest amounts of green space.

These findings were bolstered by a recent international study covering more than 20,000 people in 34 European nations which found socioeconomic inequality in mental well-being to be 40% less among respondents reporting good access to green/recreational areas, compared with those with poorer access (Mitchell *et al.*, 2015). This study was able to ask if other positive neighbourhood environmental characteristics seemed to have the same impact. None did, which suggests there is something distinctly impactful about nature.

Other population research indicates that the association between having green spaces nearby (within one kilometre) and a reduced risk of poor health, might be mediated by the way in which natural environments encourage social contacts, sense of community, and place identity. This appears to be especially true for those living in low-income households (Maas *et al.*, 2009). A recent study from England also found a relationship between better access to natural environments and reduced mortality only for those who lived in highly vulnerable areas (Litt *et al.*, 2011). These studies, and others like them, suggest that the benefits of contact with nature are greater for more vulnerable populations.

Researchers have also compared biomarkers of stress in vulnerable populations and the density of natural environments within a neighbourhood. Among vulnerable populations in Dundee, Scotland, a healthier daytime salivary cortisol pattern in conjunction with lower levels of perceived stress was recorded among those residing in areas containing greater amounts of green space (>43%) (Roe *et al.*, 2013; Ward Thompson *et al.*, 2012). The Dundee study also uncovered the stark differences in neighbourhood-level quantities of natural environments. Some of the vulnerable populations had as little as 14% of their neighbourhood comprised of natural environments, while in other still vulnerable neighbourhoods, the concentration was as high as 74% (Ward Thompson *et al.*, 2012). Such variances may have untold consequences and should definitely be considered in policies aiming to reduce health inequalities.

In addition, research shows that community gardens, structured gardening programmes, or the greening of vacant lots can improve nutritional knowledge, physical activity levels, dietary quality and/or social cohesion in vulnerable populations (Nolan *et al.*, 2012; Litt *et al.*, 2011; Garvin *et al.*, 2013). Improvements in dietary quality as a means to improve mental outlook and cognitive function are of greatest relevance to the most vulnerable (Jacka *et al.*, 2014; Logan, 2015). As highlighted in the DOHaD construct, this is particularly important for pregnant women and children with pronounced nutritional needs that have lasting impacts on health over the life course.

When considering that few factors, if any, have been shown to effectively reduce the health gap between more and less vulnerable people at a population level, these encouraging studies grow in importance. However, observational studies cannot prove a causal relationship between access to nature and reduced health inequalities, although the consistency in outcomes, and both epidemiological and experiment studies support the theory. However, for translation into policies and decisions in urban planning, longitudinal studies with large cohorts are needed to provide stronger evidence.

In addition, natural environments also offer other material benefits to vulnerable populations. These benefits are usually termed ecosystem services (Chapter 8.5 'Ecosystem services and health benefits—an urban perspective' provides additional insight into this dynamic synergy between nature and health). Given that highly vulnerable neighbourhoods have a greater likelihood of exposure to environmental contamination (Young *et al.*, 2012; Zhuo *et al.*, 2012; Woghiren-Akinnifesi, 2013), ecosystem services may play a particularly crucial role in mitigating the physical and mental health impacts associated with environmental degradation (Jennings and Gaither, 2015).

The case for more research directed towards understanding the relative benefits of natural environments, and the transforming of disadvantaged communities with 'greenness', is a strong one. The evidence so far points towards enhanced value for vulnerable individuals and neighbourhoods. While these findings have begun to find their way into policies at a variety of scales and levels, so far there are few, if any, examples of them being used to justify and inspire official implementation as a health-based intervention strategy at population scales. However, caution should be exercised before 'grey' neighbourhoods are turned 'green' with unbridled enthusiasm. Unintended consequences might include the 'paradox of urban green space', such that 'greening' leads to gentrification and potential displacement of the very population the transformation

was intended to assist (Dai, 2011; Bryson, 2012; Kabisch and Haase, 2014). This provides yet more indication that in the complex flow of health inequalities, socioeconomic circumstance is a major river into which smaller tributaries such as natural environments might contribute.

In the next section, we consider how relationships between humans and nature continue to change over time, and their pertinence for human vulnerability in the future.

Nature and vulnerable populations in the past and in the future

History may teach us something about the changing relationships between natural environments and human vulnerability as it has been defined, experienced, or addressed. The concept of 'the park' has historically been linked to feudal or private estates; formal game reserves and curated grounds for the few found their analogue in informal commons or wildlands used by the many. The park in the industrialized era served as a counterpoint to widespread mechanization and diminished environmental quality. Writers like Henry Thoreau and John Muir positioned the austere beauty of wilderness against civilization's debauchery, while urban parks preserved the memory of disappearing rural livelihoods (through nostalgia) or species (through early zoos and natural history museums) in opposition to dense, dirty, disease ridden cities (Rogers, 2001). The Garden City Movement (1900, UK), characterized by ample gardens and green belts, provides an early modern example of the deliberate use of nature to improve conditions for vulnerable populations in crowded tenements and factories. Patrick Geddes, the celebrated Scottish biologist, sociologist, and pioneer of regional-scale urban planning, called garden cities a 'Eutopia, … a place of effective health and well-being' (Geddes, 1915) where one might have a personal experience of nature and community-focused environment (Rogers, 2001).

Advances in the understanding of how diseases spread reinforced the idea that those who lived in very high density housing and neighbourhoods were vulnerable. While this new knowledge supplanted previous ideas that the density of urban areas conveyed vulnerability via miasmas, vapours, and spirits, it still supported the notion that urban parks were both a balm and refuge that helped address stressors heaped upon the most vulnerable. In many respects—as this book suggests—this relationship has only grown with time.

Today's parks also, and perhaps increasingly, act as pressure valves for unsatisfied needs that are directly subsistence or survival related for some of the most vulnerable populations. Parks often shelter those without adequate housing or sanitary facilities; alternately, they may serve as sites for political organization and visible agency. This frequently includes populations who are vulnerable by virtue of mental illness, addiction or residency status, including non-formal communities or slums (Davis, 2006a). This is particularly true of refugees and unsanctioned migrants, for whom parks may represent or be identified as a liminal space in their transition. Formal housing markets in the economically developing world rarely supply more than 20% of new housing stock; 'out of necessity, people turn to self-built shanties, informal rentals, pirate subdivisions, or the sidewalks out of desperation' (Davis, 2006b). Classical principles of urban planning, including the preservation of open space and the separation of noxious land uses from residences, are difficult to apply in these circumstances. The need to alleviate deplorable conditions in slums makes access to nature no less laudable, but arguably less urgent in situations in which basic needs are insufficiently addressed.

Spatial relationships between nature and the city expose historically embedded characterizations of vulnerability. As if taking their cue from the then-unknown metabolism of the simplest cell, the first cities were defined by a centralized core that shunted waste to the periphery. Those who lived on the internal edges (waste conduits like canals and ravines) and external edges (forests, wetlands) bore the brunt of burdens related to disease, warfare, and predation; *proximity* to nature conferred vulnerability. Climate change has inverted these spatial relationships; the value of wetlands as storm buffers, restored streams as flood conduits, and urban forests to mitigate the heat island effect has brought the outside inside (Hondula *et al.*, 2014). Now, *remoteness* from nature, or in the parlance of planners 'green infrastructure', may confer vulnerability. Read more about this topic in Chapter 8.4 'Green infrastructure—its approach and public health benefits'.

The role of natural environments in cities is projected to become even more important for vulnerable populations as the health effects of climate change increase. Cities influence a range of climate comfort parameters, many of which directly influence human comfort and health, such as precipitation patterns, wind speed, cloud cover, humidity, and evening temperatures. As is further discussed in Chapter 7.5 'Population health deficits due to biodiversity loss, climate change, and other environmental degradation', vulnerable populations including children, older people, pregnant, and chronically ill residents will bear most of the toll of the negative health effects of climate change (Gronlund, 2014).

From a life course perspective, this is particularly problematic as exposure to harsh or poor conditions during childhood and adolescence will act as cumulative biological risk factors for the individual. In Chapter 8.5 'Ecosystem services and health benefits—an urban perspective', for example, more details are provided about how natural environments can make a direct contribution to cooling the air, reducing detrimental synergies between ambient air pollution and heat, as well as improving the capacity of urban areas to absorb extreme precipitation. In addition, they might also make a particular contribution to improving psychological resilience and coping capacity in disadvantaged groups in the face of environmental challenges. A recent study examining the connection between tree coverage and health in Toronto, Canada found that people who live in neighbourhoods with a higher density of trees on their streets report significantly higher health perception and significantly less cardiometabolic conditions. The researchers went so far as to state that the number of public street trees on a city block generated proximal improvements to health perception equivalent to those resulting from a $10–20,000 increase in personal income or 1.4–7 year decrease in age (Kardan *et al.*, 2015). Although more studies like this are needed in other sociocultural and health system contexts, they suggest the potential contribution that public amenities like street trees can make to levelling health disparities.

Environmental degradation confers or compounds vulnerability and health inequalities. While much has already been said about this, the ways in which the psychological resilience of residents themselves is undermined by the degradation is less well understood. 'Solastalgia' (Albrecht, 2013) is a term with its origins in nostalgia—also place-based distress (*nostos*—return to home or native land, and *algia*—pain or suffering)—but, instead of implying separation from a loved environment, solastalgia is the experience of someone who remains in place but is no longer able to seek solace, comfort, or consolation in their environment due to its ongoing destruction. Albrecht has studied these disrupted narratives of cultural landscapes (notably in mining communities) with particular attention to mental and physical illness stemming from environmental upheaval. In some communities, vulnerability is tied to socioculturally embedded experiences of solastalgia in tandem with the diminished resilience of landscape-based ecosystem services.

Finally, even where natural environments remain in place and healthy, human interest in them may be changing over time. Given the potentially long-term social, economic, health, and developmental consequences of such problems for individuals, lack of contact with nature is increasingly believed to confer its own kind of vulnerability. Without regular contact with nature, it is hard to see how anyone can learn to appreciate and value it, and therefore engage in a lifelong bidirectional symbiotic relationship that protects biodiversity in the context of personal health. Vulnerable populations are less likely to have experience of nature from a young age (Hunt *et al.*, 2015).

Conclusion

In conclusion, vulnerable populations may be less likely to have contact with natural environments. Where they do, however, there is good reason to believe the health benefits will be profound and emerging evidence suggests perhaps relatively greater than for less vulnerable groups. Nature therefore could be central to new strategies for reducing health inequalities.

Relationships between natural environments and vulnerable groups fluctuate in meaning and importance over time, particularly for urban dwellers. However, as the global environment changes, both nature's role as a critical health amenity and its concurrent degradation may become increasingly evident for the most vulnerable in our societies. This is an important note for public health policies and should encourage incorporation of environmental resource management and green planning in public health interventions aimed at decreasing health inequalities.

References

Abercrombie, L. C., Sallis, J. F., Conway, T. L., Frank, L. D., Saelens, B. E., & Chapman, J. E. (2008). Income and racial disparities in access to public parks and private recreation facilities. *Am J Prev Med*, 34, 9–15.

Albrecht, G. (2013). Solastalgia and the Creation of New Ways of Living. In: Pilgrim, S. & Pretty, J. (eds) *Nature and Culture: Rebuilding Lost Connections*, p. 217. London, UK: Earthscan.

Astell-Burt, T., Feng, X., Mavoa, S., Badland, H., & Giles-Corti, B. (2014). Do low-income neighbourhoods have the least green space? A cross-sectional study of Australia's most populous cities. *BMC Public Health*, 14, 292.

Barbosa, O., Tratalos, J., Armsworth, P., *et al.* (2007). Who benefits from access to green space? A case study from Sheffield, UK. *Landsc Urban Plan*, 83, 187–95.

Brown, T. J., Kaplan, R., & Quaderer, G. (1999). Beyond accessibility: Preference for natural areas. *Ther Recreation J*, 33, 209–21.

Brulle, R. & Pellow, D. (2006). Environmental Justice: Human Health and Environmental Inequalities. *Ann Rev Public Health*, 27, 103–24.

Bruton, C. & Floyd, M. (2014). Disparities in built and natural features of urban parks: comparisons by neighborhood level race/ethnicity and income. *J Urban Health*, 91, 894–907.

Bryson, J. (2012). Brownfields gentrification: redevelopment planning and environmental justice in Spokane, Washington. *Environmental Justice*, 5, 26–31.

Burns, N., Paterson, K., & Watson, N. (2009). An inclusive outdoors? Disabled people's experiences of countryside leisure services. *Leisure Studies*, 28, 403–17.

Byrne, J. (2012). When green is White: The cultural politics of race, nature and social exclusion in a Los Angeles urban national park. *Geoforum*, 43, 595–611.

Byrne, J., Wolch, J., & Zhang, J. (2009). Planning for environmental justice in an urban national park. *Journal of Environmental Planning and Management*, 52, 365–92.

Cohen, D. A., Lapham, S., Evenson, K. R., et al. (2013). Use of neighbourhood parks: does socio-economic status matter? A four-city study. *Public Health*, 127, 325–32.

Dai, D. (2011). Racial/ethnic and socioeconomic disparities in urban green space accessibility: Where to intervene? *Landsc Urban Plan*, 102, 234–44.

Davis, M. (2006a). *Planet of Slums*. London, UK: Verso Publishing.

Davis, M. (2006b). Slum ecology. *Orion*, 25, 7–23.

Dobbs, C., Nitschke, C. R., & Kendal, D. (2014). Global drivers and tradeoffs of three urban vegetation ecosystem services. *PLoS One*, 9, e113000.

Garvin, E., Branas, C., Keddem, S., Sellman, J., & Cannuscio, C. (2013). More than just an eyesore: local insights and solutions on vacant land and urban health. *J Urban Health*, 90, 412–26.

Geddes, P. (1915). Paleotechnic and neotechnic. In: LeGates, R. & Stout, F. (eds) *Early Urban Planning: 1870:1940*. New York, NY: Routledge.

Ghandehari, M. R. E., Ghafouri, F., Ganjooe, F. A., & Zarei, A. (2012). Urban parks users' profile: a case study in Iran. *World Appl Sci J*, 16, 892–7.

Gronlund, C. J. (2014). Racial and socioeconomic disparities in heat-related health effects and their mechanisms: a review. *Curr Epidemiol Rep*, 1, 165–73.

Hondula, D. M., Georgescu, M., Balling, R. C. Jr. (2014). Challenges associated with projecting urbanization-induced heat-related mortality. *Sci Total Environ*, 490, 538–44.

Hunt, A., Burt, J., & Stewart, D. (2015). Monitor of Engagement with the Natural Environment: a pilot for an indicator of visits to the natural environment by children—interim findings from Year 1 (March 2013 to February 2014). Natural England Commissioned Reports Number 166 2015.

Jacka, F. N., Cherbuin, N., Anstey, K. J., & Butterworth, P. (2014). Dietary patterns and depressive symptoms over time: examining the relationships with socioeconomic position, health behaviours and cardiovascular risk. *PLoS One*, 9, 87657.

Jansson, M., Fors, H., Lindgren, T., & Wiström, B. (2013). Perceived personal safety in relation to urban woodland vegetation—A review. *Urban For Urban Greening*, 12, 127–33.

Jennings, V. & Gaither, C. J. (2015). Approaching environmental health disparities and green spaces: an ecosystem services perspective. *Int J Environ Res Public Health*, 12, 1952–68.

Jennings, V., Johnson Gaither, C., & Gragg, R. S. (2012). Promoting environmental justice through urban green space access: a synopsis. *Environmental Justice*, 5, 1–7.

Joassart-Marcelli, P. (2010). Leveling the playing field? Urban disparities in funding for local parks and recreation in the Los Angeles region. *Environment and Planning A*, 42, 1174.

Jones, A., Hillsdon, M., & Coombes, E. (2009). Greenspace access, use, and physical activity: Understanding the effects of area deprivation. *Prev Med*, 49, 500–5.

Kabisch, N. & Haase, D. (2014). Green justice or just green? Provision of urban green spaces in Berlin, Germany. *Landsc Urban Plan*, 122, 129–39.

Kardan, O., Gozdyra, P., Misic, B., et al. (2015). Neighborhood greenspace and health in a large urban center. *Science Reports*, 5, 11610.

Lachowycz, K. & Jones, A. P. (2014). Does walking explain associations between access to greenspace and lower mortality? *Soc Sci Med*, 107, 9–17.

Litt, J. S., Soobader, M. J., Turbin, M. S., Hale, J. W., Buchenau, M., & Marshall, J. A. (2011). The influence of social involvement, neighborhood aesthetics, and community garden participation on fruit and vegetable consumption. *Am J Public Health*, 101, 1466–73.

Logan, A. C., Katzman, M. A., & Balanzá-Martínez, V. (2015). Natural environments, ancestral diets, and microbial ecology: is there a modern "paleo-deficit disorder"? Part I. *J Physiol Anthropol*, 34, 1.

Logan, A. C. (2015). Dysbiotic drift: mental health, environmental grey space, and microbiota. *J Physiol Anthropol*, 34, 23.

Maas, J., van Dillen, S. M. E., Verheij, R. A., & Groenewegen, P. P. (2009). Social contacts as a possible mechanism behind the relation between green space and health. *Health Place*, 15, 586–95.

Macintyre, S., Macdonald, L., & Ellaway, A. (2008). Lack of agreement between measured and self-reported distance from public green parks in Glasgow, Scotland. *Int J Behav Nutr Phys Act*, 5, 26.

Mantler, A. & Logan, A. C. (2015). Natural environments and mental health. *Adv Integr Med*, 2, 5–12.

Mitchell, R. & Popham, F. (2008). Effect of exposure to natural environment on health inequalities: an observational population study. *Lancet*, 372, 1655–60.

Mitchell, R. & Popham, F. (2007). Greenspace, urbanity and health: relationships in England. *J Epidemiol Community Health*, 61, 681–3.

Mitchell, R. & Shaw, R. (2008). *Health Impacts of the John Muir Award*. Glasgow, UK: Glasgow Centre for Population Health.

Mitchell, R. J., Richardson, E. A., Shortt, N. K., & Pearce, J. R. (2015). Neighborhood environments and socioeconomic inequalities in mental well-being. *Am J Prev Med*, 49, 80–4.

Nolan, G. A., McFarland, A. L., Zajicek, J. M., & Waliczek, T. M. (2012). The effects of nutrition education and gardening on attitudes, preferences, and knowledge of minority second to fifth graders in the Rio Grande Valley toward fruit and vegetables. *HortTechnology*, 22, 299–304.

Pedlowski, M. A., Da Silva, V. A. C., Adell, J. J. C., Heynen, N. C. (2002). Urban forest and environmental inequality in Campos dos Goytacazes, Rio de Janeiro, Brazil. *Urban Ecosystems*, 6, 9–20.

Roe, J. J., Thompson, C. W., Aspinall, P. A., et al. (2013). Green space and stress: Evidence from cortisol measures in deprived urban communities. *Int J Environ Res Public Health*, 10, 4086–103.

Rogers, E. B. (2001). *Landscape Design: A Cultural and Architectural History*. New York, NY: Harry N. Abrams.

Seeland, K. & Nicolè, S. (2006). Public green space and disabled users. *Urban For Urban Greening*, 5, 29–34.

Strife, S. & Downey, L. (2009). Childhood development and access to nature: a new direction for environmental inequality research. *Organ Environ*, 22, 99–122.

Tregaskis, C. (2004). Applying the social model in practice: some lessons from countryside recreation. *Disability & Society*, 19, 601–11.

Ward Thompson, C., Aspinall, P., & Montarzino, A. (2008). The childhood factor: adult visits to green places and the significance of childhood experience. *Environ Behav*, 40, 111–43.

Ward Thompson, C., Roe, J., Aspinall, P., Mitchell, R., Clow, A., & Miller, D. (2012). More green space is linked to less stress in deprived communities: Evidence from salivary cortisol patterns. *Landsc Urban Plan*, 105, 221–9.

Woghiren-Akinnifesi, E. L. (2013). Residential proximity to major highways—United States, 2010. *CDC Health Disparities and Inequalities Report—United States*, 62, 46.

Wolch, J. R., Byrne, J., & Newell, J. P. (2014). Urban green space, public health, and environmental justice: The challenge of making cities 'just green enough'. *Landsc Urban Planning*, 125, 234–44.

World Health Organzation (WHO) (2008). Commission on the Social Determinants of Health. Closing the gap in a generation: health equity through action on the social determinants of health. Final report of the CSDH. Geneva, Switzerland: WHO.

Young, G. S., Fox, M. A., Trush, M., Kanarek, N., Glass, T. A., & Curriero, F. C. (2012). Differential exposure to hazardous air pollution in the United States: a multilevel analysis of urbanization and neighborhood socioeconomic deprivation. *Int J Environ Res Public Health*, 9, 2204–25.

Zhou, X. L. & Kim, J. (2013). Social disparities in tree canopy and park accessibility: A case study of six cities in Illinois using GIS and remote sensing. *Urban Forest Urban Greening*, 12, 88–97.

Zhuo, X., Boone, C. G., & Shock, E. L. (2012). Soil lead distribution and environmental justice in the Phoenix metropolitan region. *Environmental Justice*, 5, 206–13.

CHAPTER 6.4

Responses to nature from populations of varied cultural background

Caroline Hägerhäll

Nature before culture?

Do human responses to nature differ, or are there strong common preferences for nature that outweigh cultural and individual differences? Many claims have been made since the 1970s and onward that humans share a preference for nature over urban settings. This assumption of consensus rests on theoretical models referring to human adaptation during evolution (Appleton, 1975; Orians, 1980; Ulrich, 1993; Kaplan and Kaplan, 1989). Empirical studies have shown consensus in preference across different groups; however, criticism has pointed out that many of these studies have used a methodology where consensus has been more likely (see van den Berg *et al.*, 1998).

How much difference there is between cultural groups in their perceptions and use of green space is a question that has high scientific, as well as practical and policy importance (see Kloek *et al.* 2013), not least in the light of increasingly multicultural urban societies, but also in the context of rural communities being no less multicultural (Panelli *et al.*, 2009; Askins, 2009). At the same time, the complexity of a question investigating concepts like nature and culture makes clear answers illusive. This complexity may also be an explanation for the fragmented research on the topic to date.

Defining nature and culture

Definitions and the role of nature vary across populations of different countries, but also between groups within a country, such as rural and urban dwellers or groups with particular and different stakes or interests in the environment (Purcell *et al.*, 1994, O'Riordan, 1989; Kong *et al.*, 1999; Orland, 1992; Kloek *et al.*, 2013). Similarly, terminology and the definition of culture (and subculture) is problematic both politically and academically (Duncan and Duncan, 2004).

Culture has been used in the literature as a label for everything from country of origin to particular interests of groups of people, experts and non-experts, or even demographic variables like age or gender. The majority of studies on landscape perception and use suffer from the same sampling bias common to many disciplines within behavioural sciences, namely a bias towards urban Western populations and typically university students. There is an increasing awareness that using these populations for generalizing about

humans might be problematic, and that they can actually be outliers in relation to some fundamental psychological and behavioural domains (Henrich *et al.*, 2010).

Nature and culture also share the problem of being defined partly by its opposite; that is, nature and culture would also be contextually defined by the scope of the study. This is very apparent in much of the environmental preference work where natural scenes have commonly been compared to urban scenes. Although a natural versus urban dichotomy has its methodological advantages and can provide clear results, its drawback is that the simplification or polarization of content makes more elaborate relationships impossible to entangle and many of the answers then also become less useful in practice. In reality, the types of environments that have actually been studied is limited.

Apart from the environmental stimuli, there are other methodological issues that have been found to influence results in cross-cultural studies on landscape perception. The differences between groups can vary in size for different types of assessments, such as evaluative appraisals compared to preference ratings which are implying utility functions, compared to descriptive assessments, with higher consensus for the evaluative appraisals than the other two (Zube and Pitt, 1981). Preferences are more similar than perceptions (Kaplan and Herbert, 1987). This means that the exact phrasing of the preference questions that have been asked in various studies will impact results. Furthermore, concerning study design, many common factors (familiarity, typicality, preference purpose, urban or rural residence, or education level or expertise) that have been studied and proposed to influence environmental perception are intertwined with the investigation of cultural differences. For instance, a study interested in the effects of previous experiences or familiarity on preference could also be using groups from different cultures to investigate this effect (Peron *et al.*, 1998; Purcell *et al.*, 1994). A conclusion in these studies is often that most of or all factors have some impact and that they interact (Zube and Pitt, 1981; Peron *et al.*, 1998; Purcell *et al.*, 1994).

In conclusion, it is fair to say that the body of research on cultural differences in response to nature is limited, and at the same time very fragmented. Hence it is difficult to categorize or draw clear conclusions. This chapter is an attempt to point at some distinguishable patterns and lines of inquiry, when focusing more narrowly on cultural background defined as a person's origin or ethnicity and quantitative studies of general, mainly visual, preferences. A focus on visual landscape preferences is also motivated by the fact that many studies have shown that preference coincides with health outcomes and likelihood of restoration (Purcell *et al.*, 2001; Tenngart Ivarsson and Hägerhäll, 2008; Staats *et al.*, 2003; Nordh *et al.*, 2009).

Visual landscape preference across cultures

Within environmental psychology and related fields, there is a large body of research on landscape perception or general landscape preferences using quantitative methods and photos to represent the environments. Among them there are also some few studies addressing cross-cultural differences. Their results are mixed, showing both similarities and differences, often dependent on the level of analyses and the closeness of the studied cultures. In many cases, the similarities exist when looking at overall correlations, while differences appear between the cultural groups when breaking the analyses down and looking at how different cultural groups categorize the environmental stimuli and what preference means those categories receive (Herzog *et al.*, 2000). Cross-cultural consensus is generally found for content that define landscape on basic levels such as openness, smoothness of ground cover, presence of water, how dominate vegetation or signs of human influence is in the scene. How this basic content is then used and interpreted to form environmental categories varies between cultures and subcultures (Herzog *et al.*, 2000).

For natural landscapes, high overall similarities have been found between cultures that might be quite close, for example when comparing Western groups like North American, European, and Australian (Shafer and Tooby, 1973; Zube and Mills, 1976; Kaplan and Herbert, 1987; Ulrich, 1977; Herzog *et al.*, 2000), or comparing between different Asian groups (Tips and Savasdisara, 1986a). Interestingly, similarities in basic preferences have also been found when comparing Western and Asian groups, for instance Western tourists and native Balinese; both favouring natural lush or open landscapes over urban dry or enclosed (Hull and Reveli, 1989). Similarly, a study found that Western tourists and Korean citizens and students both favoured natural forms over more formal linear forms (Yang and Kaplan, 1990). Also Tips and Savasdisara (1986b) and Yu (1995) found general agreement in preferences between Western and Chinese groups, but also pointed to differences explained by other factors than ethnicity, such as education and rural versus urban residence (Yu, 1995).

There is also an example of similarities in preference between Western and African samples that Balling and Falk found while testing the savannah hypothesis. Falk and Balling (2010) repeated a previous study (Balling and Falk, 1982) of different biomes represented in photos and got similar results, showing a preference for savannah which seem to decline with age, in both North American (Balling and Falk, 1982) and West African/Nigerian (Falk and Balling, 2010) samples.

Visual landscape preference studies including indigenous peoples

The most prominent perspective in the literature on nature and health, is nature as a recreation place for urbanized populations rather than the study of responses in populations living more directly in and off the surrounding nature (i.e. rural populations and, in the more extreme case, forest-living people of tropical areas and alike). As mentioned before, there is also a bias towards Western samples and in addition, non-Western participants are often selected from urbanized and/or educated populations.

The study mentioned above by Falk and Balling (2010) was an explicit attempt to expand the inquiry to a clearly different cultural and environmental context, and hence included three Nigerian samples mainly living in (and not travelled beyond) a tropical rainforest area, although all samples were drawn from schools.

Research on indigenous people's perceptions of landscapes and nature is limited and the more common approach is to use qualitative methods. Such studies can, for instance, be found within natural resource management, where there is an interest in how management practices for production and conservation can be impacting on the native indigenous peoples inhabiting those areas (Lewis, 2008; Lewis, 2010; Lewis and Sheppard, 2005; Lewis and Sheppard, 2006). Hence, perceptions in these studies are seen and studied in a particular context, which is different from quantitative inquiries into general preferences.

Interestingly, one of the rare quantitative preference studies including indigenous peoples was conducted in the early days of this research field, when Sonnenfeld (1967) compared native Alaskan Eskimo samples with non-native subjects from various professional groups working in Alaska and college and high-school students in Delaware. Sonnenfeld hypothesized that humans' varied sensitivity to the environment was a reason for perceptual differences. Humans would likely also be more sensitive to new conditions, since new conditions require one to be sensitive. The level of contentment with an environment would be an indicator of the level of physiological and sensory adaptation. Pairwise comparisons of photos were used to test preference to live in the place depicted for a year or two. Generally, the non-native groups had higher preference than the native Alaskan Eskimos for topography and vegetation. Non-natives generally (along wih other groups who had no subsistence concerns, field scientists and youngsters) had a preference for the exotic, while contrarily the subsistence-oriented Eskimo groups preferred environments resembling their native areas. Gender differences were more pronounced in the native Alaskan Eskimo groups.

An explanation for the lack of studies including indigenous populations might be practical issues, such as lack of researchers having access to and being able to communicate with these cultural groups. More collaboration across disciplines could help overcome some of these problems and enable inclusion of populations from a much wider range of cultures and environmental conditions. One such example is a recent collaboration between landscape architecture and linguistics, where Hägerhäll *et al.* (in preparation) conducted a landscape preference study using digitally visualized landscapes of varying topography and vegetation density, with five non-Western, indigenous, and primarily rural communities in tropical areas, Jahai (Malay Peninsula), Lokono (Suriname), Makalero (Timor), Makasae (Timor), and Wayuu (Colombia), and two Western/Swedish student groups. The samples had a broad span geographically (Europe, Mainland Southeast Asia, Oceania, and South America), linguistically (the Arawakan, Austroasiatic, Indo-European, and West Trans New Guinea language families) and concerning primary subsistence mode (foraging, slash-and-burn agriculture, and industrialized). The indigenous samples were compared to the two Swedish university student samples, of which one was students in landscape architecture (i.e. students having a particular interest and expertise in landscape). Subjects were asked to choose the most preferred place to live using pairwise comparison of nine images. The overall results pointed to the two Swedish samples being clearly different from the other groups. For the Swedish samples, there were interactive effects between topography and vegetation. For all the other groups, only the main effects of the two variables were found. This indicates possible differences in the evaluation strategy. Also, there were content preference differences between Swedes and the other groups. The Swedish samples, and especially the expert landscape students, preferred the mid-levels of topography and vegetation density, while the other groups favoured the images with lower value of topography and higher value of vegetation density (i.e. flatter landscapes with dense tree cover). Furthermore, there was a difference in how much the choice was guided by familiarity (in this study preferring the image most resembling where one grew up), a factor not so important for the Swedish student samples, but highly important for some of the indigenous groups. It likely differs between the groups to what extent they have travelled beyond the areas in which they have grown up in. Apart from just having more or less experience of different landscapes, more functional aspects could also have an effect. Sonnenfeld (1967) suggested subsistence focus could be a factor explaining why indigenous groups favoured familiar landscapes.

Recreation preferences across cultures

Apart from the general landscape preference and perception work, there is a quite substantial body of research concerning recreation preferences among different cultures. North America has a fairly long tradition of research in this research area, while in Europe it is a relatively new but growing topic (Gentin, 2011; Kloek *et al.*, 2013). The majority of studies in the European context have focused on recreation in urban areas (parks or urban forests). Furthermore, the research is often focused on access, use, activities, and social interaction and inclusion in green areas (Kloek *et al.*, 2013; Gentin, 2011, Kaplan and Talbot, 1988), and not on the perceptions and responses to nature or the green areas as such. As Kloek *et al.* (2013) point out: 'Links between outdoor recreation and perceptions of green space have not been properly researched and explanatory factors are only superficially touched upon.'

Regarding the use of urban recreation areas, there seem to be some consistency pointing to non-Western ethnic minorities' use differing from the use of the mainstream Western (white) population. Non-Western immigrants seem to assign higher importance to social activities in green space and visit non-urban green spaces further away from home less often (Kloek *et al.*, 2013; Rishbeth, 2001).

Similarly, there are some consistent findings from both Europe and North America concerning preferences and responses to the content of urban green space, with studies pointing to non-urban or wild and unmanaged landscapes being less liked by non-Western immigrants than by, for instance, the native Western European/Dutch subjects (Buijs *et al.*, 2009). Kaplan and Talbot (1988) studied black versus white Americans and found, consistent with previous studies on blacks, that they favour more urbanized, open, and neat settings than whites.

Some explanations for the differences in perception of green space have been discussed, such as immigrants having a more broad definition and a more functional view of nature (Kloek *et al.*, 2013; Buijs *et al.*, 2009) The often rural background of many immigrants and religion have also been suggested to have an impact; for instance, in Islam nature is presented as ordered and well managed (Kloek *et al.*, 2013). Childhood experiences and media use could also be an influence (Jay and Schraml, 2009). The latter are factors that could differ between cultures, but which could also be seen as background variables commonly included, like age and gender.

Askins (2009), who studied perceptions and use of national parks and the English countryside, found that for all the included ethnic groups (African, Caribbean, and Asian) the countryside was understood and considered the opposite of the city, with positive attributes being assigned to the countryside, and the countryside being associated with a therapeutic value of relieving stress associated with the city. However, age and gender were found to affect the experience of the countryside across ethnic groups. For instance, the lack of interest in young people (15–24-year-olds) to visit the countryside was due to nature being conceived as being for older people. Older people were happy to visit rural areas without any planned activity, while young people wanted activities and hence also made use of more facilities and equipment than just the natural environment itself. This illustrates the problem mentioned earlier in the chapter of the many confounding factors in cross-cultural studies.

Conclusion

Current research on how populations of varied cultural background respond to nature is too limited and fragmented to draw any clear conclusions. Furthermore, the current explanations and models (i.e. the drivers behind the differences and similarities) are speculations and not properly tested. Future research needs to adopt clearer definitions and conceptualizations of culture and nature, and aim to better understand factors which interact with ethnicity. Apart from factors like age, gender, education, and expertise, the rural–urban dimension would need more attention as studies have shown notable confounding effects of rural versus urban residence. Similarly, there is a need to better understand the interactions between perceptions and use in a cross-cultural perspective.

References

Appleton, J. (1975). *The Experience of Landscape*. New York, NY: John Wiley & Sons.

Askins, K. (2009). Crossing divides: Ethnicity and rurality. *J Rural Stud*, 25, 365–75.

Balling, J. D. & Falk, J. H. (1982). Development of visual preference for natural environments. *Environ Behav*, 14, 5–28.

Buijs, A. E., Elands, B. H. M., & Langers, F. (2009). No wilderness for immigrants: Cultural differences in images of nature and landscape preferences. *Landsc Urban Plan*, 91, 113–23.

Duncan, J. S. & Duncan, N. G. (2004). Culture unbound. *Environment and Planning A*, 36, 391–403.

Falk, J. H. & Balling, J. D. (2010). Evolutionary influence on human landscape preference. *Environ Behav*, 42, 479–93.

Gentin, S. (2011). Outdoor recreation and ethnicity in Europe—A review. *Urban For Urban Greening*, 10, 153–161.

Henrich, J., Heine, S. J., & Norenzayan, A. (2010). The weirdest people in the world? *Behav Brain Sci*, 33, 61–135.

Herzog, T. R., Herbert, E. J., Kaplan, R., & Crooks, C. L. (2000). Cultural and developmental comparisons of landscape perceptions and preferences. *Environ Behav*, 32, 323–46.

Hull, R. B., IV & Reveli, G. R. B. (1989). Cross-cultural comparison of landscape scenic beauty evaluations: A case study in Bali. *J Environ Psychol*, 9, 177–91.

Jay, M. & Schraml, U. (2009). Understanding the role of urban forests for migrants—uses, perception and integrative potential. *Urban For Urban Greening*, 8, 283–94.

Kaplan, R. & Herbert, E. J. (1987). Cultural and sub-cultural comparisons in preferences for natural settings. *Landsc Urban Plan*, 14, 281–93.

Kaplan, R. & Kaplan, S. (1989). *The Experience of Nature: A Psychological Perspective*, New York, NY: Cambridge University Press.

Kaplan, R. & Talbot, J. F. (1988). Ethnicity and preference for natural settings: A review and recent findings. *Landsc Urban Plan*, 15, 107–17.

Kloek, M. E., Buijs, A. E., Boersema, J. J., & Schouten, M. G. C. (2013). Crossing borders: review of concepts and approaches in research on greenspace, immigration and society in northwest European countries. *Landsc Res*, 38, 117–40.

Kong, L., Yuen, B., Sodhi, N. S., & Briffett, C. (1999). The construction and experience of nature: Perspectives of urban youths. *Tijdschrift voor Economische en Sociale Geografie*, 90, 3–16.

Lewis, J. L. (2008). Perceptions of landscape change in a rural British Columbia community. *Landsc Urban Planning*, 85, 49–59.

Lewis, J. L. (2010). Interethnic preferences for landscape change: A comparison of first nations and Euro-Canadian residents. *Landsc J*, 29, 215–31.

Lewis, J. L. & Sheppard, S. R. J. (2005). Ancient values, new challenges: Indigenous spiritual perceptions of landscapes and forest management. *Soc Nat Resour*, 18, 907–20.

Lewis, J. L. & Sheppard, S. R. J. (2006). Culture and communication: Can landscape visualization improve forest management consultation with indigenous communities? *Landsc Urban Plan*, 77, 291–313.

Nordh, H., Hartig, T., Hägerhäll, C. M., & Fry, G. (2009). Components of small urban parks that predict the possibility for restoration. *Urban For Urban Greening*, 8, 225–35.

O'Riordan, T. (1989). The challenge for environmentalism. *New Models in Geography*, 1, 77–102.

Orians, G. H. (1980). Habitat selection: general theory and applications to human behavior. In: Lockard, J. S. (ed.) *The Evolution of Human Social Behavior*. New York, NY: Elsevier.

Orland, B. (1992). Aesthetic preference for rural landscapes: some resident and visitor differences. In: Nasar, J. L. (ed.) *Environmental Aesthetics*, pp. 364–378. New York, NY: Cambridge University Press.

Panelli, R., Hubbard, P., Coombes, B., & Suchet-Pearson, S. (2009). De-centring White ruralities: Ethnic diversity, racialisation and Indigenous countrysides. *J Rural Stud*, 25, 355–64.

Peron, E., Purcell, A. T., Staats, H., Falchero, S., & Lamb, R. J. (1998). Models of preference for outdoor scenes—Some experimental evidence. *Environ Behav*, 30, 282–305.

Purcell, A. T., Lamb, R. J., Mainardi Peron, E., & Falchero, S. (1994). Preference or preferences for landscape? *J Environ Psychol*, 14, 195–209.

Purcell, T., Peron, E., & Berto, R. (2001). Why do preferences differ between scene types? *Environ Behav*, 33, 93–106.

Rishbeth, C. (2001). Ethnic minority groups and the design of public open scape: An inclusive landscape? *Landsc Res*, 26, 351–66.

Shafer, E. L. & Tooby, M. (1973). Landscape preferences: An international replication. *J Leisure Res*, 5, 60–5.

Sonnenfeld, J. (1967). Environmental perception an adaptation level in the Arctic. In: Lowenthal, D. (ed.) *Environmental Perception and Behavior*. Chicago, IL: University of Chicago.

Staats, H., Kieviet, A., Hartig, T. (2003). Where to recover from attentional fatigue: An expectancy-value analysis of environmental preference. *J Environ Psychol*, 23, 147–57.

Tenngart Ivarsson, C. & Hägerhäll, C. M. (2008). The perceived restorativeness of gardens—Assessing the restorativeness of a mixed built and natural scene type. *Urban For Urban Greening*, 7, 107–18.

Tips, W. E. J. & Savasdisara, T. (1986a). The influence of the environmental background of subjects on their landscape preference evaluation. *Landsc Urban Planning*, 13, 125–33.

Tips, W. E. J. & Savasdisara, T. (1986b). Landscape preference evaluation and sociocultural background: a comparison among Asian countries. *J Environ Manage*, 22, 113–24.

Ulrich, R. S. (1977). Visual landscape preference: A model and application. *Man-Environment Systems*, 7, 279–93.

Ulrich, R. S. (1993). Biophilia, biophobia, and natural landscapes. In: Kellert, S. R. & Wilson, E. O. (eds) *The Biophilia Hypothesis*. Washington, DC: Island Press.

van den Berg, A. E., Vlek, C. A. J., Coeterier, J. F. (1998). Group differences in the aesthetic evaluation of nature development plans: A multilevel approach. *J Environ Psychol*, 18, 141–57.

Yang, B. E. & Kaplan, R. (1990). The perception of landscape style:a cross-cultural comparison. *Landsc Urban Plan*, 19, 251–62.

Yu, K. (1995). Cultural variations in landscape preference: comparisons among Chinese sub-groups and Western design experts. *Landsc Urban Plan*, 32, 107–26.

Zube, E. H. & Mills, L. V. J. (1976). Cross-cultural explorations in landscape perception. In: Zube, E. H. (ed.) *Studies in Landscape Perception*. Amherst, MA: Institute for Man and Environment, University of Massachusetts.

Zube, E. H. & Pitt, D. G. (1981). Cross-cultural perceptions of scenic and heritage landscapes. *Landsc Plan*, 8, 69–87.

SECTION 7

Threats, environmental change, and unintended consequences of nature—protecting health and reducing environmental hazards

[†]It is with regret we report the death of Anthony J. McMichael during the preparation of this textbook.

CHAPTER 7.1

Allergenic pollen emissions from vegetation—threats and prevention

Åslög Dahl, Matilda van den Bosch, and Thomas Ogren

Pollen biology

The reproductive function of pollen grains

A pollen grain contains the 'male', sperm-producing generation of a seed plant, the microgametophyte. Each pollen grain contains a vegetative cell and a generative cell that divides to form two sperm cells. In flowering plants, there is only one vegetative cell apart from the two sperm cells; in gymnosperms (e.g. conifers), there are a few more. The outer wall of the pollen grain, the exine, consists of sporopollenin, a very stable mixture of biopolymers extremely resistant to degradation. Sporopollenin is semi-elastic and perforated by numerous micropores that allow for the transport of water and solutes. The exine is often elaborately sculptured, and ornamentation is used to differentiate between pollen types during pollen analysis. Beneath the exine is the intine, mainly composed by carbohydrates.

Once the pollen grain is deposited on the stigma of the pistil of a compatible flower, they start a 'cross-talk'. The vegetative cell elongates into a pollen tube, which grows inside the pistil towards the ovules (containing the female reproductive parts of the plant) inside the flower, during rapid formation of tube-wall structures and enzymes to dissolve intercellular carbohydrates. When the tip of the tube enters an ovule, it bursts and delivers the two sperm cells close to the egg cell. The entire process involves many compounds with different functions, of which several, for example glycoproteins, are pre-stored in the mature pollen grain (Shi, 2010).

Adverse properties of pollen grains

Some of the stored glycoproteins are able to provoke an allergic reaction. These are called allergens. The factors that render them allergenic are largely unknown. Their most frequently identified biological functions are few; some are enzymes, some bind metal ions and lipids, some are associated with storage, and others with the cytoskeleton (Radauer et al., 2008). They are localized to various structures within the cytoplasm, and to the pollen wall. Pollen allergens are classified in only about 2% of identified protein families. Some are confined to a restricted taxon, whereas others are pan-allergens (i.e. may be common to many plant groups or even to all eukaryotes). The more closely related two species are, the larger is the probability for homology among their proteins (Radauer and Breiteneder, 2006). In medical studies, allergenic plants are often grouped into 'trees', 'grasses', and 'weeds'. This distinction is unnatural from a phylogenetic point of view, and has the disadvantage of obscuring patterns of cross-reactivity.

At hydration, pollen grains also release non-allergenic compounds with proinflammatory and immunomodulating effects (Csillag et al., 2010; Gilles et al., 2012; Shalaby et al., 2013).

The pollen may rupture, whereby the content pours out. This is common especially in pollen grains where both wall layers are thin, and when there are no intrinsic structures to cope with intense stretching during excessive hydration (Taylor et al., 2004). One example is grass pollen, which easily bursts in rainy weather. The debris contains fragmented organelles and sometimes starch grains. These 'subpollen particles' are often carriers of allergens (Motta et al., 2004). Since they are much smaller than the pollen grains, they stay longer in the atmosphere and may penetrate into lower airways.

Air pollutants may also cause rupture of the pollen grains, and subpollen particles form conglomerates with, for example, diesel and other combustion particles (Motta et al., 2006). The latter can also become carriers of allergens that diffuse from intact pollen grains in a humid environment. Air pollutants may affect pollen ontogenesis, germination rate, and protein content, as well as cause nitration of allergens, thereby potentially increasing their potency to trigger an allergic response (Rezanejad, 2007; Cuinica et al., 2014; Reinmuth-Selzle et al., 2014; Chehregani and Kouhkan, 2008). These are plausible explanations for why increased air pollution results in exacerbation of seasonal allergic rhinitis (Penard-Morand and Annesi-Maesano, 2008; Hajat et al., 2001).

Which plants are the main provokers of pollinosis?

Allergenic plants have been identified in over 70 plant families, most of which are within the composites and grasses (Lewis et al., 1983) (Table 7.1.1). Allergens are not confined to pollen from

Table 7.1.1 Plant families and genera that are reported to be significant pollen allergy provokers, globally, or at least in some parts of the world (Singh and Kumar, 2003; Pollenlibrary, 2014; Lewis, 1983). From most of Africa and South America, information is scarce, except for the occurrence of grass pollen allergy

Family	English name	Genera reported to be of substantial importance for pollinosis
Aceraceae	Maple family	*Acer negundo*
Amaranthaceae	Amaranth family	*Amaranthus, Atriplex, Bassia, Beta, Chenopodium Salsola Suaeda*
Anacardiaceae	Sumac family	*Pistacia, Rhus, Schinus*
Arecaceae	Palm tree family	*Chamaerops, Cocos, Elaeis, Phoenix, Trachycarpos*
Asteraceae	Aster family, composites	*Ambrosia, Artemisia, Baccharis, Helianthus, Iva, Parthenium*
Betulaceae	Birch family	*Alnus, Betula, Corylus*
Boraginaceae	Borage family	*Echium plantagineum*
Brassicaceae	Brassica (kale) family	*Brassica napus*
Cannabaceae	Hemp family	*Cannabis, Humulus*
Casuarinaceae	Australian Pine family	*Casuarina*
Combretaceae	Indian Almond family	*Anogeissus*
Cupressaceae	Cypress family	*Cupressus, Juniperus*
Euphorbiaceae	Spurge family	*Mallotus, Mercurialis, Ricinus, Trewia*
Fabaceae	Legume (pea) family	*Acacia, Albizzia, Cassia, Prosopis*
Fagaceae	Beech family	*Castanea, Fagus, Quercus*
Juglandaceae	Walnut family	*Carya, Juglans*
Meliaceae	Mahogany family	*Azadirachta, Melia*
Moraceae	Fig family	*Broussonetia, Maclura, Morus*
Myrtaceae	Myrtle family	*Callistemon, Eucalyptus, Melaleuca*
Oleaceae	Olive family	*Fraxinus, Ligustrum, Olea*
Papaveraceae	Poppy family	*Argemone*
Pinaceae	Pine family	*Cedrus*
Platanaceae	Plane tree family	*Platanus*
Poaceae	Grasses	Several species within subfamilies *Bambusoidae, Chloridoideae, Panicoideae, Pooideae*
Polygonaceae	Buckwheat/sorrel family	*Rumex*
Salicaceae	Willow family	*Salix Populus*
Salvadoraceae		*Salvadora*
Sapindaceae	Soapberry family	*Dodonaea*
Simaroubaceae	Quassia family	*Ailanthus*
Taxodiaceae		*Cryptomeria*
Tiliaceae	Linden (lime tree) family	*Tilia*
Ulmaceae	Elm tree family	*Celtis, Ulmus*
Urticaceae	Nettle family	*Parietaria, Urtica*

Source: data from Lewis, WH *et al., Airborne and allergenic pollen of North America*, Johns Hopkins University Press, Baltimore, USA, Copyright © 1983; Ingh AB and Kumar P, 'Aeroallergens in clinical practice of allergy in India: An overview,' *Annals of Agricultural and Environmental Medicine*, Volume 10, pp. 131–136, Copyright © 2003; and Pollenlibrary, *Allergens and Plants Research by Location*, Copyright © 2017 IMS Health Incorporated, available from http://www.pollenlibrary.com.

any pollination system. However, the probability of developing a substantial allergy problem is largest in species that use wind as a pollen vector, otherwise the pollen will not be present in ambient air. Sensitization depends on exposure, and requires that sufficient pollen is produced and dispersed by the species in question.

This varies among wind-pollinated species, according to size and degree of self-incompatibility, but also to abundance and climate. Plants living under suboptimal conditions tend to produce less pollen, and a taxon may be a problem in one country but not so in another one. Wind pollination is common when the distance between conspecifics is small, a condition typical for most temperate ecosystems (Culley *et al.*, 2002). In tropical forests, it is rare (Bawa *et al.*, 1990), except for in disturbed places and in secondary vegetation, whereas in savannahs, there is much grass. All over the world, especially as a consequence of intense urbanization, allergenic weeds with abundant pollen production thrive on ruderal ground (land where the natural vegetation cover has been disturbed by humans).

Pollen information

In many countries, the concentration of airborne pollen is monitored by collection in volumetric spore traps (Scheifinger *et al.*, 2013), often under a shaky economical foundation (Klein *et al.*, 2012). The dual impact of allergens and anthropogenic pollution shows that an integrated approach to monitoring and communicating air quality would optimize the information (Klein *et al.*, 2012). The aim of pollen monitoring is to provide healthcare workers and the public with information and short-term forecasts for improved prevention and treatment actions.

Pollen forecasting requires expertise in botany and atmospheric science, and sophisticated models are under development (Scheifinger *et al.*, 2013). The output from a monitoring station is representative for an area that as a rule of thumb have a radius of 30–70 km. This area is not absolute, and the outer limits are defined from dominating climate, vegetation, land use, and influence from external sources. Historical pollen data are used in ecological and medicinal studies.

Onset, course, and intensity of the pollen season

In order to release pollen into the air, the plants have to reach a state of maturity that has been denoted 'readiness to flower' (Dahl *et al.*, 2013). This is, in varying relative importance, determined by photoperiod (the interval during a 24-hour period when a plant is exposed to daylight), temperature, and water access. Changes in day or night length indicate the beginning or termination of favourable conditions for growth and reproduction. Temperature determines the amount of energy supply from basal metabolism to growth and development, and thus the growth rate, but also controls phenology via regulatory processes (e.g. to determine the duration of winter dormancy in temperate trees and in closing down certain genes that impede flowering in grasses and herbs). Water availability determines timing of seed germination and growth rate, and, in seasonally arid regions, induces summer dormancy (Singh and Kushwaha, 2005).

When a plant is ready to flower, certain short-term weather conditions are necessary for pollen release (Dahl *et al.*, 2013). Anthers (pollen-bearing structures on the stamen of the flower) open as a response to dehydration, either passively or by active retraction. Since pollen grains have no intrinsic mobility, wind-pollinated plants have adaptions to force them out of the calmness of the boundary layer into air currents that may carry them to conspecific stigmas. Optimal conditions for pollen transport at ground level is fairly dry and warm weather, with non-gusty winds at a speed of 2–6 m·sec^{-1}, Typically, wind-dispersed pollen grains stay in the atmosphere from for some hours to up to two or three days (Sofiev *et al.*, 2013). In the latter case, they can travel over a continent. Every year, episodes occur when considerable amounts of pollen can be traced back to sources at distances of about 1,000 km. This implies that weather at the source has been warm enough to cause a strong uplift of air parcels containing pollen to considerable height, where winds are strong (Šikoparija *et al.*, 2013). According to empirical evidence, allergenic pollen grains appear to keep their adverse potency throughout this transport. The everyday situation is rather that the bulk of the pollen registered at a certain monitoring station emanates from an area with a radius of 100–200 km, provided that the pollen trap is situated at the recommended height of 15–30 m above ground. If the pollen trap is too close to the ground, there will be an over-representation of pollen from the nearest vegetation, and the results will not be representative for more than the very spot where it is situated. Most of the pollen released from a single plant is released in its very vicinity, and only a few per cent will be dispersed on a larger scale (Faegri *et al.*, 1989). The massive impact from a single tree is very important to remember when green areas are planned close to buildings where people reside (e.g. when trees are planted to, for example, filter air pollution close to bedroom windows or for aesthetic reasons).

The pollen season, the time when a certain pollen taxon is registered at a monitoring station, is not the same from year to year. The range of the period largely reflects the flowering of local plants. But since pollen dispersal depends on meteorological factors, and distant sources often contribute to results, the reflection is seldom perfect. When all flowers of a species mature more or less simultaneously, the peak of flowering usually is a few days after start. If development of flowers is sequential, or if a pollen taxon comprises several species that flower sequentially, the peak varies more in timing and nature (Dahl *et al.*, 2013).

During the latest decades, there has been a trend towards an earlier start of the pollen season. In both hemispheres, flowering of early-flowering species appears to advance more than those that flower later in the summer, which to a larger degree are governed by photoperiod (Menzel *et al.*, 2006; Chambers *et al.*, 2013). In Europe, a stronger advance in first flowering dates has been noted for wind-pollinated species, as compared to insect-pollinated ones (Ziello *et al.*, 2012).

The change in duration of the pollen season as a result of the observed climate change (IPCC, 2014) is likely to differ between species. When inflorescences (a group or cluster of flowers arranged on a stem) mature simultaneously, as in many temperate trees, warm weather speeds up pollen release. Hence, increasing mean temperatures during the pollen period will not always prolong the pollen season, as sometimes surmised, but rather shorten it. In many grasses, on the other hand, culms that are to carry flowers mature sequentially, and they will do so for a longer period if autumn temperatures allow.

The pollen season usually varies in intensity, illustrated in comparisons of the 'seasonal pollen index', the annual sum of registered pollen at monitoring stations. Its magnitude is partly a result of the abundance of the plant group in the source areas, but also varies from year to year according to the influence of innate and environmental factors (Dahl *et al.*, 2013). External factors known to limit pollen production are observed to change (IPCC, 2014). Atmospheric carbon dioxide concentration may influence pollen production substantially, as has been shown by the explosive increase in ragweed pollen across new geographical areas (*Ambrosia artemisiifolia*) (Ziska *et al.*, 2003; Ziska and Caulfield, 2000), likewise can atmospheric nitrogen deposition. Temperatures close to those optimal for carbon assimilation during key periods of development have been shown to promote 'richer' years, which could be evident in populations living in the colder part of the species range. In seasonally arid environments, much windborne pollen emanates from annuals where seed germination depends on water availability (Dahl *et al.*, 2013). In perennial grasses, pollen index is correlated to humidity in early spring, another factor which is likely to be affected by climate change. Any external factor that has long-term effects on the vitally of the entire plant and of its abundance, such as drought, invasions of new plant pathogens, and changed land use, can reduce pollen indices over time.

Allergenic pollen's impact on human health

Allergies and asthma—prevalence and trends

Allergies and asthma were uncommon in previous times (Liu, 2015). It was not until the late nineteenth century that seasonal allergic rhinitis (AR) in response to pollen was recognized as a condition (Platts-Mills, 2015). Major changes in environment, climate, and airborne pollen, as well as in public hygiene and lifestyles are likely to have contributed to the appearance of the disease, and to its exponential increase during the later decades. Today, seasonal AR is estimated to affect between 10–30% of the population worldwide. The disease is more common in developed countries (WAO, 2011). While data on the exact prevalence of seasonal AR are hard to achieve, it is estimated that of all allergenic individuals, about 40% are affected by pollen allergies, induced by exposure to pollens from tree, grass and/or weed. In general, pollen allergens are considered a major risk factor for both AR and asthma (Asam *et al.*, 2015). Grass pollens (GP) are among the most clinically important allergen sources worldwide. Although all GP show a degree of allergenic relatedness, there are clinically important differences in immune recognition of pollen allergens from different subfamilies of grasses.

The evidence on the impact of climate change on seasonal AR is so far preliminary, but it points to a confluence of factors that favour longer growing seasons for the noxious weeds and other plants that trigger seasonal allergies and asthma attacks (Schmidt, 2016). Several factors interplay, such as precipitation patterns, temperature, and CO_2 levels in the atmosphere. When exposed to warmer temperatures and higher levels of CO_2, plants grow more vigorously and produce more pollen than they otherwise would (Ziska and Beggs, 2012; Ziska and Caulfield, 2000). A common example is the aggressive spread of ragweed over continents, a species that is invasive, hardy, noxious, and a highly prolific producer of allergenic pollen (Smith *et al.*, 2013).

There is evidence suggesting that AR prevalence is rising in many parts of the world, particularly in urban areas (Sly, 1999; Ziska and Beggs, 2012; Solé *et al.*, 2007). It is likely that climate change together with other environmental factors, such as changing diets and better hygiene, contribute to the increasing prevalence of seasonal AR and asthma by limiting early exposure to allergens and altering the immune system's normal development (Ziska and Beggs, 2012).

The relation between increasing prevalence of seasonal AR and an altered immune system development is intriguing and evidence is elusive. The issue is often framed within the 'hygiene hypothesis', which describes the importance of diverse microbial exposure during early life for immune system development (Kondrashova *et al.*, 2013; Liu, 2010; Rook, 2012). The theory discusses whether the later

century's introduction of antibiotics, improved personal hygiene, and other aspects of modern sanitized living, disrupted the immune balance between microbes and human subjects with an abruptness that did not allow for evolutionary adaptation, leading to the unintended consequence of the allergic march underlying the allergy and asthma epidemic of the past century (Liu, 2010). However, the theory is challenged by the paradox that a wide range of microbes have a well-established provocative effect on asthma symptoms. Elements that are likely to be relevant to the onset of allergy are, for example, decreased exposure to farm animals and decreased diversity of bacterial exposure, decreased exposure to soil bacteria, and water chlorination (Platts-Mills, 2015). Read more about the hygiene hypothesis and 'old friends' in Chapter 2.3 'Microbes, the immune system, and the health benefits of exposure to the natural environment'.

Mechanisms and symptoms

Allergy is induced when the immune system inadequately responds to usually harmless agents in the same way as it would respond to harmful substances, such as bacteria or virus. Individuals with pollen allergy develop specific immunoglobulin E (IgE) antibody responses to allergenic pollen with exposure over time. The specific IgE antibodies bind to high-affinity IgE receptors on mast cells and basophils (Wheatley and Togias, 2015), causing mucosal inflammation—the IgE inflammatory immune response. On re-exposure to the allergen, it is recognized by an IgE receptor and a cascade of pathways is set in motion, leading to the release of preformed bioactive mediators like histamine and lipid mediators derived from leukotrienes, prostaglandins, and platelet-activating factor, that can cause smooth muscle contraction, increased vascular permeability, and mucus secretion (Bernstein and Moellman, 2012). The release of these mediators leads to the early-phase allergic response. The mediators also attract inflammatory cells into the tissue which results in the late-phase allergic response, manifest around four to eight hours after the early response (Janeway *et al.*, 1997). These mechanisms lie behind the pharmacologic therapies which are targeted against mediators or non-specific inflammation to attenuate or ablate allergic symptoms.

Seasonal AR is associated with several bothersome symptoms, such as paroxysmal sneezing, nasal congestion, watery rhinorrhoea, conjunctivitis, itchy throat and palate, and wheezing. These symptoms may impair usual daily activities, quality of sleep, and productivity. Frequently, seasonal AR is associated with comorbidities including asthma. Overall, the quality of life is significantly impaired among patients with seasonal AR (Bauchau and Durham, 2004). Apart from the direct allergy-related symptoms, patients often describe that during the season they feel irritable, depressed, less attractive, and low in vitality and emotional functioning (Blaiss, 2007)

While nobody dies from seasonal AR alone, it is a major contributor to the total cost of health-related absenteeism (i.e. missing work) and presenteeism (i.e. showing up to work but having reduced productivity). For example, costs of hay fever and allergic conjunctivitis in the United States have been estimated at more than $6 billion per year (Blaiss, 2007). Yet, the condition can sometimes be trivialized (by the patient) and/or unrecognized (by the physician), resulting in the inadequate control of symptoms, as well as low rate of diagnosis (Bauchau and Durham, 2004; Greiner *et al.*,

2011). In addition, seasonal AR is strongly related to asthma, which still represents a potentially severe condition.

Co-morbidity

Asthma and seasonal AR frequently co-exist in the same subjects (Bousquet *et al.*, 2012). Seasonal AR has been detected in 78% of children with asthma and childhood AR has been associated with a 2–7-fold increased risk of asthma in pre-adolescence, adolescence, or adult life (Burgess *et al.*, 2007).

The first evidence about the role of allergens in asthma came between 1970 and 1980, demonstrating that chronic allergen exposure could make a major contribution to non-specific bronchial hyperreactivity (Altounyan, 1970; Cockcroft *et al.*, 1977). This has been followed by studies showing associations between asthma and elevated IgE to for example grass and ragweed pollen (Pollart *et al.*, 1988; Pollart *et al.*, 1989). Like allergies, the asthma prevalence has increased dramatically over the later decades and is now estimated to affect 300 million people worldwide (Boulet *et al.*, 2015). Both seasonal AR and asthma are increasing in urban areas at alarming rates; many call it 'epidemic'. There has been no similar rise in rural areas. Before 1960, most paediatrics textbooks did not even regard asthma as common, let alone epidemic (Platts-Mills, 2015). Not until the 1990 did it become clear that asthma was increasing in all Western countries (Haahtela *et al.*, 1990; Bråbäck *et al.*, 2004).

Interventions

Seasonal AR can be managed by three major treatment categories: (i) environmental control measures and allergen avoidance; (ii) pharmacological management; and (iii) allergen-specific immunotherapy. Environmental control is based on avoidance (i.e. avoiding exposure to pollen). This can be done by remaining indoors as much as possible when pollen counts are peaking, preferably in houses with filtered ventilation and air condition (Burge *et al.*, 2000). This approach requires, first of all, a daily life that permits such actions and also in-depth knowledge of the patterns of prevalence for each particle of concern, including seasonal, spatial, and diurnal variation patterns. Outdoor source control is another approach, based on reducing vegetation with allergenic potential. This is described in the last section of this chapter, 'What can be done?'.

Pharmacological treatments target the immune response to allergens. The options include new generation non-sedative antihistamines for mild disease, and use of intranasal steroids with low systemic bioavailability for moderate/severe disease. Treatment of seasonal AR with pharmacotherapy seems to also improve asthma control (Rotiroti and Scadding, 2016).

If the condition is severe and uncontrolled by pharmacotherapy, allergen-specific immunotherapy (SIT) is recommended. SIT is the only therapeutic modality that has a disease-modifying effect not only during the treatment period, but also in subsequent years. Moreover, it is possibly able to prevent new sensitizations and the progression of AR to asthma (Rotiroti and Scadding, 2016; Jacobsen *et al.*, 2007).

More recent treatment alternatives are, at least partly, based on the hygiene hypothesis and the importance of microbiomes. A recent systematic review (Güvenç *et al.*, 2016) provided significant evidence of beneficial clinical and immunologic effects of probiotics in the treatment of allergic rhinitis, especially with seasonal allergy.

Botanical sexism

Female trees, natural pollen-traps

The geometry of the female parts of the trees direct air currents carrying pollen toward stigmas. Pollen grains lose momentum entering the boundary layer of the stigma: at short distances, electrostatic attraction facilitates impaction. Capture is most efficient with conspecific pollen, with sperms able to fertilize the egg cells in the ovules so that these develop into seeds (Ogren, 2000; Sharma, 2015). Because females produce ('messy') seeds, horticulture has by tradition considered them as inferior, hence the preference for 'seedless' males. However, male trees all produce pollen, while female trees have the benefit of not producing any pollen.

Botanical sexism and the modern urban forest

Commercial horticulture produces vast numbers of all-male clonal selections from dioecious (producing one male plant and one female plant and not usually a single plant with both male and female parts) species. Many are patented and their value to the industry is in the billions of dollars. Close to 100% of all the ash (*Fraxinus*), poplar (*Populus*), pistache (*Pistacia*), bay laurel (*Laurus*), junipers (*Juniperus*), willows (*Salix*), ginkgo tree (*Ginkgo*), Griselinia (*Griselinia*), mulberries (*Morus*), yellowwood (*Podocarpus*), locust (*Gleditsia*) and logwoods (*Xylosma*) sold are clonal males (PolleNation, 2012). All of these trigger pollen allergies.

In California and Arizona in United States, shiny xylosma (*Xylosma congestum*) has been planted by the millions. In many cities it is the most common landscape shrub/tree and 100% of these are male.

The highest pollen count ever recorded in the United States (Nevada) came from a pollen trap on a school building (Griffith Elementary School). Approximately 60,000 grains per cubic yard of airspace were counted on one day (Las Vegas Sun, 1998; Rogers, 2010). All shrubs were male junipers and all except one of the mature trees were male ('fruitless') white mulberries.

With monoecious landscape species, there has also been a persistent trend towards plants that are more male, less female. Whenever possible, cuttings are taken only from male branches; thus the new trees are all-male. Common examples are the Mediterranean cypress (*Cupressus sempervirens*) and 'podless' honey locust (*Gleditsia triacanthos*) (PolleNation, 2012).

If property-owners have several separate-sexed trees, it is common practice to cut down the tree(s) that produces fruit/seeds (the female tree) and leave the one that doesn't (the male).

Nature, if not manipulated, has close to a 50/50 gender ratio. The sheer numbers of male trees/shrubs is increasing urban pollen counts. Commercial horticulture has unfortunately no incentive to stop this unhealthy, but highly profitable, practice of selling 'litter-free' male selections.

What can be done?

OPALS® is a criteria-based, numerical scale (1–10) with which landscape plants are ranked per allergenic potential. The scale (1 is best, 10 most allergenic) has been used by the United States Department of Agriculture (USDA) urban foresters and the American Lung Association since 1999 and 2000, respectively.

One step forward would be if plants on sale had tags that show the consumer their allergy-potential, for example by OPALS® scores. On the Isle of Guernsey, a large retail nursery is now using

OPALS® tags on all plants. Customer response has been good and there has been a preference towards the purchase of lower allergy ranked plants, and local doctors have recommended patients to shop there. Allergy tagging of nursery plants is similar to 'truth in labelling' laws that already affect packaged food in most industrialized countries.

Conclusion

Some US cities have passed pollen-control ordinances, banning the sale and planting of allergenic trees and shrubs (e.g. mulberry in the Southwestern United States). This costs little, and has great public health benefits.

Nursery plants should be allergy-ranked and labelled as pollen-control ordinances. City planners, arborists, public health professionals, and allergy organizations should engage in restoring the gender balance in urban forests.

Trees make a city great, they make it liveable, but smarter tree selection will help reduce many common and persistent human health problems.

References

Altounyan, R. (1970). Changes in histamine and atropine responsiveness as a guide to diagnosis and evaluation of therapy in obstructive airways disease. *Disodium cromoglycate in allergic airways disease.* Butterworths, London.

Asam, C., Hofer, H., Wolf, M., Aglas, L., & Wallner, M. (2015). Tree pollen allergens—an update from a molecular perspective. *Allergy*, 70, 1201–11.

Bauchau, V. & Durham, S. (2004). Prevalence and rate of diagnosis of allergic rhinitis in Europe. *Eur Respir J*, 24, 758–64.

Bawa, K. S., Ashton, P. S., Nor, S. M. (1990). Reproductive ecology of tropical forests: management issues. In: Bawa, K. S. & Hadley, M. (eds) *Reproductive Ecology of Tropical Forest Plants. Man and the Biosphere Series, 7.* Paris, France: UNESCO and The Parthenon Publishing Group.

Bernstein, J. A. & Moellman, J. J. (2012). Progress in the emergency management of hereditary angioedema: focus on new treatment options in the United States. *Postgrad Med*, 124, 91–100.

Blaiss, M. S. (2007). Allergic rhinoconjunctivitis: Burden of disease. *Allergy Asthma Proc*, 28, 393–7.

Boulet, L.-P., Fitzgerald, J. M., & Reddel, H. K. (2015). The revised 2014 GINA strategy report: opportunities for change. *Curr Opin Pulm Med*, 21, 1–7.

Bousquet, J., Schünemann, H. J., Samolinski, B., *et al.* (2012). Allergic Rhinitis and its Impact on Asthma (ARIA): Achievements in 10 years and future needs. *J Allergy Clin Immunol*, 130, 1049–62.

Bråbäck, L., Hjern, A., & Rasmussen, F. (2004). Trends in asthma, allergic rhinitis and eczema among Swedish conscripts from farming and non-farming environments. A nationwide study over three decades. *Clin Exp Allergy*, 34, 38–43.

Burge, H. A., Pierson, D. L., Groves, T. O., Strawn, K. F., & Mishra, S. K. (2000). Dynamics of airborne fungal populations in a large office building. *Cur Microbiol*, 40, 10–16.

Burgess, J. A., Walters, E. H., Byrnes, G. B., *et al.* (2007). Childhood allergic rhinitis predicts asthma incidence and persistence to middle age: A longitudinal study. *J Allergy Clin Immunol*, 120, 863–9.

Chambers, L. E., Altwegg, R., Barbraud, C., *et al.* (2013). Phenological changes in the southern hemisphere. *PLoS One*, 8, e75514.

Chehregani, A. & Kouhkan, F. (2008). Diesel exhaust particles and allergenicity of pollen grains of Lilium martagon. *Ecotoxicol Environ Saf*, 69, 568–73.

Cockcroft, D. W., Ruffin, R. E., Dolovich, J., & Hargreave, F. E. (1977). Allergen-induced increase in non-allergic bronchial reactivity. *Clin Allergy*, 7, 503–13.

Csillag, A., Boldogh, I., Pazmandi, K., *et al.* (2010). Pollen-induced oxidative stress influences both innate and adaptive immune responses via altering dendritic cell functions. *J Immunol*, 184, 2377–85.

Cuinica, L. G., Abreu, I., & Da Silva, J. E. (2014). Effect of air pollutant NO 2 on Betula pendula, Ostrya carpinifolia and Carpinus betulus pollen fertility and human allergenicity. *Environ Pollut*, 186, 50–5.

Culley, T. M., Weller, S. G., & Sakai, A. K. (2002). The evolution of wind pollination in angiosperms. *Trends Ecol Evol*, 17, 361–9.

Dahl, Å., Galán, C., Hajkova, L., *et al.* (2013). The onset, course, and intensity of the pollen season. In: Sofiev, M. & Bergmann, K.-C. (eds) *Allergenic Pollen; A Review of the Production, Release, Distribution and Health Impacts.* Dordrecht, the Netherlands: Springer Science.

Faegri, K., Iversen, J., Kaland, P. E., Krzywinski, K. (1989). *Textbook of Pollen Analysis.* London, UK: Jon Wiley and Sons.

Gilles, S., Behrendt, H., Ring, J., & Traidl-Hoffmann, C. (2012). The pollen enigma: modulation of the allergic immune response by non-allergenic, pollen-derived compounds. *Curr Pharm Des*, 18, 2314–19.

Greiner, A. N., Hellings, P. W., Rotiroti, G., & Scadding, G. K. (2011). Allergic rhinitis. *Lancet*, 378, 2112–22.

Güvenç, I. A., Muluk, N. B., Mutlu, F. S., *et al.* (2016). Do probiotics have a role in the treatment of allergic rhinitis? A comprehensive systematic review and meta-analysis. *Am J Rhinol Allergy*, 30, e157–75.

Haahtela, T., Lindholm, H., Björkstén, F., Koskenvuo, K., & Laitinen, L. (1990). Prevalence of asthma in Finnish young men. *BMJ*, 301, 266–8.

Hajat, S., Haines, A., Atkinson, R. W., Bremner, S. A., Anderson, H. R., & Emberlin, J. (2001). Association between air pollution and daily consultations with general practitioners for allergic rhinitis in London, United Kingdom. *Am J Epidemiol*, 153, 704–14.

IPCC (2014). Climate Change 2014: Impacts, Adaptation, and Vulnerability. Final Draft Report. In: II, I. W. G. (ed.). Available at: http://www.ipcc. ch/report/ar5/wg2/ [Online].

Jacobsen, L., Niggemann, B., Dreborg, S., *et al.* (2007). Specific immunotherapy has long-term preventive effect of seasonal and perennial asthma: 10-year follow-up on the PAT study. *Allergy*, 62, 943–8.

Janeway, C. A., Travers, P., Walport, M., & Shlomchik, M. J. (1997). *Immunobiology: The Immune System in Health and Disease.* New York, NY: Garland Science.

Klein, T., Kukkonen, J., Dahl, Å., *et al.* (2012). Interactions of physical, chemical, and biological weather calling for an integrated approach to assessment, forecasting, and communication of air quality. *Ambio*, 41, 851–64.

Kondrashova, A., Seiskari, T., Ilonen, J., Knip, M., & Hyöty, H. (2013). The 'Hygiene hypothesis' and the sharp gradient in the incidence of autoimmune and allergic diseases between Russian Karelia and Finland. *APMIS*, 121, 478–93.

Las Vegas Sun (1998). Mulberry Trees Produce Record Pollen Count. *Las Vegas Sun.* Las Vegas.

Lewis, W. H., Vinay, P., Zenger, V. E. (1983). *Airborne and Allergenic Pollen of North America.* Baltimore, MD: Johns Hopkins University Press.

Liu, A. H. (2010). Hygiene hypothesis for allergy and asthma. In: Martin R. J. & Sutherland, E. R. (eds) *Asthma and Infections: Lung Biology in Health and Disease.* New York, NY: Informa Healthcare.

Liu, A. H. (2015). Revisiting the hygiene hypothesis for allergy and asthma. *J Allergy Clin Immunol*, 136, 860–5.

Menzel, A., Sparks, T. H., Estrella, N., *et al.* (2006). European phenological response to climate change matches the warming pattern. *Global Change Biology*, 12, 1969–76.

Motta, A., Dormans, J., Peltre, G., LaCroix, G., Bois, F. Y., & Steerenberg, P. (2004). Intratracheal instillation of cytoplasmic granules from Phleum pratense pollen induces IgE-and cell-mediated responses in the Brown Norway rat. *Int Arch Allergy Immunol*, 135, 24–9.

Motta, A. C., Marliere, M., Peltre, G., Sterenberg, P., & LaCroix, G. (2006). Traffic-related air pollutants induce the release of allergen-containing cytoplasmic granules from grass pollen. *Int Arch Allergy Immunol*, 139, 294–8.

Ogren, T. L. (2000). *Allergy-Free Gardening*, Berkeley, CA: Ten Speed Press.

Penard-Morand, C. & Annesi-Maesano, I. (2008). Allergic respiratory diseases and outdoor air pollution. *Revue Des Maladies Respiratoires*, 25, 1013–26.

Platts-Mills, T. A. (2015). The allergy epidemics: 1870–2010. *J Allergy Clin Immunol*, 136, 3–13.

Pollart, S. M., Chapman, M. D., Fiocco, G. P., Rose, G., & Platts-Mills, T. A. (1989). Epidemiology of acute asthma: IgE antibodies to common inhalant allergens as a risk factor for emergency room visits. *J Allergy Clin Immunol*, 83, 875–82.

Pollart, S. M., Reid, M. J., Fling, J. A., Chapman, M. D., & Platts-Mills, T. A. (1988). Epidemiology of emergency room asthma in northern California: association with IgE antibody to ryegrass pollen. *J Allergy Clin Immunol*, 82, 224–30.

PolleNation (2012). PolleNation, Canadian Urban Allergy Audit 2012. Johnson & Johnson, Reactin, Toronto, Canada

Pollenlibrary (2014). Allergens and Plants Research by Location. Available at: http://www.pollenlibrary.com (accessed 2 November 2014) [Online].

Radauer, C. & Breiteneder, H. (2006). Pollen allergens are restricted to few protein families and show distinct patterns of species distribution. *J Allergy Clin Immunol*, 117, 141–7.

Radauer, C., Bublin, M., Wagner, S., Mari, A., & Breiteneder, H. (2008). Allergens are distributed into few protein families and possess a restricted number of biochemical functions. *J Allergy Clin Immunol*, 121, 847–52. e7.

Reinmuth-Selzle, K., Ackaert, C., Kampf, C. J., *et al.* (2014). Nitration of the birch pollen allergen Bet v 1.0101: efficiency and site-selectivity of liquid and gaseous nitrating agents. *J Proteome Res*, 13, 1570–7.

Rezanejad, F. (2007). The effect of air pollution on microsporogenesis, pollen development and soluble pollen proteins in Spartium junceum L.(Fabaceae). *Turk J Botany*, 31, 183–91.

Rogers, K. (2010). Pollen hangs thick in the air. *Las Vegas Review–Journal*. Las Vegas, NV.

Rook, G. W. (2012). Hygiene hypothesis and autoimmune diseases. *Clin Rev Allergy Immunol*, 42, 5–15.

Rotiroti, G. & Scadding, G. K. (2016). Allergic rhinitis–an overview of a common disease. *Paediatrics & Child Health*, 26, 298–303.

Scheifinger, H. J., Belmonte, J. B., Celenk, S., *et al.* (2013). Monitoring, modelling and forecasting of the pollen season. In: Sofiev, M. & Bergmann, K.-C. (eds) *Allergenic Pollen: A Review of the Production, Release, Distribution and Health Impacts*. Dordrecht, the Netherlands: Springer Science.

Schmidt, C. W. (2016). Pollen overload: seasonal allergies in a changing climate. *Environ Health Perspect*, 124, A70–5.

Shalaby, K. H., Allard-Coutu, A., O'Sullivan, M. J., *et al.* (2013). Inhaled birch pollen extract induces airway hyperresponsiveness via oxidative stress but independently of pollen-intrinsic NADPH oxidase activity, or the TLR4–TRIF pathway. *J Immunol*, 191, 922–33.

Sharma, J. P. (2015). *Comprehensive Biology XII*. New Delhi, India: Laxmi Publications.

Shi, D. Q. A. Y., W. (2010). Pollen germination and tube growth. In: Pua, E.-C. & Davey, M. R. (eds) *Plant Developmental Biology—Biotechnological Perspectives*. Berlin, Germany: Springer Berlin Heidelberg.

Šikoparija, B., Skjøth, C., Kübler, K. A., *et al.* (2013). A mechanism for long distance transport of Ambrosia pollen from the Pannonian Plain. *Agricultural and Forest Meteorology*, 180, 112–17.

Singh, A. B. & Kumar, P. (2003). Aeroallergens in clinical practice of allergy in India. An overview. *Ann Agric Environ Med*, 10, 131–6.

Singh, K. & Kushwaha, C. (2005). Emerging paradigms of tree phenology in dry tropics. *Curr Sci*, 89, 964–75.

Sly, R. M. (1999). Changing prevalence of allergic rhinitis and asthma. *Ann Allergy Asthma Immunol*, 82, 233–52.

Smith, M., Cecchi, L., Skjøth, C. A., Karrer, G., & Šikoparija, B. (2013). Common ragweed: A threat to environmental health in Europe. *Environ Int*, 61, 115–26.

Sofiev, M., Belmonte, J., Gehrig, R., Izquierdo, R., Dahl, A., Siljamo, P. (2013). Airborne pollen transport. In: Sofiev, M. & Bergmann, K.-C. (eds) *Allergenic Pollen: A Review of the Production, Release, Distribution and Health Impacts*. Dordrecht, the Netherlands: Springer Science.

Solé, D., Cassol, V., Silva, A., *et al.* (2007). Prevalence of symptoms of asthma, rhinitis, and atopic eczema among adolescents living in urban and rural areas in different regions of Brazil. *Allergologia et immunopathologia*, 35, 248–53.

Taylor, P. E., Flagan, R. C., Miguel, A. G., Valenta, R., & Glovsky, M. M. (2004). Birch pollen rupture and the release of aerosols of respirable allergens. *Clin Exp Allergy*, 34.

World Allergy Organization (WAO) (2011). *White Book on Allergy*. Pawanakar, R., Holgate, S. T., Canonica, G. W., Lockey, R. F. (eds). Wisconsin, US: World Allergy Organization.

Wheatley, L. & Togias, A. (2015). Clinical practice. Allergic rhinitis. *N Engl J Med*, 372, 456–63.

Ziello, C., Sparks, T. H., Estrella, N., Belmonte, J., Bergmann, K. C., & Bucher, E. (2012). Changes to airborne pollen counts across Europe. *PLoS One*, 7, e34076.

Ziska, L. H. & Beggs, P. J. (2012). Anthropogenic climate change and allergen exposure: The role of plant biology. *J Allergy Clin Immunol*, 129, 27–32.

Ziska, L. H. & Caulfield, F. A. (2000). Rising CO_2 and pollen production of common ragweed (Ambrosia artemisiifolia L.), a known allergy-inducing species: implications for public health. *Aust J Plant Physiol*, 27, 893–8.

Ziska, L. H., Gebhard, D. E., Frenz, D. A., Faulkner, S., Singer, B. D., & Straka, J. G. (2003). Cities as harbingers of climate change: common ragweed, urbanization, and public health. *J Allergy Clin Immunol*, 111, 290–5.

CHAPTER 7.2

Vector-borne diseases and poisonous plants

David Wong

Take care out there

People who engage in outdoor recreation may be exposed to a wide range of arthropod vector species—including fleas, mosquitoes, ticks, flies, and other insects—and their associated bacterial, viral, or protozoan pathogens and parasites. The World Health Organization (WHO) estimates that vector-borne diseases account for 17% of all infectious disease cases and that more than half of the world's population is at risk for exposure to at least one vector-borne pathogen (WHO, 2014). The greatest burden occurs in tropical climates where high-incidence vector-borne diseases, such as malaria, dengue, lymphatic filariasis, and leishmaniasis, each affect millions of people annually. Vector-borne diseases disproportionately impact developing countries where poor sanitation and hygiene, coupled with substandard housing, contribute to exposure risk.

Even in developed countries with primarily temperate climates, however, vector-borne diseases are significant public health problems. For example, in the United States, common vector-borne diseases include Lyme disease, West Nile virus, and spotted fever group rickettsioses (e.g. Rocky Mountain spotted fever), which collectively accounted for over 42,000 reported cases in 2013 (Adams et al., 2015). Vector-borne diseases typically have defined geographic foci, based on the distribution and abundance of vector species as well as ecologic factors such as vegetation, climate, latitude, and elevation (Reisen, 2010). Several vector-borne diseases, such as plague, present with severe clinical symptoms and are associated with high mortality rates, particularly if treatment is delayed.

It is crucial that outdoor recreationalists seeking to reap the myriad benefits from nature are also made aware of important vector-borne diseases in their geographic areas and are informed about appropriate prevention measures. The risk for acquiring a vector-borne disease is generally higher in warmer months (e.g. spring and summer), which coincides with similar increases in human outdoor activity. In most cases, exposure to vector-borne pathogens can be greatly reduced with education and simple interventions, such as wearing insect repellents and avoiding outdoor activities during the times of day when vector activity peaks.

In this chapter, I will review: (i) common vectors and vector-borne diseases by continent, with a focus on pathogens likely to be encountered by outdoor recreationalists; (ii) trends and factors influencing pathogen distribution; and (iii) personal protective measures and their effectiveness. In addition to vector-borne diseases, I will briefly highlight common poisonous plants and harmful algal blooms, which are other potential exposure risks for persons engaging in outdoor activity.

Common vectors and vector-borne pathogens

The distribution of important vector species and associated pathogens vary considerably by geography. Each vector species has preferred environmental conditions that determine its distribution and, consequently, the risk areas for vector-borne diseases. Vectors and pathogens potentially encountered in North America are distinctly different from those found in Europe, Australia, Asia, and other continents. It is also important to note that within broad geographic areas, the risk for encountering an infected vector can vary substantially, even over short distances, due to differences in micro-habitat, climate, and biodiversity—all of which can influence the prevalence of vectors and their pathogens. Some vector-borne diseases, such as tick-borne relapsing fever, are primarily associated with indoor exposure (e.g. sleeping overnight in rustic cabins) (Dworkin et al., 2002), and are not considered major risks for outdoor recreationalists. General knowledge about potential vector-borne disease risks can empower recreationalists and improve adherence to personal protective measures. In this section, I provide a high-level overview of vector-borne diseases in the Americas, Europe, Australia, and Africa/Asia.

The Americas

In the United States, the most common vector-borne disease is Lyme disease, which is caused by the bacterium *Borrelia burgdorferi* and is transmitted through the bites of infected *Ixodes* or black-legged ticks. These ticks (primarily *Ixodes scapularis*) are abundant in Northeast and Upper Midwest states, and thus 95% of confirmed Lyme disease cases in 2013 were reported from only 14 states (Adams et al., 2015). A smaller risk area for Lyme disease occurs on the northwest coast of California where *Ixodes pacificus* is the predominant vector. Typical symptoms of Lyme disease include fever, headache, fatigue, and a characteristic skin rash called erythema migrans (present in 70–80% of acute infections), which resembles a bull's eye lesion and occurs at the site of the tick bite. Most cases of Lyme disease can be treated successfully with antibiotics. Late symptoms and complications of Lyme disease include meningitis, facial paralysis, arthritis (particularly of the knee and other large joints), and an irregular heartbeat.

Rocky Mountain spotted fever (RMSF) and other spotted fever group rickettsioses are potentially fatal tick-borne diseases that are endemic in the United States (particularly North Carolina, Oklahoma, Arkansas, Tennessee, and Missouri), Central America (Mexico, Panama, and Costa Rica) and South America (Brazil, Colombia, and Argentina) (Parola *et al.*, 2013). The most common rickettsial pathogen, *Rickettsia rickettsii*, can be carried by various tick vectors, including the American dog tick, brown dog tick, and the lone star tick. Patients with RMSF experience an abrupt onset of high fever that is often accompanied by headache, nausea, vomiting, anorexia, and generalized myalgia. A maculopapular rash may develop several days later and is typically found on the wrists, ankles, and forearms. Severe symptoms of RMSF include pulmonary haemorrhage, cerebral oedema, myocarditis, and renal failure. Doxycycline is the first-line treatment for RMSF and is highly effective.

Other tick-borne diseases endemic in the Americas include tularemia, ehrlichiosis, anaplasmosis, babesiosis, and Colorado tick fever. Several tick-borne human pathogens have been recently discovered in the past 10 years, including heartland virus (south-central United States), *Borrelia miyamotoi* (northeastern United States), and Powassan virus (northeastern and Great Lake states) (Vasconcelos and Calisher 2016; Krause *et al.*, 2015). Of these, Powassan, a flavivirus, is the most virulent pathogen and is associated with meningoencephalitis and chronic neurologic problems, such as memory loss and recurrent headaches. Powassan is fatal in approximately 10% of cases (Ebel 2010).

The most commonly reported mosquito-borne pathogen in the United States is West Nile virus, which is asymptomatic in 80% of infections, causes a self-limited febrile illness in most symptomatic individuals, and in <1% of cases can lead to severe neuroinvasive disease. West Nile virus was first documented in North America (New York City) in 1999 (Nash *et al.*, 2001) and has since spread throughout the lower 48 states. The disease is carried primarily by *Culex* mosquitoes and is now widely established from Canada to Argentina (Elizondo-Quiroga and Elizondo-Quiroga 2013). Persons most at risk for acquiring West Nile virus are individuals who work or spend significant time outdoors. Neuroinvasive cases are most common in the central United States, and symptoms include headache, high fever, neck stiffness, and seizures. There is no specific treatment for West Nile virus, and no vaccine is currently available.

In tropical regions of the Americas (i.e. Caribbean, Central, and South America), the most common mosquito-borne pathogen is dengue, which is a virus carried primarily by *Aedes* mosquitoes. From 2008–2012, the Pan American Health Organization (PAHO) reported over 1.2 million cases of dengue annually from member nations; high-incidence countries include Brazil, Paraguay, Colombia, Honduras, and Mexico (PAHO 2014). Dengue can present as a self-limited febrile illness or as a severe form known as dengue haemorrhagic fever (DHF). DHF is characterized by leaky capillaries, potentially leading to ascites, pleural effusions, and shock, as well as low platelets and internal bleeding. With supportive care and proper medical supervision, the fatality rate for DHF can be reduced to <1% (Gibbons and Vaughn 2002). There is no specific treatment or vaccine, and the best prevention measure is to avoid mosquito bites.

In 2015, Zika virus—a flavivirus also carried by *Aedes* mosquitoes—emerged in the Americas in Brazil (Campos *et al.*,

2015). By January 2016, the virus had spread to 20 other countries or territories in the Americas, including South America, Central America, the Caribbean, and Mexico (Hennessey *et al.*, 2016). Zika virus infection is asymptomatic in approximately 80% of exposed persons; among those with symptoms (i.e. fever, joint pain, rash, and conjunctivitis), the clinical course is typically mild and self-limited. Zika virus, however, can cause severe birth defects, particularly microcephaly, in foetuses of infected pregnant women and has also been associated with Guillain-Barré syndrome and other neurologic complications. Zika is the first known mosquito-borne virus to cause congenital anomalies in humans (Simeone *et al.*, 2016). In multiple countries, enhanced surveillance, international coordination/research, and public awareness campaigns have been implemented to reduce the risk for Zika virus exposure, fast-track the development of a human vaccine, and learn more about Zika transmission and other potential prevention measures.

A notable flea-borne disease in the Americas is plague, which is found in the western United States (west of the 100th meridian) and parts of Peru and Brazil. Plague is caused by the bacterium *Yersinia pestis* and is thought to be maintained by reservoir rodent species, such as ground squirrels. During epizootic infection, many rodent hosts may die in large numbers and their fleas are forced to parasitize other hosts, including humans. Epizootic diseases have the highest risk for human infection. Initial symptoms of plague are non-specific (fever, headache, weakness), which then rapidly progress to more severe symptoms as the bacteria spread to other parts of the body. Bubonic plague is the most common form of plague (characterized by enlarged lymph nodes called buboes); the septicaemic and pneumonic forms of plague are more difficult to diagnosis and have fatality rates approaching 90–100% in untreated cases (Dennis and Campbell, 2004). Early treatment with appropriate antibiotics and supportive care is essential.

Europe

Tick-borne diseases are the most common vector-borne diseases in Europe. Lyme disease or Lyme borreliosis (as it is more commonly referred to in Europe) is a high-prevalence disease with at least 65,000 cases reported annually across Europe (Izzoli *et al.*, 2011). Cases have been documented from Turkey to Sweden with high-incidence countries including Germany, Austria, Switzerland, and Slovenia. The clinical presentation of Lyme borreliosis varies, depending on which of three pathogenic genospecies of the *Borrelia burgdorferi* sensu lato complex (*B. burgdorferi* senu stricto, *B. garinii*, and *B. afzelii*) is implicated in infection. All pathogenic genospecies can cause erythema migrans, but *B. burgdorferi* ss is more commonly associated with arthritis and joint pain, *B. garinii* is the predominant cause of Lyme neuroborelliosis, and *B. afzelii* infections tend to be milder and may present only with rash. *B. afzelii* is the most common genospecies in central and eastern European countries and Scandinavia. *B. burgdorferi* ss causes clinical symptoms most similar to that of Lyme disease in North America, but is the least common genospecies found in Europe (ECDC 2011).

Tick-borne encephalitis (TBE) is another important tick-borne disease in Europe. TBE is caused by the TBE virus and is spread by the bites of infected *Ixodes* ticks. There are three subtypes of TBE, of which two are found in Europe: the European subtype, which is endemic in Western, Central, and Northern Europe (e.g. Germany, Czech Republic, Sweden, Baltic states), and the Siberian subtype, which is less common and endemic in far Eastern Europe. The

European subtype of the disease is biphasic with an initial viremic phase consisting antibiotics of non-specific, flu-like symptoms, followed by (in 20–30% of patients) a second phase with signs and symptoms of meningoencephalitis and/or paralysis (Haglund and Gunther, 2003). Neuroinvasive symptoms are more common in adults than children. Males are more affected than women, and hiking has been identified as a risk factor (Kaiser, 1995). There is no specific treatment for TBE, but a vaccine is available in endemic countries.

Mosquitoes in Europe are primarily a nuisance issue with much lower numbers of reported infectious cases (compared to tick-borne diseases) and only focal outbreaks occurring in discrete regions. In 2010, a West Nile virus outbreak was reported in several Southeastern European countries, including Greece, Romania, and Hungary (Danis et al., 2011). Ongoing cases have been reported since then. In 2012, the autonomous province of Madeira in Portugal experienced a large dengue outbreak affecting over 2,000 residents and at least 78 travellers from other European countries (Franco et al., 2015). Previously, dengue had been absent from Europe for 80 years until 2010, when isolated, autochthonous cases were reported in France and Croatia (Murray et al., 2013). Patterns in distribution of mosquitoes and other vectors may change based on climate or vector importations that are sustainable in local environments; epidemiologic data are important for identifying new and emerging areas of disease risk.

Australia

In Australia, mosquitoes are the most important vector for human infections. Important mosquito-borne arboviruses include Barmah Forest Virus (BFV) and Ross River Virus (RRV), which together account for approximately 80% of vector-borne disease case reports nationwide (Fitzsimmons et al., 2010). BFV and RRV have been reported in all jurisdictions but are most common in Queensland and the Northern Territory. Symptoms of BFV and RRV include polyarthritis, fever, and rash. Another important arbovirus is Murray Valley encephalitis virus, which is rare, but potentially fatal. Currently, there are only three known tick-borne diseases in Australia: (i) Queensland tick typhus, caused by *Rickettsia australis*, is found along Australia's Eastern Coast; (ii) Flinders Island spotted fever, caused by *R. honei*, is found in Southeastern Australia, including Tasmania; and (iii) Q fever, caused by *Coxiella burnetii*, has been documented in ticks, but transmission is more common from exposure to cattle, sheep, and goats and their excreta (Lowbridge et al., 2011). Symptoms of the two rickettsial diseases are mild and treatable with antibiotics.

Africa/Asia

Countries in Asia and Africa have some of the highest incidences of vector-borne diseases. Tropical and subtropical conditions on these continents are conducive for many vectors to thrive, including mosquitoes, flies, sandflies, and other insects. For example, almost 75% of the global population exposed to dengue live in the Asia-Pacific region, with eight countries in Southeast Asia (Bangladesh, India, Indonesia, Maldives, Myanmar, Sri Lanka, Thailand, and Timor-Leste) classified as hyperendemic by the World Health Organization (Murray et al., 2013). Hotspots for plague include the Democratic Republic of the Congo, Madagascar, Myanmar, and Vietnam. Chikungunya virus, another mosquito-borne virus spread by the same *Aedes* mosquitoes that can also carry dengue, is

endemic in many countries in Africa and Southeast Asia, and has recently emerged in the Americas and southern Europe.

Malaria, a parasitic disease spread by mosquitoes, is perhaps the most well-known vector-borne disease and is associated with the highest number of annual deaths worldwide. Malaria is caused by one of five species of the *Plasmodium* parasite, of which *P. falciparum* is the most common and the most likely to cause severe malaria and death. Anopheline mosquitoes are the only known vector. In 2015, an estimated 214 million cases of malaria occurred worldwide and 438,000 people died, mostly children in sub-Saharan Africa (WHO, 2015b). Symptoms of malaria can be uncomplicated (cyclical periods of illness including high fever, chills, headache, and nausea/vomiting) or severe (life-threatening complications involving the central nervous system, lungs, red blood cells, electrolytes, and/or kidneys). Early diagnosis and treatment are key. Particularly for *P. falciparum* infections, artemisinin-based combination therapy (ACT) is the best available treatment. Currently, there is no commercially available malaria vaccine.

Other high-incidence vector-borne diseases in Asia and Africa are associated with impoverished conditions and are less likely to be encountered by outdoor recreationalists. *Lymphatic filariasis* (LF), commonly known as elephantiasis, is caused by a microscopic parasitic worm and is spread by *Culex* mosquitoes. The disease causes disfigurement and lymphedema and is estimated to affect over 120 million people worldwide, mostly in Asia and Africa (WHO, 2015a). Onchocerciasis (also known as river blindness) is a parasitic disease spread by blackflies (*Simulium*) that causes depigmentation of the skin, lymphadenitis, and visual impairment. After trachoma, onchocerciasis is the second leading cause of blindness worldwide and affects over 37 million people worldwide. Visceral leishmaniasis—the most serious form of leishmaniasis that affects the spleen, liver, and bone marrow—is caused by a parasite transmitted by phlebotomine sandflies. Approximately 300,000 new visceral leishmaniasis cases are reported each year, mostly from Africa (Ethiopia, Sudan), Asia (Bangladesh, India), and Brazil.

Trends in vector-borne diseases

Factors that increase human contact with vectors and/or the development of pathogens in vectors could increase the risk for vector-borne diseases. These potential factors are myriad and include those that primarily affect vectors (e.g. precipitation, humidity, temperature, habitat); factors based on human behaviour and population trends (e.g. land use, shifting demographics, recreational/occupational activities, socioeconomic factors); and factors associated with pathogens (e.g. disease surveillance, pathogen-host interactions, antibiotic resistance, evolving viral or bacterial strains). Given these complex dynamics, it is difficult to predict with certainty whether the incidence of specific vector-borne diseases will increase or decrease in local settings.

Changes in climate have the potential to significantly affect vector-borne disease in humans. It is estimated that average global temperatures will have risen by 1.0–3.5°C by 2100 (Githeko et al., 2000). These warming temperatures may expand vector habitats to areas that are currently inhospitable for vector survivability. As ectotherms (cold-blooded animals), vectors are unable to adapt easily to fluctuating temperatures, and thus their distribution in nature is largely dependent on environmental factors that impact their reproduction, development, behaviour, and other population dynamics. Temperatures can also affect pathogen development. Using malaria as an example, studies indicate that *P. falciparum* transmission is limited below 16–19°C; while on the other end of the spectrum, above 33–39°C, parasite development cannot occur (Gage *et al.*, 2008).

Precipitation is another important climate variable potentially affecting vector habitats. For mosquitoes, increases in precipitation may facilitate vector expansion by increasing the number of suitable breeding sites. Currently, the Sahel marks the northern limit of *P. falciparum* in Africa due to inadequate rainfall (Gage *et al.*, 2008). For ticks, both precipitation and temperature are strongly associated with host-seeking behaviour. One notable example is the *I. pacificus* tick that transmits Lyme disease in California. *I pacificus* was shown to have 82% longer peak questing times in cooler, coniferous areas compared to warmer, drier oak woodland habitats (Eisen *et al.*, 2003).

It is important to note that changes in climate are only one factor in determining vector-borne disease incidence, and these environmental variables are often influenced by human behaviours and activities. For example, global population growth may drive human communities to live in rural and semi-rural settings where potential contact with vectors is higher compared to urban areas. During droughts, the risk for mosquito-borne diseases can counterintuitively increase, if humans are more likely to store water in outdoor vessels, which can serve as peri-domestic mosquito breeding sites. Socioeconomic factors can temper vector-borne disease risk as was seen in a dengue outbreak along the United States–Mexico border in 1999 where disease incidence was lower on the United States side due to a higher prevalence of air conditioning (Reiter *et al.*, 2003). Predicting the relative impact of climate, human, and other factors on vector-borne disease incidence is difficult. Maintaining robust human-based disease surveillance systems and developing vector-based pathogen surveillance systems are critical for identifying and monitoring emerging risk areas and future trends. Read more in Chapter 7.5 about climate change and its potential effects on vector-borne diseases.

Prevention measures

Being aware of potential vector-borne disease risks and exercising appropriate personal protective measures are the most important steps for preventing vector-borne disease transmission. If educational resources are not readily available, outdoor recreationalists should research or inquire about potential risks with local health agencies and share this information with friends, family, and colleagues. Knowing about local diseases and vectors can both reinforce prevention practices and inform decisions to seek healthcare, should signs and symptoms develop.

Bites from ticks, mosquitoes, fleas, and other insects can be greatly reduced by wearing insect repellents on exposed skin. Repellents that are registered by the US Environmental Protection Agency (EPA) and that have been shown to have longer-lasting effects include DEET (recommended at up to 30% active ingredient), picaridin, oil of lemon eucalyptus, and IR3535 (Nasci *et al.*, 2016). DEET in concentrations higher than 50% does not provide additional protection. Repellents should always be used according to the label instructions. Although wearing long-sleeved shirts and long pants is a commonly cited vector-borne disease prevention measure, this practice may not be acceptable to many outdoor recreationalists, particularly in warm weather. Similarly,

permethrin-treated clothing, although highly effective for reducing tick and mosquito bites, is best implemented in combination with long sleeves and pants.

Where possible, efforts to modify activity while outdoors can reduce risk of vector exposure. Walking in the centre of hiking trails and avoiding forest edges, high grass, and leaf litter can reduce potential contact with questing ticks. Many mosquito species have peak activity during dusk and dawn, and avoiding outdoor activity during these times is recommended. Fleas carrying *Y. pestis* may be associated with rodents; recreationalists should avoid rodent burrows and other contact with wildlife.

Other prevention measures specific for tick bites include tucking pants into socks or boots, showering within two hours after coming indoors (Connally *et al.*, 2009), conducting full-body tick checks using a handheld or full-length mirror, and examining pets and recreational gear. If an attached tick is found, it should be removed carefully using fine-tipped tweezers or forceps. The tick should be grasped by its mouthparts as close to the skin as possible and then pulled upward using a continuous, steady motion. The tick can be preserved in alcohol, which can assist with identification in case symptoms (particularly fever and rash) develop. For Lyme disease and other tick-borne diseases, ticks must be attached for at least 24–48 hours before pathogen transmission can occur (Piesman *et al.*, 1987). The degree of engorgement or the time since tick exposure and discovery of the attached tick can help estimate the likely duration of attachment.

Poisonous plants and harmful algal blooms

Besides vector-borne diseases, outdoor recreationalists may be exposed to other potential environmental hazards, such as poisonous plants and harmful algal blooms. These hazards are worth highlighting, since symptoms may develop even after brief or casual exposure, as might occur while hiking or swimming.

Poison ivy, poison oak, poison sumac, and other flowering plants in the *Toxicodendron* genus are well-known poisonous plants that are found primarily in North America, but also in temperate parts of China, Japan, and Taiwan. Persons who contact the leaves or other parts of these plants may be exposed to urushiol, a natural oil that is highly toxic and causes an allergic reaction on the skin (also known as contact dermatitis). The classic presentation associated with *Toxicodendron* exposure is an itchy red rash with bumps or blisters at the site of contact. The best prevention measure is to recognize the appearance of these plants (e.g. 'Leaves of three, leave them be') and avoid contact when outdoors. If exposure occurs, the best treatment is to wash the area as soon as possible with soap and water. Topical corticosteroids and soothing measures, such as oatmeal baths, may provide symptomatic relief from the rash. Plants on other continents that may cause similar symptoms upon contact include stinging nettles and giant hogweed (broad distribution) and spurge, milky mangrove, and gympie gympie (found primarily in Australia). Stinging nettles and gympie gympie release toxins, not through sap or oils, but through tiny hollow hairs that penetrate the skin.

Recreationalists who engage in water activities are also at risk for potential toxic environmental exposures. Harmful algal blooms (HABs)—first described in the 1800s (Francis, 1878)—occur when certain species of algae overgrow in nutrient-rich marine or fresh water and produce toxins that are harmful to plants, animals, people, and the environment. In fresh water, toxins are typically associated with accumulations of cyanobacteria or blue-green algae, which may appear as green water with scum or thick, paint-like mats of algae on the water's surface. Freshwater HABs have been reported worldwide and appear to be increasing in frequency (Lopez et al., 2008).

People and animals can be exposed to algal toxins through three distinct mechanisms: (i) swallowing water contaminated with cyanobacteria or toxins may lead to gastrointestinal symptoms (e.g. vomiting, diarrhoea), liver failure, and neurologic symptoms (e.g. seizures, paralysis); (ii) skin contact with toxin-contaminated water may present as rash, itching, and/or conjunctivitis; and (iii) inhaling contaminated aerosols may lead to wheezing or difficulty breathing. Dogs, in particular, are at high risk because they are more likely to swallow contaminated water and might eat algae mats and/or lick algal toxins from their fur. Recreationalists and their pets should avoid all contact with visible algae in fresh or marine water.

Conclusion

Vector-borne diseases and other environmental hazards are potential risks for outdoor recreationalists. However, the health benefits of outdoor recreation and exposure to nature far outweigh the potential risks, which can be eliminated or greatly reduced through education and simple prevention measures. Overall, the myriad of these conditions can be avoided, particularly if users are informed, attentive, and responsible.

References

Adams, D., Fullerton, K., Jajosky, R., et al. (2015). Summary of notifiable infectious diseases and conditions—United States, 2013. *MMWR Morb Mortal Wkly Rep*, 62, 1–119.

Campos, G. S., Bandeira, A. C., & Sardi, S. I. (2015). Zika virus outbreak, Bahia, Brazil. *Emerg Infect Dis*, 21, 1885–6.

Connally, N. P., Durante, A. J., Yousey-Hindes, K. M., et al. (2009). Peridomestic Lyme disease prevention: results of a population-based case-control study. *Am J Prev Med*, 37, 201–6.

Danis, K., Papa, A., Theocharopoulos, G., et al. (2011). Outbreak of West Nile virus infection in Greece, 2010. *Emerg Infect Dis*, 17, 1868–72.

Dennis, D. T. & Campbell, G. L. (2004). Plague and other Yersinia infections. In: Kasper, D. L., Braunwald, E., Fauci, A. S., et al. (eds) *Harrison's Principles of Internal Medicine*, 16th edition. New York, NY: McGraw-Hill.

Dworkin, M. S., Shoemaker, P. C., Fritz, C. L., et al. (2002). The epidemiology of tick-borne relapsing fever in the United States. *Am J Tropical Med Hygiene*, 66, 753–8.

Ebel, G. D. (2010). Update on Powassan virus: emergence of a North American tick-borne flavivirus. *Ann Rev Entomol*, 55, 95–110.

ECDC (2011). *Second expert consultation on tick-borne diseases with emphasis on Lyme borreliosis and tick-borne encephalitis.* Stockholm, Sweden: European Centre for Disease Prevention and Control.

Eisen, R. J., Eisen, L., Castro, M. B., & Lane, R. S. (2003). Environmentally related variability in risk of exposure to Lyme disease spirochetes in northern California: effect of climatic conditions and habitat type. *Environ Entomol*, 32, 1010–18.

Elizondo-Quiroga, D. & Elizondo-Quiroga, A. (2013). West Nile virus and its theories, a big puzzle in Mexico and Latin America. *J Glob Infect Dis*, 5, 168–75.

Fitzsimmons, G. J., Wright, P., Johansen, C. A., & Whelan, P. I. (2010). Arboviral diseases and malaria in Australia, 2008–09: annual report of the National Arbovirus and Malaria Advisory Committee. *Commun Dis Intell Q Rep*, 34, 225–40.

Francis, G. (1878). Poisonous Australian lake. *Nature*, 18, 11–12.

Franco, L., Pagan, I., Serre Del Cor, N., et al. (2015). Molecular epidemiology suggests Venezuela as the origin of the dengue outbreak in Madeira, Portugal in 2012–2013. *Clin Microbiol Infect*, 21, e5–8.

Gage, K. L., Burkot, T. R., Eisen, R. J., & Hayes, E. B. (2008). Climate and vectorborne diseases. *Am J Prev Med*, 35, 436–50.

Gibbons, R. V. & Vaughn, D. W. (2002). Dengue: an escalating problem. *BMJ*, 324, 1563–6.

Githeko, A. K., Lindsay, S. W., Confalonieri, U. E., & Patz, J. A. (2000). Climate change and vector-borne diseases: a regional analysis. *Bull World Health Organ*, 78, 1136–47.

Haglund, M. & Gunther, G. (2003). Tick-borne encephalitis—pathogenesis, clinical course and long-term follow-up. *Vaccine*, 21, S11–18.

Hennessey, M., Fischer, M., & Staples, J. E. (2016). Zika virus spreads to new areas—Region of the Americas, May 2015–January 2016. *MMWR Morb Mortal Wkly Rep*, 65, 55–8.

Izzoli A., Hauffe H. C., Carpi G., et al. (2011). Lyme borreliosis in Europe. *Eurosurveillance*, 16, 1–8.

Kaiser, R. (1995). Tick-borne encephalitis in southern Germany. *Lancet*, 345, 463.

Krause, P. J., Fish, D., Narasimhan, S., & Barbour, A. G. (2015). *Borrelia miyamotoi* infection in nature and in humans. *Clin Microbiol Infect*, 21, 631–9.

Lopez, C. B., Jewett, E. B., Dortch, Q., et al. (2008). *Scientific Assessment of Freshwater Harmful Algal Blooms.* Washington, DC: Interagency Working Group on Harmful Algal Blooms, Hypoxia, and Human Health of the Joint Subcommittee on Ocean Science and Technology.

Lowbridge, C. P., Doggett, S. L., & Graves, S. (2011). Bug breakfast in the bulletin. Tickborne diseases. *N S W Public Health Bull*, 23, 31–5.

Murray, N. E., Quam, M. B., & Wilder-Smith, A. (2013). Epidemiology of dengue: past, present and future prospects. *Clin Epidemiol*, 5, 299–309.

Nasci, R. S., Wirtz, R. A., & Brogdon, W. G. (2016). Protection against mosquitoes, ticks, and other arthropods. In: Brunette, G. W. (ed.) *CDC Health Information for International Travel*, 16th edition. London, UK: Oxford University Press.

Nash, D., Mostashari, F., Fine, A., et al. (2001). The outbreak of West Nile virus infection in the New York City area in 1999. *N Engl J Med*, 344, 1807–14.

PAHO (2014). *State of the Art in the Prevention and Control of Dengue in the Americas.* Washington, DC: Pan American Health Organization.

Parola, P., Paddock, C. D., Socolovschi, C., et al. (2013). Update on tick-borne rickettsioses around the world: a geographic approach. *Clin Microbiol Rev*, 26, 657–702.

Piesman, J., Mather, T. N., Sinsky, R. J., & Spielman, A. (1987). Duration of tick attachment and *Borrelia burgdorferi* transmission. *J Clin Microbiol*, 25, 557–8.

Reisen, W. K. (2010). Landscape epidemiology of vector-borne diseases. *Ann Rev Entomol*, 55, 461–83.

Reiter, P., Lathrop, S., Bunning, M., et al. (2003). Texas lifestyle limits transmission of dengue virus. *Emerg Infect Dis*, 9, 86–9.

Simeone, R. M., Shapiro-Mendoza, C. K., Meaney-Delman, D., et al. (2016). Possible Zika virus infection among pregnant women—United States and territories, May 2016. *MMWR Morb Mortal Wkly Rep*, 65, 514–19.

Vasconcelos P. F. & Calisher C. H. (2016). Emergence of human arboviral diseases in the Americas, 2000–2016. *Vector-Borne Zoonotic Dis*, 16, 295–301.

World Health Organization (WHO) (2014). *A global brief on vector-borne diseases.* Geneva, Switzerland: World Health Organization.

World Health Organization (WHO) (2015a). *Investing to overcome the global impact of neglected tropical diseases: third WHO report on neglected tropical diseases.* Geneva, Switzerland: World Health Organization.

World Health Organization (WHO) (2015b). *World Malaria Report 2015.* Geneva, Switzerland: World Health Organization.

CHAPTER 7.3

The health impact of natural disasters

Eric K. Noji, Anas A. Khan, and Osama A. Samarkandi

Natural disasters are increasing globally

Since 1960 disasters have killed approximately five million people worldwide and injured millions more (CRED, 2015). Between 2004 and 2014, there were 4,130 disasters recorded, resulting from natural hazards around the world where 1,117,527 people perished and a minimum of US$ 1,195 billion was recorded in losses (CRED, 2016; Office of US Foreign Disaster Assistance, 2016). While developing countries are disproportionately affected, the Great East Japan earthquake and tsunami on March 2011 sent a clear message that developed countries are also vulnerable to such severe disasters. Unsustainable development practices, ecosystem degradation, poverty, as well as climate variability and extremes have led to an increase in both natural and manmade disaster risk at a rate that poses a threat to lives and development efforts (ADB, 2013; Maplecroft, 2016).

Key methods of reducing death and injury in disasters include the strengthening of buildings to withstand earthquakes and early warning systems to allow evacuation in the event of storms and floods. These measures have been extremely successful in reducing the public health impacts of disasters in high-income countries: The question is whether the measures that have proven effective in reducing deaths in high-income countries pass the benefit-cost test in developing countries (DIFD, 2015).

In many cases, building codes have been ignored, communities have been located in dangerous areas, warnings have not been issued or followed, or plans have been forgotten. In order to plan appropriate, immediate, and long-term measures to save lives or restore the physical and mental well-being of populations adversely impacted by natural disasters, governments and communities first need to understand the causal basis of the phenomena in question, characteristics, and predictability of the hazards and the factors that contribute to vulnerability of people and communities. See Table 7.3.1.

Epidemiology as the science of public health will form the core of this chapter's analysis of morbidity and mortality patterns in disasters, starting with the international impact of each type of disasters (including geographical distribution and variations of impacts across the spectrum, from developed to developing to the least developed countries). The nature of each hazard will then be explored in terms of what they do to people and presented in a systematic and consistent format: (i) scope and importance of the disaster type; (ii) predictability; (iii) factors contributing to morbidity, mortality; (iv) medical and public health consequences; (v) prevention, risk reduction and mitigation strategies; (vi) research methods; (vii) critical knowledge gaps; (viii) future directions; and (ix) recommendations for action to strengthen resiliency (Noji, 2001).

Sound epidemiologic knowledge of the morbidity and mortality caused by disasters is essential when determining what relief supplies, equipment, and personnel are needed to respond effectively in emergency situations (Saylor and Gordon, 1957). All disasters are unique because each affected region of the world has different social, economic, and baseline health conditions. Some similarities exist, however, among the health effects of different types of disasters. Recognition of these effects can ensure that the limited health and medical resources of the affected community are optimally managed (Segui-Gomez and MacKenzie, 2003).

Global magnitude and geographical distribution of the impact of natural disasters

More people and assets are located in areas of high risk. The proportion of the world's population living in flood-prone river basins has increased by 114%, while those living on cyclone-exposed coastlines have grown by 192% over the past 30 years. Over half of the world's large cities are currently located in areas highly vulnerable to seismic activity. Rapid urbanization will further increase exposure to disaster risk (UNISDR, 2014). Over the past half century, droughts have caused the largest number of disaster deaths, and most of these have occurred in Africa and Asia (Office of US Foreign Disaster Assistance, 2016). The importance of droughts as a cause of death has, however, been reduced over the past 20 years, due largely to international aid efforts.

Factors contributing to disaster occurrence and severity

Natural hazards such as earthquakes, hurricanes, floods, droughts, and volcanic eruptions usually spring to mind when the word 'disaster' is mentioned. Yet these events are in fact only natural agents that transform a vulnerable human condition into a disaster. The hazards themselves are not disasters, but rather are factors in causing a disaster. Particularly in the poorest, least developed countries,

Table 7.3.1 A framework for understanding natural disasters and related impacts for health and economy

Urban risks/Megacities	Societal/Political risks	Resilience & vulnerability	Health impacts & medical response	Economics of disasters
• Water & energy supply	• Public security • Terrorism	• Frameworks • Indicator	• Disaster • Epidemiology	• Cost-benefit analysis
• Land use/City planning	• Social unrest/Social cohesion	• Gender	• Public health in disasters	• Risk monitoring
• Early warning	• Displacement/Forced migration	• Marginalization	• Disaster medicine and surgery	• Risk assessment
• Emergency evacuation & shelter management	• Community empowement • Local action	• Social, cultural • Ecological, technical, institutional, & economic resitience	• Climate change health risks	• Risk modelling
• Mobility/Transportation/Critical infrastructure	• Gender	• Fragility • Robustness	• Environmental health risks	• Scenario building
	• Millennium Development Goals	• Exposure	• Humanitarian logistics	• Research & development
	• Culture & disasters	• Inequality		• Implications of the financial crisis to DRR

the following major factors contribute to disaster occurrence and severity (Kahn, 2005):

◆ Human vulnerability resulting from poverty and social inequality.

◆ Environmental degradation resulting from poor land use.

◆ Rapid population growth, especially among the poor.

◆ Global climate change, threats to biodiversity, and resulting environmental hazards.

The World Bank estimates that 95% of the deaths that are the result of natural disasters occur among 66% of the world's population that live in the poorest and least well-developed countries (Mechler, 2003). The poor are probably most at risk because they are (i) least able to afford housing that can withstand intense seismic activity; (ii) often living along coasts where tropical cyclones, storm surges, or earthquake-generated tsunamis strike or live in flood plains subject to extensive and cyclical inundation; (iii) forced by economic circumstances to live in substandard housing built on unstable slopes that are susceptible to landslides or are built next to landfill and chemical disposal sites; and (iv) not educated as to the appropriate life-saving behaviours or actions that they can take when a disaster occurs (United Nations General Assembly, 2005).

Exposure to future disasters has the greatest potential to be reduced if disaster risk management approach is incorporated in land use, urban and spatial planning, and in post-disaster reconstruction planning (ISDR, 1999). However, latest data shows that only 15% of low-income countries report success in using land use planning and urban development to reduce risk (Mechler, 2003). The underlying natural causes of disaster have not changed, but the human impact of disasters has increased as the world's population has grown and more people are exposed to these hazards (Shah, 1983). By the year 2030, 30 cities in the world will have populations greater than 10 million people; a significant number of these cities are located in areas that are at extremely high risk for natural disasters (United Nations General Assembly, 2005). Clearly,

people who live in wealthy, industrialized countries are buffered from natural disasters by their ability to (i) forecast severe storms; (ii) enforce strict codes for aseismic and fireproof construction; (iii) use communication networks to broadcast disaster warnings and alerts; (iv) provide skilled and widely available emergency medical services; and (v) engage in contingency planning to prepare the population and public institutions for possible disasters (Kahn, 2005).

Current state of knowledge and understanding of the public health impact of disasters

Over the past 50 years, the epidemiology of disasters has emerged as an area of special interest. In 1957, in one of the earliest reviews on the role of epidemiology during natural disasters, Saylor and Gordon considered disasters as epidemics and suggested using well-defined epidemiologic methods and parameters (Saylor and Gordon, 1957). Results of epidemiologic investigations have allowed us to target specific interventions to prevent specific disaster-related health effects (e.g. improved warning and evacuation before flash floods and tropical cyclones, the development of measures to avoid clean-up injuries following hurricanes and effective measles vaccination efforts, which have reduced the frequency and magnitude of measles outbreaks in refugee camps), to measure the effectiveness of disaster prevention and preparedness programmes, and to help local communities develop better emergency preparedness and mitigation programmes (Noji, 2001).

With natural, technological, and complex disasters becoming an increasing threat to the health of people in both industrialized and developing countries, schools of medicine and public health need to offer more training opportunities in the public health consequences of disasters. On the other hand, the relief agencies have accepted the role of epidemiology in disaster responses, their reliance on the crisis management approach has lessened, and rates of disaster-related morbidity and mortality have fallen (Zhai *et al.*, 2013).

Understanding what causes disaster-related deaths is important from the perspective of designing measures to reduce deaths. In earthquakes, the majority are caused by the collapse of buildings, causing crushing injuries to vital organs. Large numbers of building-related deaths are actually due to asphyxia, as a result of dust released (Armenian *et al.*,1997). Most storm deaths are due to drowning, as are flood deaths. In high-income countries, the majority of deaths associated with floods are motorists whose vehicles are swept away by flood waters. It is also true that more deaths are associated with flash floods (floods caused by extreme rainfall) than by riverine floods (Jonkman and Kelman, 2005).

Less is known about the distribution of deaths by age and gender. Noji (2001) reports that during earthquakes, people over 60 years of age, children, women, and the chronically ill are at increased risk of death compared to other population groups.

Deaths by gender vary by country and disaster type. In the United States and Europe, the death rate in floods and hurricanes is higher for men than women. However, in developing countries women often account for a higher proportion of disaster deaths than men (ADB, 2013)

Injuries after natural disasters are defined as those 'requiring medical attention'. It seems likely that injuries are under-reported, even if only severe injuries are counted (Association for the Advancement of Automotive Medicine, 1990). Epidemiological studies provide information about the nature of injuries suffered in disasters, as well as about the incidence of illness that may accompany the disruption of water and sanitation services following a disaster. The most serious injuries frequently suffered in earthquakes include crush injuries, fractures, and internal haemorrhage (Armenian *et al.*, 1997). Although disasters frequently disrupt water and sanitation services, which may lead to an increase in infectious disease, outbreaks of infectious diseases are rare following natural disasters, unless accompanied by overcrowding among the displaced population.

Evaluating the health impacts of disasters: challenges and opportunities

In disasters, the work of epidemiologists and governmental decision makers must be coordinated. It is virtually impossible for epidemiologists to be successful in a post-disaster setting if they operate on their own, since they must rely on governmental relief authorities for logistics support, and often the very ability to gain entry to a disaster site. Because the health component is only one part of the broad disaster problem and perhaps not the major one, epidemiologic studies of disasters require the contributions of people from a wide diversity of fields. They also require the expertise of people from all branches within the discipline of epidemiology (e.g. communicable disease, chronic disease, clinical epidemiology, and social epidemiology). Unfortunately, most natural disaster research has addressed the problem from the point of view of a single discipline, either that of epidemiologists, sociologists, or engineers. This lack of active collaboration between workers from different disciplines has been a major shortcoming of past research into the health effects of disasters (Global Pulse, 2012)

The following matrix (Fig. 7.3.1) is an overview of selected risk areas, important cross-cutting themes, and instruments for applicable solutions:

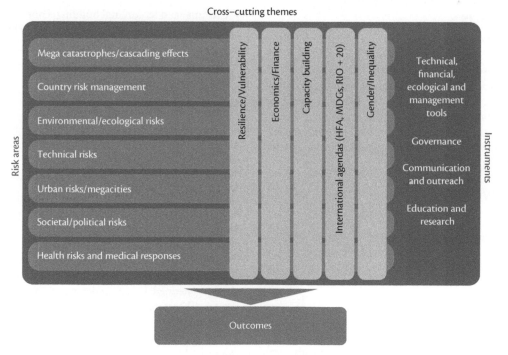

Fig. 7.3.1 Risk areas associated with natural disasters, themes cutting across the risk sectors, and instruments to approach the risks and themes. The relation between risk areas, cross-cutting themes, and instrumental approaches determines the health outcomes and other consequences of natural disasters.
Reproduced with permission from International Disaster and Risk Conference (IDRC) Davos 2012, Global Risk Forum (GRF) DAVOS, http://idrc.info.

Critical knowledge gaps

Standardized reporting methods should be developed. Unfortunately, standardized and widely accepted case definitions for disaster-related deaths or injuries do not exist. As a first step, case definitions of disaster-related diseases should be developed, agreed upon by the various agencies that are involved in relief efforts, and disseminated to the public health and emergency management communities. Case definitions must be simple and readily understandable by those who use them to ensure that the surveillance system is sufficiently sensitive at detecting the adverse health events of interest. Reporting procedures and easily modifiable standardized forms that can be used in a variety of settings should be developed. Although the emphasis in standardization here should be on flexibility and simplicity, allowance should be made for gathering sufficiently detailed information, such as the cause and circumstances of certain injuries, to guide interventions and prevention efforts.

Too often, data on the population at risk (denominator data) are not available. Without this information, epidemiologists must use other less direct measures such as proportional morbidity to estimate risk. To improve the use and interpretation of such data, public health officials should consider collecting baseline information, such as the distribution of types of illnesses and injuries at various health facilities, as a component of their preparedness activities (RIVAF, 2013). Finally, no standardized methods or indicators exist to determine rapidly the needs of disaster victims and communities. Assessment indicators and surveillance methods in disaster settings should possess all four of the attributes crucial to disaster relief activity. They should be (i) simple to use, (ii) timely, (iii) collectable under adverse field conditions, and (iv) useful.

Physical impacts of specific types of natural disasters

Populations at risk for disasters face a range of hazards within a nearly infinite set of scenarios. This unpredictability is poorly suited to scenario-based approaches to risk management (Segui-Gomez and MacKenzie, 2003). All natural disasters can markedly affect the ability of the population to maintain and access adequate shelter, water, sanitation, hygiene, healthcare, nutrition, security, public services, and utilities to maintain acceptable health during a disaster event. These factors have significant influence on morbidity following a disaster (CRED, 2015).

Geophysical events

Earthquakes

Earthquakes are among the most destructive and feared of natural hazards. They may occur at any time of year, day or night, with little warning. Within seconds, they can not only destroy entire cities but may destabilize the government, economy, and social structure of a country.

Typical adverse effects

Ground shaking can damage human settlements, buildings, and infrastructure. Aftershocks can do great damage to already weakened structures. Significant secondary effects include fires, dam failures, landslides, flooding, and tsunamis. Damage may occur to facilities that use or manufacture dangerous materials, resulting in chemical spills, and communications facilities may break down. Such destruction of property may have a serious impact on shelter needs, economic production, and living standards of community.

Depending on their level of vulnerability, many people may be homeless in the aftermath of an earthquake. Casualty rates may be even higher when quakes occur at night. In areas where houses are of lightweight construction, casualties are generally much fewer, and earthquakes may occur regularly with no serious effects on the populations (Noji, 2001).

The most widespread acute serious medical problems are bone fractures (Association for the Advancement of Automotive Medicine, 1990). Other health threats may occur with secondary flooding, when water supplies are disrupted (earthquakes can change levels in the water table).

Predictability

Earthquake warning systems currently in use warn of an earthquake that has already occurred. Examples include those that notify the high-speed trains in Japan, which if derailed would cause hundreds of deaths. One minute before the 2011 Great East Japan earthquake was felt in Tokyo, 1,000 seismometers sent out warnings that probably saved many lives. In California, it is technically feasible to develop a system that could warn Los Angeles up to a minute before the arrival of the seismic waves, allowing certain preventive actions, such as taking cover, to occur (UNISDR, 2014).

Risk reduction measures

However, because predicting the location, time, and magnitude of earthquakes is still likely many years away, warning systems and earthquake prevention measures are currently not reliable alternatives to preparedness. Preparedness actions include the following (Armenian, Melkonian, Noji and Hovanesian. 1997):

◆ Safe location of critical facilities.

◆ Creating and enforcing building codes, building earthquake-resistant structures, and retrofitting older buildings.

◆ Public education and personal adjustment to earthquake risks. Drills in schools and government buildings help to spread an attitude of preparedness.

Tsunami

Tsunami is a Japanese word meaning 'harbour wave'. Although tsunamis are sometimes called 'tidal waves', they are unrelated to the tides. The waves originate from undersea or coastal seismic activity. They ultimately encroach over land with great destructive power, often affecting distant shores.

Predictability

The majority of tsunamis occur in the Pacific Ocean, so the tsunami warning system (TWS) was developed in Hawaii shortly after the 1946 Hilo tsunami (Noji, 2001). The TWS works by monitoring activity from a network of seismic stations. A tsunami is almost always generated by an undersea earthquake of magnitude 7 or greater. Therefore, special warning alarms sound when a quake measuring 6.5 or more occurs anywhere nears the Pacific.

Lack of an effective warning system has been blamed for the extensive loss of life from the tsunami generated in the Indian Ocean in December 2004. Over 290,000 are estimated to have died in 11 countries, and tens of thousands more missing. Tsunamis have been relatively rare in the Indian Ocean, and the area has no international warning system. In Kobe, Japan, the World Conference on Disaster Reduction in January of 2005 laid the groundwork for the first TWS in the Indian Ocean. Indonesia has set up costly and sophisticated tsunami warning systems and carried out numerous drills (United Nations General Assembly, 2005). However, despite these global calls for improved tsunami warning and alert systems, 400 people were killed in an October 2011 tsunami on the Mentawai islands off the Western coast of Sumatra in Indonesia, indicating that those most at risk are not able to receive warnings through communications systems or cannot flee from a tsunami generated close to shore (RIVAF, 2013).

Vulnerability

The following major factors contribute to vulnerability to tsunamis:

◆ Growing world population urban concentration, and larger investments in infrastructure, particularly on the coastal regions, with some settlements and economic assets on low-lying coastal areas

◆ Lack of tsunami-resistant buildings and site planning

◆ Lack of a warning system or lack of sufficient education for the public to create awareness of the effects of a tsunami

◆ Unpredictable intensity

Typical adverse effects

The force of water in a bore, with pressures up to 10,000 kg/m², can raze everything in its path. The flooding from a tsunami, however, affects human settlements most. Withdrawal of the tsunami also causes significant damage.

Many people may be washed out to sea or crushed by the giant waves. Injuries occur acutely from battering by debris. Little evidence exists of tsunami flooding directly causing large-scale chronic health problems, such as malaria, contaminated water supplies, and shortage in food.

Risk reduction measures

Strategies to reduce vulnerability to tsunamis include:

◆ Warning systems: TWSs generally include a network of seismographs to determine the depth and magnitude of submarine and coastal earthquakes, tidal gauges to measure unusual rises and falls in sea level, and a network of sensors connected to floating buoys.

◆ Structural design: Improved design is needed that will allow incursion of water with minimal impact to buildings.

◆ Mapping: Tsunami run-up maps indicate the possible levels at which a tsunami can travel inland, allowing people to take precautions when they are in a potential run-up area.

◆ Education: Public education is a major lifesaver because misconceptions regarding tsunamis are likely to place people at greater risk. Lives were saved in Thailand and Indonesia in the 2004 Indian Ocean tsunami because some people recognized that the receding sea water was a warning and urged people to flee rather than stay and watch the waves (DIFD, 2015).

Volcanic eruption

A volcano is a vent to the earth's surface from a reservoir of molten rock, magma, deep in the earth's crust. Approximately 500 volcanoes are active (erupted in recorded history), and many thousands are dormant (could become active again) or extinct (not expected to erupt again). On average, about 50 volcanoes erupt every year; only about 150 are routinely monitored. Since 1000 AD, more than 300,000 people have been killed directly or indirectly by volcanic eruptions, and currently about 10% of the world's population lives on or near potentially dangerous volcanoes (CRED, 2015).

Predictability

Systematic surveillance of volcanoes, begun in the early twentieth century at the Hawaiian Volcano Observatory, indicates that most eruptions are preceded by measurable geophysical and geochemical changes. Short-term forecasts of future volcanic activity in hours or months may be made through volcano monitoring techniques (Global Pulse, 2012).

Although significant progress has been made in long-term forecasting of volcanic eruptions, monitoring techniques have not yet progressed to the point of yielding precise predictions. For the purposes of warning the public and avoiding false alarms that create distrust and chaos, ideal predictions should provide precise information concerning the place, time, type, and magnitude of the eruption.

Typical adverse effects

Deaths can be expected from pyroclastic flows, lava flows, and toxic gases. Injuries may occur from the impact of falling rock fragments and from being buried in mud. Burns to the skin, breathing passages, and lungs may result from exposure to steam and hot dust clouds. Ashfall and toxic gases may cause respiratory difficulties. Non-toxic gases of densities greater than air, such as carbon dioxide, can be dangerous when they replace normal air. Water supplies contaminated with ash may contain toxic chemicals and cause illness (Noji, 2001).

Complete destruction of everything in the path of pyroclastic or lava flows should be expected. Falling ash may be hot enough to cause fires. Communication systems could be disrupted by electrical storms developing in the ash clouds. Transportation by air, land, and sea may also be affected.

Risk reduction measures

Strengthening the forecasting of volcanic activity, creation of emergency response plans, and establishment of effective communications and warning systems are the most effective measures to reduce the risk from volcanic hazards. People may not fully accept the validity warnings because of their own perception of the likelihood of hazards and adverse effects. Even those who accept the warnings may be willing to take risks to guard their livelihoods, homes, and possessions.

Health effects due to extreme weather events

Both the direct and indirect impacts of extreme weather events can lead to impaired public health infrastructure, reduced access to healthcare services, psychological and social effects with changes in ecological systems, and human population displacement. Preparedness of a local population to extreme events is, therefore, important in affecting the disaster's impacts. Factors affecting preparedness of a local community include: exposure to natural elements, socioeconomic status, early warning capability, and cultural practices. These areas therefore are targets for mitigation efforts (Kahn, 2005).

Tropical cyclones

Tropical cyclones are the most devastating of seasonally recurring rapid-onset natural hazards. Between 80 and 100 tropical cyclones occur around the world each year. Devastation by violent winds, torrential rainfall, and accompanying phenomena, including storm surges and floods, can lead to massive community disruption. The official death and damage records for tropical cyclones include thousands of individual events.

Storm surges

The storm surge, defined as the rise in sea level above the normally predicted astronomic tide, is frequently a key or overriding factor in a tropical storm disaster.

Rainfall events

The world's highest rainfall totals over one to two days have occurred during tropical cyclones. The relationship between rainfall and wind speed is not always proportional. For instance, if the atmosphere over land is already saturated with moisture, rainfall will be strongly enhanced, and the cyclone will weaken slowly. If the atmosphere is dry, the rainfall will be greatly reduced, and the cyclone will decay faster. Thus, landfall of even a relatively weak tropical cyclone may result in extensive flooding (Jonkman and Kelman, 2005).

Predictability

Of concern is the influence that climate change might have on the frequency and severity of tropical cyclones by virtue of raising sea surface temperatures and contributing to rising sea levels. Warm sea surface temperatures influence cyclone development, and warmer ocean water will increase hurricane intensity (Maplecroft, 2016).

The locations, frequencies, and intensities of tropical cyclones are well known from historical observations and, more recently, from routine satellite monitoring. Tropical cyclones do not follow the same track, except coincidentally over short distances. Some follow linear paths, others recurve in a symmetric manner, and still others accelerate or slow down and seem stationary for a time. For this reason, predicting when, where, and if a storm will hit land is often difficult, especially with islands.

Regrettably, progress in reducing forecasting errors has remained slow in the last two decades despite huge investments in monitoring systems. However, substantial progress has been made in the organization of warning and dissemination systems, particularly through regional cooperation. The activities of national meteorological services are coordinated at the international level by the World Meteorological Organization (WMO). Unfortunately, many of the less developed countries, where most deaths from tropical cyclones occur, do not possess state-of-the-art warning systems (UNISDR, 2014).

Vulnerability

Human settlements located in exposed, low-lying coastal areas are vulnerable to the direct effects of a cyclone, such as wind, rain, and storm surges. Settlements in adjacent areas are vulnerable to floods, mud slides, or landslides from the resultant heavy rains. The death rate is higher where communications systems are poor and warning systems are inadequate and unsuitable for the building structures (Shah, 1983).

Typical adverse effects

Structures are damaged and destroyed by wind force, through collapse from pressure differentials, and by flooding, storm surge,

and landslides. Severe damage can occur to overhead power lines, bridges, embankments, non-weather-proofed buildings, and the roofs of most structures. Falling trees, wind-driven rain, and flying debris cause considerable damage.

Relatively few fatalities occur because of the high winds in cyclonic storms, but many people may be injured and require hospitalization. Storm surges may cause many deaths, but usually few injuries among survivors. Because of flooding and possible contamination of water supplies, malaria organisms and viruses may be prevalent several weeks after the flooding. Corps and food stocks may be lost or contaminated. Communication and transportation will be most likely brought down.

Risk reduction measures

The primary ways to reduce property damage from cyclones are accurate forecasting, sufficient warning, and establishment of evacuation procedures and building codes. As described earlier, significant challenges exist in forecasting the behaviour of cyclones and other severe wind storms. Another major challenge is altering the perception of people who live in coastal areas regarding the danger from cyclonic activity. People may ignore the dangers for various reasons: lack of experience in hurricanes and cyclones; insufficient understanding of the hazard; repeated false alarms; or incorrect landfall predictions that breed complacency.

Floods

Throughout history, people have been attracted to the fertile lands of the floodplains, where their lives have been made easier by proximity to sources of food and water. Ironically, the same river or stream that provides sustenance to the surrounding population also renders humans vulnerable to disaster by periodic flooding. Flooding occurs when surface water covers land that is normally dry, or when water overflows normal confinements. The most widespread of any hazard, floods can arise from abnormally heavy precipitation, dam failures, rapid snow melts, river blockages, or even burst water mains. However, floods can provide benefits without creating disaster and are necessary to maintain most river ecosystems. They replenish soil fertility, provide water for crop irrigation and fisheries, and contribute seasonal water supplies to support life in arid lands.

Flood hazard mapping supports flood management plans, land use planning, emergency evacuation plans, and increased public awareness (Zhai et al., 2013).

Predictability

Riverine flood forecasting estimates river level stage, discharge, time of occurrence, and duration of flooding, especially of peak discharge at specific points along river systems. Flooding in the catchment system, or upstream flooding is predictable from 12 hours to as much as several weeks ahead of events. Forecasts issued to the public result from regular monitoring of the river heights and rainfall observations. Flash flood warnings, however, depend solely on meteorological forecasts and knowledge of local geographic conditions. The very short lead time for development of flash floods does not permit useful monitoring of actual river levels for warning purposes (Jonkman and Kelman, 2005).

Vulnerability

Population pressure is now so great that people have accepted the risk associated with floods because of the greater need for a place to live. Urbanization contributes to urban flooding. Roads and buildings prevent infiltration of water, so run-off forms artificial streams (ISDR, 1999). Natural or artificial channels may become constricted by debris or obstructed by river facilities, impeding drainage and overflowing the catchment areas. Failure to maintain or manage drainage systems, dams, and levees in vulnerable areas also contributes to flooding. Deforestation and removal of root systems increase run-off. Subsequent erosion causes sedimentation in river channels, which decreases their capacity.

At notable risk in floodplain settlements are poor structured buildings. Infrastructural elements at particular risk include utilities, such as sewer systems, power and water supplies, and machinery and electronics belonging to industry and communications. Of great concern are lack of adequate refuge sites above flood levels and accessible routes for reaching those sites.

Typical adverse effects

Damage takes place by impact of flood waters, which is likely to be much greater in valleys than in open, low-lying areas. Flash floods often sweep away everything in their path. Mud, oil, and other pollutants carried by water are deposited and ruin crops and building contents. Saturation of soils may cause landslides or ground failure.

Currents of moving or turbulent water can knock down and drown people and animals in relatively shallow depths. Slow flooding causes relatively few direct deaths or injuries, but often increases the occurrence of snakebites. On the one hand, endemic disease will appear, but little evidence exists of floods directly causing any large-scale additional health problems besides diarrhoea, malaria, and other viral outbreaks 8 to 10 weeks after the flood (Noji, 2001). Also, normal sources of water may not be available for several days. Animals, harvest, and food stocks may be lost as well, resulting in immediate food shortages. These losses, in addition to possible loss of farm implements and seed stocks, may hinder future planting efforts; especiially when land may be rendered infertile for several years after a flood because of erosion of topsoil or salt permeation (Jonkman and Kelman, 2005).

Risk reduction measures

The major means to addressing flooding is through prevention. However, people may move to floodplains with false hopes of avoiding floods. Most dams and channels are not strong enough to withstand the heaviest water pressures and if they break down, flooding can be catastrophic. Furthermore, as levees and other physical barriers age, they become more likely to fail. European countries employ a variety of means to reduce the flood risk, such as a series of reservoirs in France called Les Grands Lacs de Seine (or Great Lakes), which help to remove pressure from the Seine during floods (during the regular winter flooding); protection from sea flooding by a huge mechanical barrier across the Thames River in London; underground canals that drain part of the flow of the Adige river in Northern Italy; and a series of flood defences in the Netherlands called the Delta Works, with the Oosterschelde dam as its crowning achievement (Guofang et al., 2013).

Since flooding may be beneficial to environmental regeneration, the challenge is to allow this while also ensuring personal and economic safety (Mechler, 2003). The concept of integrated flood management, developed by the WMO in 2004, embraces floodplain land use that does not have adverse environmental impacts (United Nations General Assembly, 2005).

Implications for policy and action

Around the world, communities are facing some of the most challenging universal trends of the twenty-first century: ageing populations coupled with non-communicable diseases, waves of pandemics, limited resources, rapid urbanization, environmental degradation, uncertainty of climate change, and poverty. The current global economic crisis, for instance, is leaving more than 100 million people in poverty every year (Mechler, 2003). At this very moment, we are yet again witnessing terrible food insecurity in the Sahel and other parts of the world. The suffering of millions of people who do not have enough to eat is a dramatic reminder that relief in the form of handouts is just not good enough. While we save lives, we must do everything we can to invest into strengthening the resilience of vulnerable people and their communities, and to contribute to eradicating the underlying causes of vulnerability. Individuals and communities facing simultaneous or repeated shocks are better supported when humanitarian action addresses the underlying vulnerabilities, and builds capacities to better respond to the medical and health needs of communities in the future (Cutter et al., 2015).

Conclusion

Resilience has been rooted in sciences and ecology, but not into medicine or public health. This must change. The term 'resilience' here means the ability of critical physical infrastructure to absorb shocks. From a more psychological point of view, it is the process of adaptation and a set of skills, capacities, behaviours, and actions in order to deal with adversity (Institute for National Security and Counterterrorism, 2009). There is a significant amount of information on what good practice is in disaster risk management and what works. There is guidance in some areas, including risk assessments with a view to eventually arriving at a common definition of disaster and risk; integration of climate change adaptation and disaster risk management; working at national and local levels; and, vulnerability of communities to the impact of hazards (Cutter et al., 2015). Attention should be given to disaster research studies that help identify solutions, and support a strategic shift in disaster risk reduction from the 'what' to the 'how' (United Nations General Assembly, 2005).

References

ADB (2013). Climate Change and Disaster Risk Management: Legislating Gender- Responsive Mitigation, Adaptation and Women's Participation. Available at: http://lib.icimod.org/record/8593 (accessed 22 October 2016) [Online].

Association for the Advancement of Automotive Medicine (1990). The Abbreviated Injury Scale 1990 Revision. Des Plaines, IL: Association for the Advancement of Automotive Medicine.

Center for Research on the Epidemiology of Disasters (CRED). (2015). Annual Disaster Statistical Review: The Numbers and Trends 2015. Brussels, Belgium: Center for Research on the Epidemiology of Disasters.

CRED (2016). EM-DAT: The International Disaster Database (CRED). Available at: http://www.emdat.be (accessed 27 October 2016) [Online].

Cutter, S. L., Ismail-Zadeh, A., Alcántara-Ayala, I., et al. (2015). Global risks: Pool knowledge to stem losses from disasters. Nature, 522, 277–9.

Department for International Development (DIFD) (2015). Natural Disaster and Disaster Risk Reduction Measures. London: United Kingdom: Department for International Development.

Global Pulse White Paper (2012). Big Data for Development: Opportunities & Challenges (May 2012). Available at: http://www.unglobalpulse.org/projects/BigDataforDevelopment [Online].

Armenian, A. K., Melkonian, A., Noji, E. K., & Hovanesian, A. P. (1997). Deaths and injuries due to the earthquake in armenia: a cohort approach. *Int J Epidemiol,* 26, 806–13.

Institute for National Security and Counterterrorism (2009). Project on Resilience and Security: Resilience in Post-Conflict Reconstruction and Natural Disasters. Workshop Report, Syracuse University, 9 March 2009.

International Strategy for Disaster Reduction (ISDR) (1999). United Nations General Assembly Resolution A/RES/54/219.

Jonkman, S. N. and Kelman, I. (2005). An analysis of the causes and circumstances of flood disaster deaths. *Disasters,* 29, 75–97.

Kahn, M. E. (2005). The death toll from natural disasters: the role of income, geography, and institutions. *Rev Econ Stat,* 87, 271–84.

Maplecroft Climate Change Risk Atlas (2016). Available at: https://maplecroft.com/ [Online].

Mechler, R. (2003). Natural disaster risk and cost-benefit analysis. In: Kreimer, A. Arnold, M., & Carlin, A. (eds) *Building Safer Cities: The Future of Disaster Risk.* Washington, DC: World Bank.

Noji EK (ed.) (2001). *The Public Health Consequences of Disasters.* Oxford, UK: Oxford University Press.

Office of US Foreign Disaster Assistance (2016). *Disaster History: Significant data on major disasters worldwide, 1900–present.* Washington, DC: Agency for International Development, November 2016.

Rapid Impact Vulnerability Analysis Fund (RIVAF) (2013). Vulnerability and Real-time Information. New York, NY: Global Pulse.

Saylor, L. F. & Gordon, J. E. (1957). The medical component of natural disasters. *Am J Med Sci,* 234, 342–62.

Segui-Gomez, M., & MacKenzie, E. J. (2003). Measuring the public health impact of injuries. *Epidemiol Rev,* 25, 3–19.

Shah, B. V. (1983). Is the environment becoming more hazardous? Global survey 1947–1980. Disasters, 7, 202–9.

UNISDR (2014). *Towards a Post-2015 Framework for Disaster Risk Reduction.* Geneva, Switzerland; ISDR (UNISDR).

United Nations General Assembly (2011). UNISDR Global Assessment Report 2011: Revealing Risk, Redefining Development. In: *Yokohama Strategy and Plan of Action for a Safer World.* General Assembly of the United Nations.

Zhai, G., Fukuzono, T., & Ikeda, S. (2013). An empirical model of efficiency analysis on flood prevention investment in Japan. *Rev Urban Reg Dev Stud,* 15, 1231–6.

CHAPTER 7.4

Risk and the perception of risk in interactions with nature

David J. Ball and Laurence N. Ball-King

Research on risk perception—some background

Risk assessment is a frequently used device for determining scientific estimates for the myriad of risks faced by humanity. However, it is now acknowledged that understanding the way that the public perceives risk may be key to answering the question: *Is this a risk that we, as a society, feel is worth taking?* The scientific estimate of the risk alone is seldom adequate for that purpose (European Commission, 2014). This realization demands knowledge of the public perception of risk. Fortunately, within the risk community, there is now a well-established body of research into how risks are perceived by the public and other stakeholders. The primary motivations for this research have been that if the stakeholders contemplating some issue have a false perception of the associated risk, then they might not act in their own best interests, the best interests of others, or of society in general. This research has implications for many activities, including the realization by the public of nature's health benefits.

One of the earliest studies of the public perception of risk was a desktop exercise by the American physicist Chauncey Starr, who sought to determine the relationship between the risk of some activity, for example, skiing, and its benefits (Starr, 1969). This research used a revealed preference approach—that is, it was conducted by examining people's actual behaviours. *Inter alia*, Starr found, as might reasonably have been anticipated, that there was a relationship between perceived risks and benefits. Thus, if the benefits of skiing were seen as high, then the associated risks were more likely to be viewed as low and hence tolerable.

Further pioneering work on the perception of risk has notably been conducted over several decades by the American psychologist Paul Slovic (2000; 2010). Part of this research utilizes an expressed preference methodology, in that members of the public are asked to rate a string of hazards and hazardous activities according to their perceived riskiness and also according to a number of other qualities such as the observability of the hazard, whether the hazard is new or old, whether the effects are immediate or delayed, and what the consequences might be. Typically, a factor analysis is then carried out on the data in order to determine if there is a lesser number of unobserved variables which accounts for the pattern of perceived riskiness.

This work, which has been replicated around the world, has generally found that there are essentially two principle factors guiding perceptions. These are commonly referred to as the 'dread' factor and the '(un)familiarity' factor. Hazards which figure high on dread and unfamiliarity are found to be more worrying and perceived as high risk. Hazards of this type typically include things like tsunamis, nuclear radiation, and pesticides. In contrast, known and personally controllable hazards, like recreational boating, swimming, cycling, mushroom hunting and the like, are regarded as low risk (Slovic, 2000).

Further research has shown that the more people are exposed to or familiar with some activity or situation, the more positive is their feeling towards it. For example, those who exercise frequently see exercise as having more positive outcomes than those who do not (Benthin *et al.*, 1995). Also increasingly recognized as important is the role of 'affect', that is, how an object or situation impacts on or feels to a person (Duncan and Barrett, 2007). Traditionally, research on how people make choices has focused upon their use of reason, and affective or emotional contributions have been disregarded since they were presumed to be in some way biased and unreliable (Peters *et al.*, 2006). However, recent research shows that affect is influential in determining people's attitudes to things and places. Thus:

' ... the relationship between perceived risk and perceived benefit was linked to an individual's general affective evaluation of a hazard. If an activity was "liked," people tended to judge its risks as low and its benefits as high. If the activity was "disliked," the judgments were opposite—high risk and low benefit'.

Text extracts from Finucane M et al., 'The affect heuristic in judgments of risks and benefits,' *Journal of Behavioral Decision Making*, Volume 13, Issue 1, pp. 1–17, Copyright © 2000 John Wiley & Sons, Ltd., reproduced with permission from John Wiley & Sons, Ltd.

Implications for engagement with nature

This body of research, although itself not focused on hazards of the natural world, suggests that as people have become more urbanized, motorized, and computerized, and their familiarity with nature has declined, in turn there will have been a shift in their perception of the natural environment and its associated riskiness. Evidence of this shift can be found in various places, some anecdotal, and some based on research. Marc Bekoff, for example, has reported that United States park rangers have observed a growing fear of nature among both children and adults (Bekoff, 2014). Bekoff quotes Judy Molland as follows: 'Rangers at National Wildlife Refuges are discovering a new phenomenon this summer: young visitors are often scared of nature, whether it's creepy crawlies, spiders, bats, snakes or sometimes even ladybugs and fish' (Molland, 2014).

This sentiment is entirely consistent with views expressed by Richard Louv in his seminal work *Last Child in the Woods*, in which he identifies the syndrome of 'nature deficit disorder' (Louv, 2005). According to this theory, while children may have academic knowledge of threats to the global environment, they no longer have personal experience of close association with nature.

Arguably, it is these early years' experiences which are most influential in determining lifelong attitudes to nature. Yet it has been known for some decades that children's freedom to move around independently has been sharply declining. An early study by Hillman *et al.* (1990) showed how, in England, the catchment area over which children could roam had become much more constrained, the primary culprit being the way in which private motor vehicles were used. Recent research by the Policy Studies Institute (2013) shows this trend to have continued to the present day and across the sixteen countries surveyed low levels of children's independent mobility were found to be common, with significant restrictions placed on the independent mobility of children across all the ages studied (7- to 15-year-olds). Countries with the lowest aggregate rank scores of children's independent mobility were, in order: France, Israel, Sri Lanka, Brazil, Ireland, Australia, Portugal and Italy (tied), and South Africa.

Impediments to realizing the benefits of nature

If anything is clear, it is that there are multiple factors responsible for what amounts to a withdrawal from encounters with nature. So far as children are concerned, a recent literature review concludes that 'Children's independent mobility is a complex phenomenon which results from a combination of factors including: children's capabilities and desires, the physical and social environment they live and move around in and parental perceptions of these factors' (Shaw *et al.*, 2013). Specific factors identified include fear of strangers, bullying, getting lost, abduction, dogs, and a parental belief that children should not be out alone. Indeed, this research found that most children felt safe in their neighbourhood and, rather, it was their parents who were the source of restrictions on children's mobility.

Although parents regularly get the blame for this situation, it would be wrong to think that other stakeholders are not implicated. For example, in 2007, Scotland's Commissioner for Children and Young People (SCCYP) published a document entitled 'Playing safe: A report on outdoor activities for looked-after children' (McGuinness *et al.*, 2007). This report noted that children and young people were missing out on a range of normal outdoor activities because their carers were afraid of being sued or blamed if an accident occurred while playing in a park or field, riding a bike, or taking trips to the beach or countryside. The Commissioner has since reiterated these concerns (SCCYP, 2010). Likewise, a recent German study of children's freedom to play without adult intrusion or oversight, considered important for developmental reasons, has identified significant differences between Germany and the United Kingdom which again points to the presence of complex and little-understood societal influences (Blinkert *et al.*, 2015).

One root of these concerns is perhaps pinpointed by Gavin Howat of the United Kingdom's Health and Safety Executive (HSE). Howat says as follows: 'There is a tendency in some sectors to take exactly the same approach to trips as they would to running a factory ... doing complicated formulaic sums rather than asking the simple question "Is the risk acceptable or unacceptable?"' (SCCYP, 2010).

The problem revealing itself here is one of competing worldviews originating from different stakeholder groups. On the one hand, there has in recent years been a major push by advocates of injury prevention, accidental and intentional, to reduce injuries, and this has resulted in the implementation of numerous safety measures, some including restrictions on the activities in which people engage. Although originally focused on workplaces, this movement has spread to encompass public life in general (Ball and Ball-King, 2011; 2013). The consequence of this has, at times, been that factory-originated procedures and restrictions have been applied across the public realm including to forests, parks, watery places, and the countryside in general. As stated in SCCYP (2010), where guidance on outdoor activities exists, it can be complicated, bureaucratic, and often based on generic guidance inappropriate for the circumstances. Many of the procedures work on the assumption of the worst possible scenario (i.e. prevention of a fatal accident). In many cases, the procedures enacted are disproportionate to the risk, but another perhaps more important issue is that they ignore the benefits, including health benefits, of a freer lifestyle and, for example, of engagement with nature.

Such situations are not unusual. They also existed in relation to, for example, the public health consequences of exposure to sunlight. As described by Mead (2008), public health messages for many years focused on the downside of sunlight exposure to the neglect of the health benefits. This was not because message formulators did not care, but because the need for a balanced approach and the inevitability of trade-offs between, for example, safety and health, went unrecognized as it has in many other contexts besides (e.g. Graham and Wiener, 1995; Margolis, 1996).

It is also well known that campaigners may deploy scare tactics in order to achieve their goals. This is quite evident in relation to hazardous activities like smoking, and many would argue that the use of scare tactics in those circumstances is morally justified. However, such campaigns may not be justifiable in all circumstances, for instance, where they support one stakeholder's preferences without any regard for those of others (Furedi, 1997). Thus, organizations whose vision is to *prevent* some kind of event, such as personal injury or death, or to reduce crime, may at times implement measures which prevent or deter persons from enjoying the natural environment. These campaigns may have long-lasting impacts on the public psyche—that, of course, being their intention.

The International Play Association (IPA) is concerned with the implementation of Article 31 of the Convention on the Rights of Children, which specifies the rights of children to play and have leisure. According to the IPA, children throughout the world face significant barriers in realizing their Article 31 rights. These include a lack of recognition for the importance of play and leisure. This can be readily observed in the way in which some educational institutions curtail playtime in an attempt to enhance educational attainment. Other factors identified by the IPA and other researchers include: resistance to children's use of public spaces; lack of access to nature; overly programmed and structured schedules; the growing influence of an electronic culture; and the marketing and commercialization of play (IPA, 2014; Valentine and McKendrick, 1997; McKendrick, 1999).

The problem of getting people outdoors and back to nature

A popular solution to influencing the public has been anchored in the premise that the problem resides in the fact that the public are ignorant and do not understand that the risks posed by, for example, nature, are really very small. The resulting solution, if you subscribe to this worldview, is that it is simply a matter of supplying data on, say, the statistical level of risk. However, research over several decades has shown that while provision of information of this kind may contribute something to a solution, it is of itself an inadequate lever for bringing about change. As long ago as 1995, Fischhoff identified eight developmental stages through which would-be risk managers had passed in attempting to influence public behaviours:

- all we have to do is get the numbers right
- all we have to do is tell them the numbers
- all we have to do is explain what the numbers mean
- all we have to do is show them that they've accepted similar risks in the past
- all we have to do is show them that it's a good deal for them
- all we have to do is treat them nice
- all we have to do is make them partners
- all of the above.

> Text extracts from Fischhoff, B, 'Risk perception and communication unplugged: twenty years of process,' *Risk Analysis*, Volume 15, Issue 2, pp. 137–145, Copyright © 1995 Society for Risk Analysis, reproduced with permission from John Wiley & Sons, Ltd.

The modern-day view is very much located at the lower, more recent end of this progression—it's about engagement and participatory decision-making as opposed to simple provision of information. The justification for this view is that lay risk perceptions, or what is interpreted as them, may be judged unfairly, leading professionals to be unduly critical of laypeople's decision-making capabilities. Further, it is now appreciated that only by understanding the decisions that individuals face can health research produce the information that people need.

Compounding the problem is that many of the hurdles to closer engagement with nature have arisen from policy choices in other sectors, such as housing, policing, the legal system, transportation, health and safety, and so on, not from an intention to bring that about, but as an unintended consequence. The realization is dawning, however, that the world we live in is an interconnected one of trade-offs and that the optimum position for humanity is invariably one of compromise and not of the single-minded pursuance of any one goal such as, for example, public safety from injury or crime, exposure to ultraviolet light or poisonous plants, or reducing the incidence of concussion.

Children and young people

Arguably, appreciation of nature is best acquired when young (Gill, 2014). Apart from education and thoughtfully orchestrated and holistic campaigns, along with information on the comparatively small risks related to nature engagement as compared to potential benefits, it is necessary to provide practical experience by reintroducing contact with nature early in children's lives. This is most likely to have a longer-term impact as it would help create familiarity with natural environments and individuals who are able to identify themselves with nature.

Two opportunities, at least, present themselves for tackling the situation of reintroducing children to nature. One is by modification of the grounds of educational establishments, and the other by altering the style of children's publicly provided play spaces. Movements are already underway to bring this about, although they still have much scope for enhancement.

Figure 7.4.1, for example, shows a playground at a Royal Society for Protection of Birds (RSPB) location in Conwy, North Wales. Although aimed at young children, the site also draws in parents by default: 'With some activities, e.g. pond dipping, where the children are fishing for small creatures in our pond, we do find that adults who at first appear to show no interest, may also become caught up by the children's excitement and wonder such that by the end we sometimes have to wrest the nets out of dad's hands so junior can have a go. Likewise, a mum with two small children became so absorbed by den building (she had never done it before) that she spent about an hour perfecting her little palace while the children had actually wandered back to the climbing frame' (Stretton, personal communication, 2014).

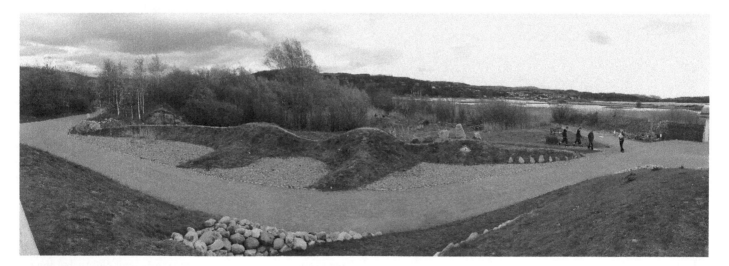

Fig. 7.4.1 Tegi the dragon at the RSPB location in Conwy.
Image reproduced courtesy of Claire Windsor.

The RSPB's initiative in Conwy is part of a broader initiative by the organization, grounded in an overall research-based policy working towards reengaging children with nature (RSPB, 2013). It is important to note that this initiative is consistent with and supported by policy initiatives at the national level emanating from other agencies concerned with children's play opportunities. Thus, the play agencies of the four nations of the United Kingdom (Play England, PlayBoard Northern Ireland, Play Scotland and Play Wales) have originated 'Design for play: a guide for creating successful play spaces', which gives much greater emphasis to the use of natural settings and materials over now traditionally conceived play space designs which are dominated by artificial, fabricated structures such as swings and climbing frames mounted on synthetic surfaces (Shackell *et al.*, 2008). See also Chapter 6.1 'Children and nature' on the value of early nature experiences for children and programmes developed for reacquainting children with outdoor natural environments.

One difficulty which the natural play movement sometimes attracts is parental resistance—parents having become accustomed perhaps to traditional play structures with their associations of 'safety', and that children will return home as clean as when they went out. One way of dealing with this, which some play providers have deployed, is to introduce nature-based play opportunities alongside traditional playgrounds so that children, and their carers, can observe the offer and think about it.

An alternative strategy is to introduce nature via an educational environment. There is a spectrum of approaches for doing this as also described in Chapter 6.1. An obvious one is by the greening of school grounds (Learning through Landscapes, 2014). Reference to children often conjures up images of the under-tens. Older children, especially teenagers, also need to be catered for and they may well wish to have more personal control over any space available to them. Britain's National Trust is one of a number of organizations which positively encourages young people to get back into nature and one route to this is via den building (National Trust, 2014). In other situations where young people have been able to commandeer a piece of derelict land for a time, they have been able to develop their own natural place. Figure 7.4.2 shows one example

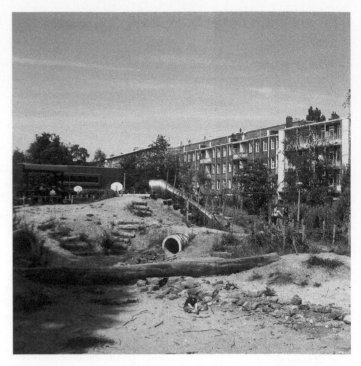

Fig. 7.4.3 In the city—space to grow.
Image reproduced courtesy of Sigrun Lobst.

whereby local teenagers have created a skateboarding facility on wasteland, entirely by their own endeavours.

City dwellers

We live in an urbanized world. If a generation of city dwellers has lost its links with nature, then an obvious remedy is to take nature to them in order to reconnect and achieve a better balanced view of risks and benefits of nature. Figures 7.4.3 and 7.4.4 show one pioneering attempt to do this within an urban area. The task is, of course, huge. It is only dwarfed by the opportunity.

Thankfully there are already many agencies now committed to this challenge all around the globe. For example, The European Green City Index is worthy of comment (EIU, 2009). This index rates cities against a number of criteria from which it generates a measure of achievement. The index is fashioned around considerations of 30 individual indicators per city, touching on a wide range of environmental matters, from environmental governance and water consumption, to waste management and greenhouse gas emissions. Greenness in terms of nature is a fairly weak contributor to overall ranking and enters directly into the equation only through environmental governance. This leads us to think that even those keen on greening may not always have grasped the full significance of the role nature could play if more strongly interwoven into the urban environment. By increasing this recognition, we may help restore a more balanced appreciation of the benefits and risks of the natural world.

Conclusion

Investigators of the perception of risk have afforded relatively little time to consideration of how people feel about nature, but the evidence suggests that over recent decades some measure of contact

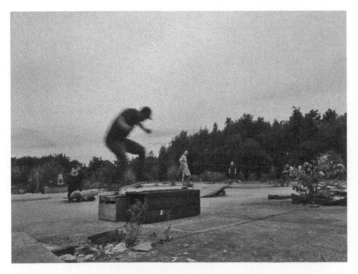

Fig. 7.4.2 Derelict land commandeered by teenagers and turned into a skate facility.
Image reproduced courtesy of Kieran Harrington-Ball.

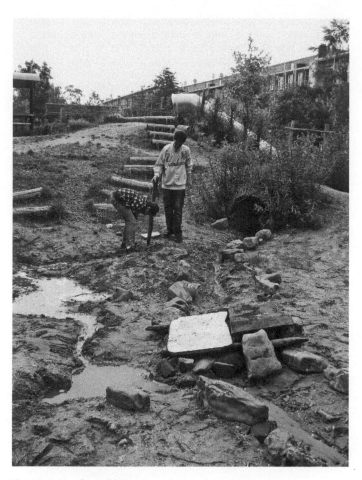

Fig. 7.4.4 An urban wild place.
Image reproduced courtesy of Sigrun Lobst.

has been lost, which may in turn have raised anxiety about encounters with nature through a loss of 'affect' or positivity towards natural things. As this book describes, there are substantial health and social welfare reasons for refamiliarizing the public with nature and counteracting the affective detriment, and the question is how this can best be achieved.

A traditionalist view might be that it is merely a matter of communicating to the lay public the imbalance between the risk perception of interacting with nature on the one hand, and the health benefits on the other. While there is something in this, it alone is unlikely to generate much change. A more fundamental issue is that society has in the past half century fragmented into a multitude of professions, each with its own priorities. This has at times created inadvertent conflict—one person's policy initiatives may trample on or subvert another's.

A simple example is, as Bekoff (2014) has suggested: 'One place to start is with the park rangers. Kids are no longer allowed to climb trees, throw rocks into the creek, or collect pine cones, all very natural, normal kid behavior. When the outdoors become a museum where nothing can be touched, you are going to see people become detached from nature. A lot of parents would love to get their kids more into nature, but it's disappearing, and what is there you aren't allowed to touch.'

While this is no doubt true, park rangers are only part of a much larger social system and in many ways are victims of it. Changes

at that level need to be tackled through lead agencies adopting appropriate policies which may then be, in time, assimilated by the professions who have the capability to bring the policies into being. Other professions with a role to play are widespread, ranging from architecture through urban design, highways, landscape architecture, water resource management, horticulture, arboriculture, and not forgetting safety and security, which have sometimes had a negative impact on exposure to nature and which may need to adjust their positions.

Acknowledgements

Text extracts from Finucane, M. *et al.*, 'The affect heuristic in judgments of risks and benefits', *Journal of Behavioral Decision Making*, Volume 13, Issue 1, pp. 1–17, Copyright © 2000 John Wiley & Sons, Ltd., reproduced with permission from John Wiley & Sons, Ltd.

Text extracts from Fischhoff, B., 'Risk perception and communication unplugged: twenty years of process', *Risk Analysis*, Volume 15, Issue 2, pp. 137–145, Copyright © 1995 Society for Risk Analysis, reproduced with permission from John Wiley & Sons, Ltd.

References

Ball, D. J. & Ball-King, L. (2011). *Public Safety and Risk Assessment: Improving Decision Making*. London/New York: Earthscan.

Ball, D. J. & Ball-King, L. (2013). Safety management and public spaces: restoring balance. *Risk Analysis*, 33, 763–71.

Bekoff, M. (2014). Who's afraid of "Big bad nature"? Far too many kids. *Psychology Today*. Available at: http://www.psychologytoday.com/blog/animal-emotions/201407/whos-afraid-big-bad-nature-far-too-many-kids (accessed 14 December 2014) [Online].

Benthin, A., Slovic, P., Moran, P., Stevenson, H., Mertz, C. K., & Gerrard, M. (1995). Adolescent health-threatening and health-enhancing behaviours. *J. Adolescent Health*, 17, 143–52.

Blinkert, B., Höfflin, P., Schmider, A., & Spiegel, J. (2015). *Raum für Kinderspiel!* Berlin, Germany: Lit Verlag.

Duncan, S. & Barrett, L. F. (2007). Affect is a form of cognition: a neurobiological analysis. *Cogn Emot*, 21, 1184–211.

Economist Intelligence Unit (EIU) (2009). *European green city index*. Available at: http://www.foresteducation.org/ (accessed 14 December 2014) [Online].

England Marketing (2009). *On childhood and nature: a survey of changing relationships with nature across generations*. London: Natural England. Available at: http://publications.naturalengland.org.uk/category/2437119 (accessed 14 December 2014) [Online].

European Commission (2014). *Future brief: Public risk perception and environmental policy*. Issue 8. Available at: http://ec.europa.eu/environment/integration/research/newsalert/pdf/public_risk_perception_environmental_policy_FB8_en.pdf (accessed 14 December 2014)

Finucane, M., Alhakami, A., Slovic, P., & Johnson, S. M. (2000). The affect heuristic in judgments of risks and benefits. *Journal of Behavioral Decision Making*, 13, 1–17.

Fischhoff, B. (1995). Risk perception and communication unplugged: twenty years of process. *Risk Analysis*, 15, 137–45.

Furedi, F. (1997). *Culture of Fear*. London, UK: Continuum.

Gill, T. (2014). The benefits of children's enjoyment with nature: a systematic review. *Children Youth and Environments*, 24, 10–34.

Graham, J. D. & Wiener, J. B. (1995). *Risk Versus Risk: Tradeoffs in Protecting Health and the Environment*. Boston, MA: Harvard University Press.

Hillman, M., Adams, J., & Whitelegg, J. (1990). *One False Move: A Study of Children's Independent Mobility*. London, UK: Policy Studies Institute.

International Play Association (IPA) (2014). Summary of UN General Comment No. 17. Available at: http://www.ipausa.org/pdf/IPASummaryofUNGCarticle31_FINAL.pdf (accessed 11 May 2016) [Online].

Learning through Landscapes (LtL) (2014). *Transforming Childhood*. Available at: http://www.ltl.org.uk/childhood/nature.php (accessed 14 December 2014) [Online].

Louv, R. (2005). *Last Child in the Woods*. London, UK: Atlantic Books.

Margolis, H. (1996). *Dealing With Risk: Why the Public and the Experts Disagree on Environmental Issues*. Chicago, IL: University of Chicago Press.

McGuinness, L., Stevens, L., & Milligan, I. (2007). *Playing It Safe? A study of the regulation of outdoor play for children and young people in residential care*. Available at: http://www.sccyp.org.uk/uploaded_docs/adult%20reports/playing%20it%20safe_sccyp%20200711.pdf (accessed 14 December 2014) [Online].

McKendrick, J. H. (1999). Not just a playground. Rethinking children's place in the built environment. *Built Environment*, 25, 5–10.

Mead, N. M. (2008). Benefits of sunlight: a bright spot for human health. *Environ Health Perspect*, 116, A160–7 and 116, A197.

Molland, J. (2014). *Why are kids afraid of nature?* Available at: http://www.care2.com/causes/why-are-kids-afraid-of-nature.html (accessed 13 December 2014) [Online].

National Trust (2014). *Family activities*. Available at: http://www.nationaltrust.org.uk/article-1355780491372/ (accessed 13 December 2014) [Online].

Peters, E., Västjall, D., Gärling, T., & Slovic, P. (2006). Affect and decision making: a "hot" topic. *Journal of Behavioral Decision Making*, 19, 79–85.

Policy Studies Institute (2013). *Children's Independent Mobility in England and Germany*, 1971–2010. Available at: http://www.psi.org.uk/site/news_article/851 (accessed 14 December 2014).

Royal Society for Protection of Birds (RSPB) (2013). *Connecting with nature*. Available at: http://www.rspb.org.uk/Images/connecting-with-nature_tcm9-354603.pdf (accessed 13 December 2014) [Online].

SCCYP (2010). *Go outdoors!: Guidance and good practice on encouraging outdoor activities in residential care*. Published by Scotland's Commissioner for Children and Young People (SCCYP) & Scottish Institute for Residential Child Care (SIRCC). Available at: http://www.playscotland.org/wp-content/uploads/assets/Go-Outdoors.pdf (accessed 14 December 2014) [Online].

Shackell, A., Butler, N., Doyle, P., & Ball, D. J. (2008). *Design for play: a guide to creating successful play spaces*. London, UK: Play England. Available at: http://www.playengland.org.uk/media/70684/design-for-play.pdf (accessed 12 December 2014) [Online].

Shaw, B., Watson, B., Frauendienst, B., Redecker, A., Jones, T., & Hillman, M. (2013). *Children's independent mobility: a comparative study in England and Germany (1971–2010)*. London, UK: Policy Studies Institute.

Slovic, P. (2000). *The Perception of Risk*. London, UK: Earthscan.

Slovic, P. (2010). *The Feeling of Risk*. Abingdon, UK: Earthscan.

Starr, C. (1969). Social benefits versus technological risk: what is our society willing to pay for safety? *Science*, 165, 232–8.

Valentine, G. & McKendrick, J. (1997). Children's outdoor play: exploring parental concerns about children's safety and the changing nature of childhood. *Geoforum*, 28, 219–237.

CHAPTER 7.5

Population health deficits due to biodiversity loss, climate change, and other environmental degradation

Anthony J. McMichael[†]

The anthropogenic era and related health risks

Humankind faces mounting risks to health and life from a range of human-driven large-scale, often global, environmental disruptions. This is a historically unprecedented circumstance that now confronts societies around the world. On many fronts the sheer weight of human pressure, due to the combination of total numbers and the intensity of industrial and agricultural activity, is perturbing, overloading, or depleting parts of Earth's operating system, the 'Earth system'. Human populations have little experience and familiarity with this category of environmental health hazard, global in span and type, and largely mediated by disruptive changes to the natural world.

The modern public health sciences, especially epidemiology (the study of the distribution, determinants, and prevention of states of poor health in populations), have not, apart from environmental epidemiologists, been particularly interested in the influences of 'the environment' on human health. Environmental exposures lack the stability, clarity, and immediate social interest that attach to individual-level 'risk factors', such as smoking, dietary choices, alcohol consumption, sexual practices and, now, variant genes. Those all fall comfortably within the purview of the health sector and the social and behavioural sciences, and all hold promise of effective intervention at the individual or family levels. Not so the more pervasive environmental exposures and, besides, the pressures of running healthcare systems, along with a general unawareness of the fundamental influence of environmental conditions and processes on health, which lead to a reflex assumption that climate change, biodiversity loss, stratospheric ozone depletion, environmental nitrification, and so on are the province of the environmental sector.

This group of changes to biogeophysical processes and ecosystems is the outward manifestation of a *syndrome* of planetary overload by the global human population (McMichael, 1993). Each of the changes poses diverse risks to human prosperity, security, health, and longevity, and to the cohesion and viability of societies.

And yet the currently prevailing, culturally-embedded, models of 'health and disease' do not extend to understanding the long-term foundations, the natural environmental life-supports, of human health. Hence we have little familiarity with the spectrum of risks to human population health from these systemic changes to the Earth's operating system, let alone the magnitude and form those risks might assume in future if our collective energy-intensive economic activities cause the natural world to deteriorate further.

Gaining that understanding is bedevilled by the complexities and uncertainties of assessing a type of outcome, human health, located at the end of an often long causal chain, or web. Glaciologists can measure the rate of sea-ice loss, fully confident that it is due to warming (Marzeion *et al.*, 2014), and they can use that knowledge base to estimate future trajectories of ice melting under specified warming scenarios. Agricultural scientists can measure the impacts on crop yield of various environmental stressors and deficits—warming, drying, nitrogen depletion, decline in pollinating species, and so on. But it is much less easy to carry the immediate consequences of these 'upstream' biological, ecological, or biophysical impacts through to estimating, for example, how losses of sea-ice around the Canadian Arctic coast or how losses of pollinators, both of which jeopardize food yields, influence the incidence of childhood undernutrition and physical and mental stunting.

Those two examples point to a main focus of interest of this chapter: How do disruptions of ecosystems and losses of species and local populations of species affect human biological and psychological functioning, the advent and progression of disease processes, and measurable health outcomes—deaths, hospitalization, disabling injuries, and serious mental health disorders? Human-driven climate change is hydra-headed in its impacts, often impinging on health by direct insult (heatwaves, intensified weather disasters, and exacerbated urban air pollution) and, as time passes and climate change advances, becomes increasingly likely to cause adverse health outcomes via less direct, often multistepped, and sometimes deferred (incubated) processes. These range from

[†] It is with regret we report the death of Anthony J. McMichael during the preparation of this textbook

climatic influences on mosquito populations, bacterial proliferation rates, crop yields, and freshwater flows and quality through to the miseries, risks, and tensions associated with job losses, enforced displacement of communities, and escalating resource conflict (Smith *et al.*, 2014; McMichael, 2013a).

Characterizing and quantifying present and future risks to health

The assessment of risks to human health from these systemic changes in and disruptions to the main components of the Earth system is necessarily of a qualitative or modelled semi-quantitative kind. If that frustrates public interest and the conventional needs of policy makers, it is because we carry a simplified, inadequate, model of 'science' in our heads. That mental model is the legacy of over three centuries of primarily experimental and reductionist research into specific physical and chemical relationships. The ghosts of Francis Bacon, René Descartes, Robert Hooke, and Isaac Newton still pervade our laboratories and journals' editorial offices.

Undoubtedly, we have learnt a very great deal about how basic, disaggregated, components of the tangible world, both animate and (particularly) inanimate, behave. But we have not yet come to terms with the urgent and challenging need to clarify the workings of the many natural complex dynamic systems that are the essence of Earth's life-supporting processes, and how those functions change in circumstances of great external stress. Nor have modern societies understood the attendant need to make prudent policy decisions under conditions of unavoidable imprecision and uncertainty.

Nine main components of the Earth's operating system are listed in Box 7.5.1. The three disruptive and large-scale environmental changes that are the main focus of this chapter are written in bold letters, but the reality for those three, and for the others shown, is that they very often mutually influence one another. This underscores the fact that the science appropriate to this realm must be weighted towards systems thinking and dynamic systems modelling. These relationships and their responses to external stressors cannot be understood via classical reductionist science.

The loss of biodiversity, as indicated in Figure 7.5.1, is the most 'downstream' of these three environmental changes in that climatic changes affect species loss, depletion of local populations, and species migration, while exposure to biotoxic persistent organic pollutants (POPs) such as the organochlorine pesticides like DDT—especially non-biodegradable chemical pollutants that permeate food chains—increases biodiversity losses and erodes the resilience and productivity of ecosystems. There are many other connections. For example, the loss of plant cover or algal populations reduces the removal, or biosequestration, of atmospheric CO_2, and a greenhouse-driven and more energetic climate system then transports volatile POPs more rapidly from low to high latitudes.

The (misconceived) 'environmentalist's paradox'

Indices of human health around the world have improved widely over the past half-century. Infant and child death rates have fallen steadily, and life expectancy has doubled for most low-income countries. Further, as the Global Burden of Disease Study 2010 (GBD2010) makes clear, most deaths in urbanizing populations in those countries are now caused, not by infectious diseases as in the long past, but by the rising incidence of chronic non-communicable diseases such as heart disease, stroke, cancer, and chronic lung

***

> **Box 7.5.1** The 9 main human-caused systemic environmental changes
>
> - **Climate change**: increased heat-trapping in the lower atmosphere due to rising concentrations of greenhouse gases and fine black-carbon particles.
>
> - Major changes to the global circulation of important elements: including (as separate problems) the nitrogen and phosphorus cycles.
>
> - **Accelerating biodiversity loss**, disrupting many ecosystems. Due to habitat loss, overharvesting, climate change, and pressures from infectious disease spread.
>
> - Destruction of stratospheric ozone (by industrial, mostly halogenated, chemicals), allowing more biologically damaging solar ultraviolet radiation to reach Earth's surface.
>
> - Aerosol accumulation (sulphates, dust, and so on) in the lower atmosphere: these pollutants alter the balance of incoming and outgoing radiation, affect air temperature, and influence cloud formation. This has a net cooling effect, currently masking around one-third of the potential warming effect of human-generated greenhouse gases.
>
> - Acidification of oceans (via increased uptake of the now-excess atmospheric carbon dioxide): a threat, with ocean warming, to the future productivity of marine fisheries.
>
> - Degradation and loss of arable land: over-exploitation, erosion, urban-industrial spread.
>
> - Depletion of freshwater supplies: aquifer emptying, diminished river flows (exacerbated by climate change: glacier melt, evaporation), and wetlands loss.
>
> - **Long-distance spread and accumulation in plants and animals of various persistent organic pollutants**: the initial local toxicity is a lesser problem than the subsequent poisoning and weakening of multiple species and ecosystems.

***

diseases (Murray *et al.*, 2013). Rates of diabetes, strongly associated with overweight and obesity, have recently surged in China as wealth and consumerism rise and modes of work, recreation, and travel become more sedentary. Other developing countries are likely to follow suit.

Herein lies the so-called 'environmentalist's paradox' (Lomborg, 2001). The presumed paradox issue is that human life expectancy has continued to increase *despite* the continuing increases in many forms of local and regional environmental pollution, human crowding, and the destruction of ecosystems and depletion of natural resources resulting from intensified industrial and agricultural practices. However, the question, while interesting, is actually misconceived. First, we cannot know how much better health gains would have been in the absence of environmental hazards, both chemical and biological. Second, the 'paradox' is generally framed in terms of exposures yesterday and health harm today. That is, it does not allow for the likely future adverse health consequences that have only recently been set in motion by systemic environmental disruption and impoverishment, especially those that will impinge on populations as these changes weaken the planet's life-support system.

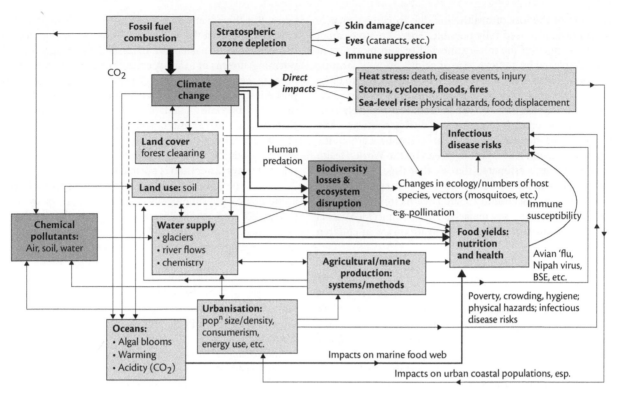

Fig. 7.5.1 Schematic representation of the many main environmental change processes and illustrative consequences that then, directly or indirectly, influence human health outcomes. The three categories of human-caused environmental change that are highlighted in this chapter are shown with darker backgrounds.
Reproduced courtesy of the author. Source: data from Ulisses Confalonieri and Anthony McMichael, (Eds.), Earth Systems Science Partnership (ESSP) Report Number 4, *Global Environmental Change and Human Health: Science Plan and Implementation Strategy*, 2006.

So, there is no real paradox (Raudsepp-Hearne *et al.*, 2010; McMichael & Butler, 2011). Instead, the environment–health relationship must be understood and assessed within a much larger socioecological frame, extending over multidecadal periods and—in particular—into the future, and thereby encompassing the consequences of large-scale *disruption* and *depletion* of crucial components of the Earth's operating system (Rockström *et al.*, 2009). Those health impacts impinge on whole communities or populations, often via circuitous and diffuse routes, and often entailing the elapse of time.

Climate change

There is, in this second decade of the twenty-first century, no serious doubt that the world's climate is changing unusually fast, nor that most of the change since mid-twentieth century has been due to human actions (Smith *et al.*, 2014). The main sources of human-generated emissions of heat-trapping greenhouse gases into the lower atmosphere, primarily carbon dioxide, have been from the burning of fossil fuels and the clearing of land, supplemented by livestock husbandry, the use of nitrogenous fertilizers, wet-rice production, and cement manufacture.

Nor is there any doubt that the consequences of changes in climatic conditions and in the variability of extremes of climate and weather that result from the higher energy levels in the circulatory systems of the lower atmosphere include serious risks to and impacts on human health (McMichael, 2013a). Some of these adverse health impacts result directly, for example, from heatwaves and thermal stress and from other weather disasters (amplified cyclones, floods, wildfires, dust storms, and others). Other impacts

arise via less direct pathways, wherein one or more aspects of climate change—warming, altered rainfall patterns, stronger winds, greater humidity, and rising sea level—affect crop yields and nutrient quality, the activity, range, and seasonality of various infectious diseases, and the flows and quality of freshwater. Even more diffuse connections occur among resource shortages, losses of livelihoods, displacement or migration, and tensions and conflict—all of which pose risks to both physical health and mental health.

At this early stage of human-driven climate change, the observable health impacts are limited in number and magnitude. Nevertheless, it is clear that heatwave-related deaths and hospitalizations have risen in many countries as warming and extremes have increased (Smith *et al.*, 2014). It is apparent from many studies around sub-Saharan Africa that cereal grain yields have been impaired and that, in many communities, nutritional sufficiency is suffering (Lobell *et al.*, 2011).

As populations grow, and if poverty and situational vulnerability persist, the adverse worldwide health toll of climate change will increase. In at least the early stages of human-driven climate change, the poor and disadvantaged will bear most of the toll of disease, injury, and deaths due to changes in climatic conditions and in weather extremes (Smith *et al.*, 2014). There will be substantial increases in the already high rates of diarrhoeal disease and cholera in disadvantaged, crowded, and unsewered communities; changes in the geographic range of malaria in much of sub-Saharan Africa; increases in undernutrition and child stunting in that continent and in South Asia; and in the vulnerability to heatwaves of countless communities with poor-quality housing in congested heat-trapping urban environments.

Quantification of the loss of healthy life due to climate change is a Herculean task, if indeed fully possible. There are no clearcut boundaries: how much of the misery, morbidity, and mortality in communities displaced by sea level rise or aridification of farming regions is attributable to the contribution of climate change to those triggering environmental conditions? The arithmetic is very difficult for relationships that differ so much from the relatively simple relationship between daily temperatures during heatwaves and daily deaths and hospitalizations (McMichael, 2013b). Early in the first decade of this century, a project overseen by the World Health Organization in Geneva estimated that, at that time, the accrued amount of climate change (surface average warming of approximately 0.5°C) was causing around 155,000 deaths from nutritional deprivation, diarrhoeal diseases, malaria, and flooding (McMichael et al., 2004). An estimated 85% of those deaths were in children below the age of five years.

That figure has recently been revised and upgraded via a project of the World Health Organization, to take account of a wider spectrum of climate-related health outcomes, and to project the likely, consequent, adverse impact on causes of death to the 2030s and 2050s. Under a base case socioeconomic scenario, the report estimates approximately 250,000 additional deaths due to climate change per year between 2030 and 2050, with a significant impact on child health and with higher rates of mortality in low- and middle-income countries (Hales et al., 2014).

Biodiversity loss

Biodiversity, spanning the multiple scales of genes, populations, species, landscapes, and biomes, is a fundamentally important resource for humanity. Indeed, biodiversity underpins and mediates many of the life-supporting processes that sustain human population health (Chivian and Bernstein, 2009). It is the prerequisite for a broad range of (so-called) 'services' provided by ecosystems.

Communities of species, within biophysical ecosystems, influence the retrieval and recycling of nutrients, the flow and quality of water (e.g. floods), the stability of infectious agents' ecology, and the impacts of climate change. For humans, biodiversity enriches well-being and is central to many cultural and other values, including recreation. Biodiversity is also crucial for food security, via processes such as pollination, pest control, and biome-level resistance to infection. Seeking synergies between biodiversity and food security holds special promise of multiple gains in human health and in social, ecological, and economic development.

Approximately nine million types of plants, animals, insects, and fungi inhabit this planet (Cardinale et al., 2012). But species, local populations, and their ecosystem communities are now disappearing unusually fast—and several thousand times faster than nature's background rate of species replacement and renewal (Pimm and Raven, 2000). Yet, on the puny timescale of an individual human life lived in one location, this ongoing loss, even if recognized, seems undramatic. This loss of biodiversity, caused particularly by habitat destruction, climate change (Parmesan and Yohe, 2003; Hannah, 2012), and the plundering of declining animal and plant stocks, has accelerated in recent centuries. Homo sapiens is causing the Sixth Extinction, that is, the sixth of the great episodes in which there was a widespread and unusually fast extinguishing of vertebrate species since the Cambrian 'explosion' around 540 million years ago. Extinction, of course, is part of life's odyssey; the average tenure of a species is around two million years. But the advent of our own species has hugely changed the equation. A rapid, human-driven, change in the world's climate this century will hasten the demise of many species. With more warming, dozens of lizard species, for example, will face extinction because their bearing of live offspring, not eggs, evolved in a cooler post-Mesozoic world. That once-successful evolutionary 'choice' may soon become maladaptive in hotter conditions (Pincheira-Donoso et al., 2013). Biological evolution cannot come to the rescue; it occurs too slowly. With the projected rates of human-driven warming, adaptive vertebrate evolution would have to occur thousands of times faster than is normal in nature (Quintero and Wiens, 2013). So, the only realistic options are for species to respond by acclimatizing physiologically or behaviourally, or by migrating to stay within a constant climatic envelope. In the Southwest United States, plants on the lower slopes have migrated several hundred metres higher over the past half-century (Brusca et al., 2013). But that option does not exist if you are already living at the coastal margin or on top of the mountain range. Many marine species are migrating towards the poles much faster than land species, which may reflect the more consistent warming signals being given by the oceans, which take up around 90% of the additional heat as the planet warms.

Approximately two-thirds of all plant foods eaten by humans require pollination. Flowering plants thus predominate in the world's food supply, and those that are not pollinated by wind require the assistance of other tiny creatures (Eilers et al., 2011). If bees, other insects, bats, and small birds go extinct, many floral species will have lost their cross-fertilizing match-makers. Pollinating and other insects also recycle nutrients and decompose organic materials, helping ensure ecosystem productivity (Dirzo et al., 2014).

Biodiversity loss has many consequences for human health, via both ecological and pharmacological paths. The depletion of major sources of staple foods, such as over-exploited fish stocks; or the commercial replacement of the many age-old potato and banana variants with just several stock species; or the declining yield of forest fruits as land is 'cleared'; all these jeopardize human nutrition and health, especially in local poorer communities. The spread of cityscapes impoverishes landscapes and creates niches for synanthropic wild species that can readily cohabit with humans. This includes bat species and their many co-evolved viruses, increasingly the cause of new and lethal epidemics in livestock and humans (McFarlane et al., 2012).

Plant and animal species are the source of many chemical compounds of medicinal, industrial, and other use. Aspirin is based on salicylates from yew bark, opiates from poppies, antimalarial quinine from the Peruvian cinchona tree, and various potent painkillers and anaesthetic agents from molluscs and sharks. Cone snail toxins are a rich source of new medicines, such as Prialt used to treat severe chronic pain not controlled by opiates.

Biodiversity, though, is much more than a count of species; it has a collective dimension. A decline in biodiversity, whether among forests, amphibians, mammals, or other groupings, can potentiate the local transmission of infectious diseases (Johnson et al., 2013; Haas et al., 2011, LoGiudice et al., 2003; Ezenwa et al., 2006). The likelihood of spread of a particular disease within, say, the one particularly susceptible species in a mixed community, is physically diluted by the presence of various non-susceptible species (Keesing et al., 2010; Ostfeld and Keesing 2012). Within the animal kingdom this may lessen the chance of a new infectious disease proliferating and then emerging from infected wildlife and being transmitted to livestock and then humans. Diversity of plant species also confers a benefit of increased productivity, including in many mixed agricultural systems, and reflecting the richer mix of micronutrients cycling in that local environment (Steudel *et al.*, 2012). For human consumers, more nutrient-rich food is thus on offer.

Biodiversity deficit can affect human biology and health in other, more subtle, ways. Research on adolescents in Finland indicates that their level of early-life exposure to bacterial biodiversity in residential, play, and learning environments influenced the development of their immune system (Hanski *et al.*, 2012). Comparisons of the range of long-term resident bacteria on each person's skin showed that the higher the level of skin-borne bacterial diversity, the less was the individual's allergic predisposition to asthma and hayfever. Other Finnish studies comparing healthy and diseased individuals show that reduced biodiversity and alterations in the composition of the gut and skin microbiota are associated with various inflammatory conditions, including asthma, allergic and inflammatory bowel diseases (IBD), type 1 diabetes, and obesity (Haahtela *et al.*, 2013). Altered indigenous microbiota and the general microbial deprivation characterizing the lifestyle of urban people in affluent countries appear to be risk factors for immune dysregulation and impaired tolerance (see Chapter 2.3 'Microbes, the immune system, and the health benefits of exposure to the natural environment' for further discussion on the importance of exposure to biodiverse environment for functional immune system development).

As scientific research clarifies the dynamic interactions within ecosystems, and the influences of cultural and socioeconomic conditions and activities, a more integrative, holistic approach to enquiry, assessment, and policymaking is emerging. This is evident, for example, in the emergence of the international EcoHealth initiative and the rejuvenation of the One Health perspective (Romanelli *et al.*, 2014). In 2012 the World Health Organization and the Convention on Biological Diversity Secretariat initiated a novel collaboration to engage both the health and biodiversity sectors in countries worldwide, in developing and applying this integrative approach—particularly in developing countries, where additional resources, experience, and scientific capacity are needed.

The domain of infectious diseases provides a good illustration. Figure 7.5.2 shows many links between environmental change and disruption, profiles of animal and plant species, patterns of contact between species, various feedback mechanisms, and the resultant changes in risks of various types and categories of infectious diseases. Clearly, achieving better surveillance and management of these infectious disease risks to humans requires the coordinated engagement of a range of research disciplines and public sectors.

One other, different, point about biodiversity and human health should also be made. Humans in most regions of the world are becoming less exposed to rural surroundings and 'wilderness' as natural landscapes have been massively transformed by urbanization, transport systems, agriculture, and forest logging. The term 'nature-deficit disorder' has been proposed by Richard Louv to describe increased rates of behavioural disorders, anxiety, and sadness in people with limited contact with 'wild' nature (Louv, 2008).

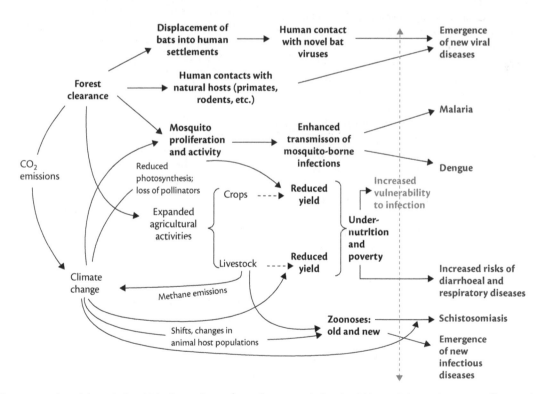

Fig. 7.5.2 Schematic representation of the paths by which climate change, forest clearance, agricultural activities, and changes in patterns of human density and mobility influence—separately and together—the risks of difference categories of infectious diseases.

Reproduced courtesy of the author. Source: data from McMichael AJ, 'Globalization, climate change and health,' *New England Journal of Medicine*, Volume 368, pp. 1335-1343, Copyright © 2013 Massachusetts Medical Society.

Toxic chemical pollutants

In 1962 American biologist Rachel Carson published *Silent Spring*, arguing that long-lasting organic pesticides like DDT were diffusing widely, bioaccumulating in food chains, and poisoning species (Carson, 1962). The reaction from the US industry, military, and government was hostile. Carson was vilified; ecology was damned as a 'subversive science'; the evidence was deemed flawed, ideologically motivated, and a threat to the economy, military technologies, corporate profits, and Cold War geopolitical dividends from bestowing chemically enhanced crop yields on poor countries.

In Western countries, concern and legislation over environmental contamination by human-generated chemical effluent and wastes peaked in the 1970s. Urban-industrial air pollution has long been a recognized health hazard, especially acting via the ozone and fine particulate components that cause increased rates of death from heart and blood vessel diseases and from chronic lung disease. Air pollutants are also implicated in exacerbating asthma and, from recent research, older-age mental decline. Meanwhile, except for acute environmental-toxin disasters such as in Japan's Minamata Bay (late 1950s) and India's Bhopal (1984), most of the rising tide of long-lasting synthetic chemicals, heavy metals, and other contaminants diffusing through the environment has been invisible. Further, the resultant ecological and health risks are not yet well understood—and hence, though not rationally, there is a widespread assumption that risks are negligible because actual exposures are presumably low.

That reasoning, inherently spurious anyway, misses the larger point that the adverse impacts are not all due to direct toxicity. The current concern about the decline of bee populations, as pollinators, underscores that point.

Two-thirds of the crops that make up the human diet, along with most wild plant species, depend on pollination by insects such as bees and hover-flies. This 'freely provided' ecosystem activity, however, is faltering. For example, after three thousand years of sustainable agriculture, farmers in Sichuan province, China, have recently had to pollinate apple flowers themselves with pollination sticks capped with chicken feathers and cigarette filters.

Many species of plant pollinators in Europe and North America are apparently in decline, both in number and geographic range. The explanation is uncertain, but one probable cause is the use of *neonicotinoid* insecticides, particularly as seed treatment (Godfray *et al.*, 2014; Lu *et al.*, 2014). First used in the 1990s, the use of these very effective pesticides now accounts for around one-third of the global insecticide market. Because the insecticide is taken up systemically by the growing plant, it is present in nectar and pollen that bees and other pollinating insects collect and consume. The neonicotinoids pose not only a serious risk to honeybees and other pollinators such as butterflies, but also to a diversity of other invertebrates including earthworms and to various birds.

Synthetic chemical production trends

Annual synthetic chemical production worldwide has increased 20-fold since 1960 (Cribb, 2014). Over 140,000 newly synthesized industrial and agricultural chemicals have been registered in North America, Europe, and Australia during those four decades. Testing and licensing is hard-pressed to keep up with this vast flow. Yet we have previously learnt how the persistent organochlorines such as DDT and polychlorinated biphenyls (PCBs), heavy metals (especially lead and mercury), and many volatile 'aromatic' hydrocarbons all have known toxic effects. And, today, what might be the unexpected risks from exposure to nano-pollutants, with their bioactivity most probably transformed by miniscule size?

Whereas climate change can cause floods, mobilize mosquitoes, and diminish harvests, and the resulting adverse human impacts are evident, long-lasting chemical contaminants act more covertly as they spread through air, soil, water, foods, and ecosystems. Some are benign, some are overtly toxic. Many act by insidious weakening or disruption of healthy biological functions—by affecting specific organ systems, altering hormonal profiles, switching genes on or off, and contributing to various cancerous, neurological, and behavioural changes.

A recent pan-European study concluded that the ecological risks from toxic chemicals in water sources greatly exceed previous assumptions. Overall, the World Health Organization estimates that around one-in-eight of all deaths are due to a form of chemical exposure, sometimes acute but mostly chronic exposure. This eclipses the annual death tolls from malaria, car crashes, and HIV/AIDS. Actual death, in this setting, is really just the 'tip of the iceberg'. Many persistent chemical contaminants have spread globally into polar-region ice, mountain glaciers, seals, and whales. Humans dine at nature's high table, often eating animals and fish that are high up in the bio-accumulating food-web, or eating industrially produced food that is grown, processed, and packaged in ways that impart traces of many chemical hazards.

Other tantalizing questions relating to chemical pollutant exposure warrant rigorous assessment. Foetal and perinatal biology and tiny bodily size renders very young humans vulnerable to toxic insult. So, is it mere coincidence that rising rates of cognitive impairment and child and adolescent behavioural abnormalities in recent decades have accompanied the increase in low-level environmental chemical exposures? Are the recent increases in allergic conditions, even autism, part of this picture (Shelton *et al.*, 2014)? In the absence of full 'cost-accounting' it is not possible to estimate the total burden of human organ dysfunction, clinical disease, or premature death caused by this great range of mostly low-level exposures.

In the meantime, to remedy this insidious environmental threat to human health, societies need, and need to share, both information and precautionary policies. Meanwhile, evidence-based changes can be made in growing, manufacturing, transporting, and consuming, and in disposing of chemical wastes. Most such changes should, anyway, already be on the policy and cultural agendas as part of the anticipated transition to an environmentally sustainable future.

Conclusion

Early in the industrial revolution, the energy-intensive process that has now encompassed much of the world, many of Western Europe's cities were crowded, smoke-enshrouded, squalid and rife with infectious diseases. However, during the nineteenth century the Enlightenment values of fairness and social responsibility helped to humanize the crude economic imperatives of laisser-faire production. England was the early front runner, forging policies to protect the population's health, particularly the health of the wealth-generating workforce. An environment of black smoke, filth, cesspits, and poverty, plus waves of urban epidemics was no way to keep the wheels of industrial capitalism turning. In a twist of history, today's environmental change predicament is the converse of the environmental problems faced during early industrialization. A primary objective, then, was to clean up the local environment to protect people's health and sustain the economic engine. Conversely, today's great challenge is to transform the working of the economy in order to sustain the natural environment and enhance human well-being and health.

Meanwhile, as many of the structures and activities of the natural world, the Earth system, remain under excess pressures from human actions and demands, the totality of adverse consequences for human health are mounting. But, of their nature, they are difficult to delineate separately from the consequences of other lesser perennial influences; their scope is unbounded and must include the consequences that accrue at the end of multistep causal-chain processes; and any attempt at full and precise quantification is simply not possible. Nor indeed could it be definitive, since the environmental, ecological, and associated social stressors impinging on human populations are changing over time.

Human-driven climate change is an obvious example; it is not possible to know what configuration of climatic conditions will exist, region by region, in the 2070s (for example), nor what social and economic consequences will flow from that configuration. And so we cannot know what the human health consequences will be half a century hence. We must rely on the approximating function of scenarios and modelled estimations. The health consequences of accruing losses of biodiversity and regional populations of species are even harder to imagine, let alone estimate.

Changes in public assumptions and expectations of 'science' and in institutional decision-making processes will be needed if the best available estimations from this domain of monitoring, modelling, and research are to be used in decision-making. The modes of scientific research into the dynamics of disrupted natural systems, their environmental and social consequences, and their remediation or stabilization must grow well beyond the bounds of classical, tightly comparative, quantitative science. A much greater understanding and application of systems science, and the use of dynamic systems modelling, is needed if we humans are to understand the risks we face now and in future, and the optimal ways of averting those risks.

References

Brusca, R. C., Wiens, J. F., Meyer, W. M., et al. (2013). Dramatic response to climate change in the Southwest: Robert Whittaker's 1963 Arizona Mountain plant transect revisited. *Ecol Evol*, 3, 3307–19.

Cardinale, B. J., Duffy, J. E., Gonzalez, A., et al. (2012). Biodiversity loss and its impact on humanity. *Nature*, 486, 59–67.

Carson R. (1962). *Silent Spring*. Boston, MA: Houghton Mifflin

Chivian, E. & Bernstein, A. (2009). *Sustaining Life: How Human Health Depends on Biodiversity*. New York, NY: Oxford University Press

Cribb, J. (2014). *Poisoned Planet*. Sydney, Australia: Allen and Unwin.

Dirzo, R., Young, H., Galetti, M., Ceballos, G., Isaac, N. J., & Collen, B. (2014). Defaunation in the Anthropocene. *Science*, 345, 401.

Eilers, E. J., Kremen, C., Greenleaf, S. S., Garber, A. K., & Klein, A. M. (2011). Contribution of pollinator-mediated crops to nutrients in the human food supply. *PLoS One*, 6, 6–10.

Ezenwa, V. O., Godsey, M., King, R. J., & Guptil, S. C. (2006). Avian diversity and West Nile virus: testing associations between biodiversity and infectious disease risk. *Proc Biol Sci*, 273, 109–117.

Godfray, H. C. J., Blacquière, T., Field, L. M., et al. (2014). A restatement of the natural science evidence base concerning neonicotinoid insecticides and insect pollinators. *Proc Biol Sci*, 281, pii: 20140558.

Haahtela, T., Holgate, S., Pawankar, R., et al. (2013). The biodiversity hypothesis and allergic disease: World allergy organization position statement. *World Allergy Organ J*, 6, 3.

Haas, S. E., Hooten, M. B., Rizzo, D. M., & Meentemeyer, R. K. (2011). Forest species diversity reduces disease risk in a generalist plant pathogen invasion. *Ecol Lett*, 14, 1108–16.

Hales, S., Kovats, S., Lloyd, S., & Diarmid Campbell-Lendrum, D. (2014). *Quantitative risk assessment of the effects of climate change on selected causes of death, 2030s and 2050s*. Geneva, Switzerland: World Health Organization.

Hannah, L. (2012). *Saving a Million Species: Extinction Risk from Climate Change*. Washington, DC: Island Press.

Hanski, I., von Hertzen, L., Fyhrquist, N., et al. (2012). Environmental biodiversity, human microbiota, and allergy are interrelated. *Proc Natl Acad Sci*, 109, 8334–9.

Johnson, P. T. J., Preston, T. L., Hoverman, J. T., & Richgels, K. L. D. (2013). Biodiversity decreases disease through predictable changes in host community competence. *Nature*, 494, 230–3.

Keesing, F., Belden, L. K., Daszak, P. et al. (2010). Impacts of biodiversity on the emergence and transmission of infectious diseases. *Nature*, 468, 647–52.

Lobell, D. B., Schlenker, W., Costa-Roberts, J., et al. (2011). Climate trends and global crop production since 1980. *Science*, 333, 616–20.

LoGiudice, K., Ostfeld, R. S., Schmidt, K. A., & Keesing, F. (2003). The ecology of infectious disease: Effects of host diversity and community composition on Lyme disease risk. *Proc Natl Acad Sci*, 100, 567–71.

Lomborg, B. (2001). *The Skeptical Environmentalist*. Cambridge, UK: Cambridge University Press.

Louv, R. (2008). *Last Child in the Woods*. Chapel Hill, NC: Algonquin Books.

Lu, C., Warchol, K. M., & Callahan, R. A. (2014). Sub-lethal exposure to neonicotinoids impaired honey bees winterization before proceeding to colony collapse disorder. *Bulletin of Insectology*, 67, 125–30.

Marzeion, B., Cogley, J. G., Richter, K., & Parkes, D. (2014). Attribution of global glacier mass loss to anthropogenic and natural causes. *Science*, 345, 919–21.

McFarlane, R., Sleigh, A., & McMichael, A. J. (2012). Synanthropy of wild mammals as a determinant of emerging infectious diseases in the Asian–Australasian Region. *EcoHealth*, 9, 24–35.

McMichael, A. & Butler, C. (2011). Promoting global population health while constraining the environmental footprint. *Ann Rev Public Health*, 32, 179–97.

McMichael, A. J., Campbell-Lendrum, D., Kovats, S., et al. (2004). Climate Change. In: Ezzati M, Lopez AD, Rodgers A, Mathers C (eds.) *Comparative Quantification of Health Risks: Global and Regional Burden of Disease due to Selected Major Risk Factors*, pp. 1543–1650. Geneva, Switzerland: World Health Organization.

McMichael, A. J. (1993). *Planetary Overload: Global Environmental Change and the Health of the Human Species*. Cambridge, UK: Cambridge University Press.

McMichael, A. J. (2013a). Impediments to comprehensive research on climate change and health. *Int J Environ Res Public Health*, 10, 6096–105.

McMichael, A. J. (2013b). Globalization, climate change and health. *New Engl J Med*, 368, 1335–43.

Murray, C. J. L., Vos, T., Lozano, R., et al. (2013). Disability-adjusted life years (DALYs) for 291 diseases and injuries in 21 regions, 1990–2010: a systematic analysis for the Global Burden of Disease Study 2010. *Lancet*, 380, 2197–223.

Ostfeld, R. S. & Keesing, F. (2012). Effects of host diversity on infectious disease. *Ann Rev Ecol Evol Syst*, 43, 157–82.

Parmesan, C. & Yohe, G. (2003). A globally coherent fingerprint of climate change impacts across natural systems. *Nature*, 421, 37–42.

Pimm, S. L., & Raven, P. (2000). Biodiversity: extinction by numbers. *Nature*, 403, 843–5.

Pincheira-Donoso, D., Tregenza, T., Witt, M. J., & Hodgson, D. J. (2013). The evolution of viviparity opens opportunities for a lizard radiation, but drives it into a climatic cul-de-sac. *Glob Ecol Biogeogr*, 22, 857–67.

Quintero, I. & Wiens, J. J. (2013). Rates of projected climate change dramatically exceed past rates of climatic niche evolution among vertebrate species. *Ecology Letters*, 16, 1095–103.

Raudsepp-Hearne, C., Petersen, G. D., Tengo, M., *et al.* (2010). Untangling the environmentalist's paradox: Why is human well-being increasing as ecosystem services degrade? *Bioscience*, 60, 576–89.

Rockström, J., Steffen, W., Noone, K., *et al.* (2009). A safe operating space for humanity. *Nature*, 461, 472–5.

Romanelli, C., Corvalan, C., Cooper, H. D., Manga, L., Maiero, M., & Campbell-Lendrum, D. (2014). From Manaus to Maputo: Toward a public health and biodiversity framework. *EcoHealth*, 11, 292–9.

Shelton, J. F., Geraghty, E. M., Tancredi, D. J., *et al.* (2014). Neurodevelopmental disorders and prenatal residential proximity to agricultural pesticides: The CHARGE Study. *Environ Health Perspect*, 122, 1104–9.

Smith, K. R., Woodward, A., Campbell-Lendrum, D., *et al.* (2014). Human health: impacts, adaptation and co-benefits. In: Field, C. B., Barros, V., Dokken, D., *et al.* (eds) *Climate Change 2014: Impacts, Adaptation, and Vulnerability. Volume I: Global and Sectoral Aspects. Contribution of Working Group II to the Fifth Assessment Report of the Intergovernmental Panel on Climate Change*, pp. 709–54. Cambridge UK and New York, USA: Cambridge University Press.

Steudel, B., Hector, A., Friedl, T., *et al.* (2012). Biodiversity effects on ecosystem functioning change along environmental stress gradients. *Ecology Letters*, 15, 1397–405.

SECTION 8

The nature of the city

[††]It is with regret we report the death of Stephen R. Kellert during the preparation of this textbook.

CHAPTER 8.1

The shift from natural living environments to urban: population-based and neurobiological implications for public health

Florian Lederbogen, Leila Haddad,
Andreas Meyer-Lindenberg, Danielle C. Ompad,
and Matilda van den Bosch

From the savannah to down-town

Humans have evolved from a rural to an urban species over millennia. A slow adaptation to this significant environmental change has occurred, but due to the exponentially escalating urbanization rate of the last century, humans' capacity for resilience has been challenged. From a biological system developed for a life in the bush, our current neurophysiological processes must cope with a daily environment full of so-called technostress and sedentary lifestyles. At the same time, those living in rural settings are facing increasing isolation and poverty as health services and work opportunities are centralized to urban areas. These are all factors that influence health and the arising disparities in health between cities and the countryside.

One causal factor for these health differences may be the mere change in physical environment. This provides an insight into how physical surroundings have a distinct impact on health. While the countryside may offer more natural experiences and possibly a sense of place and recreation, urban populations enjoy the benefits of, for example, easily accessible health resources, and a large cultural supply.

This chapter will present the phenomenon of urban–rural health disparities and discuss plausible explanations, including demographic and neurophysiological mechanisms.

The population-based perspective

The world reached a watershed moment in 2007, when for the first time in human history more than half of the global population was living in urban areas. As a result of migration and natural population growth, the rural population has decreased significantly from 70% of the global population in 1950, to 46% in 2014, and an estimated 34% by 2050. Globally, the average annual rate of urbanization is 0.9%. By country, the annual rates of urbanization range from 0.8% in Mayotte to 3.7% in Rwanda. (All numbers and information acquired from United Nations Department of Economic and Social Affairs, 2014.)

Urbanization is one of the most important demographic shifts of the twentieth and twenty-first centuries. The shift from rural to urban settings has implications for a variety of factors (e.g. socioeconomic and health changes) for both sending and receiving communities. One way in which we can examine the health impact of the rural to urban migration is analysis of urban–rural disparities.

In many cases, rural areas have poorer health outcomes relative to urban areas. In the United States, urban–rural health disparities have widened over the past four decades such that rural areas have higher mortality rates and lower life expectancies. Heart disease, unintentional injuries, chronic obstructive pulmonary disorder, lung cancer, stroke, suicide, and diabetes contributed the most to the increasing urban–rural disparity, higher rural mortality rates, and lower life expectancies (Singh and Siahpush, 2014a; Singh and Siahpush, 2014b).

However, in some countries and for some health outcomes, urban areas have poorer health outcomes on average. In the United States, youth in urban areas have higher homicide and HIV/AIDS mortality rates relative to their rural counterparts (Singh et al., 2013). Among Abuja natives in Nigeria, overweight, obesity, and hypertension were significantly higher among urban residents as compared to rural residents (Adediran et al., 2013). Mental disorders, like depression and schizophrenia, also show a higher prevalence in cities (Peen et al., 2010). These seemingly contradictory trends reflect, in part, regions at different stages of development, globalization, and the epidemiologic transition (Dagenais et al., 2016; Young et al., 2009).

We will use China and also India as case studies for exemplifying the health influence of urbanization. According to the World Urbanization Report, 'China and India will contribute more than one third of the global urban population increase between 2014 and 2050. ... Between 2014 and 2050, the urban areas are expected to grow by 404 million people in India [and] 292 million in China ... ' (United Nations Department of Economic and Social Affairs, 2014). Thus, these countries are important settings to monitor for urban–rural health disparities because they have large populations and are in the midst of substantial shifts of residents from rural to urban settings, exemplifying how the burden of disease can change by rapid environmental dislocation. In addition, many other settings have noted urban–rural differences, but have not focused on the urban environment as a possible explanation for these differences.

Diabetes is used to explore the shift from natural living environments to urban, as diabetes is a typical disease that is influenced by changes in the human ecology and living environment.

Urban–rural health disparities in diabetes

China

Over the past three decades, China has undergone rapid urbanization and economic growth. In 1980, about 20% of the population was living in urban areas, by 2010 the urban population increased to almost 50% (United Nations Department of Economic and Social Affairs, 2014). By 2050, the United Nations estimates that 76% of China's residents will be living in urban areas (United Nations Department of Economic and Social Affairs, 2014). Meanwhile, the Chinese gross domestic product (GDP) per capita (current US$) increased more than 30-fold from 1980 to 2012 (World Bank, 2014). These demographic and economic factors have been identified as key macro determinants of health in China—particularly for non-communicable diseases (Popkin et al., 2001; Tang et al., 2008; Blumenthal and Hsiao, 2005).

The prevalence of diabetes in China has dramatically increased over the past two decades, from less than 1% in the early 1980s to upwards of 3–12% in the 2010s (Yang et al., 2010; Zhang et al., 2012; Xu et al., 2013; Li et al., 2013; Pan et al., 2010; Liu et al., 2011). Urban residents generally have higher prevalence of diabetes relative to their rural counterparts (Pan et al., 2010). One analysis of the 2009 China Health and Nutrition Study examined the relation between levels of urbanization and diabetes and found a significant dose-response-type association among both men and women (Attard et al., 2012).

India

Over the past three decades, India has also undergone rapid urbanization. In 1980, 23% of the population was living in urban areas and by 2050, the United Nations estimates that this figure will rise to 50% (United Nations Department of Economic and Social Affairs, 2014). Meanwhile, the Indian GDP per capita (current US$) increased almost 6-fold from 1980 to 2012 (World Bank, 2014). Urbanization has been identified as a key macro determinant of diabetes in India.

In India, there are also significant urban–rural differentials in diabetes prevalence. Moreover, diabetes burden is expected to substantially increase in the next two decades, with 32 million people living with diabetes in 2000 projected to increase to 80 million people in 2030 (Wild et al., 2004). As in China, urban residents in many Indian settings generally have higher prevalence of diabetes relative to their rural counterparts (Anjana et al., 2011; Mohan et al., 2008).

Explanatory hypotheses and findings on urban–rural health disparities in diabetes in China and India

The transition from rural to urban living in China and India has been accompanied by changes in diet and physical activity that have resulted in increases in the prevalence of both overweight and obesity (Liu et al., 2011; Gao et al., 2009; Dong et al., 2005; Ebrahim et al., 2010; Shetty, 2012). Changes in diet are related to economic prosperity, which has resulted in increased caloric consumption as well as increases in fat and sugar intake (Alcorn and Ouyang, 2012; Popkin, 1999). This has been seen in other urbanizing low- or middle-income countries such as Nigeria (Balogun and Gureje, 2013), where more affluent individuals in urban areas have higher odds or risk of diabetes.

The links between urbanization, occupation, and physical activity have also been implicated. The transition from rural to urban living has been accompanied by a transition from agricultural, manual labour to more sedentary employment (Attard et al., 2012) particularly for men (Ng et al., 2009). Monda and colleagues (2007) have demonstrated that increases in urbanization are associated with decreasing intensity of occupation-related activity—a major source of physical activity for adults. Moreover, accessibility of home entertainment technology (i.e. television, internet, computer games, and so on) have likely contributed to more sedentary lifestyles (Gao et al., 2009), as well as a lack of healthy environments with fresh air to be out and physically active in. Finally, awareness of diabetes is relatively low in China, resulting in a significant proportion of cases going undetected (Gao et al., 2009; Dong et al., 2005; Li et al., 2013; Xu et al., 2013).

Other macro-level determinants of diabetes have also been suggested, including community economic factors, communications infrastructure, and transportation infrastructure (Attard et al., 2012). Attard and colleagues (2012) found that those living in communities with more modern markets (as defined by the number of Western-influenced business such as supermarkets, cafes, internet cafes, restaurants, and so on) and with higher wages for men and smaller percentage of agricultural workers were significantly more likely to have diabetes.

The transportation sector also plays a role in diabetes risk in China. Attard and colleagues (2012) found that those living in communities with more paved roads versus gravel or dirt roads, as well as more bus and/or train stations had higher odds for diabetes. In Qingdao, researchers speculate that a rapid increase in the number of families with cars in urban areas has decreased opportunities for physical activity (Gao et al., 2009). Bell and colleagues (2002) found increased odds for obesity among car-owners.

Van de Poel and colleagues (2012) posed the question, 'Is there a health penalty of China's rapid urbanization?' For diabetes, at least, there appears to be a notable health penalty. But, the urban health penalty has also been realized in other countries.

In an effort to understand the role urbanization plays in obesity and diabetes, Ebrahim and colleagues (2010) studied rural to urban migration in India. In a cross-section study, rural-to-urban migrant factory workers were compared to their rural-dwelling siblings as well as non-migrant urban factory workers and their non-migrant, non-factory worker urban siblings. Compared to the rural-dwellers, both urban dwellers and migrants were significantly more likely to have diabetes. Additional analyses suggested that obesity mediated the relationship between migration and diabetes and that the effect of migration on likelihood of obesity and diabetes may be stronger during the first decade post-migration.

A neuroscientific approach to investigating underlying mechanisms of epidemiological findings

Incidence and prevalence rates for psychiatric disorders have been found to be significantly higher in urban areas as compared to rural areas, particularly with increased incidence rates of schizophrenia (age-adjusted incidence rate ratio for males, 1.92, and females, 1.34) (Kelly et al., 2010) and prevalence rates of mood disorders (odds ratio (OR), 1.39) and anxiety disorders (OR, 1.21) (Peen et al., 2010). Neuroscientific work has begun to reveal some of the mechanisms that may underlie these epidemiological findings.

Urban upbringing—a risk factor for schizophrenia

Schizophrenia is a severe mental condition, characterized by a diversity of symptoms such as delusions, hallucinations, disorganized behaviour, cognitive deficits, blunted affect, and disturbed motivation (American Psychiatric Association, 2000). Although the lifetime prevalence ranges only between 0.5% and 1% (McGrath et al., 2004), schizophrenia is considered as one of the ten illnesses with the highest global burden of disease (Mathers et al., 2008). In particular, the dramatically increased suicide rates (Hor and Taylor, 2010; Palmer et al., 2005), the overall increased mortality (McGrath et al., 2008; Saha et al., 2007), and the frequent disability by mental and social impairments (Rössler et al., 2005) account for this issue, pointing at the need to further improve prevention and treatment of this disorder. The development of prevention and treatment strategies depends on, or is at least promoted by, aetiological knowledge (Kirkbride and Jones, 2011; Tost and Meyer-Lindenberg, 2012). Indeed, extensive research has provided valuable insights on aetiological factors, but also revealed the enormous complexity of the disorder and its potential risk or preventive factors, and to date left numerous questions unanswered.

The association of schizophrenia and urbanicity is a longstanding finding in the field of epidemiological research. Already in the 1930s, increased admission rates of schizophrenic patients were noticed in the inner city's hospitals of Chicago, compared to hospitals in the city's surroundings (Faris and Dunham, 1934). Evidence confirming this followed from several studies in different locations, consistently reporting elevated prevalence rates of schizophrenia in urban areas (Torrey et al., 1997; Schelin et al., 2000; Häfner et al., 1965; Vassos et al., 2012). These findings have been generated in spite of a necessarily (given the possible resolution of epidemiological studies) rather coarse definition of the urban–rural gradient; for example, using the five categories 'capital', 'capital suburb', 'provincial city with more than 100,000 inhabitants', 'provincial towns

with more than 10,000 inhabitants', or 'rural areas' in the Danish studies (Pedersen and Mortensen, 2001a; Pedersen and Mortensen, 2001b). Rigorous control for change of residence and use of data from central psychiatric registers strongly argue against the 'geographical drift' hypothesis (aggregation of subjects later diagnosed with schizophrenia in cities) and false positive findings caused by greater psychiatric resources in urban areas (Lewis et al., 1992; Pedersen and Mortensen, 2001b). In other words, the association of schizophrenia risk likely reflects a causal relationship, whatever the underlying variables may be.

Several studies have suggested a critical time window for the association of urban environments and development of schizophrenia. These data indicate that urban residence at illness onset and urban birth merely served as proxy variables for urban upbringing in a sensitive period, particularly the first 15 years of life (Marcelis et al., 1999; Pedersen and Mortensen, 2001a). Within this age period, the association with schizophrenia seems to follow dose-response patterns: incidence rates increase along rural-urban gradients and with the number of years spent in urban environments. Relocation between urban and rural environments alter schizophrenia incidence in the expected direction (Pedersen and Mortensen, 2001a). Overall, urban upbringing has turned out to be a robust risk factor, which involves an approximate twofold increase in schizophrenia incidence compared to rural upbringing.

In contrast to socioeconomic status, where selection effects have been shown to widely mediate the inverse correlation between socioeconomic positions and schizophrenia prevalence (Häfner et al., 1995), urbanicity seems to act causally on schizophrenia risk: The consistency of the association, the fact that sensitive periods for exposure precede the onset of illness, dose-response relationships, and variation of the outcome variable subsequent to changes in the degree of exposure all meet important plausibility criteria of causal risk factors (Lieb, 2005). The persistence of the effect after adjustment for many potential confounders such as age, sex, immigrant status, socioeconomic status, obstetric complications, drug use, and even genetic risk further supports the causation-hypothesis (Krabbendam and Van Os, 2005; Van Os, 2004; Harrison et al., 2003; March et al., 2008). One plausibility criterion of causality, namely insight into the risk-mediating mechanism, has nevertheless remained unfulfilled (McGrath and Scott, 2006).

Regarding the high base-rate and effect size of the risk factor urban upbringing, the resulting population attributable risk fraction of approximately 30% (Van Os, 2004), the enormous global burden of schizophrenia (Mathers et al., 2008), and worldwide tendencies towards urbanization (Dye, 2008), urban upbringing turns out to be a highly relevant mental health concern. It is, however, a complex and diverse construct with a large variety of potentially detrimental exposures. Due to this pronounced complexity, the risk-mediating factors and mechanisms cannot easily be detected. Investigation of some plausible environmental candidates did not reveal a homogeneous picture: whereas associations with increased schizophrenia risk were found for traffic air pollution (Pedersen and Mortensen, 2006a) or the family's residence place before conception (Pedersen and Mortensen, 2006b), other factors such as household crowding and infections (Brown, 2011) have not revealed unambiguous results. More consistent data, however, accumulated supporting the hypotheses that social stress and defeat mediate the effect of urban upbringing on schizophrenia incidence (Selten and Cantor-Graae, 2005). In line with this suggestion, social fragmentation, indicated by high proportions of foreigners within a municipality and single-parent households, was identified to substantially account for the association between urbanicity and non-affective psychosis in a Swedish population (Zammit *et al.*, 2010).

Although genetic and biological risk factors cover a large proportion of the variance of schizophrenia incidence, concerning urban upbringing it appears particularly worth focusing on psychosocial variables as potentially risk-mediating factors and mechanisms.

The neuroscience of urban upbringing

The advent of functional magnetic resonance imaging (fMRI) in the 1990s allowed for direct visualization of the brain areas activated during motor, emotional, or cognitive tasks. A frequent strategy in these studies is the investigation of mental risk factors in healthy samples, which enables the detection of neurobiological risk markers in the absence of potential confounders like medication or hospitalization.

Neuroscientific studies on urban upbringing are still scarce, but a number of investigations have been conducted by the authors of this chapter. In the following, this research will be presented.

Based on the presumptions of psychosocial and stress-related factors as mediators of the correlation between urbanicity and schizophrenia, a series of fMRI studies was carried out. In one of these studies (Lederbogen *et al.*, 2011) the effects of urban upbringing on social stress processing were investigated in a sample of 32 healthy individuals using a social-evaluative stress paradigm suitable for the MRI environment. Urban upbringing was quantified by scoring the size of the village, town, or city where the subject was dwelling during the first fifteen years of life, taking into account any changes of residence. A positive correlation between this variable, termed early-life urbanicity, and perigenual anterior cingulate cortex (pACC) activation under social stress induction was detected (see Fig. 8.1.1 for details). This result was replicated in an independent sample of 23 healthy students with a modified social-evaluative stress paradigm. The specificity of this result to social stress processing was furthermore demonstrated by showing the absence of an according correlation in 80 subjects who performed

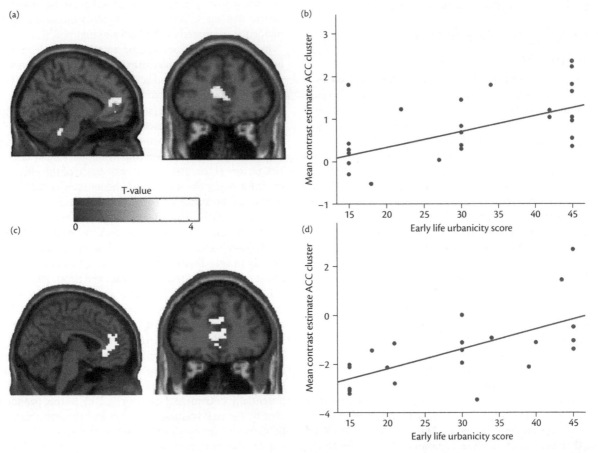

Fig. 8.1.1 Relationship between early life (birth until age 15) urbanicity scores and pACC activations in the main (a–b) and replication study (c–d). (a) First experiment: T-map of significant correlations between activations in the experimental > control contrast correlating with urbanicity scores displayed at a threshold of *p* <0.005 uncorrected. (b) First experiment: Scatterplot of urbanicity scores and mean contrast estimates of the significantly (at *p* <0.005) correlating voxels within the ACC in the experimental > control contrast. Results suggests a linear relationship between these two variables (r = 0.56, *p* = 0.001). (c) Replication study: T-map of significant correlations between activations in the experimental > control contrast and urbanicity scores (displayed at *p* <0.05, FWE corrected for the rostral ACC as ROI). (d) Replication study: Scatterplot between contrast estimates for the stress > control contrast and the urbanicity score displayed for the mean of all significantly (*p* <0.005) correlated voxels (r = 0.64, *p* <0.001).

two cognitive tasks without social stress induction. Post-hoc analyses revealed that the modulation of pACC activation by early-life urbanicity persisted, even after controlling for the potentially confounding effects of various sociodemographic and mental health-related variables. A functional connectivity analysis identified that a higher early-life urbanicity was associated with a lower functional coupling between pACC and right amygdala. The pACC is crucially implicated in the regulation of stress, particularly via its dense projections to the amygdala (Etkin *et al.*, 2006; Diorio *et al.*, 1993). The amygdala itself has strong projections to subcortical regions, such as the hypothalamus and the brain stem, and can thereby provoke biological stress responses, including physiological arousal and fight-or-flight reactions (Davis, 1992; Lang *et al.*, 1998). Further details on the neurophysiology of stress are provided in Chapter 1.4 'The physiology of stress and stress recovery'. An overactivation of the pACC under social stress and a decreased functional connectivity between pACC and the amygdala might therefore represent markers of an exaggerated sensitivity to stress in individuals who were raised in cities.

In a further MRI study (Haddad *et al.*, 2014), the effects of urban upbringing on brain morphology were investigated, applying a method called voxel-based morphometry in a sample of 115 healthy individuals. Early-life urbanicity was negatively correlated to the grey matter volume of a posterior section within the right dorsolateral prefrontal cortex (DLPFC). This result was regionally specific and not explained by confounding effects of common sociodemographic variables like age, sex, school education, and current urbanicity. The DLPFC is considerably susceptible to the effects of stress (Qin *et al.*, 2009) and early adversity (Tomoda *et al.*, 2009), and alterations of this region are present in schizophrenic patients and high-risk populations (Fusar-Poli *et al.*, 2012; Bora and Murray, 2014). The volumetric reduction in the DLPFC may consequently represent a biological embedding of an elevated exposure to stress in individuals who were raised in cities, and might contribute to their increased vulnerability for schizophrenia. In the same study, an interaction effect of sex and early-life urbanicity on grey matter volume of the pACC was found. While early-life urbanicity was inversely correlated with pACC volume in males, there was no such association in females. Interestingly, male sex is associated with an elevated schizophrenia incidence (Aleman *et al.*, 2003), earlier onsets (Eranti *et al.*, 2013), less favourable courses of disease (Thorup *et al.*, 2013), and an even more pronounced effect of urban upbringing on incidence rates (Marcelis *et al.*, 1998). This indicates a higher developmental vulnerability in males. The interaction effect of sex and early-life urbanicity might relate to these observations in terms of an indication of multiplicative risk accumulation. In line with this interpretation, decreased grey matter volumes of the ACC have been reported to be present in schizophrenic patients already at illness onset, leading to the assumption that a reduced ACC volume represents a neuroanatomical risk marker for schizophrenia (Fornito *et al.*, 2009).

A further very robust environmental risk factor for schizophrenia that interacts with urbanicity risk is ethnic minority status, which has been demonstrated for a multitude of ethnic groups and host countries with an average increase of risk by the factor 2 (Bourque *et al.*, 2011). The results patterns suggest that psychosocial stressors such as discrimination and social exclusion are critically involved in the risk-mediating mechanism. Congruent to the above-mentioned findings, a recent study reported an increased

pACC activation during social stress processing also in a sample of second-generation immigrants. Within this sample, pACC activation was positively correlated with perceived group discrimination (Akdeniz *et al.*, 2014).

In summary, the presented findings lead to the hypothesis that urban upbringing is associated with an elevated exposure to social stress during childhood and adolescence, which sensitizes affected individuals to social stress in a way that facilitates the development of schizophrenia later in life.

Current city living—a risk factor for depression and anxiety

Both depression and anxiety are common mental disorders. Globally, about 400 million people of all ages suffer from depression. More women are affected than men. Core symptoms are depressed mood and loss of interest or pleasure; additional symptoms are change in appetite, sleep difficulties, psychomotor symptoms, fatigue, feelings of worthlessness and guilt, diminished abilities to think or concentrate, and recurrent thoughts of death. The disorder often starts in the third decade of life and tends to be recurring. Thus, the burden of disease is enormous, putting major depressive disorders on rank 2 of the leading causes of disability-adjusted life years in a global perspective, projected for year 2030 (and rank 1 in high-income countries) (Mathers and Loncar, 2006). A major peril of depression is suicide, which results in premature death in approximately 10% of persons diagnosed with major depression. As also discussed in Chapter 3.2, depression is associated with exaggerated stress system activity in the majority of patients. This increased activity has been postulated to constitute a causal element in depression, as patients with persistent signs of HPA activations are prone to relapses. The prevalence of anxiety disorder figures 12.9% (11.3–14.7%) from a global perspective, making it the most frequent mental disorder (Steel *et al.*, 2014). The spectrum of anxiety disorders encompasses specific phobias, social phobia, generalized anxiety disorder, and panic disorder. Anxiety disorders are frequently co-morbid with other mental health disorders, including depression. There are two specific anxiety disorders for reactions to severe stress: acute stress reaction, and post-traumatic stress disorder.

Environmental stress seems important in the aetiology of these emotional disorders. A significant genetic contribution is also involved. Stressful life events including assault, serious marital or housing problems, death of a loved one, enduring financial problems, divorce/separation, and so on, have been identified as causal to the onset of major depressive episodes. However, it is of interest that individuals predisposed to major depression tend to select themselves into high-risk environments (Kendler *et al.*, 1999). Whether an event is perceived as stressful depends on the nature of the event, the subject's resources, and coping mechanisms.

It has been proposed that during depression and anxiety episodes, the interaction between stress and specific brain structures results in long-lasting changes in neural activity and function. Brain circuits found to be dysregulated in depression and anxiety include the prefrontal cortex and the subgenual cingulate cortex, which seem to be involved in emotion experience and processing, as well as the hippocampus and the amygdala, which are involved in emotional memory formation and memory retrieval (Ressler and Mayberg, 2007).

The neuroscience of current city living

Using a neuroscientific approach to investigate the association between exposure to the urban environment and the increased prevalence of depression and anxiety, brain circuits that include the amygdala are of high interest. The amygdala is part of the limbic system and plays an important role in learning about and remembering fear. The amygdala is functional in triggering flight responses to physical threats, even without involvement of cortical structures (Ledoux, 2000).

An enhanced functional coupling of the amygdala with a brain circuit including the dorsal anterior cingulate cortex and possibly the Locus coeruleus has been observed in the aftermath of acute stress (Van Marle et al., 2010). In addition, overactivation of the amygdala has been observed in depression and fear (Drevets, 2000), while the activation decreases with recovery of mood symptoms.

It has been proposed that anxiety disorders are associated with a particular pattern of functional network dysfunction (Sylvester et al., 2012) Amygdala activity in response to anticipatory stimuli has been found to be increased in patients with generalized anxiety disorders; and cingulate cortex activity was associated with clinical outcome eight weeks after initiation of therapy (Nitschke et al., 2009).

A cingulate-amygdala feedback circuit has been identified as target of genetic susceptibility for depression (Pezawas et al., 2005).

Furthermore, the amygdala seems to be involved in processing the demands required by a complex social life. As such, the amygdala is essential for the recognition of emotion in facial expressions (Adolphs et al., 1994) and correlates with online (Kanai et al., 2012) and real world social network sizes (Bickart et al., 2011).

A study conducted by this chapter's authors demonstrated that when exposed to a social-evaluative stressor, residents of urban environments show greater activity of the amygdala compared to inhabitants of rural areas (Lederbogen et al., 2011). Social-evaluative threat was generated by subjects' alleged failure during a mental arithmetic task in front of the study investigators. The findings were regionally and contextually specific, as the effect was observed only in this brain region and only under social-evaluative stress induction. However, peripheral stress hormones did not differentiate between subjects residing in urban or in rural areas.

These findings may indicate increased brain preparedness for fear and flight in city dwellers that is controlled by a higher order brain region in order to keep the stress reaction within normal limits. However, genetically based higher stress susceptibility or repeated and enduring stress exposure may disrupt this balance, promoting manifestation of disease. One such potential stressor which is potentially associated with current city living is unstable social hierarchy. In contrast to stable social status, the unstable hierarchy is associated with the activation of additional brain region during the processing of acute social stress-related to emotional processing (amygdala), social recognition (medial prefrontal cortex), and behavioural readiness (Zink et al., 2008). Further exploration of this environmental risk in ethnic minorities gave evidence for the importance of neural social stress processing (Akdeniz et al., 2014). This insight helps our understanding of the association between current city living and emotional disorders, as the ACC is critically involved in modulating amygdala activity (Etkin et al., 2006).

These findings shed light on a brain mechanism that is involved in the increased prevalence of depression and anxiety in city dwellers. However, there are also factors that protect from stress sequelae. Social support has been shown to be powerful in absorbing the effects of various stressors and the absence of social support is associated with increased mortality risk comparable to smoking, obesity or high blood pressure (Holt-Lunstad et al., 2010). The presence of social support is associated with diminished cortisol reactivity in response to a social stress task and seems to be mediated by decreased activity in the dorsal cingulate cortex and Brodmann's area 8 (Eisenberger et al., 2007).

Exposure to green space is associated with dampening of stress system activity (Ulrich, 1991). As discussed in Chapter 3.2, immersion in nature may protect the individual from developing affective or anxiety disorders, although it is only recently this has come to be explored neuroscientifically. In a recent study (Bratman et al., 2015), a nature walk compared to one in the urban environment improved blood flow in the same pACC region implicated in our studies of urban risk and stress, further strengthening the case for the association of this region with risk and suggesting that enhancing green space might be a useful strategy in urban environments.

Future research goals and implications

Knowledge on the impact of urbanicity on neural mechanisms that increase the risk for mental health disorders including schizophrenia, depression, and anxiety is recent and opens up new avenues of research. Several issues still need to be resolved. First, we do not know exactly whether city life is associated with increased stress levels. To tackle this question, agreement has to be reached on defining and measuring adequate stress indicators. Second, the urban environment still seems to constitute a black box containing many potential ingredients of stress, including social adversity, lack of green spaces, exposure to traffic, noise, toxins, and so on. Third, the urban environment must be spatially differentiated into finer grained areas like districts, neighbourhoods, or quarters, as the physical and social environment readily changes within small distances and intraurban health differences can be large.

Therefore, a more detailed look at the interaction between physical environment and the brain and relation to stress and mental disorders is needed. Emerging research is approaching these issues by using mobile assessment devices to allow for online analysis of mood, social stressors, type of environment, amount of nature, and may be supplemented by physiological data including heart rate, stress hormones, and so on (Abbott, 2012).

Conclusion

In general, city dwellers enjoy better health than their rural counterparts, most likely because of better economic conditions and improved infrastructure. However, specific aspects of city living may curtail these benefits, leading to profound and enduring effects on the somatic and neuropsychiatric disease spectrum. The prevalence of metabolic disorders, including diabetes mellitus, has been observed to increase along with urbanization and the same holds true for major psychiatric disorders (e.g. schizophrenia, depression, and anxiety). Science has begun to tackle the population-based and neuroscientific foundations of these associations, examining changes of health behaviour (e.g. physical activity and nutrition) and social stressors (e.g. isolation and social defeat) as potential risk factors.

A vigorous scientific approach is needed to further analyse the factors challenging the health benefit of urbanization. It seems mandatory to both study and understand the behavioural, genetic, cellular, and molecular basis of the observed shift in disease incidence. Associated factors must be classified as either circumstantial or causal, and strategies should be developed to adequately address the latter.

References

Abbott, A. (2012). Stress and the city: Urban decay. *Nature*, 490, 162–4.

Adediran, O. S., Adebayo, P. B., & Akintunde, A. A. 2013. Anthropometric differences among natives of Abuja living in urban and rural communities: correlations with other cardiovascular risk factors. *BMC Res Notes*, 6, 123–6.

Adolphs, R., Tranel, D., Damasio, H., & Damasio, A. (1994). Impaired recognition of emotion in facial expressions following bilateral damage to the human amygdala. *Nature*, 372, 669–72.

Akdeniz, C., Tost, H., Streit, F., et al. (2014). Neuroimaging evidence for a role of neural social stress processing in ethnic minority-associated environmental risk. *JAMA Psychiatry*, 71, 672–80.

Alcorn, T. & Ouyang, Y. (2012). Diabetes saps health and wealth from China's rise. *Lancet*, 379, 2227–8.

Aleman, A., Kahn, R. S., & Selten, J. P. (2003). Sex differences in the risk of schizophrenia: evidence from meta-analysis. *Arch Gen Psychiatry*, 60, 565–71.

American Psychiatric Association (2000). *Diagnostic and Statistical Manual of Mental Health Disorders*, 4th edition. Text Revision Washington, DC: American Psychiatric Press.

Anjana, R. M., Pradeepa, R., Deepa, M., et al. (2011). Prevalence of diabetes and prediabetes (impaired fasting glucose and/or impaired glucose tolerance) in urban and rural India: phase I results of the Indian Council of Medical Research–INdia DIABetes (ICMR-INDIAB) study. *Diabetologia.*, 54, 3022–7.

Attard, S. M., Herring, A. H., Mayer-Davis, E. J., Popkin, B. M., Meigs, J. B., & Gordon-Larsen, P. (2012). Multilevel examination of diabetes in modernising China: what elements of urbanisation are most associated with diabetes? *Diabetologia*, 55, 3182–92.

Balogun, W. O. & Gureje, O. (2013). Self-reported incident type—diabetes in the Ibadan study of ageing: relationship with urban residence and socioeconomic status. *Gerontology*, 59, 3–7.

Bell, A. C., Ge, K., & Popkin, B. M. (2002). The road to obesity or the path to prevention: motorized transportation and obesity in China. *Obes Res*, 10, 277–83.

Bickart, K. C., Wright, C. I., Dautoff, R. J., Dickerson, B. C., & Barrett, L. F. (2011). Amygdala volume and social network size in humans. *Nat Neurosci*, 14, 163–4.

Blumenthal, D. & Hsiao, W. (2005). Privatization and its discontents--the evolving Chinese health care system. *N Engl J Med*, 353, 1165–70.

Bora, E. & Murray, R. M. (2014). Meta-analysis of cognitive deficits in ultra-high risk to psychosis and first-episode psychosis: do the cognitive deficits progress over, or after, the onset of psychosis? *Schizophr Bull*, 40, 744–55.

Bourque, F., Van Der Ven, E., & Malla, A. (2011). A meta-analysis of the risk for psychotic disorders among first-and second-generation immigrants. *Psychol Med*, 41, 897.

Bratman, G. N., Hamilton, J. P., Hahn, K. S., Daily, G. C., & Gross, J. J. (2015). Nature experience reduces rumination and subgenual prefrontal cortex activation. *Proc Natl Acad Sci U S A*, 112, 8567–72.

Brown, A. S. (2011). The environment and susceptibility to schizophrenia. *Prog Neurobiol*, 93, 23–58.

Dagenais, G. R., Gerstein, H. C., Zhang, X., et al. (2016). Variations in diabetes prevalence in low-, middle-, and high-income countries: results from the prospective urban and rural epidemiology study. *Diabetes Care*, 39, 780–7.

Davis, M. 1992. The role of the amygdala in fear and anxiety. *Annu Rev Neurosci*, 15, 353–375.

Diorio, D., Viau, V., & Meaney, M. J. (1993). The role of the medial prefrontal cortex (cingulate gyrus) in the regulation of hypothalamic-pituitary-adrenal responses to stress. *J Neurosci*, 13, 3839–47.

Dong, Y., Gao, W., Nan, H., et al. (2005). Prevalence of Type 2 diabetes in urban and rural Chinese populations in Qingdao, China. *Diabet Med*, 22, 1427–33.

Drevets, W. C. (2000). Neuroimaging studies of mood disorders. *Biol Psychiatry*, 48, 813–29.

Dye, C. (2008). Health and urban living. *Science*, 319, 766–9.

Ebrahim, S., Kinra, S., Bowen, L., et al. (2010). The effect of rural-to-urban migration on obesity and diabetes in India: a cross-sectional study. *PLoS Med.*, 7, e1000268.

Eisenberger, N. I., Taylor, S. E., Gable, S. L., Hilmert, C. J., & Lieberman, M. D. (2007). Neural pathways link social support to attenuated neuroendocrine stress responses. *Neuroimage*, 35, 1601–12.

Eranti, S. V., Maccabe, J. H., Bundy, H., & Murray, R. M. (2013). Gender difference in age at onset of schizophrenia: a meta-analysis. *Psychol Med*, 43, 155–67.

Etkin, A., Egner, T., Peraza, D. M., Kandel, E. R., & Hirsch, J. (2006). Resolving emotional conflict: a role for the rostral anterior cingulate cortex in modulating activity in the amygdala. *Neuron*, 51, 871–82.

Faris, R. E. L. & Dunham, H. W. (1934). *Mental Disorders in Urban Areas*. Chicago, IL: University of Chicago Press.

Fornito, A., Yucel, M., Dean, B., Wood, S. J., & Pantelis, C. (2009). Anatomical abnormalities of the anterior cingulate cortex in schizophrenia: bridging the gap between neuroimaging and neuropathology. *Schizophr Bull*, 35, 973–93.

Fusar-Poli, P., Radua, J., Mcguire, P., & Borgwardt, S. (2012). Neuroanatomical maps of psychosis onset: voxel-wise meta-analysis of antipsychotic-naive VBM studies. *Schizophr Bull*, 38, 1297–307.

Gao, W. G., Dong, Y. H., Pang, Z. C., et al. (2009). Increasing trend in the prevalence of Type 2 diabetes and pre-diabetes in the Chinese rural and urban population in Qingdao, China. *Diabet Med*, 26, 1220–7.

Haddad, L., Schafer, A., Streit, F., et al. (2014). Brain structure correlates of urban upbringing, an environmental risk factor for schizophrenia. *Schizophr Bull*, 41, 115–22.

Harrison, G., Fouskakis, D., Rasmussen, F., Tynelius, P., Sipos, A., & Gunnell, D. (2003). Association between psychotic disorder and urban place of birth is not mediated by obstetric complications or childhood socio-economic position: a cohort study. *Psychol Med*, 33, 723–31.

Holt-Lunstad, J., Smith, T. B., & Layton, J. B. 2010. Social relationships and mortality risk: a meta-analytic review. *PLoS Med*, 7, e1000316.

Hor, K. & Taylor, M. (2010). Review: Suicide and schizophrenia: a systematic review of rates and risk factors. *J Psychopharmacol*, 24, 81–90.

Häfner, H., Nowotny, B., Löffler, W., & Maurer, K. (1995). When and how does schizophrenia produce social deficits? *Eur Arch Psychiatry Clin Neurosci*, 246, 17.

Häfner, H., Reimann, H., Immich, H., & Marrtini, H. (1965). Inzidenz seelischer Erkrankungen in Mannheim. *Social Psychiatry*, 4, 127–35.

Kanai, R., Bahrami, B., Roylance, R., & Rees, G. (2012). Online social network size is reflected in human brain structure. *Proc Biol Sci*, 279, 1327–34.

Kelly, B. D., O'Callaghan, E., Waddington, J. L., et al. (2010). Schizophrenia and the city: A review of literature and prospective study of psychosis and urbanicity in Ireland. *Schizophr Res*, 116, 75–89.

Kendler, K. S., Karkowski, L. M., Prescott, C. A. (1999). Causal relationship between stressful life events and the onset of major depression. *Am J Psychiatry*, 156, 837–41.

Kirkbride, J. B. & Jones, P. B. (2011). The Prevention of Schizophrenia—What Can We Learn From Eco-Epidemiology? *Schizophr Bull*, 37, 262–71.

Krabbendam, L. & Van Os, J. (2005). Schizophrenia and urbanicity: a major environmental influence--conditional on genetic risk. *Schizophr Bull*, 31, 795–9.

Lang, P. J., Bradley, M. M., & Cuthbert, B. N. (1998). Emotion, motivation, and anxiety: brain mechanisms and psychophysiology. *Biol Psychiatry*, 44, 1248–63.

Lederbogen, F., Kirsch, P., Haddad, L., *et al.* (2011). City living and urban upbringing affect neural social stress processing in humans. *Nature*, 474, 498–501.

Ledoux, J. E. (2000). Emotion circuits in the brain. *Annu Rev Neurosci*, 23, 155–184.

Lewis, G., David, A., Andreasson, S., & Allebeck, P. (1992). Schizophrenia and city life. *Lancet*, 340, 137–40.

Li, M. Z., Su, L., Liang, B. Y., *et al.* (2013). Trends in prevalence, awareness, treatment, and control of diabetes mellitus in mainland China from 1979 to 2012. *Int J Endocrinol*, 2013, 753150.

Lieb, R. (2005). Epidemiologie. *In*: Perrez, M. & Baumann, U. (eds.) *Lehrbuch Klinische Psychologie—Psychotherapie*, 3rd edition. Bern, Switzerland: Hans Huber, Hogrefe AG.

Liu, S., Wang, W., Zhang, J., *et al.* (2011). Prevalence of diabetes and impaired fasting glucose in Chinese adults, China National Nutrition and Health Survey, 2002. *Prev Chronic Dis*, 8, A13.

Marcelis, M., Navarro-Mateu, F., Murray, R., Selten, J. P., & Van Os, J. (1998). Urbanization and psychosis: a study of 1942–1978 birth cohorts in The Netherlands. *Psychol Med*, 28, 871–9.

Marcelis, M., Takei, N., & Van Os, J. (1999). Urbanization and risk for schizophrenia: does the effect operate before or around the time of illness onset? *Psychol Med*, 29, 1197–203.

March, D., Hatch, S. L., Morgan, C., *et al.* (2008). Psychosis and place. *Epidemiol Rev*, 30, 84–100.

Mathers, C., Fat, D. M., & Boerma, J. (2008). *The Global Burden of Disease: 2004 update*. Geneva, Switzerland: World Health Organization.

Mathers, C. D. & Loncar, D. (2006). Projections of global mortality and burden of disease from 2002 to 2030. *PLoS Med*, 3, e442.

McGrath, J., Saha, S., Chant, D., & Welham, J. (2008). Schizophrenia: a concise overview of incidence, prevalence, and mortality. *Epidemiol Rev*, 30, 67–76.

McGrath, J., Saha, S., Welham, J., El Saadi, O., Maccauley, C., & Chant, D. (2004). A systematic review of the incidence of schizophrenia: the distribution of rates and the influence of sex, urbanicity, migrant status and methodology. *BMC Med*, 2, 13.

McGrath, J. & Scott, J. (2006). Urban birth and risk of schizophrenia: a worrying example of epidemiology where the data are stronger than the hypotheses. *Epidemiol Psichiatr Soc*, 15, 243–6.

Mohan, V., Mathur, P., Deepa, R., *et al.* (2008). Urban rural differences in prevalence of self-reported diabetes in India--the WHO-ICMR Indian NCD risk factor surveillance. *Diabetes Res Clin Pract.*, 80, 159–68.

Monda, K. L., Gordon-Larsen, P., Stevens, J., & Popkin, B. M. (2007). China's transition: the effect of rapid urbanization on adult occupational physical activity. *Soc Sci Med*, 64, 858–70.

Ng, S. W., Norton, E. C., & Popkin, B. M. (2009). Why have physical activity levels declined among Chinese adults? Findings from the 1991–2006 China Health and Nutrition Surveys. *Soc Sci Med*, 68, 1305–314.

Nitschke, J. B., Sarinopoulos, I., Oathes, D. J., *et al.* (2009). Anticipatory activation in the amygdala and anterior cingulate in generalized anxiety disorder and prediction of treatment response. *Am J Psychiatry*, 166, 302–10.

Palmer, B. A., Pankratz, V. S., & Bostwick, J. M. (2005). The lifetime risk of suicide in schizophrenia: a reexamination. *Arch General Psychiatry*, 62, 247.

Pan, C., Shang, S., Kirch, W., & Thoenes, M. (2010). Burden of diabetes in the adult Chinese population: A systematic literature review and future projections. *Int J Gen Med*, 3, 173–9.

Pedersen, C. B. & Mortensen, P. B. (2001a). Evidence of a dose-response relationship between urbanicity during upbringing and schizophrenia risk. *Arch Gen Psychiatry*, 58, 1039–46.

Pedersen, C. B. & Mortensen, P. B. (2001b). Family history, place and season of birth as risk factors for schizophrenia in Denmark: a replication and reanalysis. *Br J Psychiatry*, 179, 46–52.

Pedersen, C. & Mortensen, P. (2006a). Urbanization and traffic related exposures as risk factors for schizophrenia. *BMC Psychiatry*, 6, 2.

Pedersen, C. B. & Mortensen, P. B. (2006b). Are the cause(s) responsible for urban-rural differences in schizophrenia risk rooted in families or in individuals? *Am J Epidemiol*, 163, 971–8.

Peen, J., Schoevers, R. A., Beekman, A. T., & Dekker, J. (2010). The current status of urban-rural differences in psychiatric disorders. *Acta Psychiatr Scand*, 121, 84–93.

Pezawas, L., Meyer-Lindenberg, A., Drabant, E. M., *et al.* (2005). 5-HTTLPR polymorphism impacts human cingulate-amygdala interactions: a genetic susceptibility mechanism for depression. *Nat Neurosci*, 8, 828–34.

Popkin, B. M. (1999). Urbanization, lifestyle changes and the nutrition transition. *World Development*, 27, 1905–16.

Popkin, B. M., Horton, S., Kim, S., Mahal, A., & Shuigao, J. (2001). Trends in diet, nutritional status, and diet-related noncommunicable diseases in China and India: the economic costs of the nutrition transition. *Nutr Rev*, 59, 379–90.

Qin, S., Hermans, E. J., Van Marle, H. J., Luo, J., & Fernandez, G. (2009). Acute psychological stress reduces working memory-related activity in the dorsolateral prefrontal cortex. *Biol Psychiatry*, 66, 25–32.

Ressler, K. J. & Mayberg, H. S. (2007). Targeting abnormal neural circuits in mood and anxiety disorders: from the laboratory to the clinic. *Nat Neurosci*, 10, 1116–24.

Rössler, W., Joachim Salize, H., Van Os, J., & Riecher-Rössler, A. (2005). Size of burden of schizophrenia and psychotic disorders. *Eur Neuropsychopharmacol*, 15, 399–409.

Saha, S., Chant, D., & McGrath, J. (2007). A systematic review of mortality in schizophrenia: is the differential mortality gap worsening over time? *Arch Gen Psychiatry*, 64, 1123.

Schelin, E., Munk-Jørensen, P., Olesen, A., & Gerlach, J. (2000). Regional differences in schizophrenia incidence in Denmark. *Acta Psychiatrica Scandinavica*, 101, 293–9.

Selten, J. P. & Cantor-Graae, E. (2005). Social defeat: risk factor for schizophrenia? *Br J Psychiatry*, 187, 101–2.

Shetty, P. (2012). Public health: India's diabetes time bomb. *Nature*, 485, S14–S16.

Singh, G. K., Azuine, R. E., Siahpush, M., & Kogan, M. D. (2013). All-cause and cause-specific mortality among US youth: socioeconomic and rural-urban disparities and international patterns. *J Urban Health*, 90, 388–405.

Singh, G. K. & Siahpush, M. (2014a). Widening rural-urban disparities in all-cause mortality and mortality from major causes of death in the USA, 1969–2009. *J Urban Health*, 91, 272–92.

Singh, G. K. & Siahpush, M. (2014b). Widening rural-urban disparities in life expectancy, U.S., 1969–2009. *Am J Prev Med*, 46, e19–e29.

Steel, Z., Marnane, C., Iranpour, C., *et al.* (2014). The global prevalence of common mental disorders: a systematic review and meta-analysis 1980–2013. *Int J Epidemiol*, 43, 476–93.

Sylvester, C. M., Corbetta, M., Raichle, M. E., *et al.* (2012). Functional network dysfunction in anxiety and anxiety disorders. *Trends Neurosci*, 35, 527–35.

Tang, S., Meng, Q., Chen, L., Bekedam, H., Evans, T., & Whitehead, M. 2008. Tackling the challenges to health equity in China. *Lancet*, 372, 1493–501.

Thorup, A., Albert, N., Bertelsen, M., *et al.* (2013). Gender differences in first-episode psychosis at 5-year follow-up—two different courses of disease? Results from the OPUS study at 5-year follow-up. *Eur Psychiatry*, 29, 44–51.

Tomoda, A., Suzuki, H., Rabi, K., Sheu, Y.-S., Polcari, A., & Teicher, M. H. (2009). Reduced prefrontal cortical gray matter volume in young adults exposed to harsh corporal punishment. *Neuroimage*, 47, T66–T71.

Torrey, E. F., Bowler, A. E., & Clark, K. (1997). Urban birth and residence as risk factors for psychoses: an analysis of 1880 data. *Schizophrenia Res*, 25, 169–76.

Tost, H. & Meyer-Lindenberg, A. (2012). Puzzling over schizophrenia: Schizophrenia, social environment and the brain. *Nature Med*, 18, 211–13.

Ulrich, R. S. (1991). Stress recovery. *J Environ Psychol*, 11, 201–30.

United Nations Department of Economic and Social Affairs (2014). World Urbanization Prospects: The 2014 Revision, Highlights. Available at: http://esa.un.org/unpd/wup/Highlights/WUP2014-Highlights.pdf (accessed 10 August 2014) [Online].

Van de Poel, E. V., O'Donnell, O., & Doorslaer, E. V. (2012). Is there a health penalty of China's rapid urbanization? *Health Econ*, 21, 367–85.

Van Marle, H. J., Hermans, E. J., Qin, S., & Fernandez, G. (2010). Enhanced resting-state connectivity of amygdala in the immediate aftermath of acute psychological stress. *Neuroimage*, 53, 348–54.

Van Os, J. (2004). Does the urban environment cause psychosis? *Br J Psychiatry*, 184, 287–8.

Vassos, E., Pedersen, C. B., Murray, R. M., Collier, D. A., & Lewis, C. M. 2012. Meta-analysis of the association of urbanicity with schizophrenia. *Schizophr Bull*, 38, 1118–23.

Wild, S., Roglic, G., Green, A., Sicree, R., & King, H. (2004). Global prevalence of diabetes: estimates for the year 2000 and projections for 2030. *Diabetes Care*, 27, 1047–53.

World Bank (2014). GDP per capita (current US$). *Catalog Sources World Development Indicators*.

Xu, Y., Wang, L., He, J., *et al.* (2013). Prevalence and control of diabetes in Chinese adults. *JAMA*, 310, 948–59.

Yang, W., Lu, J., Weng, J., *et al.*; China National, D., Metabolic Disorders Study, G. 2010. Prevalence of diabetes among men and women in China. *N Engl J Med*, 362, 1090–101.

Young, F., Critchley, J. A., Johnstone, L. K., & Unwin, N. C. (2009). A review of co-morbidity between infectious and chronic disease in Sub Saharan Africa: TB and diabetes mellitus, HIV and metabolic syndrome, and the impact of globalization. *Global Health*, 5, 9.

Zammit, S., Lewis, G., Rasbash, J., Dalman, C., Gustafsson, J. E., & Allebeck, P. (2010). Individuals, schools, and neighborhood: a multilevel longitudinal study of variation in incidence of psychotic disorders. *Arch Gen Psychiatry*, 67, 914–22.

Zhang, L., Wang, F., Wang, L., *et al.* (2012). Prevalence of chronic kidney disease in China: a cross-sectional survey. *Lancet*, 379, 815–22.

Zink, C. F., Tong, Y., Chen, Q., Bassett, D. S., Stein, J. L., & Meyer-Lindenberg, A. (2008). Know your place: neural processing of social hierarchy in humans. *Neuron*, 58, 273–83.

CHAPTER 8.2

Urban landscapes and public health

Timothy Beatley and Cecil Konijnendijk van den Bosch

The many challenges of creating healthy, resilient, and sustainable urban environments

That we are squarely in the midst of an urban age is widely understood. Global patterns of urbanization, in combination with increasing resource pressures (e.g. for food, water, energy) in combination with climate change, suggest unprecedented challenges that cities will face in the decades ahead. These trends and pressures will be overlaid onto the already unhealthy and unequally distributed levels of poverty, inadequate housing, and resource scarcity that exist in many cities. Urban environments will at once need to be more resource-efficient and sustainable, and more resilient in the face of increasing numbers of extreme weather events (flooding, storms), rising summer temperatures, and sea level rise.

Increasing urbanization patterns have resulted in significant and serious environmental health concerns. There are also a number of specific health worries associated with modern patterns of urbanization (see also Chapter 8.1 'The shift from natural living environments to urban: population-based and neurobiological implications for public health' for a discussion on urban–rural health disparities). With urbanization comes increased heat, the so-called urban heat island (UHI) phenomenon. This is a particular issue in hot climates, but the UHI phenomenon also characterizes many North American cities, for instance. A recent study of the 60 most populous cities in the United States by the organization Climate Central found that they experienced summer temperatures over the last 10 years that were on average 2.4°C hotter than rural areas (Kenward et al., 2014). Differences were much greater for some cities; for instance, it was more than 7°C for Las Vegas, around 6°C in Albuquerque, and in Denver, Portland, and Washington, the difference was close to 5°C. Climate change will severely exacerbate the problems of UHI, and cities around the world will also face serious flooding and sea level rise, and periodic drought. All raise serious public health challenges for cities.

The tendency towards urban sprawl, or growth through suburban and exurban locations, at relatively low densities, and very car-dependent societies, has carried with it significant environmental and health impacts. In American cities, a car-dependent landscape, with segregated and single-use land uses (residential separated from commercial, single-family from multi-family), has made it difficult to walk or bicycle. In just a few decades, the percentage of school-age children walking or bicycling to (American) schools has plummeted from 41% (in 1969), to 13% (in 2009) (McDonald, 2007). Distances to schools and shops are longer, and serious obstacles exist (lack of sidewalks, busy roadways). There is a general fear by parents of abduction and concern for safety of children that works against independent mobility. Studies of the mobility 'ranges' of children (how far they walk or roam) show how in just three or four generations this area has shrunk dramatically (e.g. Derbyshire, 2007). This is also influenced by an increased and perhaps unbalanced risk perception, which is further discussed in Chapter 7.4 'Risk and the perception of risk in interactions with nature'.

Few Americans get the recommended daily amounts of physical exercise (Centers for Disease Control, 2016) and the same holds true for many other populations across the world. The physical design of living and work environments often prevents and discourages active living. As unhealthy are the amounts of time people spend sitting (at work on the computer or while at home watching TV). A World Health Organization report, for example, stated that in 2010, 81% of all youths worldwide aged 11–17 were insufficiently physically active (WHO, 2015). This, in combination with changes in diet, helps explain rising obesity rates (Centers for Disease Control, 2016).

Sedentary behaviour is a health risk of its own, even for individuals getting the recommended daily amount of exercise (30 minutes per day) (Biswas et al., 2015). Overcoming our modern lifestyles where individuals, at home or at work, are sitting for extended periods of time is an important health goal and an important urban design principle—cities must be designed to make activity easy and enjoyable, a delightful experience in part because of the interesting people, art, architecture, and nature they will see when they move beyond the desk or couch. Read more about physical activity and the relation to nature and green spaces in Chapter 3.1 'Promoting physical activity—reducing obesity and other non-communicable diseases'.

In the cities of the global North, at least, sedentary lives and lifestyles may be the single greatest threat to health. Sitting in all aspects of modern life (at home as well, i.e. TV watching and increasing time on computers and phones) is emerging as a new pathology and threat to health. It is now sometimes said that 'sitting is the new smoking', and evidence is mounting that this is a serious health concern. One study of 9,000 Australians concluded that for each additional hour of TV watching, mortality rate increases by 11% (Dunstan et al., 2010). Contemporary work environments also often involve significant amounts of sitting during the day. Interventions such as standing desks have been shown to be an effective response, but so also are frequent breaks and the need for green elements and amenities (nearby parks and greenspaces) that will entice movement and physical activity.

In recognition of the need to combat sedentary lifestyles, an increasing number of cities are making greater commitments to investing in walkable neighbourhoods and the use of bicycles. Cities like Portland, Oregon, and Copenhagen, Denmark have made serious commitments to bicycle mobility, for instance. Some 45% of home to work trips in Copenhagen are made on bicycle, for example, and the city is aspiring to even great levels (Cycling Embassy of Denmark, 2015). This is a result of a remarkable investment in bike infrastructure, and of innovative initiatives like the Green Cycle Routes which provide riders the ability to commute through or alongside a park or green area.

Cubicled office environments, moreover, where workers have little or no access to windows and natural light, or to greenery or fresh air, represent further unhealthful conditions. A recent study by the company Interface highlighted that current office environments are not very healthy spaces. This survey of 7,600 offices workers in 16 countries found that almost half don't have access to natural light and nearly 60% don't have living plants in these work spaces (Interface, 2015). This despite the clear evidence that such 'green' office conditions enhance well-being and increase worker productivity.

Access to healthy and affordable food also represents a significant aspect of this problem, and emergence of 'food deserts' especially in lower-income urban neighbourhoods has emerged as a serious problem (USDA, 2009; United Nations, 2014). Urban nature and urban agriculture can help address these concerns, as for example addressed in the Food for the Cities programme of the Food and Agriculture Organization of the United Nations (FAO, undated). Many cities are encouraging and facilitating conversion of vacant spaces into orchards and community gardens, and cities such as New York and San Francisco are amending their municipal codes to allow for urban agriculture. An extensive local and regional food movement has emerged, emphasizing the view of cities as bountiful spaces that can produce at least a significant portion of food needs, and in ways that enhance diet and health (Denckla-Cobb, 2011). The rise of community gardening has changed everyday landscapes in many cities. Building on long traditions of urban agriculture, it can contribute to public health in various ways, from providing dietary supplements to encouraging physical exercise and social cohesion (Guitart et al., 2012). A literature review revealed that the large majority of these community gardens have been initiated and run by NGOs and cultural or community groups (Guitart et al., 2012). Globally, FAO stresses the need to focus on the urban poor when it comes to food security and the need to invest in urban food programmes. The supply of nutritious and safe food can be promoted by city-wide urban and peri-urban agriculture programmes (FAO, undated). According to Zezza and Tasciotti (2010), urban agriculture in developing countries is primarily geared towards consumption within the own household, although in several countries it accounts for from 15% to one-third of total agricultural production marketed.

Sprawling, car-dependent 'urbanscapes' in turn have resulted in social isolation and lower levels of social interaction and trust, all constituent elements of so-called social capital. We know that there are clear relationships between social capital, and health and happiness. (More extensive friendships have been associated

for instance with lower mortality from cancer; e.g. Holt-Lunstad et al., 2010.) Social isolation and loneliness seem to be on the rise, though planning and physical design can help to address this. Studies have shown that walkable neighbourhoods foster greater social capital. A recent study at the University of New Hampshire (Rogers et al., 2011) concludes: 'Individuals in more walkable neighborhoods have higher levels of trust and community involvement, whether that is working on a community project, attending a club meeting, volunteering, or simply having friends to one's home. Interestingly, residents in the more walkable neighborhoods indicated having excellent health and happiness more frequently than the less walkable neighborhoods.'

These social connections and relationships clearly form the basis for a healthy, meaningful life. There are many challenges to creating the conditions for human 'flourishing' and significant rates of depression, and an alarming recent rise in suicide, suggest that for many a sense of meaning and purpose may be lacking. Here nature in cities offers as well at least a partial antidote. Chapter 3.3 'Promoting social cohesion and social capital– increasing well-being' discusses the value of nature and green spaces for improved social capital in cities and neighbourhoods.

This chapter describes how we can face the challenges and develop urban environments that promote better public health, taking a landscape perspective. It stresses the need to study human–nature interactions in urban areas using a socioecological approach. After introducing an urban landscape perspective, the complex relations between different types and components of urban landscapes and public health are introduced. Next, strategic approaches to addressing healthy urban landscapes are discussed.

An urban landscape perspective

To address the above challenges and the interrelations between humans and their environment, between sociocultural and ecological factors in general, the so-called socioecological approach has gained broader following. It is based on the concept that one can only understand human behaviour when understanding people's interactions with their physical and sociocultural surroundings. In this framework, various levels of influence on a person's behaviour are distinguished; these can be divided into personal factors (e.g. age, sex, ethnic belonging, personal experiences), and social and environmental factors (e.g. physical environment, social environment, policy environment) (Foster and Giles-Corti, 2008). A socioecological approach to cities, for example, requires interdisciplinary approaches and an integrative view of urban areas (Tzoulas et al., 2007).

A useful and well-established perspective for understanding cities and towns from a socioecological perspective is that of urban landscapes. The European Landscape Convention (ELC; Council of Europe, 2000), an ambitious policy initiative adopted by the Council of Europe (2000) to promote landscape protection, management, and planning, and to organize European cooperation on landscape issues, defines landscape broadly as 'an area, as perceived by people, whose character is the result of the action and interaction of natural and/or human factors'. Thus landscapes are shaped in close interaction between nature and culture. Landscapes are not static, but change continuously, as they are the expression of the dynamic interaction between natural and cultural forces in the environment (Antrop, 2005).

The ELC recognizes urban (and peri-urban) landscapes as important focus areas. For most humans urban landscapes are everyday landscapes, the landscapes where they live, work, and play. Urban landscapes are typically highly cultural, with a large share of human-made structures and impervious surfaces. However, cities also harbour extensive open and green spaces, ranging from woodland and parks to private gardens and street tree plantations, as well as blue spaces. As discussed in for example Chapter 8.4 'Green infrastructure—its approach and public health benefits', these green (and blue) components can be regarded as a natural infrastructure that provides a wide range of ecosystem services to urban dwellers, while also making cities more resilient to environmental and other change.

Urban landscapes are the domain of landscape architects and planners, but also of a wide range of other professionals. From a public health perspective, a key question to address is how urban landscapes can be designed, planned, and managed to enhance people's health and well-being. This is the topic of the next section, building on the complex interactions between urban landscapes and public health.

Developing urban landscapes for public health

The interrelations between landscape in general and public health have been recognized for a long time. Landscapes that promote people's physical and mental health have been created for many centuries (Muir, 2005). Gesler (2005) speaks of 'therapeutic landscapes', highlighting that certain natural and built environments can promote mental and physical well-being. In these landscapes, environmental, societal, and individual factors work together to promote health. The importance of everyday landscapes, such as those urban landscapes close to people's homes, is of particular importance. In the United Kingdom for example, governments recognized the role that public parks could play in the physical and spiritual 'renewal' of the urban classes as early as the nineteenth century (Worpole, 2007). In the words of Reeder (2006): 'Nature, like art, was thought to have a morally beneficial influence as well as recuperative powers.'

In some cases urban landscapes included specific 'therapeutic' components, such as hospitals and sanatoria set in park-like environments. But the primary focus from a public health perspective has been on public parks, later broadening to creating green living environments as in garden cities, and as also reflected in for example, the American City Beautiful Movement. The importance of designing neighbourhoods with public health in mind, for example by promoting physical activity and spending time outdoors, has become recognized more widely in different parts of the world. During recent years, focus has been on the needs of specific groups, such as older people. A study among British elderly found that those who live in a 'supportive' environment tended to walk more, and high-level walkers were more likely to be in good health (Sugiyama and Thompson, 2007). Neighbourhood environments should thus be designed in such a way that they provide opportunities to be active. Moreover, more places need to be offered where people can meet with each other and enjoy nature.

This book provides a comprehensive view on how nature and landscapes impact public health, not only from a physical but also from a psychological perspective. The term 'restorative landscapes'

has also been used, referring to therapeutic landscapes that help restore emotional and physical well-being (Milligan and Bingley, 2007). Within urban landscapes, urban green and green elements such as trees have been found to play a crucial part in this respect.

Although urban landscapes are usually highly designed, with nature being more controlled and 'manicured', many cities do leave some space for wilder green spaces such as woodland, wetland, or natural vegetation on abandoned lands. Wilderness, or rather 'wildscape', has been found to carry special importance from a public health perspective, as they make specific contributions to psychological and restoration effects (e.g. Kaplan and Kaplan, 1989; Konijnendijk, 2008). Jorgensen et al. (2006) show that people need both managed and 'wilder' areas in these living and working places. They tend to prefer more managed landscapes close to their house, but also need 'wilder' green areas, including woodlands, close to their neighbourhood. Wildscapes have been suggested to be of particular importance to children and teens, functioning as 'wild adventure space' within the urban landscape where they have some form of freedom to play, experience, and learn (Thompson et al., 2006; Louv, 2008). Read about children's interactions with urban green spaces in Chapter 6.1 'Children and nature'.

An interesting case of promoting wildscapes is that of the Sihlwald forest of Zurich, Switzerland. From being a forest where timber production prevailed for centuries, it gradually became a major recreational area for the population of Zurich. Eventually, it was developed into a 'nature experience park', following new Swiss legislation that established this special category of 'smaller sisters' to National Parks. Natural processes are given ample space in the Sihlwald and forest management is limited, thus offering people a real 'nature experience' (Seeland et al., 2002; Konijnendijk, 2008).

The relation between 'wilder' nature in cities and public health is a complex one, as demonstrated by Van den Berg and Konijnendijk (2012). The authors talk about 'ambivalent' wilder landscapes with both positive connotations (such as experiencing nature and the sublime) as well as negative ones (different types of fear). Fears of different nature can be major barriers to using urban green spaces and other parts of the urban landscape, as illustrated by Sreetheran and Konijnendijk van den Bosch (2014) in a study of fear of crime in urban parks.

Barriers to using urban green space need to be overcome from a public health perspective. When people don't use green spaces, they are not exposed to potential health benefits either. Barriers can be manifold, such as the abovementioned fears as well as lack of resources and lack of knowledge, distance, mobility constraints, and social exclusion. These barriers are of particular importance in relation to people's everyday landscape and nearby nature, which consists of the natural elements and features that people encounter in and around those settings of everyday life in which they spend much of their time, including residential settings, the workplace, and schools (Nilsson et al., 2007). Brief nature experiences can produce short-term benefits, while proximity to nature can yield benefits that stand as cumulative effects of repeated brief experiences.

Strategic approaches to addressing healthy urban landscapes

While the modern city presents serious threats to health, innovative design and planning interventions offer hope for creating urban landscapes that provide the conditions for deep health and well-being. These interventions can be site- and neighbourhood-based, but also city-wide and more systematic. While there is not an exhaustive review of the options here, we present some of the main possibilities.

Green urbanism

Green urbanism offers one promising approach or paradigm. Green urbanism argues for a vision of compact urban form, dense and walkable urban neighbourhoods, and investments in public transit and alternatives to automobiles (every city can be bicycle-friendly). A central importance is given to nature and green space in urban living, and in the need to shift towards an urban metabolism that is more circular and closed-loop. Emphasis is also placed on combining the advantages of green building design—low carbon, renewable energy-powered, water and resource conserving—with the qualities of compact, walkable urbanism (see Beatley, 2000). Green urbanism also argues that opportunities for food production should be integrated into neighbourhood design.

We mentioned earlier the emergence of urban agriculture and community gardening in cities around the world builds on this idea, and there are now many compelling models of cities that have elevated food security and food systems and that are making room for the growing (and selling) of food in the city (e.g. London, San Francisco).

A new emphasis on creating healthy cities and communities represents another category of strategies. Healthy food is often as one important plank but also the application of health impact assessments. In Chapter 8.6 'The healthy settings approach: Healthy cities and environmental health indicators' you can read about the Healthy Cities Network and how it has developed around the public health principles guided by WHO.

Resilience and resilient cities

Resilience and resilient cities represent yet another set of approaches, emphasizing the ability of city residents and infrastructure to adapt and respond (to bend and not break, in the common parlance) in response to events like earthquakes and hurricanes, as well as social and economic shocks. Resilient cities have many of the same design and planning features and qualities and proposed interventions—building social capital, but also design for such things as modularity and ecosystem diversity (see Walker et al., 2006). Design for passive survivability (buildings that will be habitable in the absence of electricity), and for distributed systems of energy, for instance, are advocated.

Urban resilience has risen on the global agenda in part because of new emphasis of funders such as the Rockefeller Foundation, which has created the 100 Resilient Cities initiative (http://www.100resilientcities.org), committing to providing $1 million USD to support each chosen city. Each participating city is expected to hire a Chief Resilience Officer (CRO). Already resilience has become a key guiding principle in several cities, from New York to Rotterdam.

That we need nature in our lives, that it is essential to our health, happiness, and well-being is a key premise of biophilia, made popular by the thinking and writing of Harvard biologist E. O. Wilson. Much of the shift in city planning and design in the direction of urban greening, green infrastructure, and biophilic cities is a recognition of the immense power of nature and natural landscapes to make us healthier and happier (Beatley, 2011).

Green cities, nature-ful cities, can be more resilient, sustainable, and healthy. Finding more ways to integrate nature in and around cities is another important category of strategy. There is a renewed awareness of the important role that ecological systems and green infrastructure can play in creating a healthy city and—as illustrated by this book—of the positive health effects of trees, gardens, and the other green qualities of living environments (e.g. Donovan et al., 2011).

Biophilia and biophilic design, have emerged as important planning concepts, building on the important insights that the human species is hard-wired to need and want connections with nature, and that we are happier, healthier and more productive when nature is nearby (Kellert et al., 2008). The concept of biophilic design is described and exemplified in Chapter 8.3 'Nature in buildings and health design'. Green infrastructure has been an important framing of these issues, a way to emphasize the equally important element of forests, rivers, and other natural systems in moderating climate, delivering benefits that help create healthier urban environments (e.g. retaining storm water and addressing the combined sewer-overflow problems that exist in many cities, reducing air and water pollution, moderating urban heat, and so on).

Increasingly, these ideas have found their way into the concept of biophilic cities, that is, cities that place nature at the centre of their design and planning, and that emphasize the importance of fostering connections to the natural world (Beatley, 2011). Biophilic cities can be evaluated by the extent of nature, biodiversity, and wildness within their borders or boundaries (e.g. forest canopy coverage, percentage of urban population living with a certain distance of a green space), but also the ways in which residents connect with (or not) this nature. Biophilic urbanism has emerged as an important and different form of urban design, with the application of many new ways to design nature into urban buildings and neighbourhoods, from green rooftops, green walls, and vertical gardens, sky gardens and green balconies, and so on. The techniques and technology are advancing in ways that suggest that even in very dense, vertical cities, it will be possible to foster contact with nature.

Biophilic cities, moreover, are cities that recognize the multisensory experiences of nature, and that celebrate natural soundscapes. Bird song and natural sounds are important features, as are efforts to control and minimize human-made noise (a major health problem in its own right). More generally, biophilic cities are envisioned as spaces and places that are co-inhabited by many other species, and with an emphasis of co-existence. The potential for wonder and awe in biophilic cities is great and seen as an important health- and life-enhancing aspect (Rudd et al., 2012).

In the autumn of 2013, a global Biophilic Cities Network was launched (Beatley, 2014). Beginning with 10 initial partner cities, the Network has grown, and the idea gained traction. A protocol to guide new cities joining the Network has been unveiled (http://biophiliccities.org/wp-content/uploads/2015/03/BiophilicCitiesNetworkProtocol.pdf), and calls on them to officially adopt a biophilic cities resolution, to identify and commit to future goals and projects, and to collect and track a minimum number of biophilic indicators that will allow the assessment of progress over time. Participating partner cities will share insights and best practices, assist other cities in the Network in advancing biophilic design and planning projects, and collectively (see www.BiophilicCities.org). The Network seeks to foster organization, planning, and dialogue within cities, which is happening through grassroots efforts in

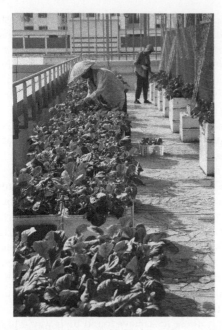

Fig. 8.2.1 The Khoo Tech Puat Hospital (KTPH) in Singapore includes many different forms of nature. The rooftop of one of the main structures boasts an urban farm, growing many different kinds of vegetables.
Image reproduced courtesy of Timothy Beatley.

a number of cities, including Washington DC (Biophilic DC) and Philadelphia (a new organization called BioPhilly).

Cities in the Network have undertaken a host of creative measures to bring nature into their urban environments. Singapore is innovating in the area of vertical greening, requiring new high-rise building to compensate for nature lost at ground level (under its Landscape Replacement Policy). San Francisco is innovating in the creation of new small green spaces, for instance 'parklets' formed from 2–3 onstreet car-parking spaces, and new sidewalk gardens. In Milwaukee, through a programme called HOME GR/OWN, vacant lots are being combined and converted into community orchards and pocket parks. Wellington, New Zealand, has an ambitious tree planting goal and efforts to bring back native species of birds in the city, as well as developing a strategy for creating a 'blue belt' (to include marine nature) to correspond to its terrestrial green belt system. Vitoria-Gasteiz, capital of the Spanish Basque region, is well known for its green ring that encircles the city. It is now extending this nature into the heart of the city, establishing an interior green ring. In a variety of creative and different ways, these cities are showing how nature can be an essential aspect of urban life.

Increasingly, the vision of biophilic cities is one that aspires to a more immersive form of urban nature, as reflected in Singapore's motto 'City in a Garden'. The leadership of the Khoo Teck Puat Hospital (KTPH; Fig. 8.2.1) in the city understands the critical importance of enlisting nature in the healing process, describing itself as a 'hospital in a garden'. (In Chapter 8.3 you can read more about the KTPH.)

Similarly, many new commercial structures in the city, adhering to and going beyond that city's design requirements, such as the new PARKROYAL Hotel, are defined as immersive nature experiences ('hotel in a garden'). The PARKROYAL, designed by the

architecture firm WOHA, includes an impressive degree of nature, including several levels of sky gardens (Beatley, 2017), and extensive hanging plants enjoyed both by hotel occupants and residents on the street. Elsewhere, the city of Melbourne (2011) has set an ambitious goal of doubling its tree canopy coverage, but even more importantly aspires to becoming a *city in a forest*. The Singapore experience is moving closer to the model of immersive urban nature—that one should not simply have to visit the garden, or the forest, or the park, but rather *live in* the garden, park, forest. The future of biophilic cities rests on understanding the need to see how green rooftops, skyparks, urban forests, parks, and greenspaces, and larger ecological and landscape features can fit together in creating a seamless green and healthy urban landscape (Figs 8.2.2 and 8.2.3).

Biophilic cities are not defined solely by the presence or absence of nature, but also by the many ways in which residents engage in that nature, and the extent to which they celebrate it, are intimately aware of it, and work to conserve and protect it. Providing opportunities to connect with and engage with nature in cities also helps to build friendships and social connections, whether through a urban nature hike, participating in a family nature club, joining a birdwatching group, or working to clean up and plant trees on vacant lots, these activities help to solidify human relationships and to forge new health-enhancing social connections. Nature and natural settings are not the only way this can happen, of course, but they seem to have special power in bringing people together. Nature, and natural urban landscapes, can also provide meaning and purpose in life. The mystery and wonder of the natural world—whether watching a diving peregrine falcon or the herculean work of a colony of pavement ants—are on display in cities, and there are now a host of creative new ways to highlight and

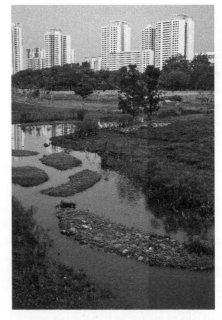

Fig. 8.2.2 The Kallang River, in Singapore, used to be little more than a concrete flood control channel. Now it has been restored back to a more natural, meandering river. Shown here, the river makes its way through Bishan-Ang Mo Kia Park, one of the city's most popular parks and an important element of natural in the middle of this dense city.
Image reproduced courtesy of Timothy Beatley.

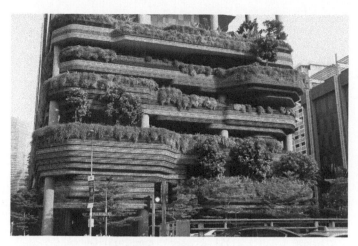

Fig. 8.2.3 The PARKROYAL at Pickering, in Singapore, is one of the most biophilic hotels anywhere. Designed by the firm WOHA, it includes extensive sky gardens, and abundant hanging plants seen from the street.
Image reproduced courtesy of Timothy Beatley.

connect urbanites to this remarkable urban nature scene. From BioBlitzes to new and growing citizen science programmes, cities from Bangalore to Los Angeles are working to engage residents with the nature around them.

Conclusion

This chapter has reviewed some of the main urban health challenges faced today, and the ways that new urban planning models can address them. Nature is a powerful elixir and can enhance health in urban settings in many ways. Trees, parks, and wildscapes can provide both direct health improvements (e.g. cooling increasingly hot urban environments), and more indirect benefits, such as encouraging more physical activity and helping to overcome sedentary lifestyles, and helping foster friendships and social connections. Investment in green and natural elements of cities, from tree planting to urban trails, is good from a societal (and economic) perspective, and one that pays considerable health dividends. These investments in nature will also help a city to be more resilient and sustainable.

An urban landscape perspective can help, as it takes an integrative view on social and ecological urban systems and networks. It recognizes the intricate links between people and place. The chapter describes some particularly promising approaches that have emerged; for example, green urbanism, resilience thinking, biophilia, and biophilic cities, and it has provided some examples of cities embracing and implementing these approaches.

The challenges faced by urban planners and decision makers advancing this urban nature agenda are substantial, however. Despite the abundance of good planning ideas (see e.g. Corburn, 2009), implementation remains a problem. Insufficient political support, and limited financial resources (and possibly perverse economic incentives), are challenges as are some larger cultural forces (long work weeks and limited time for outside nature; and a growing time sink of computers and digital media of various kinds, for instance). Moreover, even within the professional ranks, the need remains to enhance landscape thinking in urban planning, specifically for public health and well-being.

References

Antrop, M. (2005). Why landscapes of the part are important for the future. *Landsc Urban Plan*, 70, 21–34.

Beatley, T. (2000). *Green Urbanism: Learning From European Cities*. Washington, DC: Island Press.

Beatley, T. (2011). *Biophilic Cities: Urban Design and Planning that Integrates Nature*. Washington, DC: Island Press.

Beatley, T. (2014). Launching the Global Biophilic Cities Network. Nature of Cities Collective Blog. Available at: http://www.thenatureofcities.com/2013/12/04/launching-the-global-biophilic-cities-network/ (accessed 15 May 2015) [Online].

Beatley, T. (2017). *Handbook of Biophilic City Planning and Design*. Washington, DC: Island Press.

Biswas, A., Oh, P. I., Faulkner, G. E., *et al.* (2015). Sedentary time and its association with risk for disease incidence, mortality, and hospitalization in adults. Ann Int Med, 162, 123–32.

Centers for Disease Control (2016). Adult Obesity Facts. Available at: http://www.cdc.gov/obesity/data/index.html (accessed 15 May 2015) [Online].

City of Melbourne (2011). Urban Forest Strategy. Making A Great City Greener 2012–2032. Available at: http://www.melbourne.vic.gov.au/SiteCollectionDocuments/urban-forest-strategy.pdf (accessed 22 April 2016) [Online].

Corburn, J. (2009). *Toward the Healthy City: People, Places, and the Politics of Urban Planning*. Cambridge, UK: MIT Press.

Council of Europe (2000). European Landscape Convention. Strassbourg. Available at: http://www.coe.int/t/dg4/cultureheritage/heritage/Landscape/default_en.asp (accessed 5 April 2015) [Online].

Cycling Embassy of Denmark (2015). Facts about Cycling in Denmark. Available at: http://www.cycling-embassy.dk/facts-about-cycling-in-denmark/statistics/ (accessed 22 April 2016) [Online].

Denckla-Cobb, T. (2011). *Reclaiming Our Food: How the Grassroots Food Movement Is Changing the Way We Eat*. North Adams, MA: Storey Press.

Derbyshire, D. (2007). How children lost the right to roam in four generations. *Daily Mail*, 15 June 2007.

Donovan, G., Michael, Y. L., Butry, D. T., Sullivan, A. D., & Chase, J. M. (2011). Urban trees and the risk of poor birth outcomes. *Health Place*, 17, 390–3.

Dunstan, D. W., Barr, E. L., Healy, G. N., *et al.* (2010). Televison viewing time and mortality: the Australian Diabetes, Obesity and Lifestyle Study (AusDiab). *Circulation*, 121, 384–91.

FAO (undated). Food for the Cities. Brochure. Rome, Italy: FAO. Available at: ftp://ftp.fao.org/docrep/fao/012/ak824e/ak824e00.pdf (accessed 5 June 2016) [Online].

Foster, S. & Giles-Corti, B. (2008). The built environment, neighborhood crime and constrained physical activity: An exploration of inconsistent findings. *Prev Med*, 47, 241–51.

Gesler, W. (2005). Therapeutic landscapes: an evolving theme. *Health Place*, 11, 295–7.

Guitart, D., Pickering, C., & Byrne, J. (2012). Past results and future directions in urban community gardens research. *Urban For Urban Greening*, 4, 364–73.

Holt-Lunstad, J., Smith, T. B., & Bradley Layton, J. (2010). Social relationships and mortality risk: a meta-analytic review. *PLoS Med*, 7, e1000316

Interface (2015). The Global Impact of Biophilic Design in the Workplace. Available at: http://humanspaces.com/global-report/ (accessed 23 April 2016) [Online].

Jorgensen, A., Hitchmough, J., & Dunnet, N. (2006). Woodland as a setting for housing-appreciation and fear and the contribution of residential satisfaction and place identity in Warrington New Town, UK. *Landsc Urban Plan*, 79, 273–87.

Kaplan, R. & Kaplan, S. (1989). *The Experience of Nature: A Psychological Perspective*. Cambridge, UK: Cambridge University Press.

Kellert, S. R., Heerwagen, J. H., & Mador, M. L. (eds) (2008). *Biophilic Design: The Theory, Science & Practice of Bringing Buildings to Life.* Hoboken, NJ: John Wiley & Sons.

Kenward, A., Yawitz, D., Sanford, T., & Wang, R. (2014). *Summer in the City: Hot and Getting Hotter.* Princeton, NJ: Climate Central.

Konijnendijk, C. C. (2008). *The Forest and the City—The cultural landscape of urban woodland.* Berlin, Germany: Springer.

Louv, R. (2008). *Last Child in the Woods: Saving Our Children from Nature-Deficit Disorder.* Chapel Hill, NC: Algonquin Press.

McDonald, N. (2007). Active Transportation to School: Trends Among U.S. Schoolchildren, 1969–2001, *American Journal of Preventative Medicine*, 32, 509–16.

Milligan, C. & Bingley, A. (2007). Restorative places or scary spaces? The impact of woodland on the mental well-being of young adults. *Health Place*, 13, 799–811.

Muir, R. (2005). *Ancient Trees, Living Landscapes.* Stroud, UK: Tempus.

Nilsson, K., Baines, C., & Konijnendijk, C. C. (eds) (2007). *Health and the Natural Outdoors.* Final report of a COST Strategic Workshop. Brussels, Belgium: COST.

Reeder, D. A. (2006). London and green space. 1850–2000: an introduction. In: Clark, P. (ed.) *The European City and Green Space: London, Stockholm, Helsinki and St Petersburg, 1850–2000*, pp. 30–40. Hants, UK: Ashgate Historical Urban Studies.

Rogers, S. H., Halstead, J. M., Gardner, K. H., & Carlson, C. H. (2011). Examining walkability and social capital as indicators of quality of life at the municipal and neighborhoods levels. *Appl Res Qual Life*, 6, 201–13.

Rudd, M., Vohs, K. D., & Aaker, J. (2012). Awe expands people's perception of time, alters decision making, and enhances well-being. *Psychol Sci*, 12, 1130–6.

Seeland, K., Moser, K., Scheutle, H., & Kaiser, F. G. (2002). Public acceptance of restrictions imposed on recreational activities in the peri-urban Nature Reserve Sihlwald, Switzerland. *Urban For Urban Greening*, 1, 49–57.

Sreetheran, M., Konijnendijk van den Bosch, C. C. (2014). A socio-ecological exploration of fear of crime in urban green spaces—A systematic review. *Urban For Urban Greening*, 13, 1–18.

Sugiyama, T. & Thompson, C. W. (2007). Older people's health, outdoor activity and supportiveness of neighbourhood environments. *Landsc Urban Plan*, 82, 168–75.

Thompson, C. W., Travlou, P., & Roe, J. (2006). Free-range teenagers: the role of wild adventure space in young people's lives. Final report, prepared for Natural England. Edinburgh, UK: OPENspace.

Tzoulas, K., Korpela, K., Venn, S., et al. (2007). Promoting ecosystem and human health in urban areas using Green Infrastructure: a literature review. *Landsc Urban Plan*, 81, 167–78.

United Nations (2014). World Urbanization Prospects: The 2014 Revision, Highlights (ST/ESA/SER.A/352). New York, NY. Available at: https://www.compassion.com/multimedia/world-urbanization-prospects.pdf [Online].

United States Department of Agriculture (USDA) (2009). Access to Affordable and Nutritious Food: Measuring and Understanding Food Deserts and Their Consequences: Report to Congress. Available at: https://www.ers.usda.gov/webdocs/publications/42711/12716_ap036_1_.pdf?v=41055 (accessed 15 April 2015) [Online].

Van den Berg, A. E. & Konijnendijk, C. C. (2012). Ambivalence towards nature and natural landscapes. Chapter 7. In: Steg, L., Van den Berg, A. E., De Groot, J. I. M. (eds.) *Environmental Psychology: An Introduction*, pp. 67–76. Chichester, UK: BPS Blackwell.

Walker, B., Salt, D., & Reid, W. (2006). *Resilience Thinking: Sustaining Ecosystems and People in a Changing World.* Washington, DC: Island Press.

World Health Organization (WHO) (2015). Global Health Observatory Data. Available at: http://www.who.int/gho/ncd/risk_factors/physical_activity_text/en/ (accessed 15 April 2015) [Online].

Worpole, K. (2007). 'The health of the people is the highest law'. Public health, public policy and green space. In: Thompson, C. W. & Travlou, P. (eds) *Open Space: People Space: Engaging with the environment*, pp. 11–21. Conference Proceedings. London & New York: Taylor & Francis.

Zezza, A. & Tasciotti, L. (2010). Urban agriculture, poverty and food security: Empirical evidence from a sample of developing countries. *Food Policy*, 35, 265–73.

CHAPTER 8.3

Nature in buildings and health design

Stephen R. Kellert[††]

Biophilia and biophilic design

Theory backed by a growing body of evidence increasingly indicates people possess an inherent inclination to affiliate with the non-human environment—other species and the natural habitats, systems, and processes we commonly refer to as 'nature' (Kellert, 2012). This theory has been called *Biophilia* (Wilson, 1986; Kellert and Wilson, 1993, Kellert, 1997; 2008; 2012). Biophilia is essentially an understanding of human evolutionary biology, recognizing that for more than 99% of human history our species evolved in adaptive response to largely natural, not artificial, forces and stimuli. Indeed, much of what we regard as 'normal' today is of relatively recent origin—the invention of large-scale agriculture some 12,000 years ago, the creation of the city approximately 6,000 years in the past, industrial production roughly 400 years old, and electronic technology, only since the nineteenth century. As a consequence, the human body, mind, and senses evolutionarily developed under mainly the pressure of *biocentric*—not human invented or engineered—factors.

The result is that we are biologically programmed to respond to a wide variety of environmental cues and natural stimuli. Illustratively, a classic study by the Swedish psychologist, Arne Öhman (1986; Ulrich, 1993), found that people subliminally exposed to pictures of snakes, spiders, frayed electric wires, and handguns, elicited largely aversive reactions to snakes and spiders and indifference to the more modern threats. This study is both illustrative and cautionary. It demonstrates the continued emotive power of features and forces of the natural environment, but also that at least some of these reactions can be viewed as vestigial (i.e. reactions that evolved under once-adaptive circumstances, but that today have become largely irrelevant and will likely eventually atrophy over time).

Despite this possibility, a growing body of empirical data increasingly suggests many of our inherent affinities for the natural world continue to be instrumental in human physical and mental health and well-being. While the evidence supporting this relationship is not extensive and the studies often methodologically limited, the breadth of the findings across a wide variety of disciplines and human endeavours cumulatively supports the impression that certain forms of contact with nature remain important in human health, fitness, and well-being. This relationship has been revealed in studies of nature contact in educational, office, manufacturing, residential, community, and healthcare settings (Kellert, 2012).

For example, in the healthcare field, studies have reported that exposure to nature can result in stress relief, muscle relaxation, lower blood pressure, reduced cortisol levels, mitigation of pain, and healing and illness recovery (see Bowler *et al.*, 2010; Cama, 2009; Kellert, 2012; Kellert and Heerwagen, 2008; Kuo, 2010; Searles, 1960; Taylor, 2001; Townsend and Weerasuriya, 2010; Ulrich, 1993; 2008; Annerstedt and Währborg, 2011; Wells and Rollings, 2012). Further, later large-scale research projects have provided high-quality evidence for actual impact on various health states by nature contact, demonstrating both reduced morbidity and mortality (see e.g. Gascon *et al.*, 2016 and Alcock *et al.*, 2014). You can read more about this research in Section 3. In addition, other research and anecdotal evidence indicates that contact with nature can have significant healthcare operational benefits including increased comfort, satisfaction, motivation, morale, and performance of hospital staff, improved employee recruitment and retention, and reduced conflicts among patients, staff, and hospital visitors (Ulrich, 2008; Kellert and Finnegan, 2011).

Despite the apparent continuing importance of contact with nature, a number of obstacles exist in modern society to the adaptive and robust occurrence of biophilia. Of particular importance, biophilia is a 'weak'—not hard-wired—biological tendency, which like much of what makes us human is heavily reliant on learning, experience, and social support to fully and functionally develop (Wilson, 1986; Kellert, 2012). This dependence on learning is what allows humanity to be inventive and distinctive as individuals and societies, but also permits people by equal measure to behave in self-destructive and self-defeating ways. With respect to biophilia, people can either engage with the natural world in an adaptive or an inadequate and counterproductive manner. Unfortunately, for various historical and cultural reasons discussed elsewhere (Kellert, 2012), modern society has increasingly separated itself from the experience of nature, having largely concluded that the natural world is just raw material to be converted through human inventiveness to higher and better uses, or a nice but not necessary recreational amenity. This assumption is reflected in modern agriculture, manufacturing, architecture, urbanization, healthcare, and elsewhere. Unfortunately, this anthropocentric view has taken us to the situation where we are now facing decreasing biodiversity, environmental degradation, and climate change. Read more about this important issue in Chapter 7.5.

[††]It is with regret we report the death of Stephen R. Kellert during the preparation of this textbook.

With respect to modern healthcare, the prevailing medical model views illness as largely a physical malady to be remedied through mechanical means. Reflecting this bias, healthcare facilities are usually highly antiseptic and technological environments that routinely exclude non-human nature as either irrelevant or a potential threat. As a consequence, the typical healthcare facility is a featureless, sensory deprived setting devoid of natural forms and features.

The design of the built environment is especially critical in modern society as the 'natural habitat', so to speak, of contemporary humans has mainly become a constructed world. Our species may have evolved in nature, but today we spend 90% of our time indoors in a human created setting. Moreover, some four-fifths of the population in industrially developed countries now live in an urban area, historically the most environmentally transformed, degraded, and artificial of all human habitats, and where people are routinely separated from ongoing contact with nature. This contemporary shift away from the natural world has been further exacerbated by the exponential growth of electronic technology. Recent data, for example, reveals the typical American child is engaged with electronic media for more than 50 hours, while is outside involved in free play for less than one hour during a typical week (Louv 2005, Kaiser Family Foundation 2005).

Before concluding that modern humans have become largely disconnected from the natural world, it is important to recognize the experience of nature can occur in multiple ways. The most obvious form is direct contact with the natural world in outdoor settings. In addition, people experience 'indirect' contact with nature through various interactions that involve continuous human input and control such as a potted plant, a garden, aquarium, pet animals, and more. Finally, people especially in modern society experience nature vicariously and representationally through pictures, symbols, stories, recordings, television, video, computers, and more. All forms of contact with the natural world—direct, indirect, and vicarious—are important to human health and well-being, although no effective substitute exists for the unparalleled benefits of direct experience as a consequence of its particular multisensory, dynamic, unpredictable, and ambient qualities (Sebba, 1991; Kellert, 2012; Pyle, 1993).

Biophilic design of healthcare facilities

Assuming the validity of the biophilia hypothesis that people continue to rely on contact with nature for their health and well-being, a fundamental challenge in modern society is how to ensure this occurs in the built environment. This is essentially the challenge of what has been called *biophilic design*—the design of buildings and constructed landscapes that foster human health and well-being through contact with nature in places of cultural and ecological significance (Kellert and Heerwagen, 2008; Kellert and Finnegan, 2011).

The basic objective of biophilic design is to create good habitat for people as an evolved biological organism in the built environment. A number of basic principles derive from this understanding, including:

1. Biophilic design emphasizes human adaptations to the natural world that over the long course of human evolution have advanced health and well-being.

2. Biophilic design seeks to foster positive and sustained engagement with natural features and processes.

3. Biophilic design nurtures an emotional attachment to particular landscapes and places.

4. Biophilic design promotes positive interactions of people with one another and with the natural world.

5. Biophilic design involves functionally interconnected and mutually reinforcing forms of contact with nature with each application, contributing to the overall coherence of the human ecosystem.

The biophilic design of healthcare facilities emphasizes experiences of nature that contribute to patient comfort, satisfaction, and treatment, the enhanced performance and productivity of healthcare personnel, and that promote operational effectiveness and efficiency. The application of biophilic design to healthcare facilities will inevitably vary depending on particular situational circumstances, opportunities, and constraints.

A range of biophilic design tools or strategies have been identified and are roughly divided into three types focusing on the direct experience of nature, indirect contact with natural forms and processes, and characteristics of space and place. The *direct experience of nature* involves actual contact in the built environment with natural features and forces such as sunlight, air, plants, animals, water, landscapes, and more. *Indirect contact with nature* refers to the representation or image of nature, the transformation of natural materials, and particular patterns and processes of the natural world in which humans developed an affinity for over evolutionary time. Examples include artwork and pictures of nature, natural material furnishings such as wood and stone, ornamentation inspired by shapes and forms found in the natural world, and such natural processes as organized complexity, fractal geometry, and more. Finally, the *characteristics of space and place* refers to spatial features of the natural environment of particular relevance to humans such as, for example, an affinity for prospect and refuge, the former because over evolutionary time it assisted people in locating food and water and identifying sources of danger and, the latter, because it contributed to safety and security.

Related to these three categories of biophilic design are a number of specific design strategies that have been identified, although as noted, the choice of which to apply inevitably varies depending on circumstances and constraints. Also as emphasized, the choice of particular design applications should be mutually reinforcing, seeking to create an integrated whole or human ecosystem. With these cautions in mind, the following specific biophilic design applications are as follows:

Direct experience of nature

1. **Visual experience of nature**. Sight is the dominant sensory means by which humans experience the natural world. This occurs through views to the outside or visual contact with water, plants, animals, landscapes, and other natural features. Aesthetically appealing nature can enhance people's interest, curiosity, imagination, and creativity. When lacking visual contact with nature, such as windowless spaces or aesthetically displeasing nature, people are often bored, frustrated, and emotionally and cognitively impaired.

2. **Multisensory experience of nature.** Other sensory experiences of nature include sound, touch, taste, smell, and motion.

Multisensory contact with nature can enhance motivation and comfort, relieve stress, and promote better performance. Touching plants, hearing water or animal sounds, and smelling flowers can be both restful and stimulating. Conversely, unnatural sensory stimulation such as loud mechanical sounds are often disturbing and debilitating. (Read about multisensory experiences of nature in Chapter 2.5).

3. **Light.** The experience of natural light, or artificial light that mimics the dynamic and spectral qualities of natural light, foster physical and mental well-being. Access to natural light is especially satisfying, while artificial lighting that simulates the warm, cool, and dynamic properties of natural light is most beneficial. Diffuse and variable light can also evoke the dynamic and sculptural qualities of natural light.

4. **Air.** Natural atmospheric conditions such as outside ventilation, airflow, and thermal comfort enhance health and well-being. Natural and clean air, comfortable humidity and temperature levels, and variable airflow can contribute to enjoyment and satisfaction. This can be achieved through engineering or access to outside conditions, such as operable windows.

5. **Vegetation.** Vegetation and flowering plants often contribute to comfort, reduce stress, and improve performance. Single or isolated plants typically exert little effect. Vegetation in the built environment should be abundant and ecologically connected. Native rather than exotic plants are preferable, and invasive species should be avoided.

6. **Animals.** The experience of animal life such as fish in an aquarium, birds in an aviary or at feeders, butterflies in a garden, can be emotionally and intellectually pleasing and restorative. This can be achieved through enclosures, tanks, cameras, video, and creative landscape design. (Read about health benefits from contact with animals in Chapter 4.2).

7. **Water.** Water is essential to life and its positive experience in the built environment can relieve stress, enhance comfort, and promote cognitive functioning. The human affinity for water is multisensory involving sight, sound, touch, taste, and movement. The experience of water can be achieved through fountains, constructed wetlands, and other strategies. (Chapter 5.2 discusses the specific impact of water on human health and well-being).

8. **Landscapes.** Certain landscapes have been important in human evolution, such as savannah settings that include spreading vegetation, an open understory, and the presence of water. Even nonspectacular natural scenery, such as a grove of trees or grass, can be restorative.

9. **Natural systems.** Self-sustaining natural systems that support an array of environmental features and processes are often satisfying. This can occur through access to outdoor areas, or with sufficient care can be creatively designed such as a native ecosystem or green roof.

Indirect experience of nature

1. **Representational images of nature.** The image and representation of nature can be emotionally and intellectually satisfying. This can be achieved through photographs, paintings, sculptures, and other images and symbols of plants, animals, water, geological features, and landscapes.

2. **Natural materials.** Materials that involve the transformation of nature occur in furnishings, flooring, fabrics, and more. Prominent natural materials include wood, stone, wool, cotton, and leather. These materials are visually and tactility satisfying, revealing the dynamic properties of organic growth in response to environmental forces over time.

3. **Natural colours.** Colour is an attribute of people's adaptive reaction to the natural world that over evolutionary time has assisted in locating food and water, aiding movement, and wayfinding. Earth tones and hues can be especially satisfying.

4. **Organic shapes and forms.** Some of the most appealing shapes and forms are inspired by elements and features of the natural world. A fabric, decoration, or sometimes even the shape of an entire building can suggest the wings of a bird, the contours of a plant, or the geometry of a shell. (Read about the shapes and patterns of nature in Chapter 2.5.)

5. **Movement and mobility.** An essential condition of human survival has been the ability to navigate diverse settings. The presence of clear pathways and points of entry and egress are especially important, fostering comfort and security, while their absence often results in confusion and claustrophobia.

6. **Growth and time.** Nature is dynamic and continuously changing. Living and organic forms reflect patterns of growth and efflorescence. People enjoy environments that possess dynamic qualities that reflect adaptation to circumstances, and mimic the organic qualities of growth and change.

Characteristics of space and place

1. **Prospect and refuge.** Prospect provides visual access to surrounding environments, often achieved through long vistas. Within buildings this can occur by spatial connections among spaces and views to the outside. Refuge is the experience of secure and protected spaces. Especially satisfying places often possess a mix of prospect and refuge.

2. **Organized complexity.** People covet complexity in natural and human settings because it signals an environment rich in resources and opportunities. Yet, environments too complex can be confusing. What people seek are complex environments that are orderly and organized.

3. **Integrated and coherent space.** People enjoy settings with clear and discernible boundaries, and where the relationships between spaces possess overall coherence. These spaces foster a sense of familiarity and security.

4. **Simulation of natural space.** Built environments that possess qualities of exterior settings are especially satisfying. This can be achieved through expansiveness, as well as the application of natural rather than artificial geometries such as curves, sinuous patterns, and avoiding monolithic shapes and forms.

5. **Cultural and ecological connection to place.** Humans are territorial because over evolutionary time it contributed to the control of resources, enhanced mobility, and security. An attachment to place reflects a territorial propensity and can be achieved through cultural and ecological connection to local settings. Relevant designs include the use of indigenous materials, vernacular forms, and local plants and animals. A sense of place often encourages ecological and cultural conservation.

Biophilia and biophilic design in healthcare facilities

This chapter will conclude with some briefly described examples of biophilia and biophilic design in the healthcare field. This presentation should be viewed with caution for two reasons. First, the author's knowledge of the healthcare field is limited, and this will result in the omission of many relevant examples. Second, all those examples cited offer only partial illustrations of the impact of biophilia and biophilic design, as none provide a comprehensive instance of the application of biophilic design in the healthcare field.

Roger Ulrich's studies

Roger Ulrich, a professor of architecture at the Centre for Healthcare Building Research at Chalmers University of Technology in Sweden, has been in the forefront of assessing the health and healing impacts of nature in healthcare settings. Related to this examination, Ulrich contributed insightful chapters to our original volumes *The Biophilia Hypothesis* (1993) and *Biophilic Design* (2008), where he cited several relevant examples briefly described here.

The first is a frequently referenced study of patients recovering from gall bladder operations who were variably exposed to views of nature (Ulrich, 1984). Patients were demographically matched and randomly assigned to two types of room—those with a window view of trees and vegetation, the others of a brick wall. The nature view patients had significantly better physical, mental, and behavioural health outcomes. The researchers reported (1993:107): 'Patients with the nature window view had shorter post-surgical hospital stays, … fewer minor post-surgical complications, [and] far fewer negative comments in nurses notes … The wall view patients required far more potent pain killers.' While this important research provides a partial confirmation of the theory of biophilia, it does little in the way of advancing the application of biophilic design beyond underscoring the importance of views of nature.

A second Ulrich study focused on the impact of a biophilic design retrofit of a windowless hospital emergency room. The original emergency room was a largely featureless space lacking windows, having blank walls, filled with artificial furnishings, and devoid of nature. High levels of stress and aggressive behaviour occurred in this room among visitors and between visitors and staff, prompting calls for its redesign. The emergency room retrofit resulted in an attractive and colourful mural of plants and animals in a savannah-like setting, natural material furnishings and carpeting, organically designed fabrics, and potted plants. It remained a windowless room and the experience of nature was largely indirect and representational. Nonetheless, post-occupancy research found a significant decline in stress levels and aggressive behaviour. This study illustrates the importance of even indirect contact with nature, natural materials, and organic shapes and forms in helping to relieve stress and create a more healthful setting.

A third Ulrich study examined the impact of a new psychiatric facility in Gothenburg, Sweden. The building it replaced was monolithic, barren, and sensory deprived. By contrast, the new facility contained extensive gardens, plant-filled courtyards and interior spaces, widespread natural light, prospect and refuge spaces, widespread occurrence of organic shapes and forms, and natural materials. Post-occupancy research found a significant decline in hostility and aggression, the use of physical restraints dropping by more than 40%, and a 20% decline in compulsory injections used to control aggressive behaviour (Kellert and Finnegan, 2011). The calming and emotionally restorative impact of exposure to nature was again demonstrated, although the lack of a systematic approach to the application of biophilic design limits the lessons to be learned from this occurrence.

Yale-New Haven Smilow Cancer Center, New Haven, Connecticut, United States; Doernbecher Children's Hospital, Portland, Oregon, United States

Two healthcare facilities that have incorporated nature into their interior spaces are the Yale-New Haven Hospital Smilow Cancer Center in New Haven, Connecticut, and Doernbecher's Children's Hospital in Portland, Oregon, both in the United States. At the Smilow Cancer Center, the interior designer, Rosalyn Cama, incorporated several nature-related features including flowing water, extensive planting, a healing garden, tropical aquaria, and widely distributed paintings and photographs of plants, animals, and landscapes. At Doernbecher Children's Hospital, whimsical and childlike depictions of birds and other animals, colourful murals, and vegetation occurred throughout the facility. At both hospitals, anecdotal evidence indicated contact with nature exerted significant stress-relieving effects on patients and visitors alike, and contributed to staff satisfaction and morale. Still, the lack of an overall biophilic design strategy in both instances, and little focus on the external environment, limits the lessons to be learned from these applications.

Khoo Teck Puat Hospital, Singapore

An ambitious attempt at integrating nature into a hospital setting is Khoo Teck Puat Hospital in Singapore. The hospital was conceived from the outset as a 'hospital in a garden, a garden in a hospital', where 70% of the 32-acre site was designed to include gardens, verdant open spaces, and water features. The hospital complex includes an astonishing variety of plants and animals, diverse terrestrial and aquatic habitats, and thousands of identified species of birds, fish, butterflies, flowering plants and other wild animals and vegetation, as well as extensive cultivated flowers and edible and medicinal plants. The hospital has also opened its natural areas to the surrounding community, establishing a highly successful urban farm and creating a strong sense of place.

Khoo Teck Puat Hospital is an impressive accomplishment from the perspective of bringing nature into a hospital setting. Yet, the evidence of its healing, therapeutic, and operational impacts is limited and largely anecdotal. Moreover, from a design perspective, the overall biophilic approach seems somewhat fragmented. No comprehensive biophilic design strategy appeared to guide this effort or its intended health outcomes. The prevailing assumption appeared to be that any contact with nature is beneficial, with the result being a confusing array of design interventions with uncertain impacts. Additionally, contact with nature seemed to be largely confined to the direct experience of the outside environment with little approach to the biophilic design of interior spaces.

Conclusion

Theory and evidence have been cited in support of the theory of biophilia that humans possess inherent affinities for nature and natural processes that continue to exert significant physical and mental health and well-being effects. This apparent demonstration has enormous implications for the practice of medicine and the design of healthcare facilities and their associated landscapes.

This chapter identified a framework for the biophilic design of healthcare facilities. This design framework should not be applied, however, in a fragmented and checklist fashion, but rather by seeking to create an integrated and mutually reinforcing whole. Like any organism, humans function best in ecosystems that consist of linked and complementary elements where the emergent whole is greater than the sum of its parts. Not all contact with nature is necessarily biophilic. An isolated planter, a sterile water feature, or a single picture typically exerts few, if any, health impacts. The biophilic design of healthcare facilities should be engaging, ongoing, coherent, and integrated.

A brief review of examples of biophilia and biophilic design in existing healthcare settings provided some important lessons and precedents. None rose to the level, however, of a model of what can be achieved. The effective biophilic design of healthcare facilities should be guided by the principles and design strategies outlined in this chapter, and include an empirical assessment of the health and operational impacts of these interventions. A potentially revolutionary change in the design of healthcare facilities may be at hand, one that recognizes how much the human body, mind, and spirit remain deeply contingent on the quality of the connections to the world beyond ourselves of which we remain a part.

References

Alcock, I., White, M., Wheeler, B., Fleming, L., & Depledge, M. (2014). Longitudinal effects on mental health of moving to greener and less green urban areas. *Environ Sci Technol*, 48, 1247–55.

Annerstedt, M. & Währborg, P. (2011). Nature-assisted therapy: systematic review of controlled and observational studies. *Scand J Public Health*, 39, 371–88.

Bowler, D. E., Buyung-Ali, L. M, Knight, T. M., & Pulin, A. S. (2010). A systematic review of evidence for the added benefits to health of exposures to natural environments. *BMC Public Health*, 10, 456.

Cama, R. (2009). *Evidence-based Healthcare Design*. Hoboken, NH: John Wiley.

Gascon, M., Triguero-Mas, M., Martinez, D., *et al.* (2016). Residential green spaces and mortality: A systematic review. *Environ Int*, 86, 60–7.

Kellert, S. R., Heerwagen, J., & Mador, M. (2008). *Biophilic Design: the Theory, Science, and Practice of Bringing Buildings to Life*. Hoboken, NJ: John Wiley.

Kellert, S. (2012). *Birthright: People and Nature in the Modern World*. New Haven, CT: Yale University Press.

Kellert, S. (2008). *Bringing Buildings to Life: Understanding and Designing the Human-nature Connection*. Washington, DC: Island Press.

Kellert, S. (1997). *Kinship to Mastery: Biophilia in Human Evolution and Development*. Washington, DC: Island Press.

Kellert, S. & Wilson, E. O. (1993). *The Biophilia Hypothesis*. Washington, DC: Island Press.

Kellert, S. & Finnegan, B. (2011). *Biophilic Design: the Architecture of Life*. Available at: https://www.bullfrogfilms.com [Online].

Kellert, S. & Heerwagen, J. (2008). Nature and healing: the science, theory, and promise of biophilic design. In: Guenther, R. & Vittori, G. (eds). *Sustainable Healthcare Architecture*. Hoboken, NJ: John Wiley.

Kaiser Family Foundation (2005). *The Effects of Electronic Media on Children Ages Zero to Six: A History of Research*. Menlo Park, CA: H. J. Kaiser Family Foundation.

Kuo, F. (2010). *Parks and Other Green Environments: Essential Components of a Health Human Habitat*. Washington, DC: National Recreation and Parks Association.

Louv, R. (2005). *Last Child in the Woods: Saving Our Children from Nature-Deficit Disorder*. Chapel Hill, NC: Algonquin Press.

Öhman, A. (1986). Face the beast and fear the face: animal and social fears as prototypes for evolutionary analyses of emotion. *Psychophysiology*, 23, 123–45.

Pyle, R. (1993). *The Thunder Tree: Lessons from an Urban Wildland*. Boston, MA: Houghton-Mifflin.

Searles, H. (1960). *The Nonhuman Environment in Normal Development and Schizophrenia*. New York, NY: International Universities Press.

Sebba, R. (1991). The landscapes of childhood. *Environ Behav*, 23, 395–422.

Taylor, A. (2001). Coping with ADD: the surprising connection to green places. *Environ Behav*, 33, 54–77.

Townsend, M. & Weerasuriya, R. (2010). Beyond Blue to Green: the Benefits of Contact with Nature for Mental Health and Wellbeing. Available at: https://www.Beyondblue.org.au [Online].

Ulrich, R. (1984). View through a window may influence recovery from surgery. *Science*, 224, 420.

Ulrich, R. (1993). Biophilia, biophobia, and natural landscapes. In: Kellert, S. R. & Wilson, E. O. *The Biophilia Hypothesis*. Washington, DC: Island Press.

Ulrich, R. (2008). Biophilic theory and research for healthcare design. In: Kellert, S. R., Heerwagen, J., & Mador, M. (eds) *Biophilic Design: The Theory, Science and Practice of Bringing Buildings to Life*. Hoboken, NJ: John Wiley.

Wells, N. & Rollings, K. (2012). The natural environment: influences on human health and function. In: Clayton, S. (ed.) *The Oxford Handbook of Environmental and Conservation Psychology*. London, UK: Oxford University Press.

Wilson, E. O. (1986). *Biophilia: The Human Bond with Other Species*. Cambridge, UK: Harvard University Press.

CHAPTER 8.4

Green infrastructure—approach and public health benefits

Raffaele Lafortezza and Cecil Konijnendijk van den Bosch

A definition of green infrastructure

'Green infrastructure' (GI) is a term that is increasingly appearing in worldwide land conservation and development discussions (Benedict and McMahon, 2002). GI is conceptualized broadly as including natural features such as parks, forest reserves, wetlands, and marine areas, as well as man-made features (e.g. greenways and cycle paths). There is no commonly accepted or authoritative definition of the term, but GI is generally described as an interconnected network of green spaces, which together enable delivery of goods and services, and ultimately benefits to society.

The concept of GI is rooted in planning and conservation efforts dating back one hundred and fifty years. Nineteenth-century American landscape architect Frederick Law Olmsted stated that 'No single park, no matter how large and how well designed, would provide citizens with the beneficial influences of nature' (cited by Benedict and McMahon, 2002). Instead parks should preferably be linked to one another and to surrounding residential neighbourhoods.

In many major metropolitan areas, green space is rapidly disappearing. Human intervention has created fragmented development patterns that threaten native plant and wildlife communities and their associated ecological functions and processes. Social and economic consequences are also resulting from the loss of green space, which include negative impacts on public health, the depletion of biodiversity, and the increased costs of public services. To address these issues, smart conservation programmes are necessary to promote resource planning, protection, and management. GI, in particular, offers a smart solution to today's social and economic challenges because it seeks to plan land development and conservation *together* in a way that is consistent with natural environmental patterns (Naumann *et al.*, 2011).

GI originates from two important principles: (i) linking parks and other green spaces for the benefit of people; and (ii) preserving and linking natural areas to benefit biodiversity and counter habitat fragmentation (Benedict and McMahon, 2002). Given its multifunctional nature, there is no single science or discipline responsible for GI (Benedict and McMahon, 2002); the nearest integrative scientific discipline accountable for its evolution is landscape planning. Although GI has been studied since the 1970s in Germany and other countries, it is still a relatively new policy instrument, for example at the European Union level (EC, 2012a; 2012b). GI relies on the theories and practices of numerous scientific and land planning professions, such as conservation biology, landscape ecology, urban and regional planning, geographic analysis and information system, and economy.

Research into GI needs to accommodate different spatial scales since its application can range from individual buildings to neighbourhoods and cities, to entire regions (Naumann *et al.*, 2011). According to Lafortezza *et al.* (2013), GI plans should be embedded at a variety of spatial scales from the local to transnational level, with each level linked to the next. This is also supported by the European Environment Agency (EEA, 2011) which identifies three spatial groups (i): local, neighbourhood, and village scale; (ii): town, city, and district scale; and (iii): city-region, regional, and national scale. City-region appears to be a particularly useful level when planning GI, as it is large enough to be strategic with identifiable ecological hubs and links, yet not too large to be remote from community level activities and local delivery plans.

GI comprises an approach that addresses the connectivity of ecosystems, their protection, and the provision of ecosystem services (ES) while addressing mitigation of, and adaptation to, climate change. It helps ensure the sustainable provision of ecosystem goods and services while increasing the resilience of ecosystems. It also promotes integrated spatial planning by identifying multifunctional zones and by incorporating habitat restoration measures and other connectivity elements into various land-use plans and policies (EEA, 2011).

The potential health benefits of GI have been divided into three main groups: (i) increased life expectancy and reduced health inequality; (ii) improvements in levels of physical activity and health; and (iii) promotion of psychological health and mental well-being (Forest Research, 2010). The creation and management of GI in connection with territorial planning may be directed towards enhancing landscape connectivity and, hence, provide greater access to individuals to undertake green exercise. The ultimate goal of GI is to contribute to the development of a greener and more sustainable economy by investing in ecosystem-based approaches, thus delivering multiple benefits in addition to technical solutions while mitigating the adverse effects of transport and energy infrastructures.

A framework for green infrastructure

Based on the key principles of GI, the EEA report (2011) proposes that GI may: (a) act as a strategically planned network of high-quality green spaces and environmental features; (b) provide multifunctional benefits; (c) assist in place-making; and (d) deliver 'smart' conservation. It also proposes that GI benefits be presented in terms of ES, as this provides a relatively consistent and effective language that has growing resonance with policy makers and other stakeholders. Read more in Chapter 8.5 'Ecosystem services and health benefits—an urban perspective' about ecosystem services.

To support the process of developing and delivering GI, a new Green Infrastructure Framework (GIF) was proposed by Lafortezza *et al.* (2013) (Fig. 8.4.1). It represents a multifunctional, multiscale, and temporal approach that advances EEA's guiding principles while offering a new perspective on the connection between ecological and social factors contended by Weber *et al.* (2006) and Tzoulas *et al.* (2007). The GIF can support long-term plans and decisions on new GI from the local to regional, national, and trans-national level. It consists of five interconnected components, each corresponding to a specific function or cluster of functions that mark the interrelation between the different functions and benefits related to GI. Following guidance from the Millennium Ecosystem Assessment (MA, 2005), the GIF focuses particularly on the linkages between ES and human well-being. Of equal importance to the framework are the GI functions related to biodiversity, social and territorial cohesion, and sustainable development (James *et al.*, 2009; EEA, 2011). A GI that supports these elements and ES creates the environmental settings for human well-being and community health. Moreover, the GIF may assist planners and managers in developing GI plans and delivering multiple benefits to communities (Forest Research, 2010).

Key characteristics of green infrastructure

At the European scale, GI has been defined as a concept addressing ecosystem connectivity and protection, the provision of ES, as well as mitigation and adaptation to climate change (EEA, 2011). The concept is key to the overall objective of ecosystem restoration, which is currently an EU 2020 biodiversity target. Improving the functional and spatial connectivity of landscapes is a prerequisite for the ability of GI to mitigate and adapt to climate change and, in turn, to increase the value of the goods and services that ecosystems provide (Grimm *et al.*, 2008; Hodgson *et al.*, 2009). As nature's building blocks, ecosystems are important for providing species habitats and, when functioning adequately, a number of essential services to benefit humans (EC, 2012a). ES such as cleaning the air, filtering water, and cycling nutrients are provided by forest areas, wetlands, and other natural ecosystems (Weber *et al.*, 2006). GI affects the capacity of ecosystems to provide services across a range of landscape scales (Feld *et al.*, 2009). For example, GI can mitigate risks from climate change by protecting urban regions against floods and other negative effects of changing weather patterns (Krause *et al.*, 2011). However, with regard to spatial connectivity, a potential threat to ecosystem functionality and the provision of ES is the increasing fragmentation of landscapes and ecosystems. Natural ecosystems have become scattered across the landscape because of increasing urbanization and transport infrastructure. From a social perspective, landscape fragmentation intensifies social and economic divisions and the alienation of man from nature (Benedict and McMahon, 2002). Therefore, approaches and

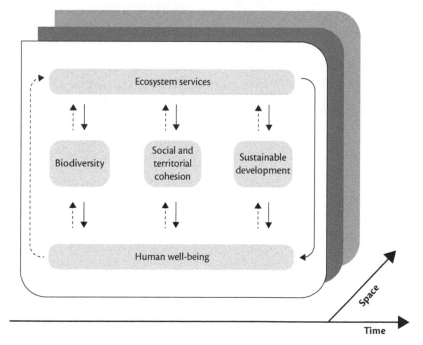

Fig. 8.4.1 A green infrastructure that supports ecosystem services, biodiversity, social and territorial cohesion, and sustainable development creates the environmental settings for human well-being and community health. The Green Infrastructure Framework (GIF) recognizes the importance of the scale at which land-use planning is undertaken and supports the idea of having a bundle of benefits at different spatial and temporal scales.

Adapted with permission from Lafortezza R *et al.*, 'Green Infrastructure as a tool to support spatial planning in European urban regions,' *iForest*, Volume 6, pp. 102-108, Copyright © 2013 by the Italian Society of Silviculture and Forest Ecology.

strategies that overcome fragmentation and enhance functionality are required.

In relation to GI's ability to protect ecosystem functions and promote ES, some researchers refer to the concept of ecosystem 'disservices' to describe the negative or unintended consequences for humans or the environment (e.g. Pataki *et al.*, 2011). Examples are increasing allergens, promoting invasive plants, hosting pathogens or pests, inhibiting human mobility and safety, or increasing fertilizer use for the management of urban trees and plants. There is little research evidence of the unwanted side effects of GI, which are labelled ecosystem disservices; however, these must be kept in mind when evaluating GI performance.

Green infrastructure and public health

As other chapters in this book show, there is a growing body of evidence to support the notion that contact with the natural environment can positively impact human health and well-being (EC, 2012a; Lafortezza *et al.*, 2009). Natural ecosystems provide a variety of services, some of which promote basic human survival, for example, by limiting the spread of disease or reducing air pollution. However, the World Health Organization (WHO, 1948) defines human health not simply in terms of lack of illness or disease but as 'a state of complete physical, mental, and social well-being' (WHO, 1948), which recognizes that a wide variety of factors contribute to overall good health. The contribution of GI to human health through its various ES is grounded in a beneficial outcome to humans resulting from the healthy functioning of ecosystems (EC, 2012a; 2012b). GI features (i.e. connectivity, multifunctionality, accessibility) provide many health benefits, including physical, psychological/emotional, and socioeconomic benefits that can be identified at both the individual and community level. To plan a GI system, its basic attributes or features must first be identified. 'One way to think about such attributes is by the benefits they provide: whether these are associated primarily with natural ecosystem values and functions or with benefits to people' (Benedict and McMahon, 2006). Needless to say, these benefits often overlap.

Several factors related to public health are closely associated with maintaining biodiversity within urban natural habitats, which is one of the roles provided by GI (EC, 2012a). In a study to assess the positive effects of urban biodiversity on the well-being of individuals visiting urban and peri-urban green areas, Carrus *et al.* (2013) concluded that the level of biodiversity and peri-urban location positively affect self-reported benefits, well-being, and perceived restorativeness. Zaghi *et al.* (2010) affirmed that species biodiversity offers protection against the spread of disease. By protecting and promoting biodiversity and ES, GI can thus contribute to these vital aspects of public health.

GI supports the health and well-being of local communities by creating more cohesive places to live, work, thrive, and connect with nature (Forest Research, 2010). Recent studies have proposed GI as a way of engaging people with the rural landscape (Espeseth and Cassens, 1996), as GI can provide cultural, ecological, and psychological linkages between people and the environment. In fact, an increasing number of epidemiological studies report that the presence of GI features (e.g. connectivity, accessibility, and functionality) increases time spent outdoors (Humpel *et al.*, 2004; Pikora *et al.*, 2003), which in turn, affects health. Furthermore, GI

creation and management in connection with territorial planning can be used to enhance landscape connectivity, accessibility, and functionality. An example is the creation of new cycleways through tree-lined corridors that link residential areas to employment sites and retail centres (Lafortezza *et al.*, 2013).

Socioeconomic health

In light of its characteristics, GI promotes health benefits not only at the individual level but also at the community, city, and regional levels. GI supports the health and well-being of local communities by providing more cohesive places (Forest Research, 2010). Natural features and open spaces play an important role in social cohesion. Kim and Kaplan (2004) reported that by encouraging pedestrianism, GI increases the likelihood of informal interactions and helps to promote a sense of community spirit. Furthermore, GI improves the appearance of an area which, in turn, influences property prices and attracts tourism and investment to the area. This leads to positive consequences for many socioeconomic aspects of a neighbourhood or city, such as employment, income, living and working conditions, access to public services, and good-quality housing (Tzoulas *et al.*, 2007).

It has been acknowledged that a healthy and well-functioning community is likely to continue to enhance ES to capitalize on the resources available, therefore initiating a positive feedback loop and reinforcing the benefits of GI (Butler and Oluoch-Kosura, 2006). Moreover, GI has been shown to reduce healthcare expenditures. In fact, an evaluation from the United Kingdom (Bird, 2004) estimated that if 20% of the population that lives within 2 km of a green space used it for 30 minutes of physical activity per day, five days per week, the savings to the National Health Service could be over £1.8 million (€2.7 million) per year. An improved understanding of the empirical links between GI and health will lead to more accurate estimates of economic implications. Read more in Chapter 10.3 'Environmental assessment and health impact assessment' on economic aspects of nature and GI.

Green infrastructure planning: public health outcomes

Applying a GI approach to spatial or territorial planning can help manage land in a more sustainable way, focusing on asset functionality, maximizing the multiple potential benefits (including health benefits) and dealing with the potential conflicting demands and pressures (e.g. housing, industry, transport, energy, agriculture, nature conservation, recreation, and aesthetics) (EEA, 2011). Spatial planning is a key tool in the development of GI. Investing in and building up GI call for smart and integrated approaches to spatial planning to ensure that limited land areas are capable of providing multiple functions for nature and society. Spatial planning can guide development away from sensitive areas and promote the restoration and enhancement of ecosystems and connections among natural areas.

Over the past 20 years, an increasing number of GI projects have been carried out at a local, regional, national, or transnational scale. Empirical evidence demonstrates that the GI approach is flexible, sound, and cost-effective. However, to optimize GI functioning and maximize its benefits, work on the different scales of GI should be interconnected and interdependent. Building at a local scale, the planning system can include local GI (e.g. green roofs and walls) as part of development projects and for promoting sustainable urban drainage schemes. For regional policy, there is a need to integrate national and regional planning authorities in projects and ensure an adequate regional framework for successful implementation. At the EU level, Member States are encouraged to develop GI strategies that would have significant social and economic benefits and aid in achieving the Europe 2020 objectives (EC, 2013). For example, the European Green Belt initiative, born in 2003 and involving 16 EU countries, aims to better harmonize human activities with the natural environment and increase opportunities for the socioeconomic development of local communities.

The GI approach shows promise for protecting the health and well-being of individuals and populations. The public health benefits that smart urban GI planning can provide are illustrated by several case studies. In one study, the city council of the Augustenborg district of Malmö, Sweden, launched an urban regeneration project that focused on flooding, waste management, and biodiversity (EEA, 2011). The project sought to create an open surface-level storm water system, green rooftops, green walls, and to improve green spaces. To further enhance the community's sense of well-being small allotments to grow food, leisure environments, and play areas for children were set up between housing blocks. The project also introduced renewable energy sources, recycling systems, sustainable construction, and local transport initiatives. Another study, conducted by Peschardt et al. (2012), demonstrated the importance of the GI characteristics of functionality and accessibility in promoting public well-being. The authors conducted a study on nine small public urban green spaces in Copenhagen, showing that these were mainly used by the local inhabitants for socializing, rest, and health restoration. Similarly, the earlier mentioned study by Carrus et al. (2013) demonstrated that the arrangement and layout of urban and peri-urban green spaces provide positive involvement through the differentiation of areas, accessibility to, and variety of activities. As a result, people tend to spend longer periods in natural settings and offered opportunities for deeper and more meaningful interactions with nature, thus leading to more positive outcomes.

Some GI features may not lead to positive outcomes for individual well-being, but rather cause health problems as well as economic setbacks when planning is not maximized. An example of the first could be park visitors who are allergic to certain plant species (Carrus et al., 2013). Read more about pollen and related allergic reactions in Chapter 7.1 'Allergenic pollen emissions from vegetation—threats and prevention' to learn more about how the issue can be approached.

Regarding economic setbacks, an interesting example is the green roof of the California Academy of Sciences Museum in San Francisco. This one-hectare 'living roof' is renowned for its innovative cooling properties, reduction of storm water run-off, and energy-saving features and provides an educational venue for communicating the importance of design and sustainability. However, its high implementation and maintenance costs have presented a major drawback. Planning GI in a manner that lends more support to the technical rather than human aspect may defeat the purpose of establishing a healthy balance between nature and human well-being and of promoting the consequent benefits discussed in this chapter.

A major factor to consider when planning improvements in the use of GI is 'accessibility' (Forest Research, 2010). The concept of accessibility refers to the quality of the green space provided, whether the area is connected to efficient and affordable public transport and has good access points away from congested roads. Availability of nearby GI therefore not only encourages people to take more physical exercise, but also to travel more sustainably, by either foot or bicycle through green spaces. This engenders an additional health benefit by reducing the CO_2 emissions produced by other transport (Moffat et al., 2010). Indeed, the GI approach is an important element for increasing accessibility to green areas and for encouraging active travel; with its focus on networking and connectivity of green spaces it can aid movement through landscapes (Forest Research, 2010).

Conclusion

Access to green space in cities has been linked to longer and healthier lives. Environmental policy is looking at these links with greater insistence.

A strength of GI is that it differs from other approaches in landscape planning because it considers ecological and social values combined with other land-use developments. In support of this view, the new Green Infrastructure Framework shows that besides the existing GI criteria of hubs, links, and multifunctionality in land-use management, consideration should be given to drivers such as ES, social cohesion, biodiversity, and sustainable development (Lafortezza et al., 2013). With careful planning, management, and community involvement at the landscape, community, and individual site levels, the public health benefits of GI can become additive and even synergistic. Community involvement should ensure that the 'top-down' and strategic perspective of GI is accompanied by a 'bottom-up' approach based on enhancing linkages between local people and local green spaces. Moreover, the relative positioning of green space within built-up areas and its connectivity with other areas are crucial to ensure that the combined benefits of GI are maximized.

While strategic GI implementation seems to be the preferred solution for today's rapidly urbanizing society, it may have negative impacts on its environment if not well planned. GI planning can be improved to better integrate public health dimensions (e.g. social and environmental health determinants of health and education).

In GI urban planning and management, GI development needs to be fine-tuned to better integrate public health aspects. Public bodies and decision makers should ensure adequate functioning of GI to tackle biodiversity loss, maintain and develop sound ecosystems, and improve the public health status within societies at all levels. In addition to health benefits, fostering appreciation of nature through positive personal experiences may lead to relevant positive outcomes, such as creating more environmentally aware citizens. The importance of urban green spaces in everyday lives may also provide inspiration for landscape architects, city planners, policy makers, and importantly health professionals for the future planning and development of our cities.

Acknowledgement

Both authors are working within the EU 7th Framework project GREEN SURGE and acknowledge financial support by the European Commission. Words of thanks also are extended to Yole De Bellis (University of Bari) for support in reviewing the text.

References

Benedict, M. A. & McMahon, E. T. (2002). Green Infrastructure: Smart Conservation for the 21st Century. *Renewable Resources Journal*, 20, 12–17.

Benedict, M. A. & McMahon, E. T. (2006). *Green Infrastructure: Linking Landscapes and Communities*. Washington, DC: Island Press.

Bird, W. (2004). *Natural fit. Can green space and biodiversity increase levels of physical activity?* A report for the Royal Society for the Protection of Birds. Sandy, UK: RSPB.

Butler, C. D. & Oluoch-Kosura, W. (2006). Linking future ecosystem services and future human well-being. *Ecol Soc*, 11, 30.

Carrus, G., Lafortezza, R., Colangelo, G., Dentamaro, I., Scopelliti, M., & Sanesi, G. (2013). Relations between naturalness and perceived restorativeness of different urban green spaces. *Psyecology*, 4, 227–44.

European Commission (EC) (2012a). *The multifunctionality of green infrastructure. Science for Environment Policy*—DG Environment News Alert Service. In-depth report, 37.

European Commission (EC) (2012b). *Guidelines on best practice to limit, mitigate or compensate soil sealing*. Commission Staff Working Document. Brussels. SWD, 101 final. pp. 1–65.

European Commission (EC) (2013). *Green Infrastructure (GI)—Enhancing Europe's Natural Capital*. Communication From the Commission to the European Parliament, the Council, the European Economic and Social Committee and the Committee of the Regions. (COM 249 final).

European Environment Agency (EEA) (2011). *Green Infrastructure and territorial cohesion. The concept of Green Infrastructure and its integration into policies using monitoring systems*. Technical report no. 18/2011. Copenhagen, Denmark: European Environment Agency.

Espeseth, R. D., & Cassens, K. M. (1996). Greenways. Those long, skinny, green parks. *Illinois Parks and Recreation*, 27, 35–6.

Feld, C. K., Martins da Silva, P., Paulo Sousa, J., *et al*. (2009). Indicators of biodiversity and ecosystem services: a synthesis across ecosystems and spatial scales. *Oikos*, 118, 1862–71.

Forest Research (2010). *Benefits of green infrastructure*. Report to Defra and CLG, Contract no. WC0807, Farnham, UK, p. 42.

Grimm, N. B., Foster, D., Groffman, P., *et al*. (2008). The changing landscape: ecosystem responses to urbanization and pollution across climatic and societal gradients. *Front Ecol Environ*, 6, 264–72.

Hodgson, J. A., Thomas, C. D., Wintle, B. A., & Moilanen, A. (2009). Climate change, connectivity and conservation decision making: back to basics. *J Appl Ecol*, 46, 964–9.

Humpel, N., Owen, N., Leslie, E., *et al*. (2004). Associations of location and perceived environmental attributes with walking in neighbourhoods. *Am J Health Promot*, 18, 239–42.

James, P., Tzoulas, K., Adams, M. D., *et al*. (2009). Towards an integrated understanding of green space in the European built environment. *Urban For Urban Greening*, 8, 65–75.

Kim, J., & Kaplan, R. (2004). Physical and psychological factors in sense of community. *Environ Behav*, 36, 313–40.

Krause, B., Culmsee, H., Wesche, K., Bergmeier, E., & Leuschnerj, C. (2011). Habitat loss of floodplain meadows in north Germany since the 1950s. *Biodivers Conserv*, 20, 2347–64.

Lafortezza, R., Carrus, G., Sanesi, G., & Davies, C. (2009). Benefits and well-being perceived by people visiting green spaces in periods of heat stress. *Urban For Urban Greening*, 8, 97–108.

Lafortezza, R., Davies, C., Sanesi, G., & Konijnendijk, C. C. (2013). Green Infrastructure as a tool to support spatial planning in European urban regions. *iForest*, 6, 102–8.

Millennium Ecosystem Assessment (MA) (2005). *Ecosystems and human well-being: synthesis*. Washington, DC: Island Press, p. 155.

Moffat, A. J., Pediaditi, K., & Doick, K. J. (2010). Monitoring and evaluation practice for brownfield regeneration to greenspace initiatives. A meta-evaluation of assessment and monitoring tools. *Landsc Urban Plan*, 97, 22–36.

Naumann, S., McKenna, D., Kaphengst, T., *et al*. (2011). *Design, implementation and cost elements of Green Infrastructure projects*. Final report. Brussels: European Commission.

Pataki, D. E., Carreiro, M. M., Cherrier, J., *et al*. (2011). Coupling biogeochemical cycles in urban environments: ecosystem services, green solutions, and misconceptions. *Front Ecol Environ*, 9, 27–36.

Peschardt, K., Schipperijn, J., & Stigsdotter, U. K. (2012). Use of small public urban green spaces (SPUGS). *Urban For Urban Greening*, 11, 235–44.

Pikora, T., Giles-Corti, B., Bull, F., *et al*. (2003). Developing a framework for assessment of the environmental determinants of walking and cycling. *Soc Sci Med*, 56, 1693–703.

Tzoulas, K., Korpela, K., Venn, S., *et al*. (2007). Promoting ecosystem and human health in urban areas using Green Infrastructure: A literature review. *Landsc Urban Plan*, 81, 167–78.

Weber, T., Sloan, A., & Wolf, J. (2006). Maryland's Green Infrastructure assessment: development of a comprehensive approach to land conservation. *Landsc Urban Plan*, 77, 94–110.

World Health Organization (WHO) (1948). *Preamble to the Constitution of the World Health Organisation as adopted by the International Health Conference*. New York, 19–22 June 1946; signed on 22 July 1946 by the representatives of 61 states and entered into force on 7 April 1948.

Zaghi, D., Calaciura, B., Spinelli, O., *et al*. (2010). *Literature study on the impact of biodiversity on human health*. Comunità Ambiente Srl, report for the European Commission (Directorate General Environment).

Ecosystem services and health benefits—an urban perspective

Elisabet Lindgren, My S. Almqvist, and Thomas Elmqvist

Defining ecosystem services

An ecosystem is a dynamic system of interacting organisms (i.e. plants, animals, and microorganisms and their physical environment). Ecosystems constitute an important part of the planet's life-supporting systems and contribute to essential needs such as food, water, pure air, shelter, and climate regulation (Corvalan *et al.*, 2005). Ecosystem services refer to services and goods provided by ecosystems that are of importance for human society and well-being (Daily, 1997; MA, 2005). The concept of ecosystem services identify the importance of nature and the benefits gained from ecosystems. Many of the outcomes of ecosystem services provide direct and indirect benefits for health (Corvalan *et al.*, 2005).

Ecosystem services are divided into four main groups (MA, 2005). Provisioning ecosystem services include products obtained from ccosystems, such as food and water. Regulating ecosystem services refer to benefits obtained from the regulation of ecosystem processes, such as regulation of local climate and air quality. Supporting ecosystem services maintain biodiversity and support other ecosystem services. Cultural and spiritual ecosystem services cover non-material benefits, such as aesthetic considerations and recreation.

Loss of ecosystem services negatively impacts health. For example, biodiversity loss tends to increase pathogen transmission and outbreaks of communicable diseases (Keesing *et al.*, 2010). On the other hand, acknowledging the beneficial direct and indirect linkages between ecosystem services and human health in, for example, city planning, leads to better health among local citizens. By the end of the day, we must realize that the basic fundament for our mere survival is functional natural ecosystems.

Provisioning ecosystem services

Provisioning ecosystem services provide essential goods for human survival, livelihoods, well-being, and health. This includes for example water and food, fibres, natural building materials, fuel for cooking and heating, as well as medicinal plants. Water is essential for life on Earth. Freshwater used for drinking, irrigation, and other human purposes is captured, filtered, and stored by vegetation cover, forests, wetlands, and lakes (MA, 2005). A rapidly growing global population will put additional pressure on the food systems, and sustainable agricultural methods will become increasingly important for future food production, both in marine and terrestrial environments.

Many plant species have medical properties and modern medicine continues to rely on biodiversity, containing the raw material for biotechnology for the development of new drugs (WHO, 2003; David *et al.*, 2015). Conservation and protection of ecosystem diversity, in particular in forest ecosystems, and sustainable collection practices are important to avoid extinction of both known and, so far, unknown medicinal plants and microorganisms (WHO, 2003).

Regulating ecosystem services

Several regulating services provided by ecosystems have direct or indirect beneficial effects on health. For example, ecosystem services provide local and global climate regulation, moderation of extreme events, water run-off mitigation, soil erosion prevention, waste treatment, air purification, noise reduction, pollination, and biological control.

Terrestrial and marine ecosystems play an important role in climate regulation, since they absorb parts of anthropogenic carbon emissions (MA, 2005). Trees act as sinks of carbon dioxide (CO_2) by storing excess carbon as biomass during photosynthesis. Biodiversity and ecosystem services are important both for climate change mitigation and adaptation, and for reducing local vulnerability and increasing resilience to climate change. Thus, ecosystem services will contribute to a reduced burden of disease from climate change, both at present and in the future.

Vegetation cover prevents against flooding, landslides, and soil erosion. Areas prone to landslides after heavy rains may be protected by the planting of trees and vegetation that stabilizes the ground. The protective capacities of many ecosystems contribute to sustainable disaster risk management and vulnerability reduction in disaster-prone areas. In coastal areas, wetlands, mangroves, deltas, and coral reefs act as natural barriers against storm surges, tsunamis, and flooding (TEEB, 2011). Restoring or replanting wetlands and mangrove close to coastal settlements can markedly reduce the risk for deaths, negative health impacts, and material damage caused by extreme events (Danielsen *et al.*, 2005).

Wetlands and aquatic ecosystems contribute to waste treatment by filtering out and decomposing organic matters in wastewaters through dilution, assimilation, and chemical recomposition (TEEB, 2011). Solid waste is treated by natural storage capacities and bacterial decomposition of ecosystems. However, wetlands used for waste water purification might create breeding sites for disease-transmitting insects, such as the Anopheles malaria mosquitos and the Culex mosquitos that are involved in West Nile virus transmission. This needs to be taken into account when restoring wetlands, as biological control measures might be required. Many ecosystems are important for regulating plant, animal, and human diseases. Larger predator mammals, birds, bats, wasps, frogs, and fungi and so on, contribute to the natural control of microorganisms, as well as of insects, arthropods, rodents, and other animals that are involved in the transmission cycles of infectious diseases.

Supporting ecosystem services

Ecosystem services depend on the functioning of local ecosystems and on biodiversity for their deliverance. Ecosystems provide habitats for living organisms and maintain genetic diversity. Maintaining biodiversity is for example of importance for controlling vector- and rodent-borne diseases, since changes in biodiversity may lead to changes in the distribution or density of species involved in disease transmission, or to invasion of new species and the risk of emergence of new disease threats.

Cultural, aesthetic, and spiritual ecosystem services

Cultural services can be described as non-material benefits obtained from ecosystems, and include recreation, mental and physical health and well-being, tourism, aesthetic appreciation and inspiration for culture, art and design; spiritual experience, and sense of place and social cohesion. Spending time in nature is proven important, and has many health benefits associated with recreational, aesthetic, and spiritual aspects.

Using nature for recreational purposes and for physical activities has many verified positive effects on health, as described in several chapters of this book. Nature plays an important role as a provider of aesthetic and psychological benefits that enrich human life with meanings and emotions (Chiesura, 2004). In many cultures, features such as specific trees, forests, caves, and mountains are considered sacred. Nature is deeply embedded in many religions and customs, and thus contributes to a sense of belonging as well as spiritual experience.

Urban ecosystem services and health

All ecosystem services are directly or indirectly of importance for urban populations (TEEB, 2011; Elmqvist et al., 2013). Several of the urban ecosystem services also have implications for the health and well-being of a city's inhabitants.

Water

Access to fresh water is essential in a rapidly growing city and may become an issue in politically unstable regions if the city depends on water sources located far from the urban area. In Europe alone (Pan-European Region as defined by UNEP, including 54 member countries) millions of people lack access to piped household drinking water supplies. In low- and middle-income countries 10 people per day die from diarrhoea caused by inadequate water or sanitation (Prüss-Ustün et al., 2014). In some areas, urban ground waters may become contaminated with toxic compounds from industrial and traffic emissions. Increases in urban green space may increase urban ground water. Well-managed peri-urban ecosystems can increase water delivery, storm water and wastewater removal, and improve water quality (Larsson et al., 2013).

Moderation of extreme events and water run-off mitigation in cities

In cities, pavements and buildings make the surface impermeable to rain water. Thus excessive rain will increase surface run-off and may cause flooding. Urban flooding will, depending on local vulnerabilities, have a range of impacts on health; from injuries, toxic exposures, and epidemics, to indirect health impacts from damaged infrastructure, non-functional societal services, and impaired livelihoods (Lindgren et al., 2010). Between 2000 and 2011 floods affected 3.4 million people in the Pan-European region and the occurrence and frequency of floods are projected to increase with climate change (Jakubicka et al., 2010).

Greenery and vegetation cover intercept rainwater and increase surface permeability, thereby reducing the risk of flooding. Preserving green space or re-establishing vegetation within a city will reduce the risk of flooding and associated health hazards.

Many coastal cities are partly protected from the impacts of storms, floods, and tsunamis and other natural events by natural barriers such as mangroves, deltas, and coral reefs. Restoring or conserving mangrove ecosystems can both decrease the impacts of coastal storms and help be an effective measure against salt-water intrusion and coastal erosion (Munang et al., 2013).

Local climate regulation

The ambient temperature in a city centre is often several degrees higher than in surrounding peri-urban and rural areas (Gill et al., 2007). This is especially prominent in cities with aggregated high-rises. This so-called urban heat island effect increases the risk of urban heatwaves. Heatwaves are especially hazardous for people with chronic respiratory and cardiovascular diseases, older people, as well as outdoor workers if temperatures are soaring (Åström et al., 2011; IPCC, 2014; Kjellström et al., 2009). Several studies have shown that deaths and the risk of cardiovascular (stroke, ischaemic heart diseases, and so on) and respiratory diseases increase during heatwave events (Michelozzi et al., 2009). The combination of heat and air pollution further increases mortality and morbidity (Ayres et al., 2009; Fischer et al., 2008). This was observed during the two heatwaves in Europe in the summer of 2003 when about 70,000 excess deaths occurred (Robine et al., 2008). In the summer of 2010, the mortality and morbidity in respiratory and cardiovascular diseases increased considerably in Moscow when a severe heatwave coincided with heavy smoke from wildfires that had hit the region after a long drought period (Shaposhnikov et al., 2014).

Urban vegetation, green areas, and waters, such as city gardens and ponds, and nearby forests, lakes, and sea, have a strong capacity to locally buffer heat extremes (Hardin and Jensen, 2007). Greenery, in particular trees, reflects solar radiation and lowers temperatures locally through evapotranspiration and shading (Bowler et al., 2010). Plant evaporation is particularly important in dry climates where the air cools by absorbing heat (McPhearson, 2011). The difference in microclimate that arises between a green space and paved surfaces gives rise to weak winds that help both to cool the surroundings and circulate the air to dilute particulates and other pollutants. Waters, including canals, lakes, streams, and coastal waters within and around a city can also help in modifying extreme temperatures (Burkart *et al.*, 2015).

In addition, urban vegetation has the potential to mitigate greenhouse gas (GHG) emissions and climate change impact. In a cooler green area, the demand for energy used by air-conditioning systems diminishes and thereby emissions are reduced. This could serve as a cost-efficient mitigation method with potentially long-term impact on the urban climate and population health.

Air purification

Air pollution, with or without concurrent heat is a major health hazard, with around seven millions premature deaths globally each year alone. Air pollution-related mortality and morbidity (e.g. respiratory and cardiovascular disease, cancer) decrease with improved air quality (Hu *et al.*, 2008; Rao *et al.*, 2014; IARC, 2013). Emissions from vehicles, home heating, and construction sites within the city, as well as from industrial sites and power plants in the vicinity of the city increase the risk for public health. Often socioeconomically disadvantaged populations live in less favourable areas close to industrial sites and heavy traffic with more air pollution and noise, contributing to increased health inequalities. City planning that maintains or introduces greenery will contribute to less air pollution exposure and, by careful planning, health inequalities can also be addressed. Vegetation and especially certain tree species contribute to improved air quality by filtering out gases and airborne particulates through their leaves; in particular, pollutants such as tropospheric ozone, sulphur dioxide, nitrogen dioxide, carbon monoxide and particulate matter smaller than 10 μm (PM10) (Bowler *et al.*, 2010). Gaseous air pollution is removed either by uptake via the leaf stomata or by the plant surface (Nowak *et al.*, 2006). Airborne particles can be absorbed, but most commonly they are intercepted (e.g. washed off by rain or dropped to the ground with leaf fall). Trees are particularly considered to be efficient in reducing concentrations of pollutants; however the capacity can vary up to 15-fold between different species (Sæbo *et al.*, 2012). In dense street canyons vertical vegetation is considered more effective (horizontal growth may even increase the pollution concentration by a trapping effect) and it has been shown to reduce street level concentrations by as much as 40% for nitrogen dioxide and 60% for PM10 (Pugh *et al.*, 2012). However, when selecting species for urban areas it is important to choose plant species with low allergenic properties in order not to increase allergic disorders. Read more about allergenic pollens and how to reduce the exposure in Chapter 7.1.

The intensity of dust and sand storms carrying particles from areas surrounding a city where land use changes have exposed the soil (causing dust storms like the ones hitting Beijing) or sand from desert areas (e.g. the sand storms blanketing many Saudi Arabian cities) may partly be reduced by establishing a vegetation zone, that helps bind both the bare soil as well as intercepting loose particles.

Noise reduction

A burden of disease assessment for noise pollution performed by the World Health Organization in 2011 showed that sufficient evidence was found to suggest relationships between noise pollution and annoyance, sleep disturbance, and cardiovascular disease (WHO, 2011). The range of disease burden is estimated to 1.0–1.6 million DALYs. Less epidemiological evidences are available for cognitive impairment and tinnitus, but still enough for assuming

an association with environmental noise pollution. One issue is that noise causes adverse molecular changes and systemic bodily changes, even without the person being annoyed and/or aware of the noise (Basner *et al.*, 2014). Preliminary health impact assessments (HIAs) suggest that the health burden from noise is similar to that from air pollution (Stansfeld, 2015). Read more about HIAs in Chapter 8.4.

Vegetation can be used to reduce noise, particularly the perception of noise (Gidlöf-Gunnarsson and Öhrström, 2007). Plant barriers can decrease noise from traffic and other sources through absorption, deviation, reflection, and refraction of sound. Trees and bushes with many branches and thick, fleshy leaves are effective in absorbing sound (Fang and Ling, 2003). Noise barriers can also cause noise to be bounced away or be reflected back toward the source. Clinging vegetation is often used on non-vegetation noise barriers and walls to refract noise. A lawn will also help refract noise. Multiple rows of trees are more effective for noise reduction than a single tree layer, preferably with smaller evergreen shrubs, plants, and grass underneath (Fang and Ling, 2003).

Biological control

Cities with large numbers of people living closely together may lead to increased transmission of mosquito-borne diseases that use humans as reservoirs, such as malaria, dengue, and chikungunya fever. Breeding sites will diminish by avoiding open waters, such as open run-off drainage systems and stagnant waters. Biological control is also used to control, for example, malaria, by adding insect larvae predators to stagnant waters. In many subtropical and tropical cities, small fishes that eat mosquito eggs and larvae are added to ponds and flower pots to control the container breeding *Aedes* species that transmit dengue and chikungunya fever.

Birds contribute to keeping insect populations down. Bird nesting opportunities could be created in city parks and gardens, and around waters, waterways, and surrounding wetlands. Cats may be kept to control rodent populations. Other predators that contribute to biological control, such as birds, snakes, and lizards are often naturally present in tropical and subtropical urban parks, gardens, and in or around waters and waterways (e.g. urban canals). In temperate zones, urban and peri-urban parks and gardens may be managed to control tick populations that are the vectors of Lyme borreliosis and tick-borne encephalitis by removing thick undergrowth and keeping lawns mown short (Gassner *et al.*, 2011).

Tourism

Ecosystems and biodiversity play an important role for many kinds of tourism and contribute to the local economy (TEEB, 2011). However, in densely populated urban environments, domestic and international tourism contribute to the spread of infectious diseases, and the rapid international trade to the introduction of exotic pathogens and species that are involved in different disease transmission cycles (Semenza *et al.*, 2016). Surveillance and an alert public health system, together with ecosystem services that provide biological control will help in reducing the risk of epidemics and the potential emergence and re-emergence of infectious diseases.

Recreation and physical and mental health

The positive health impacts of recreation and exposure to green spaces in cities are covered in several sections of this book. The importance of urban parks and gardens for recreation varies and depends on several criteria including accessibility, penetrability, privacy, comfort, and safety, but also on sensory disturbing factors such as noise pollution and heavy littering (Gómez-Baggethun and Barton, 2013).

Ecosystem services and health in different urban environments

Over the coming decades the global urban population is projected to double, which will create challenges not only for urban governance and the urban environment, but also for public health (Elmqvist et al., 2013). Many negative health effects in a rapidly urbanizing world could be avoided or reduced by urban planning, where the beneficial impacts of urban ecosystem services on health are acknowledged and integrated. In parts of the world, mainly in Europe and North America, where urban growth has slowed down, levelled out, or declined, both challenges and benefits for human health may be present. Table 8.5.1 presents a summary of ecosystem services and impacts on health in three different urban environments (i.e. affluent mature cities, affluent growing cities, and low-income growing cities). Health impacts are divided into three main groups: non-communicable diseases, communicable diseases, and mental health. The different types of urban environments exhibit either negative impacts on health from loss of local ecosystem services, or health benefits from ecosystem services that are maintained, restored, or integrated into the urban environment.

Affluent mature cities

The majority of affluent mature urban environments consist of older cities where the infrastructure, the built environment and governance are well-adapted to local conditions. The economic level has allowed the city to make decisions and take actions against many of the risk factors that may jeopardize urban population health, such as congested traffic, air and noise pollution, unsafe drinking water, poor sanitation, and natural disaster events. However, global changes such as climate change and increased travel and trade will increase the risk of negative impacts on health (McMichael and Lindgren, 2011).

Established affluent mature cities are often well-adapted to current conditions, including extreme events in disaster-prone areas. Earthquake management in Tokyo is one example; another is storm surge protection near coastal settlements in Holland. However, with climate change, the intensity and frequency of weather extremes such as storms, extreme precipitation, and periods with extreme high temperatures will increase in many areas (IPCC, 2013). Heatwave-related health effects will become an increasing problem for the public health sector, in particular since the population in affluent mature cities is becoming increasingly older. Adding greenery (street trees, green walls and roof tops, and so on) will increase both climate change adaptation and mitigation through the cooling effect of vegetation, as well as to a lesser extent, carbon storage.

In many affluent mature cities air quality is improving. This is due to strategies to reduce emissions from traffic, heating, and industrial sources within the city and its surroundings. Adding greenery will further improve urban air quality.

Urban farming is an increasing trend in many affluent mature cities, such as New York. Urban farming may contribute to a sense of place, social interaction, and to the strengthening of neighbourhood participation, as has been shown in the public access community gardens in Berlin (Bendt et al., 2013).

In some mature cities, previously lost capacities of ecosystem services are returning. Investments in conservation programmes and increases in functions and quality of public spaces are of importance for counteracting some of the impacts on health caused by urban transition and global environmental changes.

Affluent growing cities

A characteristic of many affluent growing cities is a rapid urban transition with comprehensive environmental, demographic, and socioeconomic changes that increase the demands on resources, infrastructure, and governance. Trees and greenery are often vanishing. Traffic and construction sites are increasing, and contribute to air and noise pollution. Levels of exposure to air pollution have been shown to have increased significantly in some part of the world; in particular in affluent growing urban areas with large populations (IARC, 2013). Loss of greenery and increases in the number of high-rises and asphalt areas enhance the urban heat island effect and thus increase the city's vulnerability to climate change and heatwaves, particularly if the population is growing older. Decreased surface permeability will increase the risk of flooding in flood-prone areas.

Less recreational urban green space will have negative impacts on both physical and mental health. Loss of green space and increases in traffic congestion may create an urban environment where it is difficult to move around on foot or by bicycle.

City planning that maintains or introduces green and blue areas (e.g. in the form of city parks, ponds, street trees, bushes and flowers, green walls and roof tops) will markedly decrease mortality and morbidity due to flooding, heatwaves, and air pollution; reduce conditions related to noise pollution; provide recreation opportunities, and improve mental health.

Low-income growing cities

About one-third of the current urban population in low-income countries consists of slum dwellers (UN-Habitat, 2012). In 1990 there were less than 750 million slum dwellers worldwide, a number that had grown to about one billion 15 years later, and that is expected to increase to 1.4 billion by 2020 (Lopez-Moreno and Warah, 2007).

Rapid urban growth in low-income countries is often linked to low capacity for governance and planning of the urban development (Elmqvist et al., 2013). This may create new health hazards or enhanced existing concerns. Climate change and intensification of extreme events, such as storms, floods, and heatwaves may become a challenge to poorly constructed infrastructure and buildings. Disappearing vegetation and increased traffic congestion will lead to decreased air quality and noise pollution. Vanishing peri-urban and urban farmland will affect livelihoods and food security.

The importance of urban food production varies between cities. In some low-income urban environments, locally grown vegetables and staple foods may account for a substantial part of locally consumed food (Jacobi et al., 2000). During economic and political crises, urban food production has been shown to play an important

Table 8.5.1 Urban ecosysem services and associated health risks and benefits in three different urban environments

	Affluent mature cities	Affluent growing cities	Low-income growing cities
Non-communicable diseases	**Local climate and air quality reduction**		
	Risks: An elderly population will increase the risk of mortality and morbidity from heatwaves. Adding urban vegetation, for example green roofs and walls, will reduce heat and contribute to improved air quality.	Risks: Diminishing vegetation will increase urban heat island effect and noise and air pollution. Benefits: City planning that maintain or expand urban vegetation will further improve population health.	Risks: Diminishing vegetation will increase urban heat island effect and noise and air pollution. Outdoor workers are at high risk during heatwaves. Benefits: City planning that maintain or expand urban vegetation will further improve population health.
	Moderation of extreme events		
	Risks: Climate change may increase risk of flooding and storms.	Risks: Increases in impermeable surface area will increase risk of flooding. Benefits: Planning for urban green space is important for flood prevention, as well as for natural barriers to prevent coastal storm surges or dust storms.	
	Recreation and physical health		
	Benefits: Safe urban green space facilitates physical activities and promotes stress reduction.	Risks: Urban vegetation will disappear. Benefits: Creating safe city parks—with e.g. out-door gym—will contribute to both physical and mental health.	Risks: Urban vegetation will disappear. Benefits: Creating safe green spaces will contribute to population health and social cohesion.
	Food		
	Benefits: Urban farming, e.g. rooftop gardens, may promote sense of belonging, social interactions and improve mental health.		Benefits: Urban farming is important for food security and nutrition in low-income city parts. Urban food production often becomes important during political crisis and conflicts.
	Medical resources		
			Benefits: Preserve areas for household farming and cultivation of traditional medicinal plants.
Communicable diseases	**Fresh water; waste water treatment**		
	Benefits: Urban green space may lead to increased urban groundwater.	Risks: Urban groundwater may become contaminated with toxic compounds. Benefits: Urban green space contributes to better water quality and quantity.	Risks: Urban groundwater may become contaminated with toxic compounds. Benefits: Urban green space and peri-urban wetlands contribute to better water quality and quantity and waste water treatment.
	Moderation of extreme events		
	Benefits: The risk of epidemics decrease with reduced risk of flooding and storm events.		
	Biological control		
		Benefits: Will reduce the risk of outbreaks of vector- and rodent-borne diseases.	
	Tourism		
	Risks: Increases the spread of infectious diseases.		
Mental Health	**Recreation and mental health, spiritual experience and sense of place**		
	Benefits: Access to safe urban green spaces contributes to recreation, social interactions, less stress-related symptoms, and a sense of place and belonging.	Risks: Urban green spaces will disappear. Benefits: Creating safe city parks and green spaces will promote recreation, and increase mental health.	Risks: Unsafe recreational green spaces may lead to crime and mental stress. Benefits: Important to create safe green spaces to promote social interactions, mental health, and well-being.

role for local food security (Barthel *et al.*, 2010). Reduction in urban green space will not only decrease available cultural land within a city, but also decrease the presence of pollinators that provide an important ecosystem service for food production and, thus, for food security and nutrition. Herbs, plants, and tree parts that traditionally have been used for medical purposes, may also diminish.

In a rapidly growing low-income cities it is, thus, important to keep greenery and prospecting for city parks and so on, to benefit from the range of positive effects on population health provided by associated ecosystem services. Sacred natural places and plants, such as the Bodhi tree could, if possible, be integrated in the expanding urban environment.

Conclusion

Ecosystem services are important not only for human societies and well-being, but also for human health and survival. They provide essential needs (food, water, fibres, fuelwood, medicinal plants, and so on) and help regulate the climate, moderate extremes, mitigate water run-off, prevent erosion, treat waste and wastewater, purify the air, pollinate plants, and control infectious diseases; services that are all directly or indirectly contributing to better poulation health. In addition, nature and ecosystems increase physical and mental health by providing a place for recreation, physical activity, and social interactions, as well as by having aesthetic and spiritual properties.

A rapidly growing urban population worldwide will put focus on ecosystem services and health in cities. Cities depend on the services provided by ecosystems often far from the city itself. However, several ecosystem services maintained within or in close proximity to the city have direct or indirect health benefits, such as regulation of local climate, air quality reduction, and moderation of extreme events. Planting vegetation to reduce the urban heat island effect will reduce heatwave-related health risks. Vegetation and urban green space contribute to several other beneficial effects on health, for example to stress reduction, increased physical activity with accompanying positive effects on health, and improved mental health and well-being. Tourism is important for local livelihoods, but contributes to the spread of infectious diseases and may cause emergence of new threats. Biological control can help to partly reduce urban rodent- and vector-borne disease transmission.

Assessments of ecosystem services and health benefits in a city should be based on local conditions and vulnerabilities. Affluent cities have, for example, an increasingly older population that is at high risk from heatwaves that will become more frequent and intense with climate change. Ecosystem services that affect urban water availability, water quality, and wastewater treatment play different roles of importance depending on the city's geographic location as well as other local characteristics. In many low-income urban environments, urban farming is important for food security, whereas urban farming is becoming an increasingly popular trend in many affluent mature cities, contributing to people's sense of belonging and social interactions with beneficial effects on mental health and well-being.

Acknowledging the beneficial linkages between ecosystem services and human health in city planning will lead to better health among local citizens, both in rapidly growing urban environments in affluent and low-income areas, as well as in affluent mature cities.

References

Åström, D. O., Forsberg, B., & Rocklöv, J. (2011). Heat wave impact on morbidity and mortality in the elderly population: a review of recent studies. *Maturitas*, 69, 99–105.

Ayres, JG., Forberg, B., Annesi-Maesano, I., et al. (2009). Climate change and respiratory disease: European Respiratory Society statement. *Eur Respir J*, 34, 295–302.

Barthel, S., Folke, C., and Colding, J. (2010). Social-ecological memory in urban gardens: Retaining the capacity for management of ecosystem services. *Global Environmental Change*, 20(2), 255–265.

Basner, M., Babisch, W., Davis, A., et al. (2014). Auditory and non-auditory effects of noise on health. *Lancet*, 383, 1325–32.

Bendt, P., Barthel, S., & Colding, J. (2013). Civic greening and environmental learning in public-access community gardens in Berlin. *Landsc Urban Plan*, 109, 18–30.

Bowler, D. E., Buyung-Ali, L., Knight, T. M., & Pullin, A. S. (2010). Urban greening to cool towns and cities: A systematic review of the empirical evidence. Landsc Urban Plan, 97, 147–55.

Burkart, K., Meier, F., Schneider, A., et al. (2015). Modification of heat-related mortality in an elderly urban population by vegetation (urban green) and proximity to water (urban blue): evidence from Lisbon, Portugal. *Environ Health Perspect*, 124, 927–34.

Chiesura, A. (2004). The role of urban parks for the sustainable city. *Landsc Urban Plan*, 68(1), 129–138.

Corvalan, C., Hales, S., & McMichael, A. (2005). Ecosystems and human well-being: health synthesis: a report of the Millennium Ecosystem Assessment. Geneva, Switzerland: World Health Organization.

Daily, G. C. (ed.) (1997). *Nature's Services: Societal Dependence on Natural Ecosystems*. Washington, DC: Island Press.

Danielsen, F., Sorensen, M.K., Olwig, M.F., et al. (2005). The Asian tsunami: a protective role for coastal vegetation. *Science*, 310, 643.

David, B., Wolfender, J. L., & Dias, D. A. (2015). The pharmaceutical industry and natural products: historical status and new trends. *Psychochem Rev*, 14, 299–315.

Elmqvist, T., Fragkias, M., Goodness, J., et al. (eds) (2013). *Urbanization, Biodiversity and Ecosystem Services: Challenges and Opportunities*. Dordrecht Heidelberg New York London: Springer.

Fang, C. F. & Ling, D. L. (2003). Investigation of the noise reduction provided by tree belts. *Landsc Urban Plan*, 63, 187–95.

Fischer, P., Ameling, C., and Marra, M. (2008). Effect of interaction between temperature and air pollution on daily mortality during heat-waves. *Epidemiology*, 19(6), S379.

Gassner, F., van Vliet, A. J., Burgers, S. L., et al. (2011). Geographic and temporal variations in population dynamics of Ixodes ricinus and associated Borrelia infections in The Netherlands. *Vector Borne Zoonotic Dis*, 11, 523–32.

Gidlöf-Gunnarsson, A. and Öhrström, E. (2007). Noise and well-being in urban residential environments: The potential role of perceived availability to nearby green areas. *Landsc Urban Plan*, 83, 115–26.

Gómez-Baggethun, E. and Barton, D.N. (2013). Classifying and valuing ecosystem services for urban planning. *Ecological Economics*, 86, 235–245.

Gill, S. E., Handley, J. F., Ennos, A. R., & Pauleit, S. (2007). Adapting cities for climate change: the role of the green infrastructure. *Built Environ*, 33, 115–33.

Hardin, P.J. and Jensen, R.R. (2007). The effect of urban leaf area on summertime urban surface kinetic temperatures: a Terre Haute case study. *Urban Forestry & Urban Greening*, 6, 63–72.

Hu, Z., Liebens, J., & Rao, K. R. (2008). Linking stroke mortality with air pollution, income, and greenness in northwest Florida: an ecological geographical study. *Int J Health Geographics*, 7, 20.

International Agency for Research on Cancer (IARC) (2013). Air pollution and cancer. Paris, France: IARC Scientific Publications, no. 161.

Intergovernmental Panel on Climate Change (IPCC) (2013). *The Physical Science Basis. Contribution of Working Group I to the Fifth Assessment Report of the Intergovernmental Panel on Climate Change*. Stocker, T. F., Qin, D., Plattner, G. K., et al. (eds.). Cambridge, United Kingdom and New York, NY, USA: Cambridge University Press, p. 1535.

Intergovernmental Panel on Climate Change (IPCC) (2014). Smith, K. R., et al. (2014): Human health: impacts, adaptation, and co-benefits. In: Climate Change 2014: Impacts, Adaptation, and Vulnerability. Part A: Global and Sectoral Aspects. Contribution of Working Group II to the Fifth Assessment Report of the Intergovernmental Panel on Climate Change. Field, C. B., et al. (eds.). pp. 709–54. Cambridge, United Kingdom and New York, NY, USA: Cambridge University Press.

Jacobi, P., Amend, J., & Kiango, S. (2000). Urban agriculture in Dar es Salaam: providing for an indispensable part of the diet. In: Bakker, N., Dubbeling, M., Gündel, S., et al. (eds) *Growing Cities, Growing Food, Urban Agriculture on the Policy Agenda: A Reader on Urban*

Agriculture, pp. 257–284. Germany: Zentralstelle für Ernährung und Landwirtschaft.

Jakubicka, T., Vos, F., Phalkey, R., Guha-Sapir, D., & Marx, M. (2010). Health impacts of floods in Europe: data gaps and information needs from a spatial perspective. A MICRODIS report. Brussels, Belgium: Centre for Research on the Epidemiology of Disasters.

Keesing, F., Belden, L. K., Daszak, P., *et al.* (2010). Impacts of biodiversity on the emergence and transmission of infectious diseases. *Nature*, 468, 647–52.

Kjellström, T., Kovats, R. S., Lloyd, S. J., Holt, T., & Tol, R. S. (2009). The direct impact of climate change on regional labor productivity. *Arch Environ Occup Health*, 64, 217–27.

Larson, J.H., Trebitz, A.S., Steinman, A.D., et al. (2013). Great Lakes rivermouth ecosystems: scientific synthesis and management implications. J Great Lakes Res, 39, 513–524.

Lopez-Moreno, E., and Warah, R. (2007). The state of the world's cities report 2006/2007. United Nations Human Settlements Programme. UN-HABITAT: Nairobi, Kenya.

Lindgren, E., Albihn, A., & Andersson, Y. (2010). Climate change, water-related health impacts, and adaptation. In: Ford, J. D. & Berrang-Ford, L. (eds) *Climate Change Adaptation in Developed Nations*, pp. 177–88. Dordrecht, the Netherlands: Springer.

McMichael, A. J. & Lindgren, E. (2011). Climate change: present and future risks to health, and necessary responses. *J Int Med*, 270, 401–13.

McPhearson, T. (2011). Toward a sustainable New York City: Greening through urban forest restoration. In: *Sustainability in America's Cities: Creating the green metropolis*. Slavin, M (ed.). pp. 181–204. Washington, DC: Island Press.

Michelozzi, P., Accetta, G., De Sario, M., *et al.* (2009). High temperature and hospitalizations for cardiovascular and respiratory causes in 12 European cities. Am J Respir Crit Care Med, 179(5), 383-9. Epub 2008 Dec 5.

Millennium Ecosystem Assessment (MA) (2005). *Ecosystems and Human Well-Being: Synthesis*. Washington, DC: Island Press.

Munang, R., Thiaw, I., Alverson, K., Mumba, M., Liu, J., & Han, Z. (2013). The role of ecosystem services in climate change adaptation and disaster risk reduction. *Curr Opin Environ Sustain*, 5, 47–52.

Nowak, D., Crane, D., & Stevens, J. (2006). Air pollution removal by urban trees and shrubs in the United States. *Urban For Urban Greening*, 4, 115–23.

Prüss-Ustün, A., Bartram, J., Clasen, T., *et al.* (2014). Burden of disease from inadequate water, sanitation and hygiene in low- and middle-income settings: a retrospective analysis of data from 145 countries. *Trop Med Int Health*, 19, 894–905.

Pugh, T. A., Mackenzie, R., Whyatt, J. D., & Hewitt, N. (2012). The effectiveness of green infrastructure for improvement of air quality in urban street canyons. *Environ Sci Technol*, 46, 7692–9699.

Rao, M., George, L. A., Rosenstiel, T. N., Shandas, C., & Dinno, A. (2014). Assessing the relationship among urban trees, nitrogen dioxide, and respiratory health. *Environ Pollut*, 194, 96–104.

Robine, J. M., Cheung, S. L., Le Roy, S., *et al.* (2008). Death toll exceeded 70,000 in Europe during the summer of 2003. *C R Biol*, 331, 171–8.

Sæbo, A., Popek, R., Nawrot, B., Hanslin, H. M., Gawronska, H., & Gawronski, S. W. (2012). Plant species differences in particulate matter accumulation on leaf surfaces. *Sci Total Environ*, 427–8, 347–54.

Semenza, J. C., Lindgren, E., Balkanyi, L., *et al.* (2016). Determinants and drivers of infectious disease threat events in Europe. *Emerg Infect Dis*, 22, 581–9.

Shaposhnikov, D., Revich, B., Bellander, T., *et al.* (2014). Mortality related to air pollution with the Moscow heat wave and wildfire of 2010. *Epidemiology*, 25(3), 359–364.

Stansfeld, S. (2015). Noise effects on health in the context of air pollution exposure. *Int J Environ Res Public Health*, 12, 12735–60.

The Economics of Ecosystems and Biodiversity (TEEB) (2011). TEEB Manual for Cities: Ecosystem Services in Urban Management. Available at: http://www.teebweb.org/publication/teeb-manual-for-cities-ecosystem-services-in-urban-management/ (accessed 8 December 2014) [Online].

UN-Habitat. (2012). State of the World's Cities 2012/2013, Prosperity of Cities. Nairobi: United Nations Human Settlements Programme (UN-Habitat), State of the world's cities series, HS/080/12E.

World Health Organization (WHO) (2003). WHO guidelines on good agricultural and collection practices (GACP) for medicinal plants. Geneva: World Health Organization.

World Health Organization (WHO) (2011). Burden of disease from environmental noise—Quantification of healthy life years lost in Europe. Bonn, Germany: WHO Regional Office for Europe, World Health Organization.

CHAPTER 8.6

The healthy settings approach: Healthy Cities and environmental health indicators

Evelyne de Leeuw and Premila Webster

From structural to social public health

The development of public health has been described as happening in waves; Davies *et al.* (2014) suggest four such waves:

The first wave (approximately 1830–1900) they describe as 'structural public health', concerned with classic public health interventions, such as water and sanitation, and so on, and incorporation concerns with civil and social order.

The second wave (approximately 1890–1950) is a 'biomedical public health' one, driven by scientific rationalism that generated breakthroughs in many fields including manufacturing, medicine, engineering, transport, and communications, and so on. The dominance of the germ theory in public health action led to public health revolutions stemming from vaccination approaches and epidemiological surveillance.

The third wave (approximately 1940–1980) is described by Davies *et al.* as 'clinical', but is probably better described as 'healthcare professional' in that it embeds a wider reach of healthcare systems into the welfare state and social security, social housing, and universal education, and so on.

This professionalist perspective continues in the fourth wave (approximately 1960–present) and is signified as a 'social' concern with health where effective healthcare interventions help to prolong life, a discourse around risk factors and lifestyle become of central concern to public health, and nascent concerns with social inequalities in health become a competing part of the health and welfare state agenda.

In this evolution, the 'biomedical' model of health has been contrasted with a 'social' model. Ilona Kickbusch (2007) shows, however, that both perspectives come together in a pervasive cultural, society-wide, notion of health. What was labelled the 'medical industrial complex' (Ehrenreich and Ehrenreich, 1971)—'the healthcare industry, composed of the multibillion-dollar congeries of enterprises including doctors, hospitals, nursing homes, insurance companies, drug manufacturers, hospital supply and equipment companies, real estate and construction businesses, health systems consulting and accounting firms, and banks'—is shifting to a 'health society' where deep concerns about the (social and other like environmental) causes of health and disease become engrained in a broader societal, commercial, and political discourse.

In this health society, the highly reductionist (and consequently, behaviourist and biomedical gaze) is balanced with a broader, comprehensive view of 'environments for health', including social, built, economic, and natural environments. The latter view—integral to the birth of modern public health and sanitary, as well as hygienist views of urbanization (Porter, 1994)—re-emerged from the twilight of history in a series of statements sponsored by the global community, through the World Health Organization (WHO) and its partners. The first of these was the Alma Ata Declaration on Primary Health Care (PHC) (1976), recognizing the broader context in which health is made. The original PHC approach argued for the full participation of communities in culturally appropriate and affordable actions for health, within and beyond the healthcare system (Baum, 2007).

The Alma Ata Declaration also signalled a global move towards 'Health for All by the Year 2000', in which WHO member states were to develop strategies to improve population health. In the European Region of WHO this took the shape of a number of strategic policy objectives (WHO, 1985; de Leeuw, 1985). Integral to these objectives was the recognition that health development hinges on much more than healthcare services and health behaviour modification, and an international meeting was convened in November 1986 to explore the emerging dimensions of such a new vision for public health. The Ottawa Charter for Health Promotion that resulted from this conference can be seen as a landmark statement in the evolution of the social model of health. It marked the birth of a global health promotion movement (with associated professional development, tertiary training opportunities, scholarly journals, and so on) and the introduction of a range of new ideas to the health field.

The Ottawa Charter also defined health promotion as 'the process of enabling individuals, families and communities to control the determinants of their health'. Together with critical work on health equity and social determinants of health (e.g. Marmot *et al.*, 1987; Wilkinson, 1990), this has led to significant global efforts in mapping the 'causes of the causes' of health and disease (Commission on Social Determinants of Health, 2008). Also, associated comprehensive policy responses to complex health problems were proposed, for instance Health in All Policies (Ståhl *et al.*, 2006) and a global mobilization to address non-communicable diseases (Beaglehole *et al.*, 2011). These dimensional shifts have inspired local action for health in settings such as cities, and in turn those settings demonstrate that action for global health is possible.

Settings: where people live, love, work, and play

The Ottawa Charter explicitly steps away from a risk group approach to health development. People don't live in risk groups, and rarely associate themselves with a 'risk group', but with social and environmental contexts shaped by the settings in which they live, love, work, and play. The settings approach aims to influence health through action on 'the places or social contexts in which people engage in daily activities, in which environmental, organizational and personal factors interact to affect health and well-being' (Nutbeam, 1998), as well as on people found within these settings (Poland *et al.*, 2009; Poland *et al.*, 2000).

The settings approach finds its foundation in an ecological model of health promotion, viewing health and health behaviours under the influence of multiple interacting factors, including physical (natural and built) and social (organizational, community and policy) determinants. Settings must be seen as complex, dynamic, and open systems composed of individuals, structures, and the relations between them, and have permeable boundaries (Dooris, 2004). Mark Dooris also analyses that the settings approach involves developing and changing the setting's organization and structure, and the individuals found within it, rather than focusing on the latter exclusively.

Settings can demonstrably create supportive environments for health (Dooris, 2009) but initiatives such as Health Promoting Workplaces, Healthy Universities, Healthy Prisons, Health Promoting Health Services and Hospitals, Healthy Islands, Healthy Marketplaces, Health Promoting Schools, and Healthy Cities rarely benefit from the potential synergy where one settings embraces the organizational, policy, and social benefits of another setting in which it is located or associated with.

Healthy Cities and healthy urbanization

Never before have the people of our planet moved to live in cities at the rate we are witnessing in the early years of the third millennium (Fig. 8.6.1). Half the world's population is already urbanized, and estimates are that at least 60% of the world population will live in large conurbations by 2030. More people are going to live in cities, and more will live in mega-cities. The UN technical agency for human settlements (UN-Habitat) has even adopted the term 'meta-city' for a 'heterogeneous, dynamic urban region composed of multiple dense centres, intervening suburbs, embedded green spaces, and diffuse boundaries between traditional cities, suburbs, and exurbs' (McGrath and Pickett, 2011).

Though the relationship between urbanization and health seems apparent, no unequivocal empirically validated theories are explaining causal or final correlates between 'urbanization' and 'health'. In 'focused' fields (e.g. environmental health, infectious disease public health, and increasingly lifestyle-related behavioural health) there is a considerable body of knowledge, but theories covering the complex relationship between the concepts (urbanization and health), that both at best can be defined as 'fuzzy', are yet only in the early stages of development.

In a related field, David Clark (1999) concluded a review of the literature with the statement that 'the challenge for analysts is to develop a comprehensive understanding of urban development and change so as to enable governments to act to secure a sustainable urban future'. Healthy Cities, especially in Europe, explicitly embrace this challenge.

Hugh Barton and Catherine Tsourou (2000) attempt to apply an urban planner's perspective to the complex interrelations between health, its determinants, and urban living. They apply the terminology for urban planning as compiled by the European Commission (1994): spatial planning, land use planning, town and country planning, physical planning, territorial planning, and space management systems. But none of those terms would be familiar to public health professionals, nor would probably the notion of

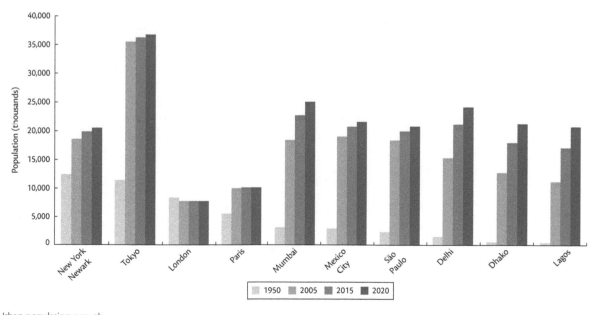

Fig. 8.6.1 Urban population growth.

From United Nations, *World Urbanization Prospects: The 2003 Revision*, Copyright © 2003 United Nations. Reprinted with the permission of the United Nations.

'determinants of health' have a profound meaning in the urban planning commons (Barton and Tsourou, 2000). Nevertheless, Barton, Grant, and Guise (2003), Barton *et al.* (2009), and Corburn (2004) show that modern public health has its roots in urban planning, and urban planning is a public health phenomenon.

Healthy Cities—phases to success

The WHO Regional Office for Europe decided to initiate an urban health promotion programme in 1986 (Hancock and Duhl, 1988; Kaasjager *et al.*, 1989; Kickbusch, 1989; WHO Healthy Cities Project, 1988a; 1988b). There was a clear conceptual link to the Ottawa Charter and a serendipity between an existing 'Healthy City' programme, the evolution of health promotion, and the challenges of urbanization in a social context.

A Toronto Healthy City programme existed since 1984, partly based on a seminal work edited by Leonard Duhl (1963). Duhl and his colleagues compared the urban environment to a living organism which could be healthy in itself, and therefore healthful for its citizens. WHO had hoped that a handful of European cities would want to volunteer in its pilot urban health promotion programme. An exploratory meeting was organized in Lisbon in 1986, and beyond any expectation, some 30 cities wished to commit themselves to the ambitious goals set. This was more than the WHO infrastructure could initially cope with, and a process of designation for European Healthy Cities was set up, as well as a series of more concrete guidelines which Healthy Cities would have to strive for. The main theme of the European Healthy City project became '... to move health high on social and political agendas' (Tsouros, 1994), not just in officially designated cities, but through a commitment by these cities to the establishment of national networks also in other European cities.

World Health Day (each year, 8 April) was officially devoted in 1996 to Healthy Cities. By this time, some 3,000 cities worldwide had in one way or another joined the international Healthy Cities Network. They go under many different labels and approaches, from a 'Healthy Urbanization' programme in the Western Pacific region of WHO, to 'Villes et Villages en Santé' in Quebec, and 'Municipios

para la Salud' in Latin America. As far as we know, the smallest town to adopt the vision is l'Isle-Aux-Grues, an island in the Fleuve St. Laurent in Quebec, Canada (with a population of 146). The largest jurisdiction to adopt a Healthy City vision is Shanghai, China (with a population of about 23,470,000). Michaela Kenzer (1999) provides an inspiring range of examples of urban health activities in a global perspective at that point in time.

Only the European Region of the WHO maintained rigorous entry requirements into its Healthy City Network. For the first (1996–1992), second (1993–1998), and third phase (1998–2002) of the Healthy City programme, cities had to demonstrate political commitment to Health for All and the Healthy City vision, appropriate resource allocations to secure a full-time project coordinator and support staff in a Healthy City Office, and commitment to specific objectives leading to the establishment of local health policies. In the first phase, among the most important of such objectives was the establishment of an urban health profile. In the second phase, designated cities were supposed to be working on the creation of City Health Plans, and the third phase committed Healthy Cities to the production of a City Health Development Plan and a process of more rigorous internal and external monitoring and evaluation.

For designated European Healthy Cities, the policy development evolution would take them from the production of Health Profiles into the development of City Health Plans, and ultimately City Health Development Plans. A City Health Plan is a policy document including the Health Profile identifying health challenges, their determinants, and roles various actors should play in targeting those challenges. A City Health Development Plan takes the process a step further; it identifies strategic development issues, incorporating also urban planning, sustainable development, and equity concerns on a long-term basis.

In recent phases (phase V ending in 2014, and phase VI starting in 2015) designated European cities are expected to commit, through council decisions and resource allocations, to a set of values and principles (e.g. equity in health, community participation, and good governance) and priority development areas with subcategories (WHO, 2009; de Leeuw *et al.*, 2014) (Table 8.6.1).

Table 8.6.1 Prioritised development areas and respective subcategories to which European Healthy Cities are expected to commit

Health and health equity in all policies	Caring and supportive environments	Healthy living	Healthy urban environment and design
	Better outcomes for all children	Preventing non-communicable diseases	Healthy urban planning
	Age-friendly cities	Local health systems	Housing and regeneration
	Migrants and social inclusion	Tobacco-free cities	Healthy transport
	Active citizenship	Alcohol and drugs	Climate change and public health emergencies
	Health and social services	Active living	Healthy urban design
	Health literacy	Healthy food and diet	Safety and security
		Violence and injuries	Exposure to noise and pollution
		Healthy settings	Creativity and liveability
		Well-being and happiness	

Adapted with permission from World Health Organization (WHO), *Phase V (2009–2013) of the WHO European Healthy Cities Network: goals and requirements*, World Health Organization Regional Office for Europe, Denmark, Copyright © World Health Organization 2009, available from http://www.euro.who.int/__data/assets/pdf_file/0009/100989/E92260.pdf

'The' Healthy City, however, does not exist. Each city is unique in its historical and social development. But more importantly, the context in which cities move towards Healthy City status is markedly different in each of the more than 10,000 cities worldwide we identify (de Leeuw and Simos, 2015). The group of designated European Healthy Cities is the core of 22 European national and language networks that each may work under their own organizational and ideological prerequisites (Tsouros and Krampac, 1997; Lafond and Heritage, 2009). In other WHO regions and countries there may be Healthy City networks as well, providing mutual support and information, but under less rigorous entry or recognition conditions.

Most, if not all, about the foundation of the Healthy City concept has been laid down in a series of WHO publications, notably the 'yellow booklets' that were published in the late 1980s (Hancock and Duhl, 1988; Kaasjager et al., 1989; Kickbusch, 1989; WHO/EURO 1988a; WHO, 1988b).

Trevor Hancock and Leonard Duhl (1988) point out that a Healthy City can only be identified by encountering it: 'It must be experienced, and we must develop and incorporate into our assessment of the health of a city a variety of unconventional, intuitive and holistic measures to supplement the hard data. Indeed, unless data are turned into stories that can be understood by all, they are not effective in any process of change, either political or administrative.' But they contend that any Healthy City ' ... that is continually creating and improving those physical and social environments and expanding those community resources which enable people to mutually support each other in performing all the functions of life and in developing to their maximum potential' should strive to provide 11 qualities:

1. A clean, safe physical environment of high quality (including housing quality)

2. An ecosystem that is stable now and sustainable in the long term

3. A strong, mutually supportive, and non-exploitive community

4. A high degree of participation and control by the public over decisions affecting their lives

5. The meeting of basic needs (food, water, shelter, income, safety, and work) to all people

6. Access to a wide variety of experiences and resources, for a wide variety of interaction

7. A diverse, vital, and innovative city economy

8. The encouragement of connectedness with the past, and heritage of citydwellers and others

9. A form that is compatible with the past, and enhances the preceding characteristics

10. An optimum level of appropriate public health and sick care services accessible to all

11. High health status (high levels of positive health and low levels of disease)

The concept of the Healthy City is firmly rooted in an understanding of the historical importance of local governments in establishing the conditions for health and a firm belief that they can and must play an important role in improving the health of their citizens. The Healthy Cities approach promotes a coalition of local governments and community organizations to address priority problems related to urban health and the environment.

One of the main differences between the WHO Healthy Cities project and other community-level health programmes is the central role of local government in the Healthy Cities concept. Another important aspect of the WHO Healthy Cities project is that it focuses on the whole community, with its strengths and problems, rather than being established under single issues or diseases such as tobacco and cancer.

The health of people living in towns and cities is strongly determined by their living and working conditions, the quality of the physical and socioeconomic environment, and the quality and accessibility of care services. The WHO Healthy Cities project aimed to translate the principles of Health for All into practice at the local level in urban settings and, as such, had a great interest in measuring urban health.

Indicators

What are Healthy City indicators?

The Healthy City indicators are numeric measures of health and well-being. Through them an overall picture of the quality of life in the participating cities can be obtained. In a sense, the indicators focus on a small, manageable, and telling piece of life in the cities to give people a sense of the bigger picture. Well-designed and carefully selected indicators can help a community determine where it is, where it is going, and how far it is from chosen goals.

While indicators are as varied as the type of systems they monitor, there are certain generally accepted characteristics that good indicators have in common. Effective indicators:

- identify the essence of the problem; they reflect something basic and fundamental and show us something about the system that we need to know;

- have a clear and normative interpretation; they are easy to understand, even by people who are not experts;

- are robust and statistically valid; we can trust the information that the indicator is providing;

- will respond to effective policy interventions;

- are measurable and based on accessible data.

City health indicators aim to measure and monitor health in cities, thus contributing to evidence-based health policies.

The rationale underpinning the development of the Healthy City indicators

Healthy City profiles and plans to improve the health of citizens were expected to cover health, social, and environmental issues. Indicators were seen as a tool to provide information towards this end.

The objectives of the collection and analysis of indicators of Healthy Cities (HC) indicators were to:

- provide a description of health in the city;

- provide a baseline of information to make comparisons over time;

+ compare and contrast cities allowing for the differing socioeconomic and cultural differences between countries in the region;

+ identify associations between selected indicators.

In order to provide a comprehensive picture of health, the indicators covered the areas of health, health services, environment, and
socioeconomic conditions. They were not intended to be a collection of comprehensive data in order to understand and explain variations. Rather, the aim of collecting such data was to facilitate more
evidence-based, rational policymaking and priority setting in relation
to health. The information was also intended to inform the development of City Health Profiles and lay the foundations of specific City
Health Plans to improve and sustain the health of citizens. Thus, HC
indicators are a part of the logical sequence, firstly collection of routinely available data in an attempt to identify those aspects of the city
that contribute to or detract from the population's health. This information could then be built on and expanded by collecting appropriate local data to develop a health profile of the city to stimulate
political and administrative action in order to create healthy public
policies based on evidence and ultimately action towards these policies. Through them, the first steps towards building an overall picture
of the quality of life in the participating cities could be initiated.

Development of the Healthy Cities' indicators

The need for Healthy Cities' indicators to monitor progress, make
comparisons within a city, and to stimulate change had been clear
from the outset of the project. However, devising indicators, which
captured a range of local initiatives addressing the wider dimensions of health, and then employ these across cities, proved to be
challenging. A working group was set up to meet these challenges
and propose a set of indicators, both objective and subjective, to
cover all aspects of city life.

An early technical challenge to the project was to devise indicators which captured a range of local initiatives addressing the wider
dimensions of health which could be used across the diverse cities in the project. The experience of using indicators at national
level in the Health for All (HFA) Programme throughout the five
WHO regions of the world had shown the variable utility of indicators in that programme. This is because of differing methods of
data collection, and difficulties in interpreting the meaning of global indicators. The WHO recognized these problems particularly
in Europe, and several cross-national consultations took place to
develop common methods and instruments. The experts on these
consultations noted the poor comparability of many broader health
indicators such as those measuring social and economic status.

In 1991, a Multi-City Action Plan on city indicators was convened
with the aim of recording a baseline of activity and measures of
health in the then 47 participating cities. Towards this end, a set of 53
indicators was developed and adopted. The indicators were devised
to reflect the HFA targets; the Ottawa Charter, adapted to a city level;
and the 11 qualities of a Healthy City. The 53 indicators covered
the areas of 'health' (including the traditional indices of mortality),
health services, environment, and social and economic conditions.

The Healthy Cities indicators were an attempt to widen the
sources of data on 'health', which has been recommended in literature (Curtice, 1995). This was the first systematic effort to collect
and analyse such a wide range of data from cities across Europe.
The analysis provided important insights into the way the indicators

were understood by different countries, the extent of the availability
of data, the reliability and validity of the information provided, and
the appropriateness of the indicators for international comparisons.
Following the analysis it was recommended that:

+ a smaller core of the indicators should be adapted from those
identified as useful in the current survey;

+ the focus nevertheless be kept as broad as possible;

+ more attention should be paid to documenting local innovations
in the project; and

+ coordinators should be trained, who would act as chief respondents to a survey in the required methods of completing the survey.

This resulted in the review of the original set of indicators in
1998, resulting in a more concise set of 32 indicators and a second
analysis was carried out near the end of Phase III.

The following are the environmental HC indicators:

Environmental indicators

+ Air pollution
+ Water quality
+ Sewage collection
+ Household waste treatment
+ Green space
+ Derelict industrial sites
+ Sport and leisure facilities
+ Pedestrianization
+ Cycle routes
+ Public transport access
+ Public transport range
+ Living space

Interestingly, green space is now defined as an indicator of a Healthy
City. The indicators for green spaces included:

1. Relative surface area of green spaces in the city. This indicator
was expected to give an idea of vegetation in the city and was
based on the surface area of green spaces relative to the total surface area of the city. The method of calculation was—total surface of green spaces in the city divided by the total surface area of
the city expressed as a percentage.

Following the first collection, it became obvious that there
was a problem with the definition. A number of cities included
only public areas, while others took a broader interpretation
of the term 'green spaces' and included school/sports grounds,
and even cemeteries (National Institute of Public Health,
Denmark. Analysis of baseline healthy cities indicators. 2nd ed.
Copenhagen: WHO Regional Office for Europe, 2001; Centre for
Urban Health, document 5027375 2001/16). The revised indicator was modified to categorize the green spaces under the following headings:

• public park
• private domestic gardens used for food growing
• unmanaged areas that may be wild vegetation or wild life havens.

2. Public access to green spaces—the indicator was expected to estimate the surface area of green spaces per inhabitant opened to the public. The respondents were asked if there was a land use survey carried out by the city and if this was the case could they give details of the survey with regards to public access to green spaces. The method of calculation was the total number of m² of green spaces with public access divided by the number of inhabitants.

Healthy City indicators and sustainable development

The report of the World Commission on Environment and Development 'Our Common Future' examined the relationships between economic development and environmental sustainability, defining sustainable development as 'development that meets the needs of the present without compromising the ability of future generations to meet their own needs'. The UN Conference on Environment and Development in 1992 moved the debate further with Agenda 21. This programme of action for sustainable development explicitly addressed the relationships between social and economic development, the need to converge and manage resources, the strengthening of the roles of major social groups, and how these are to be achieved.

Working towards sustainable development is a slow and complex process involving planning and cooperation at several levels and between a wide variety of partners. The collection of some of the HC Environmental Indicators could contribute in a small way towards gathering some baseline data on the environment. The analysis of trends could play a role in monitoring whether these indicators are moving in the right direction especially in the areas of reducing the production of pollution and waste.

Limitations of the Healthy City indicators

Valid, reliable, and comparable measures of the health states of individuals and of the health status of populations are critical components of the evidence base for health policy. Ongoing questions regarding the accuracy and validity of the data hamper comparisons and limit our understanding of the differences that exist between cities.

The inherent complexities in collecting and analysing data on health and its determinants to provide a meaningful evidence base to determine health policy and identify appropriate interventions to improve health at the city level is a problem. While work on the Healthy Cities' indicators highlights some of the complexities in collecting and analysing data at the European city level, it also illustrates the wealth of data available to measure and monitor health of people living in Europe's urban areas. However, there are still some questions that remain. Ideally indicators should provide valid, reliable information that is relevant to policy makers and practitioners. Therefore, questions about which type of indicators are most appropriate should be made on the basis of what information is likely to provide the best possible data. Often, the 'best' indicators depend to a large extent on the needs and circumstances of a given region or institution and reflect both the availability of data and local priorities. However, it is also important that indicators are not selected simply because the data is readily available.

As regards the optimal number of indicators, this depends on many factors, including the time and resources available for collection, and the specific needs of the community. While the number of Healthy Cities indicators (HCIs) has been reduced from 53 to 32, there was still much discussion among the cities as to whether this number is too few or too many. While it is true that the current 32

indicators are not comprehensive and the cities could collect additional information about other facets influencing citizens' health, there is some concern regarding the difficulty in collecting such additional data and its subsequent analysis and interpretation. This reflects the ongoing dilemma between indicators that are relevant and those where the data is readily available.

However, even in the absence of statistically reliable data, there is enough information to stimulate discussion about health status in the cities and an individual city's approaches to health. While some problems with data accuracy may be inherent in such broadly based surveys, perhaps a more systematic approach to defining and validating any future indicators, as well as working on ways of collecting comparable data in the cities, would go far in improving the quality of information collected. The most popular indicators will be those which are interpretable, avoid unnecessary complexity, are relevant to health, and are not unduly difficult to collect.

Conclusion

'Healthy Cities' embrace a value-based vision of urban health driven by a recognition of the importance of environments for health- and settings-based promotion. This vision is adapted to unique local contexts around the world and can be driven by many different actors, public sectors, and communities. The European approach is strictly codified to provide strong guidance to a select group of about 100 cities that commit to the pursuit of joint principles and thematic priorities. One of these is to measure, and progress, health and its determinants in the local context.

Essentially HC indicators are useful instruments as they provide baseline description of health and thus identify health problems. In addition, they can aid in evaluation and assess progress by analysing trends to identify whether the health of the city is going in the right direction and whether this direction is being maintained. Indicators have always played a crucial role in measuring and monitoring health status in the Healthy Cities. By turning data into relevant information for policy makers and the public, indicators help cities understand the way in which the urban environment influences population health, thus paving the way to evidence-based, rational policymaking and priority setting in relation to health, and resulting in increased visibility and public interest in such issues.

There are numerous international agencies, institutions, and other programmes that use indicators to measure and monitor urban health. In an effort to provide an integrated and comprehensive view of the urban experience, it is important to coordinate knowledge and research in these areas. This will facilitate the harmonization of indicator development methods, indicator sets, and reporting standards, thus resulting in a more integrated option for monitoring urban health.

References

Barton, H. & Tsourou, C. (2000). Healthy Urban Planning. London, UK: SPON Press.

Barton, H., Grant, M., & Guise, R. (2003). *Shaping Neighbourhoods: A Guide for Health, Sustainability and Vitality*. Oxford, UK: Taylor & Francis.

Barton, H., Grant, M., Mitcham, C., & Tsourou, C. (2009). Healthy urban planning in European cities. *Health Promot Int*, 24(Suppl 1), i91–9.

Baum, F. (2007). Health for All Now! Reviving the spirit of Alma Ata in the twenty-first century: An Introduction to the Alma Ata Declaration. *Soc Med*, 2, 34–41.

Beaglehole, R., Bonita, R., Alleyne, G., *et al.* (2011). UN high-level meeting on non-communicable diseases: addressing four questions. *Lancet*, 378, 449–55.

Clark, D. (1999). Urban development and change: present patterns and future prospects. In: *Symposia—Society for the Study of Human Biology*, pp. 46–66. Cambridge, UK: Cambridge University Press.

Commission on Social Determinants of Health (2008). Closing the gap in a generation: health equity through action on the social determinants of health: final report of the commission on social determinants of health. Geneva, Switzerland: World Health Organization.

Corburn, J. (2004). Confronting the challenges in reconnecting urban planning and public health. *Am J Public Health*, 94, 541–6.

Curtice, L. (1995). Towards the evaluation of the second phase of the WHO Healthy Cities Project. WHO Internal document, January 1995.

Davies, S., Winpenny, E., Ball, S., Fowler, T., Rubin, J., & Nolte, E. (2014). For debate: a new wave in public health improvement. *Lancet*, 384, 1889–95.

de Leeuw, E., Tsouros, A. D., Dyakova, M., & Green, G. (eds). (2014). Healthy cities. Promoting health and equity—evidence for local policy and practice. Summary evaluation of Phase V of the WHO European Healthy Cities Network. Copenhagen, Denmark: World Health Organization Regional Office for Europe.

de Leeuw, E. & Simos, J. (2015). *Healthy Cities—The Theory, Policy, and Practice of Value-Based Urban Health Planning*. New York, NY: Springer.

de Leeuw, E. J. (1985). 2000—a Health Odyssey: An Inquiry Into the Planning and Design of a Regional Strategy for Health for All by the Year 2000 in the European Region of the World Health Organization: Including a Case Study the Lifestyle Issues and the Concerned Interaction Between WHO and the Netherlands Government (Doctoral dissertation, University of Limburg, Maastricht).

Dooris, M. (2004). Joining up settings for health: a valuable investment for strategic partnerships. *Critical Public Health*, 14, 49–61.

Dooris, M. (2009). Holistic and sustainable health improvement: the contribution of the settings-based approach to health promotion. *Perspect Public Health*, 129, 29–36.

Duhl, L., ed. (1963). *The Urban Condition: People and Policy in the Metropolis*. New York, NY: Simon & Schuster.

Ehrenreich, B. & Ehrenreich, J. (1971). *The American Health Empire: Power, Profits, and Politics*. New York, NY: Vintage Books.

European Commission (1994). European Commission Expert Group on the Urban Environment; European Sustainable Cities. Office for Official Publications of the European Communities, Luxembourg. Also available at: http://courses.arch.ntua.gr/fsr/136565/EUROPEAN%20SUSTAINABLE%20CITIES_REPORT.pdf [Online].

Hancock, T. & Duhl, L. (1988). *Promoting Health in the Urban Context*. WHO Healthy Cities Papers No. 1. Copenhagen, Denmark: FADL Publishers.

Kaasjager, D. C., van der Maesen, L. J. G. & Nijhuis, H. G. J. (eds) (1989). The New Public Health in an Urban Context. Paradoxes and Solutions. WHO Healthy Cities Papers No. 4. Copenhagen, Denmark: FADL Publishers.

Kenzer, M. (1999). Healthy cities: a guide to the literature. *Environ Urban*, 11, 201–20.

Kickbusch, I. (1989). Good planets are hard to find. WHO Healthy Cities Papers No. 5. Copenhagen, DenmarK: FADL Publishers.

Kickbusch, I. (2007). Health governance: the health society. In: McQueen, D. V., Kickbusch, I., Potvin, L., Pelikan, J. M., Balbo, L., & Abel, T. (eds) *Health and Modernity*, pp. 144–61. New York, NY: Springer.

Lafond, L. J. & Heritage, Z. (2009). National networks of healthy cities in Europe. *Health Promot Int*, 24(Suppl 1), i100–7.

Marmot, M. G., Kogevinas, M., & Elston, M. A. (1987). Social/economic status and disease. Ann Rev Public Health, 8, 111–35.

McGrath, B. & Pickett, S. T. A. (2011). The metacity: a conceptual framework for integrating ecology and urban design. *Challenges*, 2, 55–72.

Nutbeam, D. (1998). Health promotion glossary. *Health Promot Int*, 13, 349–64.

Poland, B. D., Green, L. W., & Rootman, I. (eds) (2000). *Settings for Health Promotion: Linking Theory and Practice*. Thousand Oaks, CA: SAGE.

Poland, B., Krupa, G., & McCall, D. (2009). Settings for health promotion: an analytic framework to guide intervention design and implementation. *Health Promot Pract*, 10, 505–16.

Porter, D. (ed.) (1994). *The History of Public Health and the Modern State (Vol. 26)*. Amsterdam, the Netherlands: Rodopi.

Ståhl, T., Wismar, M., Ollila, E., Lahtinen, E., & Leppo, K. (2006). *Health in All Policies: Prospects and Potentials*. Helsinki, Finland: Finnish Ministry of Social Affairs and Health.

Tsouros, A. & Krampac, I. (1997). *National Healthy Cities Networks in Europe*, 3rd edition. Copenhagen, Denmark: WHO/ EURO & EURONET.

Tsouros, A. (1994). The WHO Healthy Cities Project: State of the Art and Future Plans. Copenhagen, Denmark: WHO/ EURO/ HCPO.

World Health Organization (1985) Health promotion: a discussion document on the concept and principles: summary report of the Working Group on Concept and Principles of Health Promotion, Copenhagen, 9-13 July 1984. World Health Organization Regional Office for Europe, Copenhagen.

World Health Organization—WHO Healthy Cities Project (1988a). Five-Year Planning Framework. WHO Healthy Cities Papers No. 2. Copenhagen, Denmark: FADL Publishers.

World Health Organization—WHO Healthy Cities Project (1988b). A Guide to Assessing Healthy Cities. WHO Healthy Cities Papers No. 3. Copenhagen, Denmark: FADL Publishers.

World Health Organization—WHO (2009). Phase V (2009–2013) of the WHO European Healthy Cities Network: goals and requirements. World Health Organization Regional Office for Europe. Available at: http://www.euro.who.int/__data/assets/pdf_file/0009/100989/E92260.pdf [Online].

Wilkinson, R. G. (1990). Income distribution and mortality: a 'natural' experiment. *Sociology of Health & Illness*, 12, 391–412.

Natural public health across the world

CHAPTER 9.1

Africa and environmental health trends

Emmanuel K. Boon and Albert Ahenkan

Environmental resources, livelihoods, and human health in Africa

Africa's environmental resources are at the centre of healthcare delivery, human development, and environmental protection of the continent. Health and economies both depend on well-managed natural resources and healthy ecosystems. Human health and development on the continent are largely shaped by environmental resources; their availability and quality. It is against this background that this chapter examines the role of environmental resources in improving human health and livelihoods on the continent and the emerging environmental health management challenges in Africa, with examples from a few selected countries.

Across Africa, natural resources remain central to rural people's livelihoods and health. Wild foods continue to provide the major portion of the animal fats, proteins, and minerals in the diets of millions of its people (FAO, 2016). In Nigeria, for instance, and Ghana, people living near forest reserves consume as much as 84% of their animal protein in the form of game. Although forest foods do not usually provide a complete diet, they do make a critical contribution to the food supply. People in the Congo Basin alone consume more than one million tonnes of wild meat annually (equivalent to four million cattle) (Wilkie, 2001) (Fig. 9.1.1).

Deforestation, population growth, human movement, economics, power, and diseases and health are intimately interconnected. The need to preserve forests for human health is highly evident and it is necessary to assess how forest dwellers can contribute to improving forest management. All over Africa, there is a call on community participation in natural resource management to respond to the fast rate of environmental degradation and impaired human health. However, rapid population growth, urbanization, agricultural expansion, invasive alien species, overfishing, overharvesting, and destruction of habitats are continuous threats.

Predicting the impact of specific land cover changes on human health requires analysis of local conditions (FAO, 2006). The forest resources in most parts of the continent have suffered decades of mismanagement, due mainly to the loosely defined property relations of these resources. While command and control measures have, to some extent, ensured sustainable use and management of ecosystems (UNEP, 2013), there is a need to combine these with sustained public awareness campaigns and effective management approaches to maintain and improve environmental resources in the continent.

Many aspects of natural resource and environmental management cut across the African regions: increasing beneficiary and community participation, developing and sharing environmental friendly technologies, formulating appropriate environmental policies, and promoting rural finance to encourage off-farm income-generating activities and micro enterprise to help take the pressure off environmental resources and improve public health. Other cross-cutting issues of environmental resource management include gender and indigenous knowledge. Nevertheless, the causes and effects of environmental resource degradation also vary considerably across regions, countries, and agro-ecological zones, creating a great diversity of natural resources management challenges. The various approaches to environmental resource management in Africa are the focus of the next section of the chapter.

Importance of environmental resources in Africa

The environmental services provided by forests are seldom fully valued or adequately reflected in forest planning and management decisions in Africa (FOA, 2011). Environmental resources provide social, economic, and environmental benefits in Africa as elsewhere in the world. In addition to biodiversity conservation, watershed protection, forests provide beautiful sites for tourism, recreation, spiritual healing, leisure, and religious practices. Traditionally, non-timber forest products (NTFPs), play important livelihood roles in Africa. It has been estimated that over two-thirds of the continent's 600 million people rely on forest products, either in the form of subsistence uses or as cash income derived from a wide range of timber and non-timber forest products (Timko et al., 2010; FAO, 2011; CIFOR, 2005). The importance of many NTFPs to rural livelihoods cannot be overstated, as a wide variety of forest products are used as natural subsidies by rural households across Africa. These can entail products that are collected directly for subsistence, or those that are 'transformed' through processing. NTFPs are important both for their direct subsistence value, and for their contribution to a household's cash income. Many of these people rely on NTFPs for their primary healthcare and nutritional needs. Goods and services from forests contribute immensely to the quality and standard of living of the African people. They underpin the economies of many African

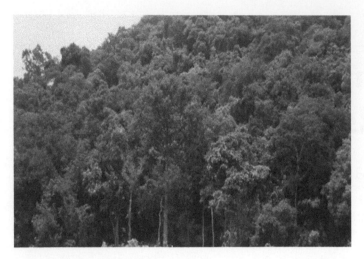

Fig. 9.1.1 Forests resources in Africa.
Image reproduced courtesy of Dr Albert Ahenkan.

countries, while enhancing the quality of the environment and people's lives (Fig. 9.1.2).

Over 70% of the continent's population depends on forest resources for their survival (FAO, 2012; Chidumayo *et al.*, 2011); NTFPs are particularly important for addressing poverty, nutrition, health and empowerment among marginalized forest-dependent communities (Ros-Tonen and Wiersum, 2005; Marshall *et al.*, 2006; Levang *et al.*, 2005; Belcher *et al.*, 2005; Cavendish, 2003; Ahenkan and Boon, 2008). They form an integral part of the livelihood strategy of rural African communities and continue to be an important component of household nutrition and health (Nkwatoh and Yinda, 2007; Sunderland and Ndoye, 2004). It is becoming increasingly obvious that deforestation, degradation of ecosystems, and poor environmental conditions cause much of the health suffering in many local communities (Rapport *et al.*, 1998). Working with communities to devise strategies to optimally use and manage NTFP resources will significantly help to support basic livelihoods and provide a strong incentive for involvement in the conservation of forests.

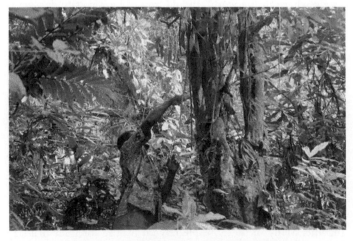

Fig. 9.1.2 Harvesting of non-timber forest products (NTFPs), SW Region, Cameroon.
Image reproduced with permission. Copyright © Christiane Badgley.

Environmental resources and traditional medicine

The use of plants as traditional medicines to treat illness has a long and venerable history in Africa. Traditional medicine is often termed 'complementary', 'alternative', or 'non-conventional' medicine (WHO, 2002). WHO (2003a) defines traditional medicine as 'the total combination of knowledge and practices, whether explicable or not, used in diagnosing, preventing or eliminating physical, mental or social diseases and which may rely exclusively on past experience and observation handed down from generation to generation, verbally or in writing'.

Plant medicines are medicinal products whose active ingredients are derived from aerial or underground parts of plants or other plant material or combination of them, whether in crude state, or as plant preparation. Plant material includes such substances as juice, gums, and oils. Herbal medicines may also contain plant materials other than the active ingredients and may even contain other non-plant organic or inorganic active ingredients (Sekagya *et al.*, 2006). Traditional medicine is also called botanical medicine or phytomedicine, and is defined as the use of whole plants or part of plants to prevent or treat illness (Lee, 2004; Lengkeek, 2004; WHO, 2002). A medicinal plant is any plant that provides health-promoting characteristics or curative properties (Musabayane, 2012). The plant parts used in treating diseases include seeds, berries, roots, leaves, bark, and flowers. Plant medicines cover a wide range of products, from traditional preparations such as teas, simple tinctures, and capsules which contain plant parts to solid dosage forms containing more concentrated dry extracts.

WHO (2002) estimates that 80% of the populations of Asia, Africa, and Latin America use traditional medicines to meet their primary healthcare needs. For many people in these countries, particularly those living in rural areas, this is the only available, accessible, and affordable source of healthcare. The use of plants was an integral part of the development of modern civilization (WHO, 2002; Lee, 2004). Much of the pharmacopoeia of scientific medicine in modern times was derived from the herbal lore of native peoples' acquired and compiled knowledge systems, which have been disseminated from generation to generation (WHO, 2002).

Today, more than 50,000 plant species are being used in various human cultures around the world for medical purposes and many of them are subjected to uncontrolled local and external trade (Schippmann *et al.*, 2002; Boon and Ahenkan, 2010). From a Western world perspective, the WHO (2002) estimates that at least 7,000 medical compounds in the modern pharmacopoeia are derived from plants. About 25% of the prescription drugs dispensed in the United States contain at least one active ingredient derived from plant material. Many conventional drugs originate from plant sources and several effective drugs are plant based, such as aspirin derived from bark of willow, digoxin derived from foxglove, quinine derived from the bark of cinchona, and morphine derived from the opium poppy (Lee, 2004). Scientific interest in medicinal plants has burgeoned due to increased efficiency of new plant-derived drugs, growing interest in natural products, and rising concerns about the side effects of conventional medicine (Lee, 2004). In tropical Africa, more than 4,000 plant species are claimed to have medicinal properties to cure, alleviate, or prevent diseases, and 50,000 tons of medicinal plants are consumed annually in the continent (Karki, 2007). Interest in environmental resources is therefore becoming more and more recognized in healthcare delivery in Africa, particularly because they are affordable, readily accepted by consumers, and locally available (WHO, 2003a; 2003b; 2003c; Falconer, 1997; Abbiw et al., 2002).

Medicinal plants and healthcare delivery in Africa

In many African countries, the significance of traditional medical practitioners is now recognized and attempts are being made to integrate Western and indigenous medicine (Brown, 1992; WHO, 2003a; 2003b; 2003c; Boon and Ahenkan, 2010). Despite the efforts of African governments and their development partners to make modern health services accessible and available in Africa, most of the health facilities are distances away from local communities and not accessible to the poor. Plant medicine has therefore remained the most affordable and easily accessible source of treatment in the primary healthcare system of poor communities in for example Ghana (Boon and Ahenkan, 2010; Abbiw et al., 2002). For instance, Falconer (1997) notes that the majority of rural households in Ghana turns first to familiar plant medicine, before seeing a doctor depending on the disease in question, access to the clinic or healer, and the family's financial situation. The importance of medicinal plants in Africa is underscored by the fact that most rural health posts in the continent are poorly equipped and are expensive to visit. It is estimated that more than half of the rural population (55%) do not consult medical personnel due to the high cost of treatment and the long distances to health posts (Heyen-Perschon, 2002). Local and indigenous plants are often the only available means of treating bacterial infections in most rural areas (Taylor et al., 2001). In order to optimize the use of medicinal plants in the treatment of diseases, many of them have been screened by medical laboratories (Rabe and van Staden, 2000; Tetyana et al., 2002).

According to WHO (2003a; 2003b; 2003c), the provision of safe and effective medicinal plant therapies could become a critical tool for increasing access to healthcare in the developing countries. Traditional medicine continues to play an important role in the healthcare systems of African countries due to its relative accessibility and affordability (WHO, 2002; Twarog et al., 2004; Sato, 2012). It is estimated that one-third of the world's population still lacks regular access to essential drugs, with the figure rising to over 50% in the poorest parts of Africa. It is estimated that in countries such as Ghana, Mali, Nigeria, and Zambia, the first line of treatment for 60% of children with high fever resulting from malaria is the use of herbal medicines at home (WHO, 2002).

Traditional medicine plays a major role in the primary healthcare of many people living in rural areas. The majority of people in Africa use plant-based traditional medicines for treating illness and ailments. Recognizing this important role of traditional medicine, WHO called for recognition of traditional healers (WHO, 1978; Kofi-Tsekpo, 2004; Sato, 2012) and declared at Alma Ata that African traditional healers should be part of primary healthcare teams. The African Regional Strategy on traditional medicine was adopted in 2000 to institutionalize and integrate traditional medicine into conventional medicine, with the aim of delivering health for all through optimization of the use of traditional medicine. The strategy emphasizes the importance of collaboration, communication, harmonization, and partnership building between conventional and traditional systems of medicine, while ensuring intellectual property rights (IPRs) and protection of traditional medical knowledge (WHO, 2003a; 2003b; 2003c). Sustainable management of medicinal plant resources in the environment is therefore important, not only because of their value as a potential source of new drugs, but the large reliance on traditional medicinal plants.

Managing environmental resources for improved healthcare delivery in Africa

Forest resource management measures are crucial in healthcare and disease mitigation in Africa. For instance, HIV/AIDS is having a large impact on woodland communities, particularly in Africa. Anyonge et al. (2006) and Timko et al. (2010) have documented an increased dependence of HIV/AIDS-affected communities on forest resources, particularly for medicines, energy, and food and have also explored the resource management implications. Weak health infrastructure and pervasive poverty continue to pose problems for the unprecedented challenge of providing and administering anti-retroviral therapy in southern African countries. In such resource-constrained settings, local communities are obliged to rely on traditional plant remedies for the management of HIV/AIDS, and traditional medicine is being institutionalized in the response to the pandemic. The forest sector therefore undoubtedly has a role to play in the prevention, care, and treatment of HIV/AIDS and the mitigation of their impact. Given these real and potential benefits of environmental resources, there is the need for African countries to ensure their sustainable management. Forestry institutions and their human resources, particularly forest managers working at the local level, have a big role to play in this direction. Forest products can play a part in income generation and other livelihood activities that can help alleviate the impact of the diseases on households.

Improving environmental resources management in Africa

Local and indigenous people have managed their environmental resources for millennia. Many farmers and hunter-gatherers throughout Africa have maintained traditional systems of collective natural resource management which help to sustain the livelihoods and cultures of millions of people (Roe et al., 2009; Kassibo, 2002). Since the 1990s, there has been a gradual shift from the predominantly centralized natural resource management towards more devolved models due to the fact that several approaches initiated to conserve forests in Africa without involving the local communities have been unsuccessful (Kassanga and Kotey, 2001; Roe et al., 2009).

It is increasingly recognized that involvement of people in forest management, apart from contributing to regeneration of degraded forest and helping in cost-effective conservation, also meets communities' subsistence needs. In Africa, natural resources have traditionally been managed collectively or communally (rather than individually) because the resources are subject to shared uses and it would be too costly to individualize the resource (Roe et al., 2009; Nelson et al., 2007).

Increasingly, debates over local communities' ability to manage their lands and environmental resources are a part and parcel of broader struggles over political and economic power and authority in African countries. During the past few decades, there has been a growing awareness of the importance of collective natural resource management practices and institutions and a recognition of the ways that historic forces have disrupted local people's ability to manage the lands and resources they depend upon. A wide range of policy makers as well as development and conservation practitioners have supported efforts to revive or bolster local natural resource management institutions in response to various economic, social, environmental, and political pressures (Roe et al., 2009). In many African countries, different approaches are being used to involve local communities in forest management. They include joint forest management (JFM), community-based natural resources management (CBNRM), collaborative forest management (CFM), and participatory forest management (PFM).

Joint forest management

Most African countries have moved towards a decentralized and participatory forest management programme called joint forest management. For instance, in Burkina Faso various policy reforms have been introduced to devolve use and management rights to local communities since the 1980s (Pascaline, 2011; Roe et al., 2009; Odera, 2004). The JFM seeks to promote local communities' involvement, collective decision-making, social fencing, empowerment of the village community, sharing of authority, and focus on NTFP and sustained harvest of usufructs. Efforts at involving local people in management of forest resource have produced encouraging results with respect to conservation and regeneration.

Community-based natural resources management

Community-based natural resources management, as a forest management concept, crystallized in the past two decades as an effective approach for the management of tree and forest resources. The concept emerged as a result of manifold trends, ideas, and crises which led to a broad rethinking of both development and conservation fields during the 1980s.

Experiences from various countries have shown that when communities are empowered with responsibility and legally secured rights for the management of forest resources, and receive benefits from them, the rate of degradation is substantially reduced (Odera, 2004). CBNRM is a term that refers to *local* and *collective* resource governance arrangements and practices. Given the great diversity of both human communities and resources, CBNRM covers a wide range of resource use practices. It describes the management of resources such as land, forests, wildlife, and water by collective local institutions for local benefit and may involve attempting to reinstitute local resource governance measures. For example, the involvement of a community in wildlife management following decades of progressive loss of local rights over wildlife due to colonial and post-colonial conservation policies (Roe et al., 2009; Jones and Mosimane, 2007). CBNRM equally applies to traditional resource management arrangements such as the collective regimes governing rangelands and pastoralists grazing reserves and communally managed forests. CBNRM can be formal or informal and often straddles both realms, particularly given the contemporary social and institutional transformations occurring across much of sub-Saharan Africa.

The emergence of CBNRM in southern and eastern Africa often had deep locally derived roots. In the late 1960s, user rights over wildlife on freehold lands in Zimbabwe, South Africa, and Namibia was through a series of legislative reforms, devolved to landowners (Jones and Murphree, 2001). This dramatic shift away from strictly centralized governance of wildlife fundamentally changed

wildlife's status on private lands from an economic liability to an asset and led to profound recoveries of wildlife on freehold lands and the growth of wildlife-based industries in all three countries (Bond et al., 2004). Local involvement occurs in diverse forms, but is broadly encompassed by the term 'participatory forest management'. The generic term 'forests' is used to encompass diverse types, from dry woodlands to moist tropical forests, coastal mangroves, and plantations. 'Community' in the context of PFM refers to people living within or next to forests. Forest management is itself primarily a matter of governance.

The Community Forestry Management system in Ghana in 1992 sought to promote the creation of community forestry committees as a contact point for consultation in forest reserve planning (Odera, 2004; Kassanga and Kotey, 2001). Boundary maintenance contracts are issued to adjacent communities and the *Taungya* regime has been modified to allow foresters to pay farmers who tend seedlings in planted areas. In cases where local people are involved only to regulate their own forest use and where the forest has few non-product values of use to the wider community (such as water catchment functions), the founding of management or user groups may be workable. However, this is decreasingly the purpose of PFM development, which looks more and more to wider managerial functions on the one hand and the organization of significant income generation and/or revenue receipt on the other.

Emerging environmental health management challenges in Africa

Despite the use of various approaches to ensure a sustainable management of environmental resources in Africa, the continent still faces a number of fundamental challenges. Overall, there are very few cases of communities obtaining formal authority over lands and the natural resources found on those lands. Centralized control over natural resources persists despite the ubiquitous change in the rhetoric over land and resource management (Roe et al., 2009). African environmental resources may be doomed to extinction by over-exploitation resulting from excessive commercialization, habitat destruction, and other natural and man-made destructive influences unless energetic conservation measures are taken to ensure their continued availability (Rukangira, 2002). Political interferences and rapid deforestation due to poor farming methods, uncontrolled logging, over-exploitation of the resources, bushfires, and climate are additional challenges (Fig. 9.1.3).

Political interference is a complex and challenging issue in environmental resources management in Africa. The existing institutional, legal, and governance environment is probably not effective enough to cushion the professionals against such political and social pressures. Yasmi (2007) notes that natural resource management is almost always characterized by conflict, particularly because stakeholders have competing interests, perceptions, and ideas about how natural resources should be managed. Also, the implementation of decentralization policies gives rise to conflict between local and central government and among local stakeholders in Africa.

In Africa, medicinal plants are obtained primarily from home gardens, agricultural fields, marginal lands, forests, and markets. The forests are increasingly threatened by various environmental, socioeconomic, and institutional problems. Many medicinal plants in Africa are in jeopardy due to rapid deforestation. It is estimated that 117 species of medicinal plants are threatened by extinction in

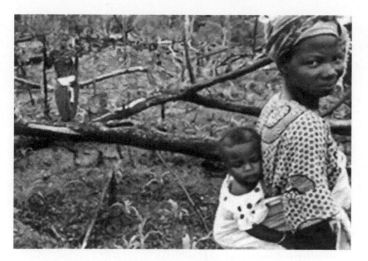

Fig. 9.1.3 Deforestation through poor farming practices.
Image reproduced courtesy of Dr Albert Ahenkan.

Ghana (IUCN, 2005; MES, 2005). Although it is difficult to have reliable data on the actual rate of deforestation because of the different methods of forest resources assessment used and the lack of uniform and generally accepted definitions (Appiah *et al.*, 2009), most recent reports by FAO estimated that in several African countries, the rate of deforestation exceeded the global annual average of 0.8%. This suggests that natural resources in Africa face an ever-increasing set of pressures resulting in the loss of forest and biodiversity.

The demand by most of the people in developing countries for medicinal plants has been met by indiscriminate harvesting of spontaneous flora, including those in forests. As a result, many plant species have become extinct and some are endangered. The threat posed by over-exploitation of medicinal plants has serious implications on the survival of several plant species, many of which are faced with extinction. South Africa for instance is a home to over 30,000 species of higher plants and 3,000 of these species have been found to be used in traditional medicine across the country. South African medicinal plants are decreasing at an alarming rate as a result of over-exploitation. Today many medicinal plants face extinction, but detailed information is lacking. Over 90% of medicinal and aromatic plants (MAPS) in developing countries are harvested and collected in the wild (Karki, 2007).

The impacts of deforestation are widespread and are affecting not only the livelihoods of local people, but also destroying important plant species. For instance, in Ghana although there are insufficient records or indications of the state of medicinal plants, many research findings (Abbiw *et al.*, 2002; Falconer, 1997; Ahenkan and Boon, 2010) and the results of consultations with key informants, health professionals, botanists, and traditional healers indicate that medicinal plants are gradually being depleted due to frequent bushfires, poor farming practices, over-exploitation of forest resources, uncontrolled logging, and mining activities. The high rate of deforestation would have a detrimental effect on medicinal plants and traditional heath care delivery system in Africa (Abbiw *et al.*, 2002).

Sustainable forest management is central to human health because it provides the resource base for the provision of ecosystem services such as food and medicines in Africa. Unfortunately, land degradation caused by inappropriate land use practices, vegetation cover loss, contamination by heavy metals, and soil depletion are undermining productivity of food and nutrition security in the continent (UNEP, 2013). The continued loss of habitat caused by deforestation will remain a big threat to many medicinal plants in Africa if effective measures are not taken. Implementing policies that prevent environmentally detrimental land use changes and inequitable landholding structures will significantly help to enhance food and nutrition security, especially for the vulnerable segments of the population which hold land under traditional tenure systems (UNEP, 2013). Climate change is another important emerging environmental health challenges in Africa. Environmental resources are vulnerable to climate change. Africa is one of the most vulnerable regions in the world to climate change. Climate change is affecting medicinal and aromatic plants and could ultimately lead to losses of some key species. One-third of the people in Africa lives in drought-prone areas and are very vulnerable to the impacts of drought. Climate change is likely to impact the availability of environmental resources as well as the vulnerability of medicinal plants.

Conclusion

This chapter regards high-quality environmental health to be a fundamental element of human health in Africa. Forest ecosystem services such as NTFPs and medicinal plants contribute significantly to human health in the continent. Sustainable management of environmental resources is therefore crucial in healthcare and disease prevention in Africa. During the past decades, many African countries adapted various approaches and strategies to facilitate sustainable environmental resources management. To a large extent, the continent has visibly shifted from the predominantly centralized environmental resource management approach, to more devolved models such as joint forest management, community-based natural resources management, collaborative forest management, and participatory forest management. Despite the gains achieved through the use of these approaches, environmental health and natural resources management in Africa continue to face fundamental challenges, including remaining centralized control over natural resources, political interferences, and rapid deforestation due to poor farming methods, uncontrolled logging, over-exploitation, frequent widespread bushfires, and the depletion of environmental goods such as NTFPS and medicinal plants. The formulation and implementation of appropriate environmental resource policies and effective community participation will significantly help to enhance environmental health in the continent.

References

Abbiw, D., Gillett, H., Agbovie, T., Akuetteh, B., Amponsah, K., & Owusu, A. (2002). *Conservation and Sustainable Use of Medicinal Plants in Ghana.* UNEP-WCMC/Darwin Initiative: pp. 3–32

Ahenkan, A. & Boon, E. (2008). Enhancing food security, poverty reduction and sustainable forest management in Ghana through Non-Timber Forest Products farming: Case study of Sefwi Wiawso District, GRIN Publishing. Available at: http://www.grin.com/en/e-book/86653/enhancing-food-security-and-poverty-reduction-in-ghana-through-non-timber (accessed 8 August 2014) [Online].

Ahenkan, A. & Boon, E. (2010). Commercialization of non-timber forest products in Ghana: Processing, packaging and marketing. *JFAE*, 8, 962–9.

Anyonge, C. H., Rugalema, G., Kayambazinthu, D., Sitoe, A., & Barany, M. (2006). Fuelwood, food and medicine: the role of forests in the response to HIV and AIDS in rural areas of southern Africa. *Unasylva*, 57, 20–3.

Appiah, M., Blay, D., Damnyag, L., Dwomoh, F. K., Pappinen, A., & Luukkanen, O. (2009). Dependence on Forest Resources and Tropical Deforestation in Ghana, Environ Dev Sustain, 11, 471–87.

Belcher, B., Ruiz Pérez, M., & Achdiawan, R. (2005). Global Patterns and Trends in the Use and Management of Commercial NTFPs: Implications for Livelihoods and Conservation, *World Development* 33, 1435–52.

Boon, E. and Ahenkan, A. (2010). Assessing the Impact of Forest Policies and Strategies on Promoting the Development of Non-Timber Forest Products in Ghana. *J Biodiversity*, 1(2), 85-102.

Bond, I., Child, B., De La Harpe, D., Jones, B., Barnes, J. & Anderson, H. (2004). Private land contribution to conservation in South Africa. In: Child, B. (ed.). *Parks in Transition: Biodiversity, Rural Development, and the Bottom Line*. pp. 29–61. London: Earthscan.

Brown, K. (1992). Medicinal Plants, Indigenous Medicine and Biodiversity in Ghana. Global Environmental Change Working Paper, 92-36, Centre for Social and Economic Research on the Global Environment, University of East Anglia and University College London.

Cavendish, W. (2003). *How Do Forests Support, Insure and Improve the Livelihoods of the Rural Poor? A Research Note*. Bogor, Indonesia: Center for International Forestry Research, pp. 3–23.

Chidumayo, E., Okali, D., Kowero, G., & Larwanou, M. (eds.). 2011. *Climate Change and African Forest and Wildlife Resources*. Nairobi, Kenya: African Forest Forum.

CIFOR. 2005. Contributing to African development through forests strategy for engagement in sub-Saharan Africa. Center for International Forestry, Bogor, Indonesia.

Falconer, J. (1997). Developing research frames for non-timber forest products: experience from Ghana. In: Ruiz Pérez, M. & Arnold, J. E. M. (eds) *Current Issues in Non-timber Forest Products Research*, pp. 143–160. Bogor, Indonesia: Centre for International Forestry Research.

Food and Agricultural Organization (FAO) (2006). Forests and human health, Unasylva, Vol 57, 224. Available at: ftp://ftp.fao.org/docrep/fao/009/a0789e/a0789e.pdf [Online].

Food and Agriculture Organization (FAO) (2016). Forest foods vital for food and nutritional security in Congo Basin. Available at: http://www.fao.org/forestry/news/92779/en/ (accessed 20 December 2016) [Online].

Food and Agriculture Organization of the United Nations (FAO) (2011). The State of Forests in the Amazon Basin, Congo Basin and Southeast Asia. A report prepared for the Summit of the Three Rainforest Basins, Brazzaville, Republic of the Congo, 31 May–3 June 2011. Rome.

Food and Agriculture Organization of the United Nations (FAO) (2012). State of the World's Forests, FAO Research and Extension, FAO Rome, Italy.

Heyen-Perschon, J. (2002). Report on current situation in the health sector of Ghana and possible roles for appropriate transport technology and transport related communication interventions, Institute for Transportation and Development Policy (ITDP), pp. 4–32.

International Union for Conservation of Nature and Natural Resources (IUCN). (2005). *2004 IUCN Red List of Threatened Species*. IUCN: Gland, Switzerland. Available at: http://www.redlist.org/info/tables/table5.html (accessed on July 2009) [Online].

Jones, B. and Murphree M. (2001). The evolution of policy on community conservation in Namibia and Zimbabwe. In: Hulme, D. and Murphree M. W. (eds.) *African Wildlife and African Livelihoods: the promise and performance of community conservation*. James Currey. Oxford.

Jones, B. & Mosimane, A. (2007). Promoting Integrated Community Based Natural Resource Management as a Means to Combat Desertification: The Living in a Finite Environment (LIFE) Project. Namibia, Africa: USAID.

Karki, M. (2007). Medicinal plants: Resources and Distribution, Global NTFPs Partnership. Kathmandu, Nepal: International Centre for Integrated Mountain Development (ICIMOD), pp. 4–12.

Kassanga, K. & Kotey, N. (2001). *Land Management in Ghana: Building on Tradition and Modernity*. London, UK: DFID.

Kassibo, B. (2002). Participatory Management and Democratic Decentralization Management of the Samori Forest in Babye Commune, Mopti region, Mali. Conference on Decentralization and the Environment, 18–2 February, 2002. Bellagio, Italy: World Resources Institute.

Kofi-Tsekpo, M. (2004). Institutionalization of African traditional medicine in health care systems in Africa. *Afr J Health Sci*, 11(1–2), i–ii.

Lee, J. K. (2004). Medicinal plants: a powerful health aid? *The Science Creative Quarterly*, 3, 1–8.

Lengkeek. (2004). Trees on farm to mitigate the effects of HIV/AIDS in SSA. Available at: http://www.agroforestry.net/pubs/LengkeekHIV.pdf (accessed May 2009) [Online].

Levang, P., Dounias, E., & Sitorus, S. (2005). Out of the forest, out of poverty? *Forests, Trees and Livelihoods*, 15, 211–37.

Marshall, E., Schreckenberg, K., & Newton, A. C. (eds) (2006). Commercialization of Non-timber Forest Products: Factors Influencing Success. Lessons Learned from Mexico and Bolivia and Policy Implications for Decision-makers. UNEP World Conservation Monitoring Centre, Cambridge, UK. pp 1–20

Millennium Ecosystem Assessment (MES) (2005). Ecosystems and Human Well-being: Current State and Trends, Volume 1. Washington, DC, Island Press, pp. 1–18.

Musabayane, C.T. (2012). The effects of medicinal plants on renal function and blood pressure in diabetes mellitus. *Cardiovasc J Afr*, 23, 462–468.

Nelson, F., Nshala, R., & Rodgers, W. (2007). The evolution and reform of Tanzanian wildlife management. *Conservation & Society*, 5, 232–61.

Nkwatoh, A. F. & Yinda, G. S. (2007). Assessment of non-timber forest products (NTFPs) of economic potentials in the Korup National Park, of South West Cameroon. *Global Journal of Agriculural Science*, 6, 41–8.

Odera, J.A. (2004). The state of secondary forests in Anglophone Sub-Saharan African countries: challenges and opportunities for sustainable management in Africa. A thematic paper presented at the FAO/ECHNV/GTZ workshop on secondary forest management in Africa, 9-13 December, 2002. Rome, Italy.

Pascaline, C. L. (2011). Appraisal of the Participatory Forest Management Program in Southern Burkina Faso. (Doctoral Thesis submitted to the Swedish University of Agricultural Sciences).

Rabe, T. & van Staden, J. (2000). Isolation of an antibacterial sesquiterpenoid from *Warburgia salutaris*. *J Ethnopharmacol*, 73, 171–4.

Rapport, D. J., Christensen, N., Karr, J. R., & Patil, G. P. (1998). *Sustainable Health of Humans and Ecosystems*, unpublished report.

Roe D., Nelson, F., & Sandbrook, C. (eds) (2009). Community management of natural resources in Africa: Impacts, experiences and future directions. Natural Resource Issues No. 18. London, UK: International Institute for Environment and Developmen.

Ros-Tonen, M. A. F. & Wiersum, K. F. (2005). The scope of improving rural livelihoods through non-timber forest products: An evolving research agenda. *Forests, Trees and Livelihoods*, 15, 129–48.

Rukangira, E. (2002). *Medicine in Africa: Constraints and Challenges*. Nairobi, Kenya: Conserve Africa International, pp. 179–84.

Sato, A. (2012). Revealing the popularity of traditional medicine in light of multiple recourses and outcome measurements from a user's perspective in Ghana. *Health Policy Plan*, 27, 625–37.

Schippmann, U., Leaman, D. J., & Cunningham, A. B. (2002). Impact of cultivation and gathering of medicinal plants on biodiversity: global trends and issues. Inter-Department Working Group on Biology Diversity for Food and Agriculture. Rome, Italy: FAO, pp. 1–10.

Sekagya, Y. H., Finch, L., & Garanganga, E. (2006). *A Clinical Guide to Supportive and Palliative Care for HIV/AIDS in Sub-Saharan Africa*.

Part 3: Psychology/Spiritual and Traditional Care. Alexandria, Virginia: Foundation for Hospices in Sub-Saharan Africa, pp. 9–221.

Sunderland, T. & Ndoye, O. (2004). *Forest Products, Livelihoods and Conservation. Case Studies of Non-Timber Forest Products Systems. Vol. 2–Africa.* Bogor, Indonesia: CIFOR, pp. 1–55.

Taylor, J. L. S., Rabe, T., McGaw, L. J., Jäger, A. K., & van Staden, J. (2001). Towards the scientific validation of traditional medicinal plants. *Plant Growth Regulation*, 34, 23–37.

Tetyana, P., Prozesky, E. A., Jäger, A. K., Meyer, J. J. M., & van Staden, J. (2002). Some medicinal properties of *Cussonia* and *Schefflera* species used in traditional medicine. *South Afr J Botany*, 68, 51–4.

Timko, J. A., Kozak, R. A., & Innes, J. L. (2010). HIV/AIDS and forests in Sub-Saharan Africa: Exploring the links between morbidity, mortality, and dependence on biodiversity. *Biodiversity*, 11, 45–8.

Twarog, S. & Kapoor, P. (eds) (2004). *Protecting and Promoting Traditional Knowledge: Systems, National Experiences and International Dimensions.* Geneva, Switzerland: UNCTA, pp. 1–23.

United Nations Environment Programme (UNEP) (2013). Africa Environment Outlook 3: Our Environment, Our Health: Summary for Policy Makers. Nairobi, Africa: UNEP, p. 40.

Wilkie, D. S. (2001). Bushmeat hunting in the Congo Basin—a brief review. In: Bakarr, M. I., da Fonseca, G. A. B., Mittermeier, R. A., Rylands, A. B., & Painemilla, K. W. (eds) *Hunting and Bushmeat Utilization in the African Rain Forest*. Washington, DC: Conservation International.

World Health Organization (WHO) (1978). The promotion and development of traditional medicine. WHO, Technical representative series, 622. Geneva, Switzerland: WHO.

World Health Organization (WHO). (2002). WHO Traditional Medicine Strategy 2002–2005. Geneva, Switzerland: WHO, pp. 10–74.

World Health Organization (WHO). (2003a). Priorities for promoting the use of traditional medicines. WHO fact sheet No. 134. Geneva, Switzerland: WHO

World Health Organization (WHO) (2003b). Traditional Medicine: Facts Sheet No 134 Revised. Geneva, Switzerland: WHO. Available at: http://www.who.int/mediacentre/factsheets/2003/fs134/en/ (accessed 22 June 2010) [Online].

World Health Organization (WHO) (2003c). Traditional Medicine: Our Culture, Our Future. African Health Monitor Magazine of the World Health Organization Regional Office for Africa, Volume 4, No.1. Geneva, Switzerland: WHO.

Yasmi, Y. (2007). Institutionalization of conflict capability in the management of natural resources: theoretical perspectives and empirical experience in Indonesia. Wageningen University, Wageningen, Netherlands. p.188.

CHAPTER 9.2

Latin America and the environmental health movement

Ana Faggi, Sylvie Nail, Carolina C. Sgobaro Zanette, and Germán Tovar Corzo

A complex legacy

Public green spaces (GS) across Latin America (LA) have traditionally been favourite meeting places for people from all walks of life and all ages, as places associated with air, light, and nature, as well as culture and multiculturalism. Today, more than ever before and in common with the rest of the world, they cater to a wide range of needs and provide society with social, environmental, and economic benefits.

By the late nineteenth century, green spaces began to be relevant urban areas in social life in Latin America. Large public parks arose under the influence of French and English landscaping models coinciding with the hygienist movement in its attempts to relieve the burden of urban living. These transformations in the urban matrix produced large changes in Latin American cities that gradually departed from their colonial past, with tiny dry plazas between blocks, to striking landscaped big parks playing a central role as places for social integration (Faggi and Ignatieva, 2009).

LA is presently the most urbanized region worldwide and public green spaces are intensively used as more than 80% of the population lives in cities (United Nations, 2012). However, its occupancy patterns and urban development are far from sustainable. The physical growth of cities causes a loss of plant cover as well as the fragmentation of ecosystems which, added to waste pollution and water contamination, cause irreparable damage to biodiversity. Such a pressure is expected to continue to grow due to intensive rural-urban migration and to the decrease in the home sizes, as family homes are pulled down to build blocks of smaller flats. Moreover, social inequality in Latin America leads to strongly divided and segregated cities, many of them displaying an uneven distribution of green space availability, as well as disparity in their quality within cities (Siemens, 2010). Data collected between 2003 and 2008 from 16 cities in the region show that almost half of them exceeded the recommendation of the World Health Organization regarding green space, put at 9–11 m^2 per inhabitant. However, the variety of criteria for green areas and its irregular distribution in cities complicates the calculation of the actual average. Many cities have grown haphazardly without taking environmental criteria on board. Often included in the calculations are green areas actually located on the outskirts, which are not part of most of the population's immediate surroundings, much less of everyday urban life. Frequently, low-income neighbourhoods are typically either interspersed with the natural habitats in peri-urban areas or completely lacking green spaces, while high-income quarters have normally a higher concentration of well-kept green areas (Barbosa et al., 2007; Reyes and Figueroa, 2010).

In many cities, urban green has suffered in the last decades from inadequate maintenance without systematic planning for urban trees and permeable surfaces, as a culture of concrete as a symbol of modernity persists. In addition, run-down or poorly planned public spaces have promoted antisocial and violent behaviour, being seriously compromised by insecurity, which has turned to be one of the main concerns of citizens in the region, along with unemployment, corruption, and poverty (Latinobarómetro, 2011).

Nevertheless, across the region, cities are trying to change the current models of urbanization, making urban centres more inclusive and sustainable. In line with this, there is an increasing attention by Latin American planners on the need to revitalize existing green spaces and to create new ones for the physical well-being of the growing urban population (Pauchard and Barbosa, 2013; Caula et. al., 2013). However, as the Latin American City index—a study which included most major urban areas—showed, policies on GS are widespread and they tend to retain existing GS rather than to create new ones (Siemens, 2010).

Over the last decades, Latin American parks have taken on a new role that has gone beyond the traditional meeting places and places for leisure (Breuste et al., 2013), or that of social identity of the neighbourhood. Today, they are valued as habitats for biodiversity, for enhancing the air quality and the urban climate (and as sources of restoration from a stressful life). Nevertheless, studies on how GS, well-being, and health interplay in Latin American cities are difficult to find. Indeed, most research recognizing that mental health, which is an essential part of well-being, can also be improved through natural environments, originates mainly from the United States and Europe. It has deepened the grounds laid by Stephen and Rachel Kaplan's seminal work on restorative natural environments to fight against mental fatigue and restore competence and attention (Kaplan and Kaplan, 1989; 2003; Kaplan et al., 1998). Abundant literature today suggests that GS promote health by restoring mental fatigue (Kaplan, 2001, Kaplan and Kaplan, 2005), while also serving as a resource for outdoor life and physical activities (Björk et al., 2008), and reducing the mortality (Mitchell and Popham, 2008) related to physical inactivity, overweight, bad nutrition and stress (World Health Organization, 2007). Although this aspect of the health–nature relationship seems more difficult to elicit in this region and is notably absent from grey literature—which may reflect the so far rather weak influence of environmental psychology in LA on policy and practice—some activities which have developed over the past few years seem to partake of that need to preserve/restore one's mental health through nature's hidden benefits (Kaplan, 2004).

This chapter shows some trends in Latin American cities that reveal the role of GS for the health and well-being of urban-dwellers. Indeed, health as defined by the World Health Organization consists of being in the capacity to make the most of one's potential, which entails physical, mental, as well as social well-being. It is along those lines that the different initiatives carried out in natural settings in LA show a growing change towards quality, equity, and sustainability.

Curitiba, a showcase in Latin America

Over the last four decades, green spaces have become major actors in the profound urban changes that led Curitiba, Brazil, to fame. Indeed, it has become an international model for sustainable development and social regeneration. Since the early 1970s, Curitiba, with its 64.5 m² of green area per capita (Fermino et al., 2013; Prefeitura Municipal de Curitiba) has emerged as a smart model of an ecologically sustainable city. Its success was based on the vision of Mayor Lerner, an architect and the city's mayor for three terms beginning in 1972. The success of his policy plan was greatly influenced by social and political foundations on both the local and national stages that were laid long before he arrived in office. He applied a win-win strategy to solve environmental, social, and economic problems, and established a multifaceted strategy to promote a healthier life through sport and the prevention of illnesses. Parks were major players in this strategy and turned Curitiba into an example to be followed by developed urban centres all around the world.

By the 1970s, concern about public GS was aired and Curitiba's landscape was transformed by the first parks, such as Barigui, Barreirinha, and São Lourenço. In 1996, there were eight more great GS: the Pope woodland, the Botanical Garden, the Zaninelli woodland, the Wire Opera House, the Passaúna, the Germán, the Tangua, and the Tingui parks (Dudeque, 2010). Due to the implementation of a new public transportation system and of waste management, Curitiba was awarded the title of 'Ecological Capital City' and became known worldwide for the improvement in its quality of life as a consequence of the GS growing process (Oliveira, 2000).

Currently, there are 21 parks, 15 woodlands, 451 public squares, and 444 pocket gardens in this city, a very different picture from the traditional colonial cities of Latin America, with their scarce green urban areas. The Public Park created at the end of the nineteenth century was the first one in the city. Thanks to it, citizens re-established their relationship with domesticated nature, doomed to

aesthetic contemplation, to sidewalk, and to the urban atmosphere. Nowadays, its 69.285 m² of green space represents an urban oasis in the heart of the city for 1,850,000 inhabitants (IBGE, 2013).

Initially, many GS have been increased and conceived as water reservoirs for flooding remediation. They were valued as ideal places to protect nature and some were part of rehabilitation projects on degraded areas destroyed by mineral exploitation.

However, as time passed by, these actions represented a lot more for the Curitiba citizens. Nowadays, they are closely related to the promotion of public health. GS contribute not only to environmental improvement, but also as places for socialization and the practice of sports (Moysés and Krempel, 2004). As great leisure venues or meeting points for the population, green areas can be compared to great islands within the urban web, which offer constant contact with nature and encourage outdoor activities. Indeed, many of the GS offer 'healthy stations', sports centres, multifunctional courts, bike lanes, among other features, where more than 150,000 people spend their weekends (Krempel et al., 2004). Still, more than representing a high quality of life and the balance between the city and the environment relationship, these places contribute to community welfare. Contrary to cities that offer natural attractions, such as Rio de Janeiro or Porto Alegre, downtown parks embedded in great urban centres may promote the population's mental health.

A new start in Bogotá's urbanism

Bogotá has also been honoured, thanks to the city's successful recovery of public space, its network of cultural equipment, and its advanced public transportation system (Tixier et al., 2010). The city became the 'Golden Lion Award to cities' at the 2006 Venice Biennale. Concerning GS, much has been done for the implementation of regulations and to improve knowledge. Inventories in urban public areas, which include trees, green areas, and gardens, report that Bogotá boasts 1,175,000 trees, 4,900 ha of green spaces and gardens, 10,8738 ha all round. A municipal project for an urban forest was announced in 2013 aiming to plant 115,000 more hectares of woodland to connect already existing forest reserves in the Eastern hills with wetlands and the Bogotá River.

The care of GS is undertaken through the implementation of regulations that seek to guarantee the existing green area, through a Council Agreement (327-2008), requesting any public construction requiring hard surfacing over green areas to compensate for it with the same amount.

However, indicators of green areas per capita currently show an imbalance between the northern and southern parts of the city, at 7.73 m² and 5.97 m², respectively, mirroring the socioeconomic distribution of the population. Just as remarkable is the imbalance in the number of inhabitants per tree—4.67 in the North and 11.35 in the South.

A carbon sequestration model validated experimentally in several regions of the country, with clear-cut standard mathematical methods and models developed by FAO (Brown et al., 1996) estimated that in Bogotá, the tree cover has captured throughout its development 98286.6 T of CO_2, especially through species that exhibit greatest average height such as eucalyptus species, silver wattle (*Acacia decurrens*) and Mexican weeping pine (*Pinus patula*).

A greater knowledge of urban green was accompanied by public health policies aiming to link indicators of respiratory, cardiac, nervous, and mental diseases with environmental policies.

The main role of public policies in Bogotá over the past three decades in terms of public health has been focusing on preventing injuries and promoting behavioural change towards active living (Heath et al., 2012). Territorial planning, which became compulsory according to Law 388 of 1997, has allowed a new urban model to be envisaged for the future in Bogotá, stressing among its main components a common use of public spaces (Tixier et al., 2010). Teaching respect between motorists and pedestrians and the promotion of a healthy environment, among others, have been part of the Mayors' priorities, with so much apparent success that 11 years after Mayor Peñalosa set out to make life easier for cyclists and pedestrians (Fig. 9.2.1), Professor Martin Wiseman of the World Cancer Research Fund argued that London should take a leaf out of Bogotá's book in order to make urban-dwellers more active, thanks to cycle paths, pedestrian zones, and better parks, thus improving public health and possibly reducing the risk of cancer (Wiseman, 2009; Heggie et al., 2003).

Indeed, in Bogotá, the recreational cycling programme stands out as being the longest network in the world available for leisure cycling on Sundays and public holidays, with its 90 km of streets taken over by bikers, skaters, and walkers. This contributes in a significant way to the physical health of those who regularly take part, not only because it partakes in their physical fitness (up to an estimated level of 5% of needed physical activity) (Sarmiento et al., 2010), but also because during the time when the streets are closed to traffic, air pollution diminishes, with positive effects on the whole population's health.

However, in this well-documented initiative, the natural component is absent. The streets put at the disposal of the population are the same that irrigate the city, not greener ones. This comment applies to many programmes around physical health: they provide spaces, but often fail to make the connection with natural elements to make the most of the health potential in its widest remit.

The role that green spaces play in the physical health of urban-dwellers in a metropolis such as Bogotá is thus better exemplified through other projects.

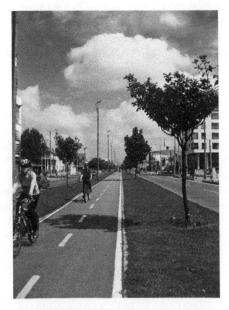

Fig. 9.2.1 Bike path in Bogotá.
Reproduced courtesy of Gilberto Meija.

The Eje Ambiental ('Environmental Axis'), a 2.8-km long pedestrian route in the city's historic centre, has replaced heavy traffic since the late 1990s. This pedestrian zone, with benches placed under the shade of native trees, is now well frequented at all times. There, pedestrian space has since 2002 been shared by the Transmilenio, a Bus Rapid Transit System. Following the present architectural fashion of reintroducing water in urban regeneration projects worldwide, a water canal has been designed in the middle of the pedestrian zone as a series of connecting fountains, reminiscent of the Rio San Francisco that used to flow along this road and was channelled in the 1930s.

As part of the urban regeneration that has characterized Bogotá over the past 20 years, public parks have played a greater part in providing specific infrastructures for physical activity. On top of the numerous 'pocket parks' that can be found at the bottom of many housing developments, where many people walk briskly on a regular basis or walk their dog, games for children and fitness installations for adults have become more frequent in public parks. They are particularly well used at weekends by young and old alike and provide permanent structures for regular exercise in a more pleasant environment than the innumerable gyms that dot the capital city.

Regarding mental health, new initiatives have emerged. One of them is parajiando (birdwatching) in the wetlands of the city. Birdwatching is indeed a typical activity that allows one to pay attention without effort, which leads to mental restoration, even though the wetlands in Bogotá are often far from idyllic places and have in some cases become little better than open sewers. They constitute contested landscapes between builders and the preservationists who want to save these remnants of natural ecosystems for their multifarious benefits. They have therefore become the focus of much public attention, not least because they represent some of the last surviving natural ecosystems in Bogotá, and so far 540 ha of them have been saved (Brodzinsky, 2014).

Such natural spaces as the wetlands and urban forests can also contribute, although only empirical evidence exists to this day, to promote social health in the form of social interaction, providing a counterweight to the anomie of big cities (Coley et al., 1997). This may lead to stronger neighbourhood social ties and to 'a greater sense of safety and adjustment' (Kuo et al., 1998).

On top of natural settings, one must evoke the growing importance of urban agriculture in gardens and on rooftops, especially since the launch in 2004 of the 'Bogotá Without Hunger' strategic programme. It provides physical health through exercise and better food, but also mental health through the relief from daily fatigue and the satisfaction of growing one's own food. Last but not least, urban agriculture promotes social health through the development of networks. An academic study (Barriga Valencia and Leal Celis, 2011) produced unexpected results. On top of food security for matters conducive to better health was the mental and the social health component that came to the fore in the results: among the effects noted by the participants, a case of resolved autism was mentioned, as well as an increased capacity to face the future with trust and a valuable contribution to the participants' social capital, especially among elderly people.

Improving health in the Buenos Aires parks

Inspired by Curitiba's example, Buenos Aires recognized the importance of GS to the outdoor life of the population. The mega city Buenos Aires—the largest city in Argentina—is the second largest metropolitan area in South America after São Paulo in Brazil. Approximately three million people live there, while every day over three to four million more people enter in the city from the metropolitan area to get to work.

For the last 10 years, municipal authorities have set up a revitalization programme and established a multifaceted strategy to promote a healthier life through sport and the prevention of illnesses. These actions aim at guaranteeing good, easily accessible places for social interaction, for walk or sports, or simply to come close to nature. As the attractiveness of parks improved and the number of users increased significantly, the city council has used parks as ideal venues to promote healthy habits, following the WHO (2007) call for implementation of health-promoting environments.

In Argentina, recent studies show that more than half of the population over age 18 (53.4%) was overweight, a figure that is increasing significantly year by year, while one in three people die of stroke or other cardiovascular diseases (Ministerio de Salud de la Nación, 2011). In Buenos Aires city, half of the population is not physically active and does not consume fruits and vegetables, while over 40% of school-age children are overweight because of an excess intake of sweets and junk food. To cope with this situation, the city council has established a strategy to promote a healthier lifestyle through sport and the prevention of illnesses. Among the many programmes offered, the following actions stand out:

◆ Outdoor gyms free to use have been set up in several parks in order to increase the number of people getting physically active. They contain high quality fitness equipment suitable for people of all ages. In addition, professional instructors give a wide range of aerobics sessions, yoga classes, and different recreational activities.

◆ Use of bicycles: As in Bogotá, a programme promoting the use of bicycles has been implemented. It was achieved through a coordinated effort of planning, engineering, policy development, and public education, as a win-win action against sedentary lifestyles and to reduce the use of individual cars. First, the bike lanes were designed to interconnect several parks, and then the circuit was extended to 78 km to link many neighbourhoods. Today, there are 12 bike stations in downtown parks. To make the program more attractive, the city administration offered Buenos Aires'

residents the opportunity to purchase bicycles in small monthly instalments. At present, more and more people ride a bike not only for recreation, but for daily travel (Macri et al., 2009).

◆ 'Healthy Stations': At several parks and plazas there are 25 'Healthy Stations' (Fig. 9.2.2), which are municipal points of prevention of chronic diseases where free basic health checks (measurement of weight, height, waist circumference, blood pressure, blood glucose level, cholesterol level of carbon monoxide in exhaled air) and counselling on healthy eating are carried out. The 'Healthy Stations' programme started in 2011 and today more than 50,000 people have benefited from it.

Conclusion

In the recent decades, Latin American GS have become areas par excellence for the promotion of healthy habits for all, as well as for an education to ecology and an encouragement to physical and cultural activities. Most of these actions have been undertaken in existing GS, in old and forgotten public spaces being taken over by the population or in new places being created by the community, such as Sofia woodland and the bikers' pocket park in the historical town of the Curitiba city. Although this city is regarded as a model of an ecologically sustainable city today, it is interesting to note that few of its original policies are explicitly environmental in their purpose, but rather were the results of creative cost-cutting measures. However, increasing urbanization also offers great opportunities for sustainable development if handled correctly, a chance to turn deficits into opportunities. Arguably it is this assets-focused mindset that has made Curitiba, Brazil, globally noteworthy in matters of sustainable development and turned it into a model for innumerable actions throughout the subcontinent, where green spaces have become vibrant places for the enactment of health-promoting actions. Many cities all over Latin America are now carrying out programmes based on multiple strategies to promote a healthier life through sport and the prevention of illnesses in green spaces.

Nevertheless, although a turn has clearly been taken in favour of public action using green spaces as objects and backdrops, objective measures as well as epidemiological research are still needed to turn these observations into factual assessments likely to weigh on policy development in most cities.

References

Barbosa, O., Tratalos, J. A., Armsworth, P. R., et al. (2007). Who benefits from access to green space? A case study from Sheffield, UK. Landsc Urban Plan, 83, 187–95.

Barriga Valencia, L. M. & Leal Celis, D. C. (2011). Agricultura Urbana en Bogotá. Una evaluación externa-participativa. Proceedings from the X Congreso Nacional de Sociología, Universidad ICESI, Cali, Colombia. Available at: http://www.icesi.edu.co/congreso_sociologia/images/ponencias/9-Barriga%20Leal-Agricultura%20urbana%20en%20 Bogota.pdf (accessed 18 January 2016) [Online].

Björk, J., Albin, M., Grahn, P., et al. (2008). Recreational values of the natural environment in relation to neighbourhood satisfaction, physical activity, obesity and wellbeing. J Epidemiol Community Health, 62, e2.

Breuste, J., Schnellinger, J., Quereshi, S., & Faggi, A. (2013). Urban Ecosystem services on the local level: Urban green spaces as providers. Ekologia (Bratislava), 32, 290–304.

Brodzinsky, S. (2014). A Tale of Two Cities: Bogotá, America's Quarterly, [Online] February. Americas Society/Council of the Americas.

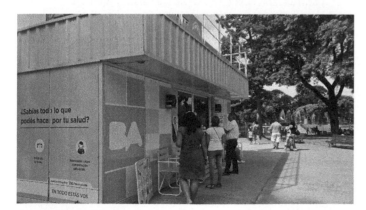

Fig. 9.2.2 Healthy station in a highly visited park in Buenos Aires city where free health checks are offered.
Reproduced courtesy of Ana Faggi.

Available at: http://www.americasquarterly.org (accessed 10 May 2014) [Online].

Brown, S., Sathaye, J., Cannell, M., & Kaupp, P. F. (1996). Management of forests for mitigation of greenhouses emissions. In: Watson, R. T., Zinyowera, M. C., & Moss, R. H. (eds), *Climate Change 1995: Impacts, Adaptations and Mitigation of Climate Change: Assessment Report of the Intergovernmental Panel on Climate Change*, Cambridge and New York: Cambridge University Press.

Caula, S., Florez, G., & Álvarez-Iragorry, C. V. (2013). Venezuela. In: Macgregor-Fors. I & Ortega-Alvárez, R. (eds) *Ecología Urbana. Experiencias en América Latina*. Available at: http://www1.inecol.edu.mx/libro_ecologia_urbana/ecologia_urbana_experiencias_en_america_latina.pdf (accessed 10 August 2014) [Online].

Coley, R. L., Kuo, F. E., & Sullivan, W. C. (1997). Where does community grow? The social context created by nature in urban public housing, *Environ Behav*, 29, 468–94.

Dudeque, I. (2010), Nenhum dia sem uma linha: uma história do urbanismo em Curitiba. São Paulo, Brazil: Studio Nobel.

Faggi, A. & Ignatieva, M. (2009). Urban green spaces in Buenos Aires and Christchurch. *Municipal Engineer*, 162, 241–50.

Fermino, R., Reis, R. S., Hallal, P. C., & de Faria, J. C. Jnr. (2013). Perceived environment and public open space use: a study with adults from Curitiba, Brazil. *Int J Behav Nutr Phys Activity*, 10, 35.

Heath, G. W., Parra, D. C., Sarmiento, O. L., *et al.* (2012). Evidence-based intervention in physical activity: lessons from around the world. *Lancet*, 380, 272–81.

Heggie, S. J. *et al.* (2003). Defining the state of knowledge with respect to food, nutrition, physical activity, and the prevention of cancer. *J Nutr*, 133, 3837–42.

IBGE (2013). *Curitiba*. Available at: http://cidades.ibge.gov.br/xtras/perfil.php?lang=&codmun=410690 (accessed 24 August 2014) [Online].

Kaplan, R. (2001). The nature of the view from home: Psychological benefits. *Environ Behav*, 33, 507–42.

Kaplan, S. (2004). Some hidden benefits of the urban forest. In: Konijnendijk, C. C., Schipperijn, J., & Hoyer, K. H. (eds) *Forestry Serving Urbanised Societies*. Vienna, Austria: IUFRO World Series, 14. pp. 221–32.

Kaplan, R. & Kaplan, S. (1989). *The Experience of Nature: A Psychological Perspective*. New York, NY: Cambridge University Press.

Kaplan, R. & Kaplan, S. (2003). Health, supportive environments, and the Reasonable Person Model. *Am J Public Health*, 93, 1484–9.

Kaplan, R. & Kaplan, S. (2005). Preference, restoration, and meaningful action in the context of nearby nature. In: Barlett, P. F. (ed.) *Urban Place: Reconnecting with the Natural World*. Cambridge, MA: MIT Press.

Kaplan, R., Kaplan, S., & Ryan, R. L. (1998). *With People in Mind: Design and Management of Everyday Nature*. Washington, DC: Island Press.

Krempel, M. C., Moysés, S. T., & Freitas, R. E. (2004). Projeto-Âncora Vida Saudável: A Cidade como Espaço de Promoção de Saúde. In: Vilarta, R. (ed.). *Qualidade de Vida e Políticas Públicas: Saúde, Lazer e Atividade Física*. Campinas, Brazil: Ipes.

Kuo, F. E., Sullivan, W. C., & Coley R. L., (1998). Fertile ground for community: Inner-city neighborhood common spaces. *Am J Community Psychol*, 26, 823–51.

Latinobarómetro (2011). Available at: http://www.latinobarometro.org (accessed 8 April 2014) [Online].

Macri, M., Chain, D., & Lastri, H. (2009). Modelo territorial Buenos Aires 2010–2060 Buenos Aires: Ministerio de Desarrollo Urbano del Gobierno de la Ciudad Autónoma de Buenos Aires. Available at: http://www.ssplan.buenosaires.gov.ar/MODELO%20TERRITORIAL/WEB/modelo_territorial.html (accessed 18 April 2014) [Online].

Ministerio de Salud de la Nación (2011). *Segunda Encuesta Nacional de Factores de Riesgo para Enfermedades No Transmisibles*, Buenos Aires, Argentina: MSL.

Moysés, S. T. & Krempel, M. C. (2004). Avaliando o processo de construção de políticas públicas de promoção de saúde: a experiência de Curitiba. *Ciência & Saúde Coletiva*, 9, 627–41.

Oliveira, D. (2000). *Curitiba e o mito da cidade modelo*. Curitiba, Brazil: UFPR.

Pauchard, A. & Barbosa O. T. (2013). Regional Assessment of Latin America: Rapid Urban Development and Social Economic Inequity Threaten Biodiversity Hotspots In: ELMQVIST *et al.* (eds.), *Urbanization, Biodiversity and Ecosystem Services: Challenges and Opportunities:A Global Assessment*. Springer Open Access Book. Available at: http://www.springer.com/life+sciences/ecology/book/978-94-007-7087-4 (accessed 24 August 2014) [Online].

Prefeitura Municipal de Curitiba, Secretaria Do Meio Ambiente. *Curitiba*. Available at: http://www.curitiba.pr.gov.br/noticias/indice-de-area-verde-passa-para-645-m2-por-habitante/25525 (accessed 24 August 2014) [Online].

Reyes, S. & Figueroa, I. (2010). Distribución, superficie y accesibilidad de las áreas verdes en Santiago de Chile. *EURE*, 26, 89–110.

Sarmiento, O., Torres, A., Jacoby, E., Pratt, M., Schmid, T. L., & Stierling, G. (2010). The Ciclovía-Recreativa: A Mass-Recreational Program With Public Health Potential. *J Phys Act Health*, 7, 163–80.

Siemens (2010). *Latin American Green City Index. Assessing the environmental performance of Latin America's major cities* [Online] Available at: http://www.siemens.com/entry/cc/features/greencityindex_international/all/en/pdf/report_latam_en.pdf (accessed 8 April 2014) [Online].

Tixier, N., Assefer, I., Cifuentes, C., *et al.* (2010), *Bogotá: case study. Research 2009–2010*. Available at: http://cressound.grenoble.archi.fr/fichier_pdf/librairie_ambiance/Tixier_2010_bogota.pdf (accessed 16 April 2014) [Online].

United Nations Department of Economic and Social Affairs/Population Division (2012). *World Urbanization Prospects: The 2011 Revision*. New York, NY: United Nations.

Wiseman, M. (2009). *Make London like Bogota*. Available at: http://news.bbc.co.uk/2/hi/health/8102621.stm (accessed 1 April 2014) [Online].

World Health Organization (WHO) (2007). *Diet and physical activity: a public health priority*. Available at: http://www.who.int/dietphysicalactivity/en/ (accessed 27 July 2007) [Online].

CHAPTER 9.3

Healthy Islands

Evelyne de Leeuw, Erik Martin, and Temo Waqanivalu

Programmes and declarations for small island developing states

One particular environment where nature and ecosystem health meet population health is the nation-state island. These environments are typically characterized as small, remote, isolated, dependent on limited national resources, and vulnerable to natural disasters (Briguglio, 1995). This was recognized as early as 1994 when the UN-sponsored Global Conference on the Sustainable Development of Small Island Developing States determined that sustainable development was the only option for the development of such nations. The conference subsequently adopted the Barbados Programme of Action for the Sustainable Development of Small Island Developing States (SIDS).

Where the Barbados Programme of Action continues to work toward sustainable economic and ecological development (see www.sidsnet.org), the Yanuca Island Declaration (1995) squarely connects development with health. The Declaration adopts a settings-based health promotion agenda, recognizing that (Healthy Pacific) islands are places where children are nurtured in body and mind; environments invite learning and leisure; people work and age with dignity; ecological balance is a source of pride; and the ocean which sustains people is protected. As a key action programme, the Yanuca Island Declaration advocates for a strengthening of healthcare and the healthcare workforce with the emphasis that primary healthcare is one of the main means of achieving the vision of Healthy Islands. Collaborative efforts between SIDS with further development of expertise and technology to address the unique challenges to these group of countries is part of the challenge.

The WHO Healthy Islands Programme

The formal WHO Healthy Islands Programme governed by the Yanuca Declaration extends to countries and territories in the Pacific Ocean (American Samoa, Cook Islands, Fiji, French Polynesia, Guam, Kiribati, the Marshall Islands, the Federated States of Micronesia, Nauru, New Caledonia, Niue, the Commonwealth of the Northern Mariana Islands, Palau, Papua New Guinea, the Pitcairn Islands, Samoa, Solomon Islands, Tokelau, Tonga, Tuvalu, Vanuatu, and Wallis and Futuna). There is considerable diversity among these islands in terms of demography (most have Melanesian/Micronesian/Polynesian core populations, but there have been considerable European and Chinese influences), geography (some nations like Vanuatu are highly volcanic, others like Kiribati consist of numerous coral reefs and atolls, and a few like Pitcairn or Nauru are singular rocky outcrops), and 'development'

(Palau ranks 52 on the Human Development Index—above Russia—and the Solomon Islands occupies 143d—Malik, 2013).

All of these islands find themselves in the vast expanse of the Pacific Ocean (Fig. 9.3.1), and those that occupy territorial areas of several million square kilometres (like Kiribati or the Cook Islands) suffer from an 'internal tyranny of distance' as much as the smaller ones do with their most direct neighbours. To travel from the outer islands to the administrative centre may well take weeks, and acute health issues are often hard to address promptly. This challenge, of course, is also exacerbated by low population sizes and a smattering of expertly trained professionals, including public health and health promotion specialists.

Numbers alone may deceive, though. Pacific islands have a rich cultural history and established systems of navigating the high seas through 'wayfaring' long before European (and Chinese) technologies enabled the colonization of the area (Pyrek, 2011).

In the subsequnt biennial meetings, health ministers of Pacific islands continue to confirm their commitment to the Hcalthy Islands concept (Galea *et al.*, 2000; Nutbeam, 1996), and discuss its key issues of implementation. For example in 1997, the Rarotonga Agreement stated that: 'The Healthy Islands concept involves continuously identifying and resolving priority issues related to health, development and well-being by advocating, facilitating and enabling these issues to be addressed in partnerships among communities, organizations and agencies at local, national and regional levels.'

The following priority areas and concerns are listed in the Agreement:

- adequate water supply and sanitation facilities;
- nutrition, food safety and food security;
- waste management;
- housing;
- human resources development;
- communicable and non-communicable disease prevention and control;
- lifestyle and quality of life issues;
- reproductive and family health;
- promotion of primary healthcare;
- social and emotional well-being;
- population issues;
- ecological sustainability;
- information management;

- tobacco or health;
- alcohol and substance abuse; and
- environmental and occupational health.

The initial three-point focus of the 1995 meeting (i.e. communicable diseases, non-communicable diseases (NCDs), and human resource for health) continues to be the key challenge in the following years with resurgence of communicable diseases including new global ones, while the NCD epidemic has increased to an extent that the same ministers recommended declaration of a health crisis due to NCDs in 2011. The main cause of death for the Pacific population of about 11 million people was NCD, with 75% of deaths attributable to it and most of the deaths occurring before the age of 60 years, providing real challenges to development of the islands. Also, the human resource issue remains unresolved for the most part.

The most serious threat to health (apart from NCDs) and the very existence of these islands, however, is climate change. The International Panel on Climate Change, IPCC, forecasts that some of these '... may face serious threat of permanent inundation from sea-level rise. Among the most vulnerable of these island states are the Marshall Islands, Kiribati, Tuvalu, Tonga, the Federated States of Micronesia, and the Cook Islands' (Smith et al., 2001, p. 935). This effectively means the annihilation of human existence on those islands (Nunn, 2013) and although some island governments have pre-empted this future (e.g. Kiribati purchasing land in Fiji for possible relocation of its residents, Office of the President, 2014), it will have profound

impacts on the health of these nations. The Paris Agreement of the Conference of Parties to the Framework Convention on Climate Change (United Nations, 2015) clearly stipulates specific actions and consideration for least developed nations and in particular SIDS—they are given special consideration in reporting and implementation measures and have achieved a firm position on the climate change action agenda. Although the climate change phenomenon is of recent times, the subject of ecological balance and sustainable environment was already enshrined in the vision of Healthy Islands more than two decades before the IPCC identified its ecological threat.

Some of the more traditional health challenges in Pacific SIDS are summarized in Table 9.3.1. This material shows that some Pacific islands are surprisingly urbanized, and would merit a Healthy City programme on their own (e.g. as Suva on Fiji has declared, although there is very little documentation—Fig. 9.3.2).

Islands, and in particular SIDS, seem proverbial 'settings for health' and as Mark Dooris (2004) has written, the range of settings (healthy market places, health promoting schools, healthy villages, health promoting health services) could benefit from consistency in value systems across the scope of the extent in which they are places where people 'live, love, work and play' (WHO, 1986) and create health. This vision has been adopted in the Pacific in the Yanuca Island Declaration (WHO, 1995) which builds on a heritage of global conferences around health, sustainability, and development in the latter half of the twentieth century.

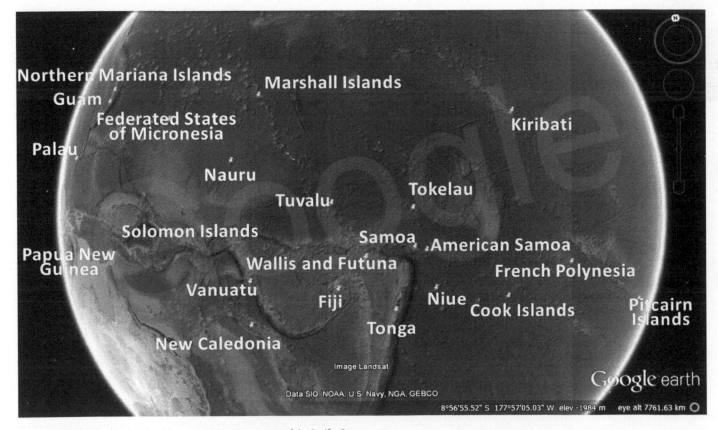

Fig. 9.3.1 Pacific island nations/territories occupy a vast expanse of the Pacific Ocean.
Source: Google Earth.

Table 9.3.1 Pacific island nation/territory demographic information and health expenditure (WHO/WPRO, 2012—WHO Multi-Country Cooperation Strategy for the Pacific 2013–2017)

Country or territory	Population			Per capita GDP		Health expenditure			General government expenditure on health (% of total government expenditure)
	year	Population (in'000s)	Urban population (%)	Year	US$	Year	Per capita US$	As % of GDP	
Melanesia									
Fiji	2010 e	854.0	51.9	2009	2978.95	2009 p	130.40	3.60	9.30
New Caledonia	2009 p	245.6	57.4	2008	36758.00	2008	3420.76	9.5	...
Solomon Islands	2009	515.9	18.6	2008	1014.00	2009 p	71.84	5.30	16.80
Vanuatu	2009	234.0	25.6	2009	2685.10	2009	104.00	3.90	13.60
Papua New Guinea	2011 i	677.4	12.5	2011	1767.24	2011 i	75.98	4.28	12.75
Micronesia									
Federated States of Micronesia	2010 p	102.6	22.7	2008	2223.00	2009 p	333.33	13.80	20.60
Guam	2010 e	180.7	93.2	2005	22661.00	...	...	...	8.71
Kiribati	2010	103.5	48.3	2010	1307.40	2009 p	204.80	12.20	8.70
Marshall Islands	2012	54.4	71.8	2007	2851.00	2009 p	419.35	16.50	20.10
Nauru	2010 e	10.0	100.0	2006–07	2071.00	2009 p	625.00	10.85	18.50
Northern Mariana Islands	2010 e	63.1	91.3	2005	12638.00	2007	...	...	25.40
Palau	2010 e	20.5	83.4	2007	8423.00	2009 p	1000.00	11.20	16.70
Polynesia									
American Samoa	2010 e	65.9	93.0	2005	9041.00	2003	500.00	...	14.00
Cook Islands	2010 e	23.3	75.3	2009	10298.00	2009 p	503.60	4.50	10.60
French Polynesia	2010 e	268.8	51.4	2006	16803.36	2008	3361.57	13.09	29.00
Niue	2010 e	1.5	37.5	2006	8208.20	2009 p	1866.55	16.94	15.81
Pitcairn Islands	2009	.05	n	...	...	...	...	...	...
Samoa	2010 e	184.0	20.2	2009–10	2908.02	2009 p	161.04	5.30	14.50
Tokelau	2006	1.5	0.0	2003	612.50	2001–09	3705.64	...	10.46
Tonga	2010 e	103.4	23.4	2008–09	2988.00	2009 p	161.04	5.30	14.50
Tuvalu	2010 e	11.2	50.4	2002	1139.32	2009 p	312.50	10.50	11.00
Wallis and Futuna	2010 e	13.3	0.0	2004	3800.00	2008	...	...	24.00

e = estimated; p = provisional; i = http://hiip.wpro.who.int/portal/countryprofiles/PapuaNewGuinea.aspx GDP = Gross Domestic Product.

Source: data from WHO Country Health Information Profiles (CHIPS) 2011.

Reproduced with permission from World Health Organization, *WHO Multi-Country. Cooperation Strategy for the Pacific 2013–2017*, Copyright © World Health Organization 2012, available from http://www.wpro.who.int/southpacific/who_pacific_mccs.pdf. Source: data from World Health Organization, *Wester Pacific Country Health Information Profiles (CHIPS)*, Copyright © World Health Organization 2011, available from http://www.wpro.who.int/health_information_evidence/documents/CHIPS/en/.

Over the ensuing years, the Ministers of Health from the Pacific in their biennial meetings have discussed and made decisions on key health issues either enhancing or hindering the achievement of Healthy Islands. These were recognized in the ministers' meeting in 2009, where they called for the revitalization of the Healthy Islands programme. The Pacific Forum agreed on a programme of recognition of successful and worthy projects in Healthy Islands.

Formal Healthy Island Recognition Programme

The WHO Healthy Island Recognition Programme explicitly connects with the visionary ideas from the Ottawa Charter on Health Promotion (WHO, 1986) and the work that was initiated by the Yanuca Declaration (Fig. 9.3.3).

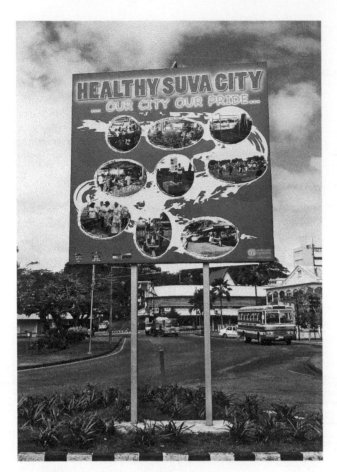

Fig. 9.3.2 Suva, capital of Fiji: a Healthy City billboard.
Image reproduced courtesy of Evelyne de Leeuw. Copyright © E de Leeuw 2014.

The WHO Healthy Island Recognition Programme was called for at the 2009 Pacific Ministers of Health Meeting as part of the call for Revitalization of Healthy Islands. Since the conception of Healthy Islands, WHO has over the years worked with its member countries and organizations to provide support for project and programme planning, implementation, and evaluation for the improvement of health and quality of life of Pacific islanders. It was soon obvious that such initiatives fell on fertile ground and a diversity of Healthy Island initiatives have been developed and progressed. To encourage further development and building on this momentum, WHO member states found that the sterling and pioneering work involved needs formal recognition.

With the main purpose to encourage communities and countries to continue to innovate and demonstrate effective and efficient ways of promoting and protecting health of populations, a formal recognition programme to recognize and award outstanding work in certain defined areas was developed. In particular, the focus was on good practices or proposals for Healthy Islands. These would have been based on community actions or efforts, would engage across different sectors, and have strong governmental support. Entries into the programme were open to all Pacific island countries and organizations. Applications were to be submitted either in the form of a report of current work in progress or completed for the Best Practice category. The Best Proposal category required the submission of a detailed proposal for intended work to be initiated. Award

monies could be used to start the proposed actions. The concept and proposal was endorsed in May 2010 during the Healthy Island Forum in Geneva, and Recognition Awards have been issued since at every Pacific Ministers of Health Meeting after receiving applications from a wide range of governments, non-governmental organizations (NGOs), and civil society organizations. A formal review of the process revealed that the countries applauded the program as a great measure of recognition of Healthy Island practices which resulted in more and better quality proposals and reports in the second round. Awards were presented for this round at the 9th Pacific Ministers of Health Meeting in Apia, Samoa, and later at the twentieth anniversary of the Healthy Islands, which was held in Fiji in 2015 where the first Pacific Ministers of Health Meeting was held initially in 1995.

Tobacco control policy in small island developing states

In addition to the importance of priority-setting through promoting sustainable development in the Healthy Islands setting, it is also crucial to recognize how public health responses to local and global health concerns can be shaped by the island environment (e.g., Rasanathan & Tukuitonga, 2007). A priority area in the Rarotonga Agreement is tobacco, one of the leading causes of death in the Pacific region. The health policy response to the global tobacco epidemic and the first international public health treaty, the Framework Convention on Tobacco Control (FCTC), has been ratified by all Pacific island nation-states, as well as all countries in the Western Pacific Region of the WHO. Adoption and ratification of the FCTC by all small island developing states in the region is an indication of the political commitment of governments to social, economic, health, and ecological development as the treaty is wide-ranging in nature, going far beyond 'traditional' tobacco control measures.

Since ratifying the FCTC, many Pacific island countries have developed tobacco control legislation and introduced key provisions such as increasing taxes on tobacco products, banning smoking in public places, and banning tobacco advertising, promotion, and sponsorship. However, numerous challenges exist in the Pacific islands that act as a barrier to implementing such provisions, some of which are attributable to the environment of small island developing states. For example, tobacco control activities in public health departments and NGOs are shaped by the small administration (with few staff undertaking many roles), a limited expertise base to draw upon, and tobacco control activities may not always infiltrate very remote islands and communities (Martin and de Leeuw, 2013; Martin, 2014). The small island environment does not always result in challenges though; some opportunities have been identified. For example, small and tightly-knit institutional and tobacco control networks can result in lean structures where decision makers are readily known and can be particularly influential, if supportive of tobacco control (Martin, 2014). This analysis of tobacco control efforts indicates that such challenges and opportunities are translatable and may similarly shape public health policy responses to other NCD-related concerns such as inadequate nutrition, physical inactivity, alcohol use, and environmental health. It is crucial that public health and health promotion professionals and agencies are cognizant of this, especially if desired policies are based on practices elsewhere.

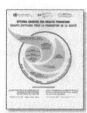
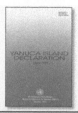
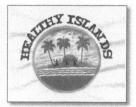

Ottawa Charter for Health Promotion	Yanuca Island Declaration Healthy Island Forum	Healthy Island Recognition
Fundamental conditions for health (peace, shelter, education, food, income, a stable ecosystem, sustainable resources, social justice, equity)	**An island-based development agenda**	**Healthy Island vision**
	Healthy places, where	**Relevance to local need**
	• Children are nurtured in body and mind	**Originality and innovation**
Adaptation to local need	• Environments invite learning and leisure	
	• People work with age and dignity	**Supported by evidence**
	• Ecological balance is a source of pride	
Enable, mediate, advocate	**Common features in Pacific islands**	**Transferability**
Reorient health services	**Flexible collaborative efforts**	**Community ownership**
Create supportive environments	**Strengthen health services (workforce)**	**Stakeholder engagement**
Strengthen community action	**Joint action environmental health**	**Government support**
Develop personal skills	**Further develop expertise and technology**	**Mass and targeted approach**
Build healthy public policy		**Overall balance**

Fig. 9.3.3 Linking the Ottawa Charter, the Yanuca Island Declaration, and the WHO Healthy Island Recognition Programme.
Reprinted from *Ottawa Charter for Health Promotion*, WHO Regional Office for Europe, Copenhagen, Copyright © 1986, available from http://www.euro.who.int/__data/assets/pdf_file/0004/129532/Ottawa_Charter.pdf.

Conclusion

The natural and social environments of small island developing states and territories in the Pacific are challenging health and equity. Climate change and the continuing crisis of NCDs add to the still existing challenges of infectious disease and inclement natural events such as storms, floods, and volcanic events. In this chapter we have discussed these challenges and two themes in which considerable progress has been made: systemic and comprehensive settings-based Healthy Island programmes, and tobacco control efforts. In spite of the adverse circumstances for many Pacific islanders and their countries, international networking efforts and agreements to recognize and support health development and sustainability are making a significant impact. It is important to continue these in a spirit of building on local assets and opportunities.

References

Briguglio, L. (1995). Small island developing states and their economic vulnerabilities. *World Development*, 23, 1615–32.

Dooris, M. (2004). Joining up settings for health: a valuable investment for strategic partnerships?. *Critical Public Health*, 14, 49–61.

Galea, G., Powis, B., & Tamplin, S. A. (2000). Healthy Islands in the Western Pacific—international settings development. *Health Promot Int*, 15, 169–78.

Malik, K. (2013). Human development report 2013. The rise of the South: Human progress in a diverse world. New York, NY: UNDP Human Development Report Office.

Martin, E. & de Leeuw, E. (2013). Exploring the implementation of the Framework Convention on Tobacco Control in four small island developing states of the Pacific: a qualitative study. *BMJ Open*, 3, e003982.

Martin, E. (2014). Implementing an International Health Treaty in Small Pacific Island Nations (Doctoral thesis, Deakin University).

Nunn, P. D. (2013). The end of the Pacific? Effects of sea level rise on Pacific Island livelihoods. *Singapore Journal of Tropical Geography*, 34, 143–71.

Nutbeam, D. (1996). Healthy Islands—a truly ecological model of health promotion. *Health Promot Int*, 11, 263–4.

Office of the President (2014). Kiribati buys a piece of Fiji. Kiribati Climate Change. Available at: http://www.climate.gov.ki/2014/05/30/kiribati-buys-a-piece-of-fiji/ [Online].

Pyrek, C. C. (2011). The Vaeakau-Taumako Wind Compass: A Cognitive Construct for Navigation in the Pacific (Doctoral dissertation, Kent State University).

Rasanathan, K. & Tukuitonga, C. F. (2007). Tobacco smoking prevalence in Pacific Island countries and territories: a review. *N Z Med J*, 120, U2742.

Smith, J. B., Schellnhuber, H. J., Mirza, M. M. Q., *et al.* (2001). Vulnerability to climate change and reasons for concern: a synthesis. In: McCarthy, J., Canziana, O., Leary, N., Dokken, D., White, K. (eds) *Climate Change 2001: Impacts, Adaptation, and Vulnerability*, pp. 913–67. New York, NY: Cambridge University Press.

United Nations (2015). Framework Convention on Climate Change. Adoption of Paris Agreement. Available at: https://unfccc.int/documentation/documents/advanced_search/items/6911.php?priref=600008831 (accessed 2 February 2016) [Online].

World Health Organization. (1984). Health promotion: a discussion document on the concept and principles: summary report of the Working Group on Concept and Principles of Health Promotion, Copenhagen, 9-13 July.

World Health Organization. (1986). Ottawa charter for health promotion: an International Conference on Health Promotion, the move towards a new public health, November 17–21, 1986. Ontario, Canada. World Health Organization, Health Canada, Canadian Public Health Association, Copenhagen/Ottawa.

World Health Organization. (1995). Yanuca Island Declaration. Regional Office for the Western Pacific, Manila.

SECTION 10

Bringing nature into public health plans and actions

CHAPTER 10.1

The role of the health professional

Robert Zarr and William Bird

Engaging doctors with nature therapy as a form of treatment that reflects good medicine

An ever increasing part of a healthcare provider's job is to help patients manage their chronic disease, and to focus on prevention. According to the US Centers for Disease Control and Prevention (CDC), more than one-third of Americans (133 million) currently suffer from non-communicable disease (NCD) like coronary heart disease, stroke, high blood pressure, type 2 diabetes, and mental health conditions (http://www.cdc.gov/healthyweight/effects/).

This chronic disease epidemic is true not only for the United States, but for many developed, and now developing countries. Globally, approximately 44% of all NCD deaths occur before the age of 70. In low- and middle-income countries, a higher proportion (48%) of all NCD deaths are estimated to occur in people under the age of 70 with 29% under the age of 60, compared with high-income countries (26% under the age of 70 and 13% under the age of 60).

Healthcare professionals have several tools to combat chronic disease, but many of the current treatment options run risks, which must be weighed carefully. Prescribing nature to prevent and treat chronic disease and promote wellness is slowly becoming an acceptable option for many health providers, looking for ways to help patients, while limiting side effects and adverse reactions. Health care providers' first duty to patients is to provide sound advice to promote health and healing and prevent disease.

As we have seen in other chapters of this book, there is a rapidly growing body of scientific literature that illustrates the effects of spending time in nature on human health. This evidence has to be 'sold' to other healthcare professionals in a way that makes prescribing nature a mainstream activity that reflects good medicine. The acceptance of nature as part of healthcare should strengthen with increasing scientific evidence. However, as also described in this book, the complexity of global health in relation to the environment may also call for an acceptance of other kinds of evidence-based medical practice. It may be that we need to conduct science and seek for knowledge around these complex issues through other kinds of studies other than randomized controlled trials. See, for example, Chapter 7.5 'Population health deficits due to biodiversity loss, climate change, and other environmental degradation' for further discussion on this matter. As evidence increases, healthcare providers can and should start incorporating nature prescriptions into their daily practice.

Parks can be prescribed as part of the daily routine of providing healthcare, in a diversity of settings, to a diversity of patients. Just as patients are asked about daily routines, including sedentary behaviour, smoking, and alcohol consumption, sleep schedules, seatbelt use, a question or two about time spent outside in natural settings can easily be inserted. Patients are often asked about their readiness and willingness to make a change in behaviour, and this can also be done in the context of asking about time spent in nature. These questions can be initiated by registration clerks, medical assistants, nurses, or other members of the healthcare team.

Healthcare providers are naturally adept at incorporating new modalities or new treatment options into the patient's treatment plan. Just as medications are prescribed, referrals to specialists initiated, and sleep hygiene recommended, professionals can write a prescription for patients to engage in physical activity or simply to spend more time outside in a park. Prescribing a park may be thought of as a small tweak in the care already delivered. Depending on the practice setting, a park prescription may be made through an electronic health record, and linked to an electronic database of parks, or it may be a paper prescription. As other prescriptions and recommendations are already done, risks and benefits shall be weighed and shared with patients. The degree of specificity and detail of the park prescription depends on the willingness or readiness of the patient, physical and mental capacity, and the likelihood of incorporating a change into their daily or weekly schedule. As with any treatment modality, follow-up is necessary to gauge the failure or success of the intervention, and to provide insight into how best to make changes that might better suit the needs of the patient. In this way, a prescription for a park is no different than any other treatment option, in that it often requires minor changes more amenable to the patient's likelihood to follow through.

All health interventions require evaluation to determine whether it has been effective and whether it remains cost-effective when compared to another similar intervention. The data collected can be objective, such as body mass index, peak flow, haemoglobin A-1 C, and blood pressure; or subjective, such as validated physical activity or mental health questionnaires asked at baseline, and at intervals up to a year. This combination of subjective and objective evaluation helps confirm whether prescribing parks brings about the desired outcome in patients' health and well-being.

The medical model is not suited in treating the global rise of depression, diabetes, obesity, and other NCDs. The causes are too complex and the problem too broad for healthcare to be able to adequately reverse the rising trend. Even public health schemes to increase physical activity and diet struggle to make inroads to changes in whole population health behaviour. There needs to be a structural change in thinking in order to shift this epidemic.

In the following, the authors of this chapter share insights from their own healthcare practice and experience of nature prescription. Four schemes are outlined where nature is used as part of the overall treatment for patients or as health promotion. These schemes can be seen as part of what is sometimes termed the third revolution of healthcare. The first revolution in the nineteenth century was the introduction of public health principles, such as improved sanitation, better housing, and working conditions. Many of our urban parks were created during this period, to improve the health of the people in the neighbourhood. The second revolution in the twentieth century was based on technology, using drugs and anaesthetics to create new cures. During this era, the sense of environment and nature as healthy places was, at least partly, lost and many parks and nature areas were sacrificed. The third revolution, currently starting, is the democratization of health by communities through increased knowledge, support, and development of healthier places and self-care.

Park Rx America

As a primary care public health paediatrician in Washington DC, I was inspired by Richard Louv's bestseller *Last Child in the Woods* (2005), to create a programme to help doctors and other healthcare professionals connect their patients to parks and other protected areas, through an actual park prescription. An often under-recognized social determinant of health, access to green space can and should play a vital role in creating and maintaining our physical, mental, and emotional health, while at home, work, school, or play.

The average person living in a developed nation spends approximately 90% of any 24-hour period indoors (Matz *et al.*, 2014). Much of this time is spent sedentary and in front of a screen, many times while eating. This indoor, and often sedentary lifestyle, is an ever increasing factor in developing chronic disease, which leads to poor health outcomes and premature death. In the United States, for every dollar spent on healthcare, 86% is spent on patients with one or more chronic disease. We also know that 70% of our world population will be living in an urban area by 2030, just 13 years away. Given the current burden of chronic disease and the density of the human population in urban areas, the relevance of urban parks is beginning to take centre stage in public health, medicine, and health economics. The urgency and gravity of this public health epidemic motivated my colleagues and I to find a way to make it easy to connect our patients to green spaces.

Park Rx America is a non-profit organization whose mission is to decrease the burden of chronic disease, increase health and happiness, and foster environmental stewardship, by virtue of prescribing Nature during the routine delivery of healthcare.

The success of Park Rx America is in large part due to the partnerships among healthcare providers, health centre and hospital administrators, public health officials, academic institutions and their students, local health departments, local and federal land management agencies, and several national organizations with either a vested environmental or health interest.

With such robust partnerships, we have identified and catalogued green space in Washington DC, several metropolitan areas of Maryland, Anchorage, Alaska, and Bellingham, Washington. We have created clear and concise one-page summaries, called Park Pages, for over 2000 parks. As such, a national searchable park database (www.ParkRxAmerica.org) (see Fig. 10.1.1) has been created and linked to the electronic health records of community health centers, hospital systems, and group practices around the country. The uniqueness of Park Rx America is that it has been created by health providers for health providers. We have paid particularly

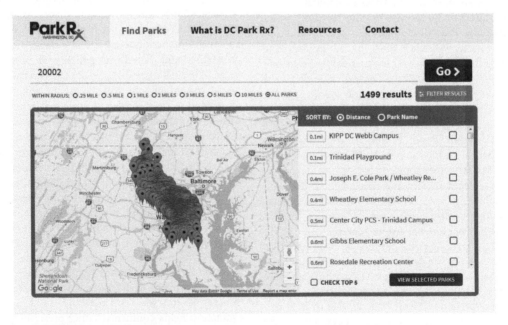

Fig. 10.1.1 Screenshot of the Park Rx America 'Park Formulary'.
Reproduced with permission from Park Rx America, Washington DC, Copyright © 2017 Park Rx America.

close attention to make sure that Park Rx America is not only relevant to the work of health providers, but that it is easy to use.

Since 1 July 2013, as a growing group of health providers, we have been prescribing parks to people of all ages to prevent and treat chronic disease, as well as promote wellness. Park Rx America has been integrated into the culture of several provider organizations across the US. Since its inception, over 2,000 Park prescriptions have been prescribed. At subsequent visits to the initial park prescription, providers are also highly encouraged to ask six follow-up questions, fully embedded into the electronic health record. The answers to these questions both guide clinical management for how best to modify subsequent park prescriptions, as well as generate data for quality improvement purposes.

Park Rx America is rapidly expanding across the US. Close partnership with US National Park Service's Healthy Parks Healthy People Initiative, as well as funding from a local family foundation has allowed us the opportunity to: (i) expand nationally; (ii) maximize technology (bidirectional communication between providers and patients, portability via mobile device apps, social media capacity) to enhance ease of use of park database for health providers, patients, and the public at large; (iii) measure change in chronic disease health outcomes; and (iv) partner with organizations well positioned to expand Park Rx nationally. Given the current endeavour of the United States Geological Survey in creating a Protected Areas Database of the United States (http://gapanalysis.usgs.gov/padus/), it is quite possible that within the next few years, we will grow our nascent national park database, relevant to health providers and the public at large, that can ultimately be hard-coded into electronic health record packages as a standard feature, just as they currently provide for drug formularies. Park Rx America may contribute to creating a new paradigm in which parks are not just seen as places to recreate, but as an essential part of individual and public health.

Health Walks, Green Gym, and Beat the Street

In the United Kingdom, about 30% of the adult population do less than 30 minutes of physical activity a week. Levels of walking continue to decline. As a family physician in the United Kingdom, I have been working to increase levels of physical activity in patients who are inactive and whose lives are increasingly been confined to indoors because of poverty, illness, or poor mental health. However, a significant reason for low levels of inactivity is that patients have little opportunity to walk in supportive surroundings, particularly when they live in hostile urban environments often characterized by antisocial behaviour, fast traffic, and poor aesthetics.

Walking for Health (https://www.walkingforhealth.org.uk/) was set up 1996 in Oxfordshire, UK as scheme where patients lead other patients on short walks often in parks designed for those who are inactive. There are now over 100,000 Health Walks a year in the United Kingdom with 850,000 participants. The key factors that get people started are that the walks are short, regular, and local using the local natural environment, and recommended by a friend or health professional. Women make up 60% of participants and they especially benefit from the group walks as they feel safer walking in a group. The concern about personal safety appears to reduce after participating in Health Walks (Dawson et al., 2007).

Patients can be referred by their family doctor or nurse to the free local walk group where they join the introductory walks in green space that are less than 1.5 km, walked at a slow speed, which means that at this level of intensity there are no health contraindications to start. Each new person then fills in a Physical Activity Readiness Questionnaire (PAR-Q; a 1-page form to see if you should check with your doctor before becoming much more physically active) (Cardinal et al., 1996). If this is positive for any risk factor such as chest pain or palpitations, then the leader explains to the new walker that they should seek medical advice, but the responsibility remains with the patient so they are free to participate if they choose.

The family doctor has a key role in recommending Health Walks. First, they explain the importance of walking as an exercise that carries virtually all the benefits of gym-based exercises. Second, they give permission for the patient to be active which is particularly important if they have an existing medical condition. Third, they encourage the patient to be active by signposting and recommending them to the walking scheme (or park or other exercise scheme). This endorsement by the doctor or nurse is important to link the healthcare setting with a community setting.

Although the patient may see health as the initial motivating factor, the social interaction and experience of walking through local green space become powerful motivating factors for continuing walking (Sugiyama et al., 2013). These factors further enhance the health effect, as both social interaction and access to green space are important health factor.

There is good evidence that nature-based Health Walks lead to significantly less depression, perceived stress, and negative affect compared to non-participation (Marselle et al., 2014). It seems to be the improvement in mental health that is important in preventing physical illnesses. Patients with long-term conditions such as diabetes, obesity, dementia, cancer, and cardiovascular disease are more likely to have associated mental illness (Patten et al., 2005).

Nature-based Health Walks prevent the annual decline in function usually seen in older people. Keeping active is of significant importance in maintaining independence and preventing ageing diseases such as dementia, cardiovascular disease, and falls (Dawson et al., 2006).

The Green Gym

Despite the strong evidence linking local green space with good health, it is unclear how we can engage a community to improve their own green space. The Green Gym (http://www.tcv.org.uk/greengym) is a UK National Scheme which I set up in 1997 with the Trust for Conversation Volunteers (TCV) where the family physician refers patients with mental health problems or other chronic diseases into conservation work supervised by trained conservationists. Yerrell (2008) found numerous fitness benefits (in strength, flexibility, stamina, and enhanced daily activity levels) gained from working outdoors in an evaluation of the Green Gym. Findings suggested that activities were of sufficient duration and intensity to improve general cardiovascular fitness among participants, promoting significant improvements in physical health scores after six months of regular involvement.

Birch (2005) found that in addition to improving fitness, the participants valued the scheme as a means of enhancing mental well-being, being stimulated by nature and enjoying social contact, and as a flexible way in which to attain a valued productive role. In particular, the flexibility and diversity of tasks at the Green Gym suggest that it has the potential to enable occupationally deprived individuals, including those who have experienced social exclusion through mental ill-health, to access a productive occupation in the community.

There are many areas where the National Health Service uses Green Gyms and outdoor exercise to treat and look after their patients (see for example: http://www.nhs.uk/Livewell/fitness/Pages/free-fitness.aspx#couch). Social Prescribing is being rolled out across the NHS in England so that every family doctor will eventually have the ability to refer patients to walks, parks, cookery lessons, fitness events as part of normal medical care.

Beat the Street

Beat the Street is an initiative created by Intelligent Health (www.intelligenthealth.co.uk) and funded by local health organizations that uses gamification to get more people to become active and visit parks and green spaces. Gamification is defined as 'The use of game design elements in non-game contexts' (Deterding et al., 2011). It was highlighted by the UK Government's behavioural insights team as an example of the 'nudge' theory of behaviour change (Mitlon and Oliver, 2010). Beat the Street originated in Hyde Park, London (Rashid et al., 2008) and then as a walk to school programme (Hunter et al., 2015). By now, it works as a programme where every family doctor in a defined geographic area can take part by handing a smartcard to patients. At the same time, all school children and their parents are issued with a card and are then instructed to touch their radio frequency identification (RFID) cards on card readers placed in parks and on lampposts. Children and their parents and grandparents are therefore encouraged to walk or cycle into parks, along rivers and into greenspace to touch their card on the units and create journeys. Each person is a member of a team that is a community group or a school. The more journeys made between the RFID units, the more points go to teams, and the higher up the leader board they go. In some towns, up to 39% of the entire population play at the same time for a period of seven weeks. This means that in many towns and cities between 20,000 and 40,000 people participate, of which 50% are children and the remaining 50% are made up of parents, grandparents, neighbours, and patients. In the city of Reading, United Kingdom, 15,074 participants (8,416 children and 6,658 adults) played Beat the Street accumulating 244,537 miles. Some 35% of adults reached the Government's recommended physical activity levels and this increased to 45% at the end of the scheme and 53% after three months. Twelve per cent (12%) of the participants of Beat the Street had a long-term condition such as diabetes (Meredith and Wagstaff, 2016). The return on investment using the National Institute of Clinical Excellence and Health (NICE) criteria means that for every one dollar spent there is a return of $3.53 in transport savings, $14.58 in extra productivity (workplace benefits), and $16.39 savings in healthcare costs based on a quality-adjusted life year (QALY) model (Mallender et al., 2013).

The main impact from Beat the Street is connecting people to their local area and to parks and green spaces that they haven't been to before. The extrinsic reward to the 'game' is then converted to the intrinsic reward of the experience in the park, often with friends or a family that the person had not experienced before. This connection to place and the associated sense of place and purpose brings communities together and helps individuals become a part of the community, while also being physically active.

Conclusion

Healthcare is changing to deal with the mass epidemic of chronic, non-communicable diseases. The natural environment is a health resource that remains largely underused by health providers. Even with clear evidence that confirms and sometimes quantifies the benefits of nature, there is very poor evidence as to how this can be best used and delivered in healthcare. The schemes demonstrated in this chapter are examples that will create an evidence base to help us know what works best in harnessing the health benefits of nature to both prevent and help treat patients with long-term conditions. There are many more schemes around the world that are engaging patients with nature and over time the evaluation and research will expose the weaker initiatives and promote the effective ones. Although these are early days, it may be the first steps to a systematic inclusion of nature into healthcare delivery for the health benefit of coming generations.

References

Birch, M. (2005). Cultivating wildness: three conservation volunteers' experiences of participation in the Green Gym scheme. *Br J Occupational Ther*, 68, 244–52.

Cardinal, B. J., Esters, J., & Cardinal, M. K. (1996). Evaluation of the revised physical activity readiness questionnaire in older adults. *Med Sci Sports Exerc*, 28, 468–72.

Dawson, J., Boller, I., Foster, C., & Hillsdon, M. (2006). Evaluation of changes to physical activity amongst people who attend the walking the way to health initiative (WHI). Cheltenham, UK: Oxford Brookes University, the Countryside Agency.

Dawson, J., Hillsdon, M., Boller, I., & Foster, C. (2007). Perceived barriers to walking in the neighborhood environment: a survey of middle-aged and older adults. *J Aging Phys Act*, 15, 318.

Deterding, S., Dixon, D., Khaled, R., & Nacke, L. (2011). From game design elements to gamefulness: defining gamification. In: Proceedings of the 15th international academic MindTrek conference: Envisioning future media environments, pp. 9–15. ACM.

Hunter, R. F., de Silva, D., Reynolds, V., Bird, W., & Fox, K. R. (2015). International inter-school competition to encourage children to walk to school: a mixed methods feasibility study. *BMC Research Notes*, 8, 1.

Louv, R. (2005). *Last Child in the Woods: Saving Our Children from Nature-Deficit Disorder*. Chapel Hill, NC: Algonquin Books.

Mallender, J., Bertranou, E., Owen, L., Lester-George, A., Jhita, T., & Roberts, S. (2013). *Physcial Activity Return on Investment Tool*. London, UK: National Institute for Health and Care Excellence.

Marselle, M. R., Irvine, K. N., & Warber, S. L. (2014). Examining group walks in nature and multiple aspects of well-being: A large-scale study. *Ecopsychology*, 6, 134–47.

Matz, C. J., Stieb, D. M., Davis, K., et al. (2014). Effects of age, season, gender and urban-rural status on time-activity: Canadian Human Activity Pattern Survey 2 (CHAPS 2). *Int J Environ Res Public Health*, 11, 2108–24.

Meredith, S. & Wagstaff, C. (2016). Evaluating stealth motivation interventions to promote exercise referral scheme engagement and adherence. In: Scott, A. & Gidlow, C. (eds) *Clinical Exercise Science*, pp. 285-303. Abingdon, UK: Routledge.

Milton, A. & Oliver, L. (2010). Applying behavioural insight to health. Cabinet Office Behavioural Insights Team. Crown copyright. Available at: https://www.gov.uk/government/uploads/system/uploads/attachment_data/file/60524/403936_BehaviouralInsight_acc.pdf [Online].

Park Rx America. Available at: www.ParkRxAmerica.org [Online].

Patten, S. B., Beck, C. A., Kassam, A., Williams, J. V., Barbui, C., & Metz, L. M. (2005). Long-term medical conditions and major depression: strength of association for specific conditions in the general population. *Can J Psychiatry*, 50, 195–202.

Rashid, O., Coulton, P., & Bird, W. (2008). Using NFC to support and encourage green exercise. In: 2008 Second International Conference on Pervasive Computing Technologies for Healthcare, pp. 214–17. IEEE.

Sugiyama, T., Giles-Corti, B., Summers, J., du Toit, L., Leslie, E., & Owen, N. (2013). Initiating and maintaining recreational walking: a longitudinal study on the influence of neighborhood green space. *Prev Med*, 57, 178–82.

The Green Gym. Available at: http://www.tcv.org.uk/greengym [Online].

United States Geological Survey. Protected Areas Database of the United States. Available at: http://gapanalysis.usgs.gov/padus [Online].

US Centers for Disease Control and Prevention (CDC). The Health Effects of Overweight and Obesity. Available at: http://www.cdc.gov/healthyweight/effects/ [Online].

Walking for Health. Available at: https://www.walkingforhealth.org.uk/ [Online].

Yerrell, P. (2008). *National Evaluation of TCV's Green Gym*. Report for the School of Health and Social Care, Oxford Brookes University. Oxford UK: Oxford Brookes University.

The role of environmental law

Cinnamon P. Carlarne and Jeffrey M. Bielicki

Environmental law: an overview

'Environmental law' is an expansive term frequently used to discuss the legal and regulatory strategies used to control pollution, manage natural resources, and generally mediate how humans interact with the natural environment. The laws creating the National Park System and the National Forest System in the United States and elsewhere are early examples of environmental laws. The modern field of environmental law is a product of the 1960s and 1970s, when the field emerged rapidly in response to the increasing visibility of environmental degradation and increasing awareness of the negative impacts of environmental degradation on human and natural systems. At the domestic and international levels, environmental law evolved in tandem with the rapid growth of the global economy and the concomitant growth in consumption and the associated negative impacts these changes sometimes brought both for the environment and the humans that depended upon it. Polluted waterways, smog-filled air, and disappearing species created a backdrop against which scientists, civil society, and politicians called for regulations to address environmental concerns. The development of environmental law proceeded apace, and almost all developed and many developing countries implemented parallel systems of domestic environmental law. Similarly, at the international level, countries developed the corpus of international environmental law, which now includes more than 1,100 multilateral, 1,500 bilateral, and 250 'other' environmental treaties—the vast majority of which have been negotiated since 1960 (Mitchell, 2014).

Objectives of environmental law

The shape, intent, and goals of environmental law are complex and vary within and across jurisdictions. Among others, these varied goals include: integrating environmental considerations into decision-making; improving environmental conditions (e.g. air quality, water quality); minimizing loss of biodiversity; and preserving natural ecosystems. Environmental law is directly and indirectly tied to human health and well-being, and many instruments of environmental law have explicit human health objectives, including many *pollution control laws, natural resource laws*, and *mineral resource laws* that exist under the broad umbrella of environmental law.

Pollution control laws

Pollution control laws focus on improving environmental quality by controlling the release of substances into the environment. The United States' Clean Air Act and Clean Water Act (and their counterparts in other jurisdictions) are classic pollution control statutes that reflect diverse objectives, including direct and indirect justifications for preserving and improving human health and well-being. The US Clean Air Act, for example, seeks 'to protect and enhance the quality of the Nation's air resources so as to promote the public health and welfare and the productive capacity of its population' (42 U.S.C.A. § 7401(b)(1). (2012)). And, while the US Clean Water Act does not directly emphasize human health in its preamble, the Act uses human health as the primary criterion for establishing Water Quality Standards, one of the cornerstones of the Act.

Natural resource laws

Natural resources laws focus on managing the way that humans directly interact with the environment by designating how certain lands and resources can be used. For example, laws creating national parks and forests characterize certain ecosystems as special and then dictate the ways in which humans can interact with these lands. These limitations have multiple goals, ranging from maintaining ecosystem services, preserving rare species or habitats, providing recreational opportunities, to protecting a space perceived to be important because of its beauty and uniqueness. Many of these goals are intimately linked with concerns for human well-being. For example, setting aside land for parks and forests preserves ecosystem services that are vital to human well-being because of the ecosystem services that they provide (e.g. flood control, water filtration, fuel and fibre production). Further, since the early days of the US Natural Park System, lawmakers have recognized that natural spaces are important to human well-being in part because these areas provide spaces not only for recreation, but also for mental and spiritual renewal.

Mineral resource laws

Mineral resource laws frequently control access to, and use of land with minerals on or under them, dictating who can extract those minerals and how extraction can take place. These laws also regulate how the materials can be transported, converted, combusted, and disposed of—processes that often also fall under the purview of one or more pollution control laws. Issues of access and extraction (at the beginning of the supply chain) involve interactions between property laws, zoning laws, and natural resource laws; public lands and the relevant laws are likely to be applied from the top down, whereas when private lands are involved an array of national and local laws may apply.

The underlying objective of most mineral resource laws has typically been to maximize production and minimize waste; concerns for human well-being do not tend to be primary drivers or underlying goals. Explicit consideration of human well-being tends to focus on the details of the particular operations (e.g. safety standards, limitations on air and water emissions). But the human well-being implications of the extraction and subsequent use of these minerals are profound and complex, and mineral resource laws thus link the environment to human well-being in direct and indirect ways. For example, laws that facilitate access and extraction of energy resources support a primary foundation of developed economies: affordable and reliable energy. Access to affordable and reliable energy allows people to stay cool, to stay warm, and to travel to the jobs that provide them with the income they need to enhance their well-being.

There are definite benefits to human well-being from laws that encourage access to mineral resources, but the negative impacts to human well-being of using them—especially fossil fuel resources—are abundant as well. From local air pollution, to land degradation, to water contamination, to climate change, the downsides of easy access to energy resources and minimal control over their subsequent use are well documented.

Beyond environmental law

Many fields of law outside of the traditional umbrella of environmental law influence how environmental law functions, whether and how environmental objectives are met, and thus the direct and indirect effects of nature and the environment on human well-being. Environmental law exists alongside and interacts with numerous other areas of law that influence the ways in which humans interact with the environment, including: energy law, public health law, property law, disaster law, and tax law.

As important as environmental laws are in influencing the quality of the natural environment—with direct and indirect effects on well-being—land use laws, for example, are often equally important in shaping how humans interact with, and are affected by, the environment. Land use law interacts with larger rules of property law and environmental law to determine what the natural and built environment looks like. Broadly understood, land use law 'encompasses the full range of laws and regulations that influence or affect the development and conservation of the land' (Pace Law School, 2008). These laws determine whether land can be developed, how that land can be used (e.g. industrial, agricultural, commercial, residential), and what types of general restrictions will be placed on the land in the context of the designated use. Land use laws affect population density, transportation, levels of light, levels of noise, ease of access to food, and ease of access to public spaces—all of which have important ramifications for human well-being.

Within this larger context, it becomes evident that understanding how environmental law influences human health requires multipart analyses of how law directly and indirectly influences at least three environmental and social conditions:

1. the quality of the environment (e.g. air, water, biodiversity);

2. the accessibility of the environment (e.g. parks, forests, open spaces); and

3. background conditions (e.g. access to affordable and reliable energy that underpins daily comfort and existence).

These factors—and the laws that influence them—cannot be viewed in isolation if the hope is to fully understand the interplay between law, nature, and human well-being.

Environmental law—human well-being in context

Environmental law often exists in a complicated relationship with other fields of law, with complex implications for human well-being. The case of hydraulic fracturing, for example, provides a contemporary example of the complexity involved in understanding the relationship between environmental law, other areas of law, nature, and human well-being. In the United States, as described in the following section, a federal energy law exempts this new production technique from a key provision of existing environmental law. This exemption, alongside numerous other pre-existing exclusions from environmental law for oil and gas exploration and production wastes, removes regulatory barriers. These regulatory exemptions enabled the rapid expansion of the use of horizontal drilling for hydraulic fracturing. This new wave of drilling presents a series of questions concerning the human and environmental risks and benefits associated with hydraulic fracturing and related activities. The risks and benefits are direct and indirect, and understanding the full range of risks and benefits is critical to understanding the relationship between the role of law and the nature–human health and well-being dynamic.

Unconventional oil and gas development with hydraulic fracturing

Hydraulic fracturing is a process that injects a mixture of large volumes of water, sand, and chemicals under high pressure to create fractures in impervious geologic formations (typically shale). This fracturing creates new pathways for oil and natural gas to flow and thus be cost-effectively produced. Since the early 2000s, hydraulic fracturing in combination with deep horizontal drilling have provided the technological means that facilitated the rapid expansion of unconventional oil and gas development in the United States; the use of these techniques has spread to other countries (e.g. the United Kingdom, Australia, China, and Poland). The US Environmental Protection Agency (EPA) frames the many benefits and concerns of unconventional oil and gas development thusly: 'Natural gas plays a key role in our nation's clean energy future. The United States has vast reserves of natural gas that are commercially viable as a result of advances in horizontal drilling and hydraulic fracturing technologies enabling greater access to gas in shale formations. Responsible development of America's shale gas resources *offers important economic, energy security, and environmental benefits*. EPA is working with states and other key stakeholders to help ensure that natural gas extraction does not come at the *expense of public health and the environment* ... The Agency is investing in improving our scientific understanding of hydraulic fracturing, providing regulatory clarity with respect to existing laws, and using existing authorities where appropriate to enhance health and environmental safeguards' (emphasis added). (US EPA, 2015).

The rapid expansion of unconventional oil and gas development was enabled in key part by the 2005 US Energy Policy Act, which amended the Safe Drinking Water Act to exempt hydraulic fracturing from primary provisions of this environmental law (US Congress, 2005). The hydraulic fracturing technique has also been exempted or excluded from numerous other environmental and public health laws, regulations, and forms of governance and oversight, including: the Clean Water Act; the National Environmental Policy Act; the Resource Conservation and Recovery Act; the

Comprehensive Environmental Response, Compensation, and Liability Act; the Clean Air Act; and the Emergency Planning and Community Right-To-Know Act (Brady, 2012; GAO, 2012; Vann *et al.*, 2014).

These exemptions and exclusions have removed oversight and allowed the horizontal drilling and hydraulic fracturing technologies to expand widely in the United States. The widespread and increasing use of these technologies for unconventional oil and gas development has potential upsides and potential downsides to human well-being across the three themes. We next briefly introduce some of these potential benefits and drawbacks:

Potential benefits of unconventional oil and gas development with hydraulic fracturing

1. **Expanding the supply of affordable and reliable energy.** Using hydraulic fracturing, oil and gas can be produced from shale resources that are not otherwise economically recoverable using conventional approaches. Affordable and reliable sources of energy are economic cornerstones in most developed countries. Cheap and reliable energy increases human well-being in various ways, including by facilitating human mobility, enabling people to more affordably heat or cool their environment to be safe and comfortable, and by allowing people to have more money left-over to provide for other needs and wants.

2. **Decreasing dependence on foreign energy sources.** Unconventional oil and gas development also supplements domestic energy production. This reduced dependence on foreign sources of energy benefits the domestic economy, reduces security risks associated with relying on unstable areas for fuel, and improves the United States' overall position in the global energy economy.

3. **Reducing emissions and negative by-products of use.** Expanded supplies of affordable, reliable, and abundant natural gas have reduced the amount of coal used to generate baseload electricity in the United States. Compared to coal, natural gas emits less carbon dioxide, sulphur dioxide, nitrogen oxides, and virtually no particulates or mercury when it is burned. The direct, immediate, and local threats to human well-being from using coal (e.g. particulates create and exacerbate respiratory conditions, mercury is toxic and impedes senses and coordination) are avoided or minimized when natural gas is substituted for coal, and the pace of long-term global threats to human well-being from issues like climate change, arguably, are slowed. Further, natural gas does not produce physical by-products when it is burned. Burning coal produces 'coal combustion by-products', including fly ash. Fly ash disposal is poorly regulated, and mismanagement creates substantial risks to human well-being, property, and the terrestrial and aquatic ecosystems that humans rely upon and appreciate (US EPA, 2010; WHO, 2005).

4. **Encouraging penetration of renewable energy technologies in the electricity system.** To avoid blackouts and brownouts, the amount of electricity that is supplied must equal the amount that is demanded; natural gas power plants can generate electricity when needed to fill in generation from variable renewable sources, like wind and sunlight; coal power plants can only provide relatively constant baseload power. As a result, natural gas can be a fuel that enables penetration of wind and solar energy technologies by providing electricity that is demanded when these renewable resources are not generating electricity (e.g. no

wind, night-time). Human well-being is increased when energy technologies that have less environmental impacts and fewer human health hazards than fossil fuel energy technologies, especially coal, are increasingly utilized.

5. **Decreasing surface environmental footprints.** Horizontal wells have smaller surface environmental footprints than conventional vertical wells because each horizontal well runs along the subsurface formation and thus contacts more of the formation than does a vertical well. In addition, multiple horizontal wells in the subsurface can emanate in different directions from the surface wellpad. This reduced surface area decreases the amount of land that is impacted, with concomitant benefits for the quality of the local environment including less sedimentation, less surface runoff, and reduced areas where ecosystems and biodiversity may be affected, among others. Similarly, where natural gas is displacing coal, the extraction footprint is smaller and has fewer negative consequences as compared to surface mining and mountaintop removal, as well as minimizing hazards to human well-being associated with working in mines and around the heavy machinery that is required for coal extraction.

6. **Developing local economies.** Unconventional hydrocarbon production develops industries and creates jobs, provides royalty and lease income, and generates activity that infuses money into areas that are typically rural and, often, in-need of economic investment (Hefley and Wang, 2015; Paredes *et al.*, 2015; Weinstein and Partridge, 2014). Much of the development targets shale resources that are located underneath economically depressed areas (e.g. Eastern Ohio), the jobs, incomes, and monetary infusions can have positive effects on human well-being in those areas.

Potential drawbacks of unconventional oil and gas development with hydraulic fracturing

1. **Consuming increasingly scarce water.** The hydraulic fracturing process consumes vast amounts of water—3–5 million gallons per well, on average, but some operators have reported up to 10 million gallons or more—which is often acquired from surface water or municipal water sources. Given that tens of thousands of wells have already been hydraulically fractured, the aggregate demand for water is enormous. Many environmental groups and community organizations have expressed concerns and objections to the use of these public waters for private use, including in terms of competition for increasingly scarce water resources due to other demands, and changing supplies due to droughts and altered precipitation patterns resulting from climate change. Consuming extensive amounts of water poses important questions about who has access to, and who benefits from, using this water.

2. **Managing flowback water disposal.** The flowback water that is produced early in the hydraulic fracturing process is contaminated with numerous constituents, some of which may be toxic and hazardous to human health and others of which may be radioactive (Adgate *et al.*, 2014; US EPA, 2012). This water is often so contaminated after use that it cannot be treated or reused by others outside the oil and gas industry. Flowback water that is not reused for subsequent hydraulic fracturing is often disposed through deep injection wells, which, in the United States, are regulated under the EPA's Underground Injection

Control programme. Onsite spills, accidents during transportation, or mismanagement and improper disposal of this flowback water may contaminate ecosystems and groundwater (US EPA, 2012), and thus affect human well-being by decreasing the function and utility of these natural resources.

3. **Potentially contaminating groundwater.** The fracturing process itself is typically deep underground and isolated from groundwater resources, but it is possible that the well casing or cementing that penetrates through groundwater aquifers could leak, and thus groundwater could become contaminated by chemicals and other hazardous and toxic constituents of the fracturing fluids, the flowback water, or the produced oil or gas (Darrah et al., 2014; Jackson et al., 2013; Zoback and Arent, 2014).

4. **Creating seismic hazards.** There is growing evidence that hydraulic fracturing and deep well disposal of flowback water can induce seismicity. Some of the largest earthquakes in areas without much history of seismic activity have recently occurred where hydraulic fracturing is widely deployed (e.g. Ohio) or where flowback water is being disposed in deep injection wells (e.g. Oklahoma) (USGS, 2015; Wines, 2015). Measurements also indicate a significant increase in low-level earthquakes in areas where deep well disposal is taking place, and the number and timing of these seismic episodes correlates with the rapid expansion of hydraulic fracturing activities. Earthquakes endanger human well-being in numerous ways, including by damaging property and infrastructure, and creating the potential for human injury or death.

5. **Exacerbating climate change.** In addition to producing a hydrocarbon that emits carbon dioxide when combusted, hydraulic fracturing may release methane—a more potent greenhouse gas than carbon dioxide—into the air, in part because the production process may not fully capture all of the natural gas (typically about 93% methane) that is liberated from the shale. Rates of fugitive emissions of methane directly at the wellpad are presently uncertain, but studies have reported up to 3.3% (Howarth, 2014; Howarth et al., 2011). Ageing infrastructure, such as pipelines, that is increasingly relied upon to transport natural gas produced by hydraulic fracturing is another major source of leakage. An early study suggested that 1.4% of natural gas flowing through pipelines in Russia leaked to the atmosphere (Lelieveld et al., 2005), but recent studies have shown that emissions from infrastructure and other facilities and activities in US cities is much higher (Jackson et al., 2014; Mckain et al., 2015; Phillips et al., 2013). Methane emissions create local, short-term hazards to human health through ambient air contamination and global, long-term hazards to human health by exacerbating climate change.

6. **Increasing exposure to toxic and hazardous substances are adversely affecting air quality.** Many of the chemicals used in hydraulic fracturing fluids are known to be toxic and hazardous to human health (Colburn et al., 2011; Wattenberg et al., 2015), and public concerns have been raised about the lack of transparency in what is being used. While the potential for public exposure to these chemicals is low, transporting and mixing and using these chemicals on site at the wellpad creates occupational exposure hazards (Adgate et al., 2014; Wattenberg et al., 2015). Due to the emissions of ozone precursors, particulates, and air toxics throughout the lifecycles of oil and natural gas production, unconventional oil and gas development can produce or exacerbate local and regional air quality issues (Adgate et al., 2014; Moore et al., 2014).

7. **Creating local community disruption.** The increase in activity and the influx of jobs and money associated with hydraulic fracturing can engender layers of problems for human well-being. The typically rural communities where unconventional hydrocarbon development is occurring tend to lack adequate road, healthcare, hotel, restaurant, and other infrastructure sufficient to support the influx of activity. Residents have also voiced concerns about increased heavy truck traffic and the resulting degradation of roads and bridges, noise and air pollution, and general disruption to their rural way of life (Willow, 2015). The influxes of people and money are often associated with increased drug and alcohol abuse, as well as prostitution due to the large numbers of typically male workers migrating to the area (Hennesy-Fiske, 2014; Horowitz, 2014). Social stress may also result because some residents may benefit more than others (e.g. royalties from lease vs. no lease; differences in lease terms) or there may be mixed feelings about the presence of the industry or deployment of the hydraulic fracturing technique in the community. Property near hydraulic fracturing sites may lose value (Gopalakrishnan and Klaiber, 2014). In addition, concerns have been voiced about the potential for the extreme economic lows that typically follow the extreme economic highs in the boom-bust cycles that are often associated with extractive industries like unconventional oil and gas development (Weinstein and Partridge, 2014). When the boom dissipates, local communities can be left socially fragmented and economically dependent on an industry that is no longer there. If planning has not adequately addressed and prepared to mitigate these issues during the boom, the fallout can be devastating for social relations and human well-being. Overall, these challenges put additional physical and mental stressors on local communities (Adgate et al., 2014).

The potential benefits and drawbacks of unconventional oil and natural gas development with hydraulic fracturing reveal the challenges that law and policy makers face when devising laws to meditate the relationship between humans and the environment. Understanding is increasing about the degree to which these potential outcomes are benefits and drawbacks of the hydraulic fracturing enterprise, but the related regulatory regimes remain in their infancy, with many of these activities still excluded from, or exempted from oversight. Human well-being is influenced by economic conditions, access to energy, access to social and health services, the existing quality of the local environment, and the state of the global climate. Even if environmental laws ensure that humans have access to green space, their health may be poor if the land, the air, or the water is polluted, or if they return to a home that is too cold or too hot, or if they live in a depressed region where they cannot find a job that allows them to afford adequate food and healthcare. Equally, if the law permits liberal energy extraction, this many have certain positive short-term, localized effects on human health through job creation and affordable energy, but also negative long-term, local, and global effects on human well-being as a result of growing income inequalities, new forms of pollution and pathways for them, and exacerbating climate change.

National parks

The role that law plays in creating parks, conservation areas, and other 'set-aside' natural areas is another way of examining the complex ways in which nature conservation law can influence human well-being. The US Congress began the first era of formal nature conservation during the late 1800s (Baritz, 1961; Fussell, 1966; Nash, 2001). In 1872, legislation created the world's first official National Park: Yellowstone National Park. By 1890, Congress had established three more national parks—Sequoia, Yosemite, and General Grant—and by the mid-twentieth century had designated a further 58 areas as national parks, and allocated some level of protected status to over 390 different sites nationwide. Other nations soon followed: Australia established the Royal National Park in 1879; Canada created Banff National Park in 1885; New Zealand set up its first national park in 1887; and Sweden became the first European nation to protect some of its land with its set of nine national parks in 1909. By the turn of the century, over 44,000 protected areas covered 13,630,616 km^2 worldwide (IUCN, 2015).

Different legal designations for protected areas include national parks, national forests, nature reserves, and other formal designations that accord varying levels of legal protection depending on the country and the type of landscape. Some systems, such as the US National Park System, prohibit most types of economic activity in the protected area. By contrast, other systems, such as the US National Forest System[1], allow limited economic activities, such as logging, in the designated area.

Prompted in part by early preservationist and conservationist leaders such as Henry David Thoreau, George Perkins Marsh, John Muir, and Gifford Pinchot, many of the early laws emerged as a result of Romanticist art and Transcendentalist writing and reflected notions of the intrinsic value of nature to human well-being. The perpetual existence of these areas allowed humans to know that these areas exist, to visit them, and to trust that they would exist in the future. Today, much is known about the benefits to human well-being associated with spending time outdoors. In many locations, parks and preserves provide invaluable opportunities to do so. From this perspective, using law to designate these protected areas enhances the nature–human connection and offers opportunities for enriching human well-being.

But the early approach to creating protected areas emphasized centralized planning and generally excluded local people from planning and management processes (Brown, 2002; Mehta and Kellert, 1998; Neumann, 2002). During this era, especially in the developing world, the interests and priorities of the people living around and within conservation areas were generally viewed as obstacles and in conflict with nature conservation goals. Sometimes people were excluded from decision-making processes; sometimes they were displaced to create protected areas; and sometimes their ability to use the land for alternative purposes was constrained or eliminated. These early approaches often alienated people who depended on the natural resources in the now-protected areas for their lifestyles, and led to a myriad of park-versus-people conflicts (Agrawal and Gibson, 1999). Over time, there was increasing recognition that many of these projects failed to consider the ways in which environmental conservation laws might undermine social development and human well-being (Durham, 1995), and many policy makers began to emphasize the importance of integrating human and cultural concerns into conservation planning (Larson and Wyckoff-Baird, 1997; Mehta and Kellert, 1998).

In 1980, the World Conservation Union's (IUCN) *World Conservation Strategy* started a new era in conservation planning by emphasizing the 'importance of linking protected-area management with the economic activities of local communities' (Larson and Wyckoff-Baird, 1997). In 1982, the World Congress on National Parks followed suit, calling for increased support for local populations living in and around parks and protected areas. The Parks Commission supported community development through education, revenue sharing, and participation in decision-making where such activities would be compatible with conservation priorities. This heightened emphasis on 'meeting local resource needs and development objectives' gradually became a central objective for organizations such as IUCN, World Wildlife Fund, and UNESCO, as well as a central tenant in international agreements, including The Convention on Wetlands, and the Convention on Biological Diversity (Calheiros *et al.*, 2000; Inamdar, 1999; Perreault, 1996; Vojnovic, 1995)[2].

In many countries, designating an area as protected continues to restrict human inhabitation and limit or prohibit economic activity. This creates many benefits to human—recreational, physical, emotional, and spiritual—but it may also create costs. Beyond direct human displacement, where the costs for human health are high and well understood, there are indirect costs associated with the creation of these protected areas, including: limiting access (e.g. visitor costs or limits), limiting economic activity (e.g. access to timber, fish, or game), limiting development abilities in the area (e.g. limiting road developing, prohibiting airports within a certain distance) or allocating substantial resources to protecting single large areas instead of funding more widely dispersed environmental projects.

Conclusion

In the end, one might decide that the benefits of regulating or banning hydraulic fracturing or creating parks and other protected natural areas outweigh the costs, but in order to answer the question, 'What role does/can environmental law play in mediating the relationship between nature–human health and well-being?' one must delve more deeply into the ways that environmental law, as it intersects with other areas of law, influences the quality of the natural environment and the quality of the human environment in varied and complex ways. How does environmental law affect the air we breathe, the water we drink, the spaces we inhabit? How does environmental law shape that physical, social, and economic systems that surround and support us in the short and long term? How can we better appreciate and use environmental law as a tool for responding to the competing short- and long-term, local and global, physical and economic factors that influence human health and well-being? These are the questions that must be asked and analysed in order to appreciate the role that environmental law does and can play in improving human health and well-being.

Notes

1 The US Congress passed the Forest Reserve Act in 1891, which empowered the President to designate areas as 'forest reserves', creating the legislative foundation for what is now known as the National Forest System.

2 For a fuller discussion of the history and development of natural conservation law, see Cinnamon Carlarne, *Putting the 'And' Back in the Culture-Nature Debate: Integrated Cultural and Natural Heritage Protection*, 25 UCLA JOURNAL OF ENVIRONMENTAL LAW AND POLICY 153 (2006–2007).

References

Adgate, J. L., Goldstein, B. D., & Mckenzie, L. M. (2014). Potential public health hazards, exposures and health effects from unconventional natural gas development. *Environ Sci Technol*, 48, 8307–20.

Agrawal, A. & Gibson, C. C. (1999). Enchantment and Disenchantment: The Role of Community in Natural Resource Conservation. *World Dev*, 27, 629–49.

Baritz, L. (1961). The Idea of the West. *Am Hist Rev*, 66, 618–40.

Brady, W. J. (2012). Hydraulic fracturing regulation in the United States: The laissez-faire approach of the federal government and varying state regulations. *Vt J Environ Law*, 14, 39.

Brown, K. (2002). Innovations for conservation and development. *Geogr J*, 168, 6–17.

Calheiros, D. F., Seidl, A. F., & Ferreira, C. J. (2000). Participatory research methods in environmental science: local and scientific knowledge of a limnological phenomenon in the pantanal wetland of Brazil. *J Appl Ecol*, 37, 684–96.

Carlarne, C. (2006). Putting the 'and' back in the culture-nature debate: integrated cultural and natural heritage protection. *UCLA J Envt'l Law & Policy*, 25, 153–224.

Colburn, T., Kwiatkowski, C., Shultz, K., & Bachran, M. (2011). Natural Gas Operations from a Public Health Perspective. *Hum Ecol Risk Assess*, 17, 1039–56.

Darrah, T. H., Vengosh, A., Jackson, R. B., Warner, N. R., & Poreda, R. J. (2014). Noble gases identify the mechanisms of fugitive gas contamination in drinking-water wells overlying the marcellus and barnett shales. *Proc Natl Acad Sci*, 111, 14076–81.

Durham, W. H. (1995). Political ecology and environmental destruction in Latin America. In: Painter, M. & Durham, W. H. (eds) *The Social Causes of Environmental Destruction in Latin America*, pp. 249–65. Ann Arbor, MI: University of Michigan Press.

Fussell, E. (1966). *Frontier: American Literature and the American West*, 3rd edition. Princeton University Press, Princeton, NJ.

GAO (2012). Unconventional Oil and Gas Development: Key Environmental and Public Health Requirements. Washington, D. C.

Gopalakrishnan, S. & Klaiber, H. A. (2014). Is the shale energy boom a bust for nearby residents? evidence from housing values in Pennsylvania. *Am J Agric Econ*, 96, 43–66.

Hefley, W. E. & Wang, Y. (eds.) (2015). *Economics of Unconventional Shale Gas Development: Case Studies and Impacts*. New York, NY: Springer.

Hennesy-Fiske, M. (2014). Fracking Brings Oil Boom to South Texas Town, For a Price. *Los Angeles Times*.

Horowitz, S. (2014). Dark Side of the Boom. *Washington Post*.

Howarth, R. W. (2014). A bridge to nowhere: methane emissions and the greenhouse gas footprint of natural gas. *Energy Sci Eng*, 2, 47–60.

Howarth, R. W., Santoro, R., & Ingraffea, A. (2011). Methane and the Greenhouse-Gas Footprint of Natural Gas from Shale Formations. *Clim Change*, 106, 679–90.

Inamdar, A. (1999). Capitalizing on nature: protected area management. *Science*, 283, 1856–7.

IUCN (2015). World Database on Protected Areas. Available at: http://data.unep-wcmc.org/pdfs/12/WCMC-016-WDPA-Metadata.pdf?1437132301 (accessed 16 May 2015) [Online].

Jackson, R. B., Down, A., Phillips, N. G., *et al.* (2014). Natural gas pipeline leaks across Washington, DC. *Environ Sci Technol*, 48, 2051–8.

Jackson, R. B., Vengosh, A., Darrah, T. H., *et al.* (2013). Increased stray gas abundance in a subset of drinking water wells near marcellus shale gas extraction. *Proc Natl Acad Sci U S A*, 110, 11250–5.

Larson, P. & Wyckoff-Baird, B. (1997). *Lessons From the Field: A Review of the World Wildlife Fund's Experience with Integrated Conservation and Development Projects*. Washington, DC: World Wildlife Fund, pp. 5–59.

Lelieveld, J., Lechtenbohmer, S., Assonov, S. S., *et al.* (2005). Low methane leakage from gas pipelines. *Nature*, 434, 841–842.

Mckain, K., Down, A., Raciti, S. M., Budney, J., Hutyra, L. R., & Floerchinger, C. (2015). Methane emissions from natural gas infrastructure and use in the urban region of Boston, Massachusetts. *Proc Natl Acad Sci*, 112, 1941–6.

Mehta, J. N. & Kellert, S. R. (1998). Local attitudes toward community-based conservation policy and programmes in Nepal: A case study in the Makalu-Barun conservation area. *Environ Conserv*, 25, 320–33.

Mitchell, R. B. (2014). International Environmental Agreements Database Project,. Available at: http://iea.uoregon.edu (accessed 6 November 2014) [Online].

Moore, C. W., Zielinska, B., Pétron, G., & Jackson, R. B. (2014). Air Impacts Of Increased Natural Gas Acquisition, Processing, And Use: A Critical Review. *Environ Sci Technol*, 48, 8349–59.

Nash, R. F. (2001). *Wilderness and the American Mind*, 4th edition. New Haven, CT: Yale University Press.

Neumann, R. P. (2002). *Imposing Wilderness: Struggles Over Liveliehood and Nature Preservation in Africa*. Berkeley, CA: University of California Press.

Pace Law School (2008). *Beginner's Guide to Land Use Law*. New York, NY: Land Use Law Center, Pace University Schoool of Law.

Paredes, D., Komarek, T., & Loveridge, S. (2015). Income and employment effects of shale gas extraction windfalls: evidence from the Marcellus region. *Energy Econ*, 47, 112–20.

Perreault, T. (1996). Nature Preserves and Community Conflict: A Case Study in Highland Ecuador. *Mt Res Dev*, 16, 167–75.

Phillips, N. G., Ackley, R., Crosson, E. R., *et al.* (2013). Mapping urban pipeline leaks: Methane leaks across Boston. *Environ Pollut*, 173, 1–4.

US Congress (2005). Energy Policy Act of 2005, Public Law. United States of America.

US EPA (2010). Human and Ecological Risk Assessment of Coal Combustion Wastes. Washington, DC.

US EPA (2012). Study of the Potential Impacts of Hydraulic Fracturing on Drinking Water Resources. Washington, DC.

US EPA (2015). Natural Gas Extraction—Hydraulic Fracturing. Availabe at: http://www2.epa.gov/hydraulicfracturing (accessed 15 May 2015) [Online].

US Federal Register (2012). Congressional Findings and Declaration of Purpose. United States.

USGS (2015). Earthquakes Hazard Program: Induced Earthquakes. Available at: http://earthquake.usgs.gov/research/induced/ (accessed 17 May 2015) [Online].

Vann, A., Murrill, B. J., & Tiemann, M. (2014). Hydraulic Fracturing: Selected Legal Issues. Washington, DC.

Vojnovic, I. (1995). Intergenerational and intragenerational equity requirements for sustainability. *Environ Conserv*, 22, 223–8.

Wattenberg, E. V., Bielicki, J. M., Suchomel, A. E., Sweet, J. T., Vold, E. M., & Ramachandran, G. (2015). Assessment of the acute and chronic health hazards of hydraulic fracturing fluids. *J Occup Environ Hyg*, 12, 611–24.

Weinstein, A. & Partridge, M. (2014). Economic implications for unconventional fossil fuel production. In: Albrecht, D. (ed.) *Our Energy Future: Socioeconomic Implications and Policy Options for Rural America*, pp. 19–39. London, UK: Routledge.

World Health Organization (WHO) (2005). Ecosystems and Human Well-Being—Health Synthesis. Geneva, Switzerland: WHO.

Willow, A. (2015). Wells and well-being: neoliberalism and holistic sustainability in the shale energy debate. *Local Environ Int J Justice Sustain*, 21, 768–788.

Wines, M. (2015). New Research Links Scores of Earthquakes to Fracking Wells Near a Fault in Ohio. *New York Times*.

Zoback, M. D. & Arent, D. J. (2014). Shale gas development: Opportunities and challenges. *Bridg*, 44, 16–23.

CHAPTER 10.3

Environmental assessment and health impact assessment

Salim Vohra, Marla Orenstein, Francesca Viliani, Ben Cave, Ben Harris-Roxas, and Filipe Silva

The role of impact assessment

Impact assessment is the name given to a range of systematic approaches and methodologies. Its purpose is to identify the future consequences of, and make recommendations to strengthen, a proposed project, programme, plan, or policy. Impact assessment can look at effects ranging from social, cultural, economic, and health effects to effects on the physical environment. These consequences can be either positive or negative; intended or unintended.

Impact assessments are often conducted as part of a policy development or regulatory process in order to inform decision makers about whether and how a project, programme, plan, or policy should be implemented. For example, a company may submit a proposal to government to explore for natural gas near a national park, or near a town or city, using hydraulic fracturing (fracking) methods. An impact assessment would identify the likely potential effects of the development on local ecosystems including flora, fauna, air, water, and soil. It would also identify how the project could affect social conditions, economic opportunities, and health status of human populations. And finally, it would suggest recommendations on how to avoid or minimize potential harms from the project. Another example, focusing on the review of a policy rather than a project, would be the assessment of a local greenspace strategy or the strategic redevelopment of unused green spaces in a district for private housing (City of London, 2014; Palerang Council et al., 2006; Health Scotland et al., 2008).

As indicated above, impact assessments identify and prioritize potential effects (impacts) of a project or policy proposal, as well as recommend mitigation and enhancement measures. These measures may focus on how the design of the proposal could be improved, or how best it could be implemented to avoid or minimize harms and maximize benefits. Examples of mitigations include: minimizing air emissions through the use of alternative technologies that reduce air emissions at source; suggesting how local hiring could be undertaken so that affected communities can also benefit from a proposal; or outlining how agricultural land and natural spaces could be protected and enhanced as part of a housing development or a transport strategy.

While impact assessments characterize effects and develop potential mitigation and enhancement measures, these assessments do not comprise decision-making itself. Rather, a decision-making body such as a regulatory authority, permitting authority, or government (local or national) will take the results of the impact assessment under advisement when making a decision about whether or how to allow the proposed project or policy to proceed.

Impact assessments are prospective, meaning they are undertaken when a proposal is being developed and before it is implemented, as this is the time where there is the greatest scope for changes to be easy to make to a proposal. Even so, for an impact assessment to influence decision-making, the commitment of decision makers to implement recommendations and the timing of the assessment in relation to the wider social and economic environment are crucial.

This chapter focuses on two broad types of impact assessments relevant to public health: environmental assessment (environmental impact assessment and strategic environmental assessment) and health impact assessment (HIA)[1]. Environmental assessment (EAs) and HIA approaches, and processes, can help to protect and enhance public health by:

- critically analysing proposals;

- analysing how the proposals are likely to be implemented; and

- examining how the proposals are likely to be operationalized in real-world contexts.

The best assessments bring people together: proponent, decision-makers, communities, academia, and other stakeholders. The process therefore should be rigorous and scientific and, at the same time, encourage the participation of stakeholders with different competencies and interests. This requires a multidisciplinary team that has community and stakeholder engagement skills, communication skills, as well as technical subject-specific assessment expertise. A well-conducted impact assessment can help to foster working relationships between organizations and develop a consensus on shared priorities. Public health professionals and the health sector in general therefore need to understand, engage with, and participate in both EAs and HIAs. By not doing so they abdicate responsibility to other groups who quite reasonably focus on their own priorities at the expense of public and environmental health issues.

Environmental impact assessment

Environmental impact assessment (EIA) is the oldest and most established form of impact assessment. The requirement for EIA was originally mandated in the United States in 1969, with the passing of the National Environmental Policy Act (NEPA). This was an important landmark for EIA, as it influenced the development of similar requirements in most other countries of the world (Alm, 1988).

One of the simplest definitions of EIA is that it is 'an assessment of the impacts of a planned activity on the environment' (United Nations Economic Commission for Europe, 1991). A more nuanced definition is that:

'... EIA is a ... systematic process that examines the environmental consequences of development actions, in advance. The emphasis, compared with many other mechanisms of environmental protection, is on prevention.Of course planners have traditionally assessed the impacts of developments on the environment, but invariably not in the systematic, holistic and multidisciplinary way required by EIA.'

Text extracts from Glasson J, Therivel R and Chadwick A, *Introduction to Environmental Impact Assessment*, Second Edition, University College London (UCL) Press, London, UK, Copyright © 2015, reproduced with permission from Taylor and Francis Ltd.

EIAs generally focus on potential effects across the following topic areas: water, air and soil quality/quantity; flora and fauna; archaeology and heritage; noise; landscape and visual amenity; and socioeconomic environments. The core steps of the process are shown in Figure 10.3.1.

The requirements for conducting EIA are embedded within the laws and regulations of national and cross-country authorities. Although the main intent of EIA, of identifying and mitigating in advance the potential adverse environmental consequences of a planned action, is the same, procedural elements vary across jurisdictions.

Though EIA encompasses impacts on human populations, the way in which health has been approached in EIAs[2] has traditionally

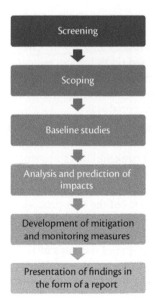

Fig. 10.3.1 Core steps of the environmental impact assessment (EIA) process.
Source: data from Morris P and Therivel R, (Eds), *Methods of Environmental Impact Assessment*, Second Edition, Spon Press, Taylor and Francis Group, Oxford, UK, Copyright © 2001 Peter Morris and Riki Therivel.

been very narrowly defined as the potential for negative impacts on biophysical health outcomes (Harris *et al.*, 2015). This is often specifically framed in terms of the hazards and risks of exposure to chemicals in the air, water, or soil that are associated with a project. As will be discussed later, this narrow focus within EIA was one of the reasons for the rise and development of HIA in some countries (and social impact assessment, SIAs, in others) (Kemm *et al.*, 2004; Dendena and Corsi, 2015).

Some countries, international lending institutions, international industry sector associations, and transnational businesses have either mandated or recommended that EIAs have strong social and health components (Harris-Roxas *et al.*, 2012). These assessments are often described as environmental, social, and health impact assessments (ESHIAs). ESHIAs are part of a family of assessments called integrated impact assessments (IIA) or integrated assessments (IA), because they bring together separate types of assessments in order to produce a more integrated understanding of the potential impacts, an integrated set of mitigation and enhancement measures, and an integrated set of monitoring indicators (Bond *et al.*, 2001; Milner *et al.*, 2005).

Strategic environmental assessment

The term 'EIA' is generally reserved for the assessment of projects. When the same type of analysis is conducted on strategies, plans, or programmes—such as an open space strategy or an oil and gas leasing programme—the term 'strategic environmental assessment' (SEA) is applied. SEA is most often undertaken or commissioned by national or local governments, because these are the entities that are concerned with the types of wide-ranging future strategies or policy actions that SEA assesses.

For example, an SEA would assess whether the vision and objectives of the policy are sound from an environmental, social, economic, and health perspective; what criteria should be used to decide on where future developments should be situated; what green and blue spaces would be 'no go' areas for development, and the kinds of approaches and technologies that should be considered by any future development in order to protect human health and the environment. The SEA helps to ensure that the strategy is sound from an environmental, social, and health perspective. An example of this is an SEA for an open space strategy (Dumfries and Galloway Council, 2014).

Only after the SEA has assessed a policy or strategy would an EIA then be conducted, on a case-by-case basis, as proposals come forward seeking approval from decision makers to implement specific projects within the policy or strategy boundaries. An example of this is a transport strategy which sets out a vision for an updated transport system involving a rapid bus transit scheme, a road bypass, and a new rail scheme. Only after the SEA is completed on the transport strategy, and the transport system, would an EIA be undertaken on the outline or detailed plans of the rail scheme.

Health impact assessment

A widely accepted definition of HIA is that: 'Health impact assessment may be defined as a combination of procedures, methods and tools that systematically judges the potential, and sometimes unintended, effects of a policy, plan, programme or project on the health of a population and the distribution of those effects within the population. HIA identifies appropriate actions to manage those effects' (Quigley *et al.*, 2006).

HIA has developed from three main strands of thinking (and their associated frameworks and processes) (Kemm *et al.*, 2004):

1. Epidemiological and quantitative health risk assessment;

2. Healthy policy and health promotion; and

3. Social determinants of health.

From risk to impact

Starting in the 1950s, developments in epidemiology led to approaches that quantified the potential adverse impacts of exposure to man-made chemicals in the air, water, soil, and food. These approaches, and associated methodologies, are known as *health risk assessment*. From the 1970s and 1980s, the healthy public policy and health promotion movements recognized that promoting health and preventing ill health were as important as treating disease, and that health and well-being were not just about good quality healthcare. They were also about good quality and affordable access to the natural environment, housing, education, transport networks, and public and private goods and services. From the 1980s and 1990s, there was a growing recognition of the need to incorporate the social determinants of health into EIA. This was accompanied by two realizations; firstly, the limited value of the health risk assessment approach used in most EIAs and secondly, the need to address, and promote, more equitable social and health outcomes (Harris-Roxas and Harris, 2011).

HIA is undertaken in many countries around the world, though it has not been embedded in regulatory processes to the same extent as EIA. Several countries have adopted requirements for stand alone HIA; some have endorsed better consideration of health in their national EIA processes; while others have developed national-level guidance on undertaking HIA or better considering health in EIA (Winkler *et al.*, 2013; Ross *et al.*, 2014; Fehr *et al.*, 2014).

Steps for health impact assessment

The steps of an HIA are similar to EIA and are described in Box 10.3.1 (Birley, 2011).

HIA has an explicit set of values that frame the HIA process. These values are that the HIA be: democratic and participatory; equitable, sustainable, transparent, and ethical in the use of evidence (European Centre for Health Policy and World Health Organization Regional Office for Europe, 1999; Bhatia *et al.*, 2014; Martuzzi *et al.*, 2014). One additional underlying value of HIA is that the maximization of health opportunities for all is an important societal good and a priority societal goal (Hurley and Vohra, 2010). Health impacts are contextual and are linked to a specific natural and socioeconomic environment. HIA, like EIA, therefore aims to develop a set of evidence-based, locally implementable, legislatively appropriate, and culturally relevant recommendations for dealing with the potential impacts that are identified.

A key feature of HIA is that it considers both positive and negative impacts on community health and well-being. This is different than EIA, which generally only considers potential adverse effects. HIA systematically considers a wide range of environmental and social determinants of health as shown in Figure 10.3.2. Those impacts may be direct or indirect. Direct impacts are those generated by a project and its activities (e.g. traffic injuries from lorries going to and from a project or changes in employment status from the provision of project-related jobs). Indirect impacts are those which occur as a result of the project changing other social, economic, and

---

Box 10.3.1 The key steps in a health impact assessment (HIA) process

Screening: deciding if a proposal could generate potential health consequences and whether a HIA should be undertaken.

Scoping: setting the scope of the impact assessment by identifying the potential health impacts of concern, what issues do not need to be considered, what sources and types of evidence will be considered, what qualitative and quantitative methods will be used, whether there will be an expert steering or advisory group, and what the assessment's temporal, spatial, and population boundaries will be (i.e. what time period, geographical area and communities, and population subgroups, will be considered in the assessment). The findings and judgements made during scoping will be written up either as a Scoping Report or a Terms of Reference for the HIA.

Baseline assessment or community profile: collecting and analysing a range of desktop and fieldwork information to understand the existing health and well-being status of the affected populations and the current state of the environmental and social determinants of health influencing them. This provides the baseline from which predictions on possible and likely health impacts are made. Information types that are used include demographic, health, environmental, and socioeconomic statistics; scientific and other credible literature on health impacts; existing policies; expert opinion; and community feedback and other stakeholders' views, including public health practitioners and healthcare providers.

Impact analysis: identifying, characterizing, assessing the significance of and prioritizing the potential health and well-being impacts.

Formulating recommendations: developing feasible mitigation and enhancement measures to minimize the potential negative impacts and maximize the potential positive impacts. These measures are written up can be written up in a separate impact management plan.

Decision and subsequent implementation: the authority responsible for the HIA process will decide whether a proposal goes ahead and, if it goes ahead, what changes need to be made to the proposal based on the recommendations of the HIA. The proponent of a proposal will take responsibility for ensuring that the impact management plan is implemented alongside the implementation of a proposal.

Follow-up: monitoring and evaluation of both the implementation of a proposal and, less often, the HIA process.

The findings of stakeholder engagement and consultation should inform the HIA process and its findings. Many guides recommend stakeholder engagement and consultation be undertaken at all steps of the HIA process. More often than not, consultation is undertaken at one or two points in time: during scoping and during the analysis steps.

The above description of the steps of HIA makes it look like a linear process but, in reality, the process is more iterative (i.e. as changes to the design of the proposal are occurring, the scope of the assessment, the baseline information that is needed and the findings of the preliminary analysis have to be reviewed and revised).

Source: data from Birley M, *Health Impact Assessment: Principles and Practice*, Earthscan/ Routledge, London, UK, Copyright © 2011.

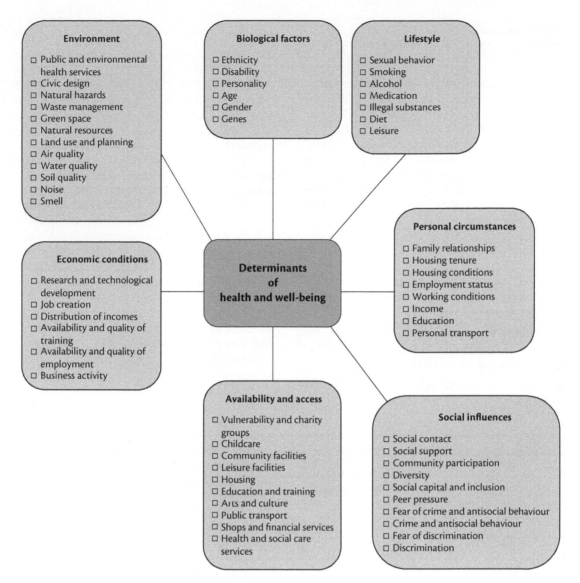

Fig. 10.3.2 The wider environmental and social determinants of health and well-being.
Source: data from Harris A, *Rapid health impact assessment: A guide to research*, Copyright © 2003.

cultural factors (e.g. an increase in demand for local goods and services leading to a rise in local prices and resultant food insecurity or housing affordability). Not all determinants apply in all cases; each HIA will focus on those determinants most likely to be affected by the proposed project or policy.

To give a sense of the types of issued examined in an HIA and the types of recommendations that may be made, Boxes 10.2.2 and 10.2.3 present a high-level summary of two HIAs that were undertaken on greenspace project proposals. Although the findings and recommendations presented may appear somewhat self-evident to those familiar with the determinants of health, they highlight the way in which HIA can be a useful approach and process to systematically bring forward health-related issues into decision-making processes that would not otherwise consider health.

Impact assessment and decision-making

Impact assessment fits into the broader evidence-based policy movement. Hence, the general consensus is that the purpose

of impact assessment is to support policy and decision-making in institutions such as national and local governments, private sector businesses, and international lending agencies and institutions (Senécal *et al.*, 1999; International Finance Corporation, 2012 and 2009; International Council on Mining and Metals, 2010).

Impact assessments often generate a range of expectations and aspirations that the impact assessment practitioner, team or advisory committee needs to take into account and manage (Kemm, 2000; Peterson, 2004; LaBouchardiere *et al.*, 2014).

The legislative mandate under which EIA operates means that EIA has become part of the accepted process by which policies, plans, programmes, and projects are permitted. This in turn has ensured that, to varying degrees, most countries and key international institutions have an institutional infrastructure for EIA. In most countries around the world, HIA does not enjoy a legislative mandate similar to that of EIA. This in turn means that there is often an associated absence of institutional infrastructure for HIA ranging from an absence of accepted forms of practice to

---

Box 10.3.2 A HIA of park, trail, and green space planning in the west side of Greenville, South Carolina, United States

This HIA was undertaken by the South Carolina Institute of Medicine and Public Health to inform urban and greenspace planning in three economically depressed and physically fragile neighbourhoods on the west side of Greenville, South Carolina (South Carolina Institute of Public Health, 2013). The HIA focused on six priority areas: physical activity; social cohesion/capital; community and family economic stability; food access; individual and community safety; and air and water quality.

The HIA concluded that the park had the potential to increase physical activity, leading to an improvement in mental and physical well-being and addressing the high obesity and chronic disease rates in the community. The HIA also found that the proposed park would increase social cohesion among residents by providing a venue for them to gather.

The HIA made a number of specific recommendations to the city to support positive health during the park development process. These recommendations included the following:

- Provide opportunities to walk and bike to and from the potential new park (*e.g. sidewalks and bike lanes as well as good signage and community education*)

- Provide access to healthy and affordable food sources (*e.g. community garden and/or farmer's market in the potential new park*)

- Provide opportunities for interaction between community members (*e.g. community garden and/or event space in the park*)

- Provide safe paths and signs to encourage utilization of the potential park (*e.g. connection from the west side to potential new park, signage in English and other languages*)

- Provide opportunities to strengthen the relationship between the potential new park and the surrounding community (*e.g. integrate history and culture of local community in the design of the potential new park, encourage partnerships with local artists*)

- Provide opportunities to improve mental health of community residents (*e.g. design in places for relaxation and meditation, such as open green space with benches and swings*)

Source: data from South Carolina Institute of Medicine and Public Health, *A health impact assessment (HIA) of park, trail, and green space planning in the west side of Greenville, South Carolina,* Copyright © 2013 South Carolina Institute of Medicine and Public Health, http://imph.org/wordpress/wp-content/uploads/2013/03/27843-REV-HIA-FULL-REPRT.pdf.

Box 10.3.3 A HIA of the Garden City Project in Yala City, Thailand

This HIA was undertaken by the Thailand Ministry of Public Health. The city of Yala is a Buddhist-Muslim community in the south of Thailand (Thailand Department of Health, 2004). The Yala Garden City Project is an ongoing effort intended to make Yala City a healthy place to live and to provide a learning environment for residents. As part of the project, 19 km^2 of space in various municipal areas have been developed as gardens, parks, and green areas surrounding the city. Five subprojects including gardens and parks for different functions such as recreation, exercise, and social activities have been completed and opened to the public. The HIA hypothesized that the 'Garden City' approach would have various impacts on the health of individuals, families, and the community at physical, psychological, social, and spiritual levels. The HIA used participatory action research to provide recommendations to the local authority, the Yala Municipality, for further increasing the positives and reducing the negative impacts of the project.

The HIA used a variety of methods to understand how the Garden City Project was influencing the health of local community members, including a survey of park users, food and drink vendors, and local residents; observations of park use; and interviews with key authorities.

The HIA found that the Garden City Project had a number of positive health impacts. The gardens provided recreation areas for outdoor activities and exercises, beautiful scenery in the city, and among the residents of Yala City, it enhanced the sense of security and care by the local government. Local people reported an increase in physical strength and a decrease in fatigue, as well as an increase in joyfulness and a reduction in irritation. In terms of social health, local people identified that there were more opportunities to join with friends and to see other people. However, the HIA did not find a quantitative change in the rates of participation in social activities held in the parks and gardens, and there was no change identified in objective measures such as the use of routine medication and the frequency of visits to primary care.

This HIA reinforced for the decision-maker—in this case, the municipality—that investments that were made in improving the physical environment could simultaneously result in improved health and well-being for the local population. As a result, the policy makers have taken the public recommendations for project development into account and assigned responsible authorities for implementation. In addition, local experts and specialists formed a multidisciplinary research and development network to continue impact assessments for the sustainable development of local public health policy.

Source: data from Thailand Department of Health, *The health impact assessment for healthy public policy: a case study of "Garden City Project" Yala City, Thailand,* Ministry of Public Health, Thailand, Copyright © 2004.

---

mechanisms for assuring HIA quality and pathways for educating public health, environmental, and planning professionals in HIA.

A review of voluntary and regulatory approaches to HIA at the national, subnational and international levels concluded that there is considerable untapped potential for HIA to be used more widely and effectively (Winkler *et al.*, 2013).

Methodological challenges to the development of HIA include questions about its usefulness, the evidence and frameworks that it uses, and the values that inform an assessment of health and well-being (Cashmore *et al.*, 2004; Parry and Stevens, 2001; Krieger *et al.*,

2010; Vohra *et al.*, 2010). Scrutiny and review is welcomed and is an essential way of improving HIA. However, critics often overlook the value HIA provides and the constraints under which it operates. HIA practitioners are advocating for health and well-being outside the health sector and would benefit from the support as well as the critique of their peers. HIA is a pragmatic approach and uses a range of sources of evidence. For health impacts caused by biophysical changes, such as air pollution, there is epidemiological evidence that can help with the identification and quantification of health impacts for a specific intervention. For health impacts caused by social or political changes, the relationship is more complex, or less amenable to focusing on the particular effects of a single policy or project. In particular, there is a lack of evidence on the efficacy of interventions on the social determinants of health in real-world contexts.

The process of impact assessment involves engaging a range of stakeholders in discussion and negotiation (Birley, 2011). Stakeholders usually include, as a minimum, the proponent, the policy development, or decision-making authority and communities. It is also a process of applied science that uses the best available evidence, a systematic and transparent approach to reduce bias, a range of sources of evidence, and a variety of qualitative and quantitative methods of prediction to ensure that the findings are as accurate as they can be (Hurley and Vohra, 2010).

The success or the effectiveness of an HIA can occur at two broad levels (Quigley and Taylor, 2004). Firstly, successfully altering a specific proposal so that it is more likely to improve community health outcomes, reduce inequalities, and enhance equity. Secondly, helping to build health partnerships and relationships; for example, fostering interagency working relationship or increasing the visibility of health in the political agenda (Haigh *et al.*, 2015). This is most likely to happen when the experts and practitioners involved are pragmatic, tactical, and technical (Harris *et al.*, 2014).

By reviewing past HIA reports and processes, researchers have developed a series of recommendations to make HIA more effective (Haigh *et al.*, 2015; Bourcier *et al.*, 2015):

* Consider if HIA is the right process for the proposal to be examined in the early phases;

* Clarify early in the process: purposes, goals, values and expected outcomes;

* Select an appropriate team to conduct the HIA with a mix of competences; as well as identify key stakeholders and their relative points of influence within policy development and decision-making processes;

* Involve stakeholders as early as possible;

* Ensure HIA processes include potentially affected communities and pay attention to the needs of vulnerable subgroups;

* Craft clear, actionable recommendations, with the support of the involved decision makers, affected stakeholders and the proponent of the proposal;

* Be both technical and tactical: understand the context and the actors, proactively engage, and where needed utilize a more flexible though still structured HIA process.

Impact assessment, health, and the precautionary principle

There are two broad formulations of the Precautionary Approach or Principle (Ahteensuu, 2007). The first is the 1992 Rio Declaration on Environment and Development. This states that: 'In order to protect the environment, the precautionary approach shall be widely applied by States according to their capabilities. Where there are threats of serious or irreversible damage, lack of full scientific certainty shall not be used as a reason for postponing cost-effective measures to prevent environmental degradation' (United Nations, 1992, Principle 15).

The second is the 1998 Wingspread Statement. This states that: 'When an activity raises threats of harm to human health or the environment, precautionary measures should be taken even if some cause and effect relationships are not fully established scientifically' (Science and Environmental Health Network *et al.*, 1998). The latter is a more proactive definition advocating action to minimize harm. The Wingspread Statement also puts the burden of proof on the proponent of a proposal. It advocates that the process of applying the principle must be open, informed, democratic, include potentially affected parties and involve reviewing the full range of alternatives, including not taking any action. The Wingspread Statement closely echoes the values that are embedded within impact assessment and HIA especially.

In relation to applying the precautionary principle, environmental health regulatory systems, generally make a determination on a potential threat, the 'reasonable grounds for concern', based on preliminary scientific assessments that provide information and evidence of the potential for something being a hazard to the environment or human, animal, and plant health (European Commission, 2000; Martuzzi and Tickner, 2004). Environmental, social, and health impact assessments can be seen as a form of 'preliminary assessment'.

Impact assessments are inherently precautionary because they assess and recommend measures to reduce harm and, wherever possible, enhance benefits. They do so in a context of uncertainty in relation to baseline information on the status of affected communities and natural environments, both in the present and over the life of a proposal. They consider both how a proposal will be implemented and how the proposal is likely to operate over its life. Most importantly, they examine who is likely to be worst affected, as well as how and when. High-quality impact assessments gather the best available information and evidence within time and resource constraints, address uncertainty clearly, consider worst case scenarios, and develop mitigation measures to enable these worst case scenarios to be minimized. They also leverage opportunities to enhance, maximize, and equitably share out the beneficial impacts to all the communities that are involved or affected.

However, there are challenges in applying the precautionary principle because different stakeholders and some proponents, whether governments or businesses, can frame the impact assessment, and the policy and decision-making process in ways that preclude the use of the precautionary principle to its fullest extent. A key issue is the defensibility of predictions and statements made in an impact assessment in judicial and quasi-judicial settings. This is particularly the case in the following three contexts (European Commission, 2000; Martuzzi and Tickner, 2004; Hardstaff, 2000):

* Where there is a lack of, or inconclusive, evidence for an impact that is theoretically possible;

* Where there is no scientific consensus on the causal mechanism for the impact; and

* Where there the likelihood of the impact occurring cannot be qualitatively or quantitatively estimated.

Deciding when and how to invoke the precautionary principle is also not straightforward. An example of this are the opposing views on the potential environmental and health impacts from projects using high-volume hydraulic fracturing (fracking) for the extraction of natural resources (Kovats *et al.*, 2014; Cotton, 2015). International opinion is divided not only between project proponents and communities, but also between national and state governments in different countries (and even within the same country). The scientific evidence is also not clear-cut. Some jurisdictions have allowed extensive use of this technology (California Fracking, 2016). Others have mandated a moratorium until further research is undertaken, the potential impacts associated with this technology are sufficiently understood, and a satisfactory regulatory framework is in place (Scottish Government, 2015; Keep Tap Water Safe, 2016).

Ultimately, the precautionary principle needs to be embedded in, and be a part of, policy and decision-making processes for its use to be fully effective within impact assessment. This is because, as stated in the previous section ('Impact assessment and decision-making'), impact assessments most often support and inform the decision-making process and advise how to improve the design of a proposal, rather than fighting for, or against, a particular decision.

Conclusion

HIA and EA are approaches and processes that support better, healthier, and more sustainable policy development and decision-making. When undertaken well, and when valued and applied, they can also help to support better, more informed, transparent and democratic policy development and decision-making processes. However, they are not a panacea; rather, they constitute one important piece of the policy development and decision-making puzzle.

Public health practitioners need to increase their knowledge and understanding of EA and HIA. They should improve their links with EA and HIA specialists. They also need to proactively and consistently undertake and commission assessments of health either within EA or as stand alone HIAs. Public health practitioners would also do well to oversee and scrutinize the scope of work for, and the findings of, EAs and HIAs that are commissioned and undertaken by others in the localities in which they work. By doing so, public health practitioners can help to advance the agenda of improving health for all by acting on the upstream determinants of health and bringing together key actors across society.

Acknowledgements

Text extracts from Glasson, J., Therivel, R., and Chadwick, A., *Introduction to Environmental Impact Assessment*, Second Edition, University College London (UCL) Press, London, UK, Copyright © 2015, reproduced with permission from Taylor and Francis Ltd.

Text extracts from United Nations, 1992, Principle 15, © 1992 United Nations. Reprinted with the permission of the United Nations.

Notes

1   Health impact assessment can often be stated as human health impact assessment or community health impact assessment to identify that the focus is on humans rather than the health of flora and fauna. In this chapter, the discussion of health is related to the health and well-being of individuals and groups in human communities and settlements.

2   'Health component' is used here to mean the whole range of assessments that consider human health and include elements such as the air quality assessment, land contamination assessment, water quality assessment, and socioeconomic assessment, as well as a health impact assessment that considers the implications of changes to the social environment because of a proposal.

References

Ahteensuu, M. (2007) 'Rationale for taking precautions: normative choices and commitments in the implementation of the precautionary principle', SCARR (Social Contexts and Responses to Risk) *Risk & Rationalities*, Queens' College, Cambridge, 29-31 March 2007. Available at: https://www.kent.ac.uk/scarr/events/ahteensuu.pdf (accessed 1 June 2017) [Online].

Alm, A. L. (1988). NEPA: Past, Present and Future. *EPA Journal*, January/February.

Bhatia, R., Farhang, L., Heller, J., *et al.* (2014). *Minimum Elements and Practice Standards Document: Minimum Elements and Practice Standards for Health Impact Assessment*. Version 3, September, 2014.

Birley, M. (2011). *Health Impact Assessment: Principles and Practice*. London, UK: Earthscan.

Bond, R., Curran, J., Kirkpatrick, C., & Lee, N. (2001). Integrated impact assessment for sustainable development: a case study approach. *World Development*, 29, 1011–24.

Bourcier, E., Charbonneau, D., Cahill, C., & Dannenberg, A. L. (2015). An evaluation of health impact assessments in the United States 2011–2014. *Preventing Chronic Disease*, 12, 140376.

California Fracking (2016). Fracking in California: where is fracking occurring. Available at: http://www.cafrackfacts.org/fracking-in-california/where-is-fracking-occurring (accessed 1 May 2016) [Online].

Cashmore, M., Gwilliam. R., Morgan, R., Cobb, D., & Bond, A. (2004). The interminable issue of effectiveness: substantive purposes, outcomes and research challenges in the advancement of environmental impact assessment theory. *Impact Assessment and Project Appraisal*, 22, 295–310.

City of London (2014). *Draft City of London Open Space Strategy: Supplementary Planning Document Rapid Health Impact Assessment*. London, UK: City of London Department of the Built Environment.

Cotton, M. (2015). Stakeholder perspectives on shale gas fracking: a Q-method study of environmental discourses. *Environ Plan*, 47, 1944–62.

Dendena, B. & Corsi S. (2015). The environmental and social impact assessment: a further step towards an integrated assessment process. *Journal of Cleaner Production*, 108, 965–77.

Dumfries & Galloway Council (2014). Dumfries and Galloway draft open space strategy SEA environmental report. Available at: http://www.dumgal.gov.uk/CHttpHandler.ashx?id=17595&p=0 (accessed 1 May 2016) [Online].

European Centre for Health Policy and World Health Organization Regional Office for Europe (1999). *Health Impact Assessment: Main Concepts and Suggested Approach*. The Gothenburg consensus paper. Brussels, Belgium: WHO.

European Commission (2000). *Communication from the Commission on the precautionary principle*. Brussels, Belgium: Publications Office of the European Union.

Fehr, R., Viliani, F., Martuzzi, M., & Nowacki, J. (2014). *Health in Impact Assessments: Opportunities Not to be Missed*. Brussels, Belgium: World Health Organization Regional Office for Europe, European Association of Public Health and International Association for Impact Assessment.

Glasson, J., Therivel, R., & Chadwick, A. (2005). *Introduction to Environmental Impact Assessment*, 2nd edition. London, UK: University College London (UCL) Press.

Haigh, F., Harris, E., Harris-Roxas, B., *et al.* (2015). What makes health impact assessments successful? Factors contributing to effectiveness in Australia and New Zealand. *BMC Public Health*, 15, 1009.

Hardstaff, P. (2000). *The precautionary principle, trade and the WTO.* A discussion paper for the European Commission Consultation on Trade and Sustainable Development. Bedfordshire, UK: Royal Society for the Protection of Birds.

Harris, P., Sainsbury, P., & Kemp, L. (2014). The fit between health impact assessment and public policy: Practice meets theory. *Soc Sci Med*, 108, 46–53.

Harris, P., Viliani, F., & Spickett, J. (2015). Assessing health impacts within environmental impact assessments: an opportunity for public health globally which must not remain missed. *Int J Environ Res Public Health*, 12, 1044–9.

Harris-Roxas, B. & Harris, E. (2011). Differing forms, differing purposes: a typology of health impact assessment. *Environ Impact Assess Rev*, 31, 396–403.

Harris-Roxas, B., Viliani, F., Bond, A., *et al.* (2012). Health Impact Assessment: the state of the art. *Impact Assessment and Project Appraisal*, 30, 43–52.

Health Scotland Greenspace Scotland, Scottish Natural Heritage and Institute of Occupational Medicine (2008). *Health Impact Assessment of Greenspace: A Guide.* Stirling, UK: Greenspace Scotland.

Hurley, F. & Vohra, S. (2010). Health Impact Assessment. In: Ayres, J. G., Harrison, R. M., Nichols, G. L., & Maynard, R. L. (eds) *Environmental Medicine.* London, UK: Edward Arnold.

International Council on Mining and Metals (2010). *Health Impact Assessment: summary of the good practice guidance.* London, UK: International Council on Mining and Metals (ICMM).

International Finance Corporation (2009). *Introduction to Health Impact Assessment.* Washington, DC: International Finance Corporation (IFC), World Bank Group.

International Finance Corporation (2012). *Performance Standards on Environmental and Social Sustainability.* Washington, DC: International Finance Corporation (IFC), World Bank Group.

Keep Tap Water Safe (2016). *List of bans worldwide.* Available at: http://keeptapwatersafe.org/global-bans-on-fracking (accessed 1 May 2016) [Online].

Kemm, J. (2000). Can health impact assessment fulfil the expectations it raises?. *Public Health*, 114, 431–3.

Kemm, J., Parry, J., & Palmer, S. (2004). *Health impact assessment.* Oxford, UK: Oxford University Press.

Kovats, S., Depledge, M., Haines, A., *et al.* (2014). The health implications of fracking. *Lancet*, 383, 2211–12.

Krieger, G. R., Utzinger, J., Winkler, M. S., *et al.* (2010). Barbarians at the gate: storming the Gothenburg consensus. *Lancet*, 375, 2129–31.

LaBouchardiere, R. A., Goater, S., & Beeton, R. J. S. (2014). Integrating stakeholder perceptions of environmental risk into conventional management frameworks: coal seam gas development in Queensland. *Australasian Journal of Environmental Management*, 21, 359–77.

Martuzzi, M. & Tickner J. A. (2004). *The Precautionary Principle: Protecting Public Health, the Environment and the Future of Our Children.* Copenhagen, Denmark: World Health Organization, Regional Office for Europe.

Martuzzi, M., Cave, B., Nowacki, J., Viliani, F., & Vohra, S. (2014). *Health Impact Assessment.* Fastips No. 8. Fargo, ND: International Association for Impact Assessment.

Milner S. J., Bailey, C., Deans, J. and Pettigrew, D. (2005). 'Integrated impact assessment in the UK—use efficacy and future development', *Environmental Impact Assessment Review*, 25(1) pp. 47–61.

Morris, P. and Therivel, R. (ed.). (2001). *Methods of Environmental Impact Assessment.* 2e. Spon Press. Oxford.

Palerang Council, Greater Southern Area Heath Service (NSW Health) and University of New South Wales (2006). *Bungedore health impact assessment: a rapid health impact assessment of two development scenarios in Bungedore, New South Wales.* Center for Health Equity Training, Research and Evaluation.

Parry, J. & Stevens, A. (2001). Prospective health impact assessment: pitfalls, problems, and possible ways forward. *BMJ*, 323, 1177–82.

Peterson, K. (2004). The role and value of strategic environmental assessment in Estonia: stakeholders' perspectives. *Impact Assessment and Project Appraisal*, 22, 159–65.

Quigley, R., den Broeder, L., Furu, P., Bond, A., Cave, B., & Bos, R. (2006). *Health Impact Assessment: International Best Practice Principles.* Special Publication Series No. 5. Fargo, ND: International Association for Impact Assessment.

Quigley, R. J. & Taylor, L. C. (2004). Evaluating health impact assessment. *Public Health*, 118, 544–52.

Ross, C. L., M. Orenstein, M., & Botchwey, N. (2014). *Health Impact Assessment in the United States.* New York, NY: Springer-Verlag.

Science and Environmental Health Network, Johnson Foundation, W. Alton Jones Foundation, C. S. Fund and Lowell Center for Sustainable Production, University of Massachusetts-Lowell (1998). *Wingspread consensus statement on the precautionary principle: Wingspread Conference on the Precautionary Principle.* Johnson Foundation, Racine, 23–25 January. Racine: Science and Environmental Health Network.

Scottish Government (2015). *Moratorium on fracking.* Available at: http://news.scotland.gov.uk/News/Moratorium-called-on-fracking-1555.aspx (accessed: 1 May 2016) [Online].

Senécal, P., Goldsmith, B., Conover, S., Sadler, B., & Brown, K. (1999). *Principles of Environmental Impact Assessment: Best Practice.* Special Publication Series No. 1. Fargo, ND: International Association for Impact Assessment and Institute of Environmental Assessment.

South Carolina Institute of Public Health (2013). *A Health Impact Assessment (HIA) of park, trail, and green space planning in the west side of Greenville, South Carolina.* Greenville, SC: South Carolina Institute of Public Health.

Thailand Department of Health (2004). *The Health Impact Assessment for Healthy Public Policy: A Case Study of "Garden City Project" Yala City, Thailand.* Nonthaburi Province, Thailand: Thailand Ministry of Public Health.

United Nations (1992). Report of the United Nations Conference on Environment and Development, Annex 1: Rio Declaration on Environment and Development. Rio de Janeiro, 3–14 June 1992.

United Nations Economic Commission for Europe (UNECE). (1991). Policies and Systems for Environmental Impact Assessment. Geneva, Switzerland: UNECE.

Vohra, S. Cave, B., Viliani, F. Harris-Roxas, B. F., & Bhatia, R. (2010). New international consensus on health impact assessment. *Lancet*, 375, 2010.

Winkler, M. S., Krieger, G. R., Divall, M. J., *et al.* (2013). Untapped potential of health impact assessment. *Bulletin of the World Health Organization*, 91, 237–312.

CHAPTER 10.4

Quantifying and valuing the role of trees and forests on environmental quality and human health

David J. Nowak

Valuing nature

Nature provides numerous services that affect the lives and well-being of people across the globe. Understanding impacts and benefits of nature will lead to better management decisions and designs in sustaining nature within society. One of the most dominant aspects of nature in many areas of the globe is vegetation, and one of the most dominant elements of vegetation in many areas are trees and forests. In addition to environmental quality, these trees and forests, particularly when within urban areas, have substantial impacts on human population health and well-being.

Understanding the myriad of potential services and costs associated with trees and forests is critical to estimating net benefits of vegetation and for guiding appropriate vegetation management plans. However, while many of the ecosystem services and costs of vegetation cannot be adequately quantified or valued at this time, it is important to understand within decision-making processes that these services or costs do exist. Discounting nature or vegetation as having no value leads to uninformed decisions regarding nature (e.g. Costanza *et al.*, 2014). Quantifying or understanding monetary and non-monetary values of nature in a given context, though difficult, will lead to more informed environmental and economic decisions.

Services provided by trees and forests

Trees provide numerous economic and ecosystem services that produce benefits to a community, but also incur various economic or environmental costs. Through proper planning, design, and management, trees can improve human health and well-being in urban areas by moderating climate, reducing building energy use, and atmospheric carbon dioxide (CO_2), improving air quality, mitigating rainfall run-off and flooding, and lowering noise levels (Nowak and Dwyer, 2007). However, inappropriate landscape designs, tree selection, and tree maintenance can increase environmental costs such as pollen production, chemical emissions from trees and maintenance activities that contribute to air pollution,

and can also increase building energy use, waste disposal, infrastructure repair, and water consumption (Escobedo *et al.*, 2011). These potential costs must be weighed against the environmental and health benefits in developing natural resource management programmes.

The Millennium Ecosystem Assessment (Hassan *et al.*, 2005) describes four categories of ecosystem services: (a) supporting (e.g. nutrient cycling, primary production); (b) provisioning (e.g. food, fuel); (c) regulating (e.g. climate regulation, water purification); and (d) cultural (e.g. aesthetic, spiritual). While science continues to advance in understanding and quantifying the relationships between forest structure and many of these services, several of these services can be currently quantified based on local forest, environmental, and human population data. Read more in Chapter 8.5 'Ecosystem services and health benefits—an urban perspective' for a full understanding of the ecosystem service concept.

Specific attributes of the vegetation resource such as abundance, size, species, health, and location affect the amount of services and costs provided by vegetation. Many of the services and costs provided by vegetation and their management affect human health. Thus, designing nature and management to maximize these benefits and minimize the costs can help improve human health.

There are four main steps needed to quantify ecosystem services and values from forests (or other ecosystem elements):

1. Quantify the forest structural attributes that provide the service for the area of interest (e.g. number of trees, tree cover). These structural data are essential as they quantify the resource attributes that provide the services.

2. Quantify how the structure influences the ecosystem service (e.g. tree density, tree sizes, and forest species composition are significant drivers for estimating carbon storage).

3. Quantify the impact of the ecosystem service. In many cases, it is not the service itself that is important, but rather the impact that the service has on human health, or other attributes of the environment that provide value to society.

4. Quantify the economic value of the impact provided by the ecosystem service.

There is an interdependence between forest structure and ecosystem services and values. Valuation is dependent upon good estimates of the magnitude of the service provided and the service estimates are dependent upon good estimates of forest structure and how structure affects services. The key starting point to valuing services provided by forests is quality data on forest structure. Services and values cannot be adequately estimated without good forest data. Combining accurate forest data with sound procedures to quantifying ecosystem services will lead to reliable estimates of the magnitude of ecosystem services provided by the forest. Finally, with sound estimates of forest ecosystem services, values of the services can be estimated using valid economic estimates and procedures. Thus, three critical elements in sequence are needed to value forest ecosystem services: structure → services → values. Errors in precursor elements will lead to errors in subsequent estimates (e.g. errors in forest structure will lead to errors in estimating services and valuation). All current estimates and means of estimation can be improved to varying degrees.

By understanding how vegetation affects services and values, better decisions can be made relating to landscape management to improve environmental quality and human health. To this end, tools are being developed that use local data to estimate ecosystem services and its economic value to help guide management and sustain optimal vegetation structure through time.

Modelling vegetation ecosystem services

Various models exist that quantify and value ecosystem services. InVEST (www.naturalcapitalproject.org/invest/) is a suite of free, open-source software models used to map and value the goods and services from nature that sustain and fulfil human life. InVEST enables decision makers to assess quantified trade-offs associated with alternative management choices and to identify areas where investment in natural capital can enhance human development and conservation. The toolset currently includes 18 distinct ecosystem service models designed for terrestrial, freshwater, marine, and coastal ecosystems (Natural Capital Project, 2016).

Another modelling system that assesses local vegetation structure and its associated ecosystem services and economic values is i-Tree (www.itreetools.org). This free suite of tools was developed through a public-private partnership and has been used across the world. The model requires users to enter local vegetation data, either through an inventory or sample, and combines the vegetation data with local meteorological and pollution data to simulate various ecosystem services: air pollution removal; carbon storage and sequestration; VOC emissions; reduced run-off; and effects on building energy use (Nowak et al., 2008). The model focuses on estimating the magnitude of services received (e.g. tons removed) and relies on economic valuation (e.g. $/ton removed) to estimate a value of the service. These values can vary depending upon how the receivers of the benefits (e.g. humans) are distributed across the landscape relative to the trees. Not all ecosystem services are, or can be, evaluated due to scientific limitations (Fig. 10.4.1).

Other valuation toolkits exist, for example Ecosystem Valuation Toolkit (Earth Economics, 2016) with more models likely to be developed in the coming years.

Estimating the economic values of services and human health impacts

Once the services from nature are quantified, then economic values may be estimated using various methods. Some valuing procedures use direct market costs. For example, for altered building energy use, the local cost of electricity ($/kWh) and heating fuels ($/MBTU) can be applied to changes in energy use due to local vegetation. For other ecosystem services, proxy values often need to be used, as many of the services derived from trees are not accounted for in the cost of a market transaction (e.g. externality costs). An externality arises whenever the actions of one party either positively or negatively affect another party, but the first party neither bears the costs, nor receives the benefits. Externalities are not reflected in the market price of goods and services. A classic example of a negative externality is air pollution, where the health and clean-up costs are paid by society and not the producer of the pollutant. Trees often produce positive externalities (e.g. cleaner air). There are various ways to estimate these non-market-price-based values, including general systems analysis, the social fabric matrix, direct cost, contingent valuation, travel cost, hedonic pricing, mitigation and avoided cost methods, and the property approach (Hayden, 1989; Pascual et al., 2010; TEEB 2010). Each method has its own strengths and weaknesses (Pascual et al., 2010).

The various approaches to estimating the value of ecosystem services may or may not include health valuation. Some studies have estimated health impacts from vegetation by linking vegetation effects on pollution concentrations to human health impacts and values. Various models exist that estimate health values and impacts—for example, the Environmental Benefits Mapping and Analysis Program (BenMAP) (US EPA, 2012) and Air Quality Benefits Assessment Tool (AQBAT) (Judek et al., 2006). These models use population data and concentration-response functions to estimate the change in adverse health effects due to change in air pollutant concentrations. Valuation functions calculate the associated monetary value from health effects. These calculations are based on meta-analyses of epidemiological studies and clinical experiments. Economic valuation is based on estimates of healthcare expenses and productivity losses associated with specific adverse health events, and on the value of a statistical life in the case of mortality. Changes in hourly air pollution concentration combined with population data can be used to estimate health impacts and values.

Based on a national assessment, trees and forests in the conterminous United States were estimated to remove 17.4 million metric tons of air pollution in 2010, with human health effects valued at $6.8 billion (range: $1.5–13.0 billion) (Nowak et al., 2014) (Fig. 10.4.2). Most of the pollution removal occurred in rural areas, while most of the health impacts and values were within urban areas. Health impacts included the avoidance of more than 850 incidences of human mortality and 670,000 incidences of acute respiratory symptoms. Using median air pollution cost factors from Europe that include health costs, building and material damage, and crop losses (van Essen et al., 2011), pollution removal by US trees would jump to over $86 billion, a 13-fold increase over the $6.8 billion health value.

Other studies that have linked pollution removal and health effects include one in London, UK, where a 10 × 10 km grid with 25% tree

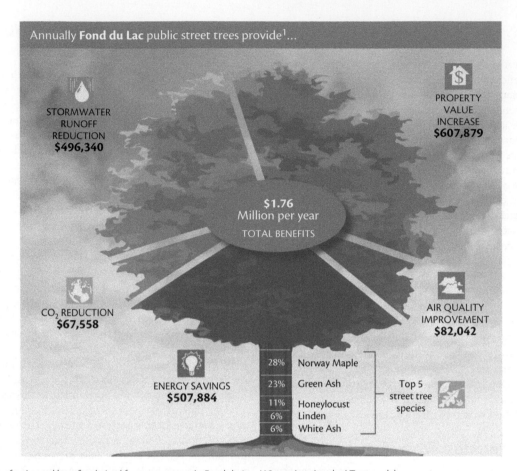

Fig. 10.4.1 Example of estimated benefits derived from street trees in Fond du Lac, Wisconsin using the i-Tree model.
Reproduced courtesy of The Wisconsin Department of Natural Resources, available from https://www.itreetools.org/resources/reports/WDNR_Fond_du_Lac_reports.pdf.

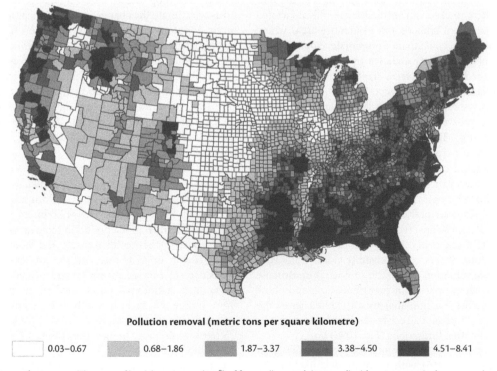

Pollution removal (metric tons per square kilometre)

0.03–0.67	0.68–1.86	1.87–3.37	3.38–4.50	4.51–8.41

Fig. 10.4.2 Estimated removal per square kilometre of land (metric tons km⁻²) of four pollutants (nitrogen dioxide, ozone, particulate matter less than 2.5 microns, sulphur dioxide) by trees per county in the conterminous United States in 2010.
Reprinted from *Environmental Pollution*, Volume 193, Nowak DJ *et al.*, 'Tree and forest effects on air quality and human health in the United States,' pp. 119–129, Copyright © 2014 published by Elsevier Ltd, with permission from Elsevier, http://www.sciencedirect.com/science/journal/02697491.

Table 10.4.1 Summary of total monetary value per ecosystem biome in international $ per hectare per year, 2007 price levels

Ecosystem biome	Annual value per hectare
Coral reefs	$352,249
Coastal wetlands	$193,845
Coastal systems	$28,917
Inland wetlands	$25,682
Tropical forests	$5,264
Fresh water (lakes and rivers)	$4,267
Temperate forests	$3,013
Grasslands	$2,871
Woodlands	$1,588
Open ocean	$491

Source: data from De Groot R et al., 'Global estimates of the value of ecosystems and their services in monetary units,' *Ecosystem Services*, Volume 1, Issue 1, pp. 50-61, Copyright © 2012 Elsevier B.V. Published by Elsevier B.V.

cover was estimated to remove 90.4 t of PM_{10} annually, which equated to the avoidance of two deaths and two hospital admissions per year (Tiwary et al., 2009). In addition, Nowak et al. (2013) reported that the total amount of $PM_{2.5}$ removed annually by trees in 10 US cities in 2010 varied from 4.7 t in Syracuse to 64.5 t in Atlanta. Estimates of the annual monetary value of human health effects associated with $PM_{2.5}$ removal in these same cities (e.g. changes in mortality, hospital admissions, respiratory symptoms) ranged from $1.1 million in Syracuse to $60.1 million in New York City. Mortality avoided was typically around one person per year per city, but was as high as 7.6 people per year in New York City. These are just a few examples of linking ecosystem services to health impacts and values. These studies focus on tree effects on air pollution, often in cities, but there are numerous other studies, ecosystems, and ecosystem services and values that can be derived from nature.

The estimated total annual value per hectare from ten ecosystem biomes ranges from $490 international dollars for open oceans to $350,000 international dollars for coral reefs (de Groot et al., 2012, Table 10.4.1). These average values vary among ecosystem type and are mostly outside the market and best considered as non-tradable public benefits. The total values include provisioning, regulating, habitat, and cultural services. Numerous other estimates of ecosystem values exist (e.g. TEEB 2010), yet many services remain to be adequately quantified and valued.

While valuing ecosystem services in monetary terms can be complex and controversial, natural resources are economic assets, whether they enter the marketplace or not, and could be accounted for in land management decisions (TEEB, 2010). The Economics of Ecosystems and Biodiversity report (TEEB, 2010) provides several recommendations to analysing and structuring the valuation of ecosystem services.

Even though models can calculate some ecosystem and health benefits and costs, there are multiple benefits and costs yet to be quantified. More research is needed to quantify the numerous health and environmental benefits provided by vegetation and other ecosystems. In addition, the potential environmental and maintenance or management costs associated with vegetation and ecosystems need to be quantified to facilitate vegetation

management that optimizes economic, environmental, and health benefits from vegetation.

Conclusion

By understanding and accounting for the ecosystem and health benefits provided by nature, better planning, design, and economic decisions can be made toward utilizing nature as a means to improve human health. InVEST, i-Tree, and other tools offer a means to assess and value the impact of trees, forests, and other ecosystem elements at varying scales for several key ecosystem services. While more research is needed regarding several ecosystem services and impacts on human health, landscape management plans and designs should incorporate the role of vegetation and nature to lower costs and improve human health and environmental quality, and thereby provide substantial economic savings to society.

Disclaimer

The use of trade names in this article is for the information and convenience of the reader. This does not constitute any official endorsement or approval by the United States Department of Agriculture or Forest Service of any product or service to the exclusion of others that may be suitable.

References

Costanza, R., de Groot, R., Sutton, P., et al. (2014). Changes in the global value of ecosystem services. *Global Environmental Change*, 26, 152–8.
de Groot, R., Brander, L., van der Ploeg, S., et al. (2012). Global estimates of the value of ecosystems and their services in monetary units. *Ecosystem Services*, 1, 50–61.
Earth Economics (2016). Ecosystem Valuation Toolkit. Available at: http://esvaluation.org/ (accessed February 2016) [Online].
Escobedo, F.J, Kroeger, T., & Wagner, J. (2011). Urban forests and pollution mitigation: Analyzing ecosystem services and disservices. *Environ Pollut*, 159, 2078–87.
Hassan, R., Scholes, R., & Ash, A. (2005). *Ecosystems and Human Well-being: Current State and Trends, Volume 1*. Washington, DC: Island Press.
Hayden, F. G. (1989). *Survey of methodologies for valuing externalities and public goods*. EPA-68-01-7363. Washington, DC: Environmental Protection Agency.
Judek, S., Stieb, D., & Jovic, B. (2006). Air Quality Benefits Assessment Tool (AQBAT) release 1.0. Ottawa, Canada: Health Canada.
Natural Capital Project (2016). InVEST: *Integrated valuation of ecosystem services and tradeoffs*. Available at: http://www.naturalcapitalproject.org/invest/ (accessed January 2016) [Online].
Nowak, D. J. & Dwyer, J. F. (2007). Understanding the benefits and costs of urban forest ecosystems. In: Kuser, J. (ed.) *Urban and Community Forestry in the Northeast*. New York, NY: Springer.
Nowak, D. J., Hirabayashi, S., Bodine, A., et al. (2013). Modeled PM2.5 removal by trees in ten U.S. cities and associated health effects. *Environ Pollut*, 178, 395–402.
Nowak, D. J., Hirabayashi, S., Ellis, E., et al. (2014). Tree and forest effects on air quality and human health in the United States. *Environ Pollut*, 193, 119–29.
Nowak, D. J., Hoehn, R. E., Crane, D. E., et al. (2008). A ground-based method of assessing urban forest structure and ecosystem services. *Arboriculture and Urban Forestry*, 34, 347–58.
Pascual, U., Muradian, R., Brander, L., et al. (2010). *Chapter 5: The economics of valuing ecosystem services and biodiversity*. TEEB document. Available at: http://www.teebweb.org/wp-content/uploads/2013/04/

D0-Chapter-5-The-economics-of-valuing-ecosystem-services-and-biodiversity.pdf (accessed February 2016).

TEEB (2010). *The Economics of Ecosystems and Biodiversity: Mainstreaming the Economics of Nature: A synthesis of the approach, conclusions and recommendations of TEEB*. Malta: Progress Press.

Tiwary, A., Sinnett, D., Peachey, C., *et al.* (2009). An integrated tool to assess the role of new planting in PM_{10} capture and the human health benefits: A case study in London. *Environ Pollut*, 157, 2645–53.

U.S. Environmental Protection Agency (US EPA) (2012). *Environmental Benefits Mapping and Analysis Program (BenMAP)*. Available at: https://www.epa.gov/benmap (accessed May 2012) [Online].

van Essen H., Schroten A., Otten M., *et al.* (2011). *External Costs of Transport in Europe, Update Study for 2008*. Delft, the Netherlands. Available at: http://www.cedelft.eu/?go=home.downloadPub&id=1258&file=CE_Delft_4215_External_Costs_of_Transport_in_Europe_def.pdf [Online].

CHAPTER 10.5

The role of civil society and organizations

Matilda van den Bosch, Cathey E. Falvo, Génon K. Jensen, Joshua Karliner, and Rachel Stancliffe

First do no harm

Non-governmental (NGOs) and civil society organizations (CSOs) play a special role in engaging the public and policy makers for actions linking environment and health in a sustainable and healthy manner. Such organizations can serve as, for example, knowledge brokers, lobbyists, and advocates. They can also shape policy recommendations, support development of education and educational tools, provide evidence-based information to the public, act as a watchdog, and be involved in concrete projects serving as case studies by taking good examples of ecosystem-based solutions into practice. This reinforces the notion that, following the oath of 'first do no harm', doctors and health professionals have a specific ethical duty to protect human health in current and coming generations from negative impacts of environmental degradation and changes. This includes maintaining and creating natural environments for everyone to enjoy and to stay healthy in contact with nature.

In particular, health organizations with an environmental perspective are important for recognizing the crucial role healthcare professionals and researchers in medicine and healthcare play in influencing the future health agenda, which must to a much greater extent than currently is the case, incorporate environmental and sustainability knowledge, both in terms of health promotion and disease prevention.

Bridging the science-policy gap

With their independent status, NGOs and CSOs are efficient tools for engaging civil society and individuals outside a political or ideological arena.

Any healthcare system is based on a structural organization with a built-in latency in adapting to changed needs and requirements. For example, the recognition of environmental and climate change impacts on health is often relatively minor in the medical curriculum, as are the opportunities for health promotion that can be realized through interactions with natural environments. The education and training in these topics is often insufficient for both physicians and other healthcare professionals (Prasad *et al.*, 2011), in spite of the scientific consensus regarding environmental impact on health, having now reached major medical journals (Wang and Horton, 2015; Watts *et al.*, 2015; McMichael, 2013; Hartig, 2008; Hartig *et al.*, 2014).

Through persistent, often voluntary, work by professional organizations, the awareness and necessary changes can be enforced and strengthened. This is reflected especially through collaborations and consultative statuses with major established international health organizations and networks. These are all good examples of ways to improve science-to-policy communication.

This chapter presents four central health organizations with environment and climate at their core, giving some examples of their work and actions. These organizations have contributed to putting the environment-related health opportunities and threats on the medical and public health agenda. Globally, there are many other important organizations working towards the same goals. These four organizations, however, serve as representative examples.

International Society of Doctors for the Environment, ISDE

Cathey E. Falvo, MD, MPH, past President of ISDE

◆ Website: http://www.isde.org/

The International Society of Doctors for the Environment (ISDE), a not-for-profit, non-governmental organization registered in Switzerland in 1990, is a federation of national associations of physicians and other NGOs whose programmes include environmental health (see Fig. 10.5.1).

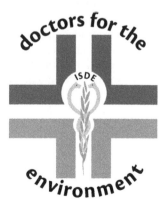

Fig. 10.5.1 International Society of Doctors for the Environment (ISDE) logo. Reproduced courtesy of International Society of Doctors for the Environment (ISDE).

Vision and mission

ISDE's goals are to promote human health through the protection and restoration of the environment, to alert physicians, other professionals, decision makers, and the public to the health effects of environmental degradation locally and worldwide, and to promote sustainable development. To achieve these aims at the international level, ISDE works with and has official collaborative status with the United Nations (UN) Economic and Social Council (ECOSOC), the World Health Organization (WHO) and works closely with the United Nations Environmental Program (UNEP). The particular issues focused upon are decided by the ISDE directing board, and implementation is supervised by the International Secretariat.

On the regional, national, and local levels, the areas of focus are chosen by the national organizations working within and among themselves. Collaborations with other regional organizations such as the Health and Environment Alliance (HEAL) and Health Care Without Harm (HCWH) in Europe and the Washington DC, USA Green group are ongoing and encouraged.

History

ISDE began as a group of physicians discussing ways to help their patients have healthier lives by modifying their behaviour in relation to their environment; for example, riding a bicycle or walking instead of motoring, eating organic foods, or growing their own food to avoid toxic chemicals. It became clear that many actions could not be carried out by individuals because of lack of appropriate policy, as well as their individual situation. Further, many issues of environmental health were being decided in the public press without clear scientific evidence. Thus was born ISDE and the independent ISDE Scientific Office based in Arezzo, Italy as a tool for educating and updating physicians and the general public, and stimulating awareness and initiatives by public and private bodies, in particular governmental agencies, about the positive and negative interactions between the environment and human health.

Collaborations, channels, and functioning

ISDE has a long working relationship with WHO for creating educational tools for health and training lay personnel on children's environmental health (World Health Organization, Children's Environmental Health Training Packages).

At the UN, ISDE works in collaboration with other health-oriented organizations to keep environmental health in focus during deliberations as varied as climate change, sustainable development, human rights, arms trade, and nuclear weapons proliferation. One example was the inclusion of three paragraphs on environmental health in the final outcome document from the 2012 UN meeting, Rio+20, setting the UN direction on development for the next decades (UN, 2012). The original draft document from the UN Commission on Sustainable Development hardly mentioned the word 'health'.

In conjunction with the WHO and UNEP, ISDE members participated in the Intergovernmental Forum on Chemical Safety (IFCS) (now part of the Strategic Alliance for International Chemical management (SAICM)) working groups on nanoparticles, lead, mercury, and cadmium. ISDE submitted a proposal to add environmentally persistent pharmaceutical pollutants to the SAICM agenda of emerging issues, which was adopted at the International Conference on Chemicals Management (ICCM4) in October, 2015.

Activities

Key country activities include major campaigns in the United States, Canada, and Australia on coal-fired power plants because of the immediate health effects on respiratory systems and long-term climate change. ISDE USA is updating the Children's Environmental Health Toolkit (http://www.psr.org/resources/pediatric-toolkit.html) endorsed by the American Academy of Pediatrics (AAP) to reflect these changes.

The ISDE organizations in Australia, Ireland, and the United Kingdom are focusing their activities on climate change.

Doctors for the Environment Australia (DEA) helped launch a successful lawsuit to require a new coal-fired power plant in Victoria to adhere to the highest/cleanest world standard (DEA, 2013). Sustainable Development Policy Institute (SDPI), the partner in Pakistan, is leading international efforts to control mercury pollution with major input from Argentina.

ISDE Austria has recently published guidelines for policy makers on electromagnetic fields. Several country organizations including Ireland are working with their governments on various aspects of climate change (see country websites).

The German organization is working with the government on a website portal to educate on biocides including nanosilver (Peterson et al., 2013a; Peterson et al., 2013b).

The ISDE Scientific Office in Italy maintains a Listserv for all interested to keep physicians abreast of the latest research findings pertinent to environmental/toxics effects on human health. Recent topics have included the important research on pesticides and other chemical toxins in relation to epigenetic changes affecting foetal development, risk factors for autism and other central nervous system dysfunction, and a variety of chronic diseases.

National member organizations with websites

- Argentina: Asociación Argentina de Médicos por el Medio Ambiente, http://www.aamma.org/
- Australia: Doctors for the Environment (Australia) Incorporated (DEA), http://dea.org.au/
- Austria: Ärztinnen und Ärzte für eine Gesunde Umwelt (ÄGU) - ISDE Austria, http://www.aegu.net/
- Belgium 2: HECTOR asbl—Health and Environment Care Technical Organization, http://www.hector-asbl.be/
- Canada: Canadian Association of Physicians for the Environment (CAPE), http://www.cape.ca/
- Ecuador: Corporación para el Desarrollo de la Producción y el Medio Ambiente Laboral, http://www.ifa.org.ec/
- France: L'Association pour la Recherche Thérapeutique Anti-Cancéreuse, ARTAC, http://www.artac.info/
- Germany: Ökologischer Ärztebund, http://www.oekologischer-aerztebund.de/
- Italy: Associazione Medici per l'Ambiente—ISDE Italia, http://www.isde.it/
- Pakistan: Sustainable Development Policy Institute, http://www.sdpi.org/

- Netherlands: Nederlandse Vereniging voor Medische Milieukunde (NVMM), http://www.nvmm-mmk.nl/
- Sweden: Läkare för Miljön, http://www.lakareformiljon.org/
- Switzerland: Ärztinnen und Ärzte für Umweltschutz, Mèdecins en Faveur de l'Environnement, Medici per l'Ambiente, http://www.aefu.ch/aktuell/
- United Kingdom: British Society for Ecological Medicine, http://www.ecomed.org.uk/
- United States: Physicians for Social Responsibility (PSR), http://www.psr.org/
- Uzbekistan: Center Perzent—The Karakalpak Center for Reproductive Health and Environment, http://www.friends-partners.org/ccsi/nisorgs/uzbek/perzent.htm

Health and Environment Alliance, HEAL

Génon K. Jensen, Founder and Executive Director of HEAL

- Website: http://www.env-health.org/

The Health and Environment Alliance (HEAL) is a European non-governmental organization with a paid-up membership of more than 70 member organizations in 28 countries representing not-for-profit health insurers, doctors, nurses, cancer and asthma groups, citizens, women's groups, youth groups, environmental NGOs, scientists, and public health research institutes (see Fig. 10.5.2).

Vision and mission

The vision of the Health and Environment Alliance (HEAL) is a world in which today's and future generations can benefit from a clean environment to enjoy long and healthy lives; a world that is free of health-harming chemicals, where the air we breathe and food we eat are health promoting; and a future in which we have transitioned to a non-toxic, de-carbonized, climate resilient, and sustainable economy and way of life.

Rather than looking at how nature positively affects public health, the focus is on harm to health from environmental stressors, such as polluted air from exhaust associated with fossil fuel energy generation or road vehicles; from harmful toxics in food and everyday products; and on health threats resulting from climate change. HEAL also highlights the co-benefits to health of reducing pollution and promoting a cleaner, physical environment.

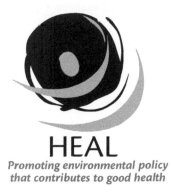

Fig. 10.5.2 Health and Environment Alliance (HEAL) logo.
Reproduced courtesy of Health and Environment Alliance (HEAL).

In response to these health concerns, HEAL formulates environmental, climate, and energy policy recommendations to share with European and international decision makers, thus playing a major role in promoting 'health in all policies' at the European level. To help persuade policy makers of the need for action, HEAL often highlights the 'win-win-win' aspects of a proposal, as well as the health costs of inaction.

HEAL's overall mission is to provide the health voice in environment, climate, chemicals, and energy policy in Europe and worldwide. This includes:

- Work to ensure that health evidence and health voices are heard by politicians and policy makers in Europe and beyond. The aim is to protect those most harmed by pollution, such as the foetus, children, pregnant women, and older people, and those with existing health problems or living in especially exposed environments.

- Having strong relationships with our European members and partnering with organizations around the world to raise awareness and share evidence, change laws, and defend and improve people's health and well-being.

- Helping to shape laws on chemicals, pesticides, air quality, climate change, and energy by sharing real life stories on the health harm of pollution, and making the economic case for environments that promote health. We focus particularly on building knowledge about the opportunities for reducing cancer, lung and heart disease, allergies and asthma, diabetes, obesity, Alzheimer's disease, Parkinson's disease, autism and attention deficit and hyperactivity disorder (ADHD), genital birth defects, premature puberty, and infertility.

History

HEAL was created in late 2003 when the 'health and environment' section of the leading umbrella organization, the European Public Health Alliance (EPHA) was expanding rapidly and required a separate structure. At about that time, both the World Health Organization (WHO) and the European Union (EU) were setting up programmes to address the relationship between human health and the environment, which prompted growing interest from many health groups within civil society.

Collaborations, channels, and functioning

Members include international and Europe-wide organizations, as well as national and local groups. HEAL also works closely with hundreds of partner organizations around the world to defend people's health and well-being.

HEAL receives substantial recognition and trust from, for example, the WHO, the European Commission, the European Parliament, UNEA, and participates in many EU and international expert groups such as the WHO European Environment Health Task Force.

HEAL has built its status not only on the basis of groups it represents (such as European Respiratory Society representing more than 10,000 health professionals) but also on how the views of members and partners are represented and shared to external audiences. Each year, HEAL holds an annual general meeting in which members have the opportunity to bring emerging issues to the table and to agree on the annual work programme. HEAL's second highest decision-making body is its Executive Committee who guides the organizational development during the course of the year as well as exchange on issue specific internal and public virtual working groups.

Because HEAL is based in Brussels, the Secretariat can reach policy makers directly through personal contact or by organizing or attending key events. Close contact with European journalists helps ensure a media profile for the organization and its policies in respected newspapers and EU policy websites.

HEAL works closely with public health and other doctors and health professionals who are highly influential spokespeople in relaying information to politicians and policy makers. This important role helps to increase political pressure to speed up necessary action to protect people and environments. Health experts and advocates, including medical professionals, civil society groups, and young people, have contributed substantially to many recent policy advances in Europe. The more health professionals become involved, the sooner the much-needed sense of urgency for prioritizing environmental policy change to boost children's and adults' health will be created.

The materials produced by HEAL bring attention to key environmental concerns identified by members and partners as they relate to different policy discussions. The information is substantiated by the latest science, trends in the related health conditions, and cost estimates of the health benefits that could be reaped from a change in policy. HEAL's media and communication's track record includes over 1000 hits annually in major media across Europe and increasingly globally, as well as a prominent social media strategy which provides toolkits for members and partners to share info and actions on a daily basis, translate, and rebrand for their own purposes.

Activities

Three recent campaign reports demonstrate the 'win-win-win' approach that HEAL brings to policy makers:

1. **Cleaner air.** A large body of scientific evidence now exists consolidating the various health effects of air pollution. While air quality has generally improved in Europe over the last decades, evidence is ever-expanding on the seriousness and the range of health effects. For example, WHO's recent 'Review of evidence on health aspects of air pollution' showed that long-term effects of exposure to outdoor air pollution had again been underestimated. Diabetes was added to the existing list of respiratory and heart disease consequences in adults, and new findings pointed to effects on the neurodevelopment and cognitive function of children. This evidence underpins the need for strengthened efforts to reach 'clean air everywhere', as people in many cities still breathe in air that is considered harmful to health.

   HEAL chose to focus on the harm to health from coal-generated electricity in Europe in its current campaign. The report, 'The Unpaid Health Bill—How coal power plants make us sick' (2013) showed €43 billion annual 'wins' for public health from moving to cleaner energy sources. The calculation took into account the respiratory and some cardiac effects resulting from air pollution associated with coal power plants. The 'wins' were not only for human health and the environment, but also for the economy in terms of improved productivity and lower healthcare spending. National versions of the Unpaid Health Bill now exist

in Germany, Poland, Romania, United Kingdom, Turkey, and the Western Balkans, as well as a vibrant health energy network.

2. **Fewer carbon emissions.** The future burden on public health resulting from climate change (due to rising carbon dioxide and other greenhouse gas emissions) are challenging to measure. However, many policies aimed at combating climate change have indirect benefits for health aside from the direct benefits that avoiding global warming would bring. For example, 'active transport' where people walk or cycle more and use their cars less, reduces greenhouse gas emissions and leads to reductions in cardiovascular disease and cancer through improved fitness.

   HEAL's climate change report 'Acting NOW for better health' (HEAL, 2010) was able to make the case for the European Union stepping up its target on reductions of greenhouse gas emissions on health grounds alone. The report began by pointing to the health benefits that were already accruing due to improvements in air quality associated with fewer carbon and greenhouse gas emissions. The report then calculated the additional health benefits that could be achieved by increasing the target of a 20% reduction in emissions to a 30% target for 2020. The benefits were estimated at up to €30.5 billion per year by 2020.

   The report was important in reframing the climate debate from a focus on what climate action would 'cost' to a perspective focused on the 'benefit' for health. It also highlighted the 'wins' for health, the environment, the economy, and climate change mitigation.

3. **Reducing environmental toxics: hormone disrupting chemicals in consumer products.** HEAL's campaign for stronger regulation on endocrine disrupting chemicals (EDCs) has also demonstrated the huge likely 'wins' from removing these substances from cosmetics, food packaging, paints and solvents, pesticides, and electronics.

   Evidence is growing fast that spiralling rates of certain chronic conditions, such as hormone-related cancers, diabetes, and obesity, infertility, and certain neurological conditions, may be due to exposure to hormone-mimicking synthetic chemicals found in food, drink, and everyday products.

   The alarm bells for human health risks associated with EDCs only began to ring once bird, reptile, and animal life had been affected. HEAL's latest report shows that 31 billion Euros could be avoided each year if just a small proportion of the hormone-related conditions are conclusively shown to be the result of exposure to hormone disrupting chemicals. The likely 'wins' are for health, productivity and healthcare spending.

Health Care Without Harm

Josh Karliner, Director of Global Projects and International Team Coordinator

◆ Website: https://noharm.org/

Health Care Without Harm (HCWH) is an international coalition of hospitals and healthcare systems, medical professionals, community groups, health-affected constituencies, labour unions, environmental and environmental health organizations and religious groups (Fig. 10.5.3).

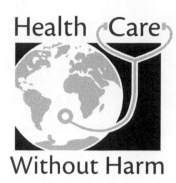

Fig. 10.5.3 Health Care Without Harm (HCWH) logo.
Reproduced courtesy of Health Care Without Harm (HCWH).

Vision and mission

HCWH works to transform the health sector worldwide, without compromising patient safety or care, so that it becomes ecologically sustainable and a leading advocate for environmental health and justice across the globe. HCWH has a vision of a healthcare sector that does no harm, and instead promotes the health of people and the environment. To that end, HCWH is working to implement ecologically sound and healthy alternatives to healthcare practices that pollute the environment and contribute to disease.

History

Health Care Without Harm began in 1996 after the US Environmental Protection Agency identified medical waste incineration as the leading source of dioxin, one of the most potent carcinogens.

In response to this serious problem, 28 organizations came together in Bolinas, California to form the coalition Health Care Without Harm (HCWH). Since then, HCWH has grown into a broad-based international coalition of hundreds of organizations in 52 countries, with offices in Arlington, VA, Brussels, Buenos Aires, and Manila.

Collaborations, channels, and functioning

HCWH has significant experience working around the world. HCWH works globally with health professionals, hospitals, health systems, architects, and ministries of health, and international organizations in dozens of countries to promote environmentally sustainable healthcare and protect public health. The HCWH Network includes partner organizations in numerous countries including Australia, Brazil, China, India, Indonesia, Nepal, and South Africa.

Activities

HCWH has developed a broad diversity of initiatives. For instance, HCWH co-created the Green Guide for Health Care, which formed the basis of Leadership in Energy and Environmental Design (LEED) for Health Care—a major green building system for hospitals. HCWH also created a sister organization in the United States, Practice Greenhealth (https://practicegreenhealth.org/) which supports implementation and has more than 1,200 paying hospital members (2016). In 2012, HCWH mobilized 11 of the largest US health systems representing $20 billion in purchasing power to create the Healthier Hospitals Initiative, in order to commit to and rigorously document the reduction of their environmental footprint and its cost-effectiveness (www.healthierhospitals.org). In 2014 HCWH U.S. launched the Climate and Health Care Council, which is mobilizing 17 leading US health systems as vocal advocates on climate change.

From 2008 to 2015, HCWH managed a joint initiative with the WHO to substitute mercury-based medical devices globally (www.mercuryfreehealthcare.org) that helped lay the groundwork for the phase-out of mercury thermometers and blood pressure devices via the Minamata Convention on Mercury.

HCWH was a principle cooperating agency in a seven-country UNDP-GEF Global Healthcare Waste project that promoted sustainable healthcare waste management, and is playing a similar role in a new project being executive four African countries (http://www.gefmedwaste.org/).

In Europe, HCWH works on a broad diversity of issues, including advocating for policies to phase-out endocrine disrupting chemicals in medical devices, addressing the environmental health impacts of pharmaceuticals, as well as the promoting more climate friendly healthcare systems.

In 2011, HCWH took the lead in organizing the First Global Climate and Health Summit in Durban, which was the first worldwide gathering of health leaders on climate change. The summit participants, which included major global health federations such as the World Medical Association, the World Federation of Public Health Associations, and the International Council of Nurses, issued the Durban Call to Action, which is a mutually agreed upon framework for global health sector organizing on climate. Emerging from this effort, HCWH helped found the Global Climate and Health Alliance, a worldwide network working to engage the health sector on climate change. This Alliance has since organized annual health summits at the climate negotiations. Also emerging from this experience was HCWH's Healthy Energy Initiative (http://www.healthyenergyinitiative.org/), an effort designed to address the health impacts of energy choices in key countries around the world, and to engage the health sector in advocating for policies that foster a shift away from fossil fuels, particularly coal, which harm human health during extraction, transport and combustion, and towards clean, renewable energy.

In 2011 HCWH released a pragmatic 10-step guide called the Global Green and Healthy Hospitals Agenda, a comprehensive environmental health framework for hospitals and health systems around the world. Based on this guide, in 2012 HCWH launched the Global Green and Healthy Hospitals Network (http://www.greenhospitals.net/), a collaborative worldwide effort to reduce the health sector's environmental footprint. Today, institutions representing the interests of more than 20,000 hospitals and health centres in 35 countries are members of Global Green and Healthy Hospitals and are working to promote greater environmental health both via their own organizations' actions. They are also becoming adovates for local, national, and international policy thereby contributing to the broader worldwide movement for environmental health. For instance, many are participating in the 2020 Health Care Climate Challenge, which is mobilizing healthcare systems around the world to reduce their carbon footprint, become more resilient in the face of climate change, and take leadership action.

The Centre for Sustainable Healthcare

Rachel Stancliffe, Founder and Director

♦ Website: http://sustainablehealthcare.org.uk/

The Centre for Sustainable Healthcare, CSH, is a British independent, non-profit charity organization, helping current healthcare systems in the transformation from resource-intensive interventions downstream to upstream prevention and promotion, partly through the wider determinants of health. It is now one of the foremost institutions in the world working on sustainable healthcare in research and practice (Figs 10.5.4 and 10.5.5).

Mission and goals

CSH's overall goal is to support patients, healthcare professionals, and organizations to develop a healthcare system which is sustainable not just financially, but also environmentally and socially.

One key element of this goal is to see more joined-up thinking whereby health and well-being are supported by all relevant sectors and through all projects and interventions, including the wider

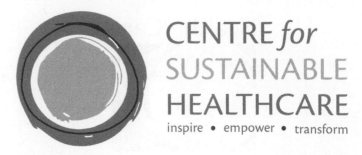

Fig. 10.5.4 The Centre for Sustainable Healthcare.
Reproduced courtesy of the Centre for Sustainable Healthcare. The figure may be copied freely with acknowledgement.

infrastructure of society. For example, it would be national policy for outdoor therapeutic environments to be incorporated into overall hospital or ward design and for green prescriptions to be routinely prescribed by GPs to address chronic health problems. This could create good value for money and better long-term health for everyone.

The mission is to support this to happen through strategic work at national and international level, changing policies of key institutions, and research and projects to demonstrate the value of such an approach.

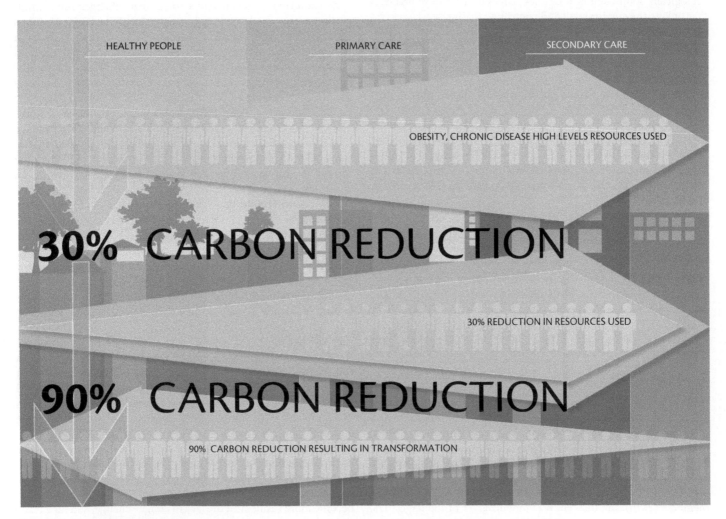

Fig. 10.5.5 Transforming arrow.
Reproduced courtesy of the Centre for Sustainable Healthcare. The figure may be copied freely with acknowledgement.

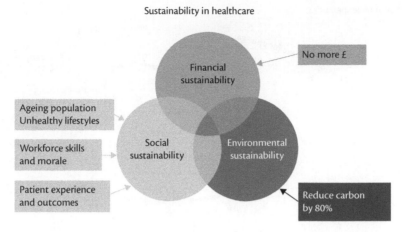

Sustainability in healthcare

"Sustainable healthcare delivers the highest possible value to patients from a radically reduced resource input." *Green Nephrology Summit 2012–position statment*

Fig. 10.5.6 Sustainability in healthcare.
Reproduced courtesy of the Centre for Sustainable Healthcare. The figure may be copied freely with acknowledgement.

History

The CSH (formerly known as The Campaign for Greener Healthcare) is a registered charity set up in 2008 to support the British National Health Service (NHS) and other healthcare organizations to become sustainable. This includes helping them to fulfil the legal requirement to reduce the carbon footprint by 80% by 2050 and transforming systems within healthcare so that patients have better outcomes and fewer resources are used (Fig. 10.5.6). The Trustees are legally responsible for overseeing the strategic development of the charity and for decisions about finance and employment, but in practice, many of these decisions are made by the Director together with the whole team. The small team of eight includes several part-time staff and is collaborative and open. There is a very low staff-turnover, with five staff having been there since the first year. CSH welcomes interns and has been lucky to enjoy working with many committed people who have volunteered as interns from the United Kingdom, Canada, Brazil, and Australia.

Collaborations, channels, and functioning

CSH believes that the best way to implement and embed sustainable practices in healthcare is by partnering with government, industry, third-sector organizations, and people who work on the ground in different areas of healthcare. These include:

♦ Clinical specialties

♦ Public health and local authorities

♦ Medical education

♦ Patient groups

♦ Procurement and industry

♦ Commissioners of health and social care services

The people CSH works with include patients, researchers, behaviour change experts, carbon footprinting groups, healthcare economists, architects and engineers, estates and energy managers, and many healthcare professionals from different clinical areas.

The Centre also collaborates with other health and environment organizations globally such as Healthcare Without Harm (of which

it is a member), Healthy Planet, The Climate and Health Council, and HEAL (Health and Environment Alliance).

CSH is working with Public Health England and the Faculty of Public Health in the United Kingdom to support work on sustainability in these organizations, primarily through its Fellowship Programme which trains public healthcare professionals in sustainability and works alongside them to embed it in their organizations both top-down via policy and strategy and bottom-up from a network of people and case studies. Our work also focuses on transformation across existing silos, and so wherever we start in the system we try to draw people and projects upstream and are interested in developing methodologies and metrics to do this more systematically.

Activities

CSH pursues its goals by:

♦ developing a range of programmes that will inspire, empower and support people to change;

♦ working with key partners to engage healthcare professionals, patients, and the wider community in understanding the connections between health and environment;

♦ exploring methodologies and metrics that can help to transform models of care; and

♦ researching and highlighting best practice that reduces healthcare's resource footprint, while also improving health outcomes.

The Centre's main focus is on finding ways to mainstream sustainability so that it is integral to the planning of health systems and the practice of healthcare professionals. Recognizing that the natural community of practice in healthcare is most often its specialty, the Centre has developed a clinical specialties transformation programme. Alongside this, CSH develops tools such as the Sustainable Commissioning Guide (CSH, 2013) and carries out research projects in particular areas to develop leaner care pathways and low carbon alternatives.

Clinical specialties are uniquely placed to address the sustainability of services—from the design of the clinical pathway to the organization and delivery of care. The CSH specialty-led approach

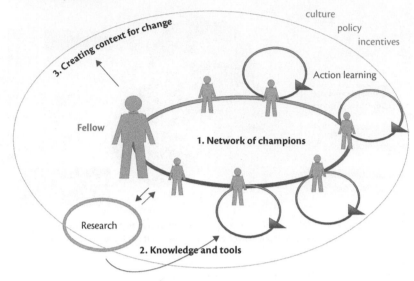

Fig. 10.5.7 Sustainable specialties.
Reproduced courtesy of the Centre for Sustainable Healthcare. The figure may be copied freely with acknowledgement.

Marston Green Health Route Map - Length 2.5 miles approx

The Centre for Sustainable Healthcare has developed the Marston Green Health Route to take in the various nature reserves, schools, church and coffee shops of the Marston area.

Opposite is the Marston Green Health Route map. Please look out for the maps at the Resident Association displays throughout Marston and for signs along the route.

The route is flat and manageable with trainers or sturdy shoes and is suitable for wheelchairs or buggies. You can also stop off for coffee at the local cafe on Cherwell Drive or the 'Over 50's Cafe' at the Scout Hall on a Tuesday morning.

So go on get outside and try to do three walks a week enjoying the fresh air and the great green space in Marston.

NHS FOREST
growing forests for health
www.nhsforest.org

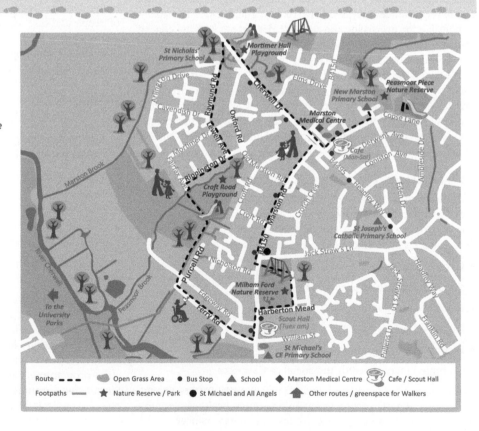

Fig. 10.5.8 Health Walk Map.
Reproduced courtesy of the Centre for Sustainable Healthcare. The figure may be copied freely with acknowledgement.

combines research with support for local change, underpinned by wider engagement with patients, and relevant industry and clinical bodies. The programmes benefit from a range of in-house resources, including web-based networking tools, online case libraries, and the Sustainable Action Planning toolkit for clinical teams.

CSH has pioneered the Sustainable Specialty Research Fellowship, seconding a clinician to work full-time on sustainability for one to two years before returning to clinical practice. The approach was successfully demonstrated in kidney care in 2009–2011 and is now being extended to other specialties including public health. The work includes fellows who establish a national network of local representatives in the United Kingdom and abroad, supported by a programme of research, annual awards, and practical initiatives. The flexibility of the Sustainable Specialty model makes it suitable for all clinical disciplines, ensuring that strategic interventions are rooted in engagement and practical experience on the ground (Fig. 10.5.7).

CSH works with education providers, professional bodies, and healthcare organizations to deliver programmes and develop resources for education and training in sustainable healthcare. This is run through the Sustainable Healthcare Education Network and has included developing priority learning outcomes for including sustainability in the medical curriculum.

The Centre has pioneered several concepts including the four principles of sustainable healthcare: Prevention, Patient-centred care, Leaner care pathways, and Choice of low carbon treatment alternatives (Mortimer, 2010).

The Centre also runs the NHS Forest, to engage staff, patients, and the wider community with the links between health and the environment. CSH is currently supporting people working on the interface between health and the natural environment at national and local levels (Fig. 10.5.8).

References

Centre for Sustainable Healthcare (CSH) (2013). Sustainable Commissioning Guide. In: NHS Institute, F. F. T. F., CSH (ed.). NHS Institute for Innovation and Improvement.

Doctors for the Environment Australia (DEA) (2013). The health factor: Ignored by industry and overlooked by government. Adelaide, Australia: Doctors for the Environment Australia.

Hartig, T. (2008). Green space, psychological restoration, and health inequality. *Lancet*, 372, 1614–15.

Hartig, T., Mitchell, R., Vries, S., & Frumkin, H. (2014). Nature and Health. *Annu Rev Public Health*, 35 207–28.

Health and Environment Alliance (HEAL) (2010). *Acting NOW for Better Health*. In: Jensen, G., Leetz, A. (eds). Brussels, Belgium: Health and Environment Alliance and Health Care Without Harm Europe.

Health and Environment Alliance (HEAL) (2013). *The Unpaid Health Bill—How coal power plants make us sick*. Brussels, Belgium: Health and Environment Alliance.

McMichael, A. (2013). Globalization, climate change and health. *N Engl J Med*, 368, 1335–43.

Mortimer, F. (2010). The sustainable physician. *Clin Med*, 10, 110–11.

Peterson, E., Gartiser, S., Smolka, S., Jahn, B., Wieck, S. (2013a). Alternatives to biocides—a contribution to a healthier indoor environment. In: *Abstracts of the 2013 Conference of the International Society of Environmental Epidemiology (ISEE), the International Society of Exposure Science (ISES), and the International Society of Indoor Air Quality and Climate (ISIAQ)*. Abstract 3311. Research Triangle Park, NC: Environmental Health Perspectives.

Peterson, E., Gartiser, S., Smolka, S., Jahn, B., Wieck, S. (2013b). Nanosilver in Medical and Consumer Products: Risks for Health and Environment? In: *Abstracts of the 2013 Conference of the International Society of Environmental Epidemiology (ISEE), the International Society of Exposure Science (ISES), and the International Society of Indoor Air Quality and Climate (ISIAQ)*. Abstract 3312. Research Triangle Park, NC: Environmental Health Perspectives.

Prasad, V., Thistlethwaite, W., & Dale, W. (2011). Effect of clinical vignettes on senior medical students' opinions of climate change. *Southern Medical Journal*, 104, 401–4.

United Nations (UN) (2012). The future we want. Resolution adopted by the General Assembly on 27 July 2012. RIO+20 United Nations Conference on Sustainable Development, 20–22 June 2012. Rio de Janeiro, Brazil.

Wang, H. & Horton, R. (2015). Tackling climate change: the greatest opportunity for global health. *Lancet*, 386, 1798–9.

Watts, N., Adger, W. N., Agnolucci, P., Blackstock, J., Byass, P., & Cai, W. (2015). Health and climate change: policy responses to protect public health. *Lancet*, 386, 1861–914.

Index

Notes
vs. indicates a comparison
Tables, figures and boxes are indicated by an italic, *t*, *f* and *b* following the page number